THE
JOURNEY OF AN
INDIAN-AMERICAN
PEDIATRIC
CARDIOLOGIST

A   M   E   M   O   I   R

*With Emphasis on Scientific
Contributions to the Medical Literature*

P. Syamasundar Rao
MD, DCH, FAAP, FACC, FSCAI

Professor of Pediatrics & Medicine
Emeritus Chief of Pediatric Cardiology
UT Health McGovern Medical School
Houston, Texas, USA

Published by BookBaby, 7905 N. Crescent Blvd., Pennsauken, NJ 08110

Library of Congress Cataloging-in-Publication Data

The journey of an Indian-American pediatric cardiologist /P. Syamasundar Rao p. cm.

Includes bibliographical references.

ISBN No. 978-1-54398-768-3

1. Congenital heart disease-treatment. 2. Electrocardiography. 3. Echocardiography. 4. Cardiac catheterization. 5. Cardiac surgery. I. Rao, P. Syamasundar, 1941-

[DNLM: 1. Balloon valvuloplasy/angioplasty - methods. 2. Trans-catheter occlusion-methods. 3. Cardiac surgery-methods. 4. Cardiac catheterization-methods. 5. Heart diseases-in infancy, childhood & adulthood. 6. Heart diseases-surgery.

While the author and publisher believe that the drug selection and the dosage and specifications and usage of diagnostic catheters, balloon valvuloplasy/angioplasty catheters, occluder and other devices, and other equipment, as set forth in this book, are in accord with current recommendations and practice at the time of publication; they accept no legal responsibility for any errors or omissions, and make no warranty, express or implied, with respect to material contained herein. In view of ongoing research, equipment modifications, changes in governmental regulations and the constant flow of information relating to drug therapy, drug reactions and the use of equipment and devices, the reader is urged to review and evaluate the information provided in the package insert or instructions for each drug, piece of equipment or device for, among other things, any changes in the instructions or indications of dosage or usage and for added warnings and precautions.

Some drugs and devices and other equipment presented in this book have Food and Drug Administration (FDA) clearance for limited use in restricted research settings. It is the responsibility of the health care provider to ascertain the FDA status of each drug or device planned for use in their clinical practice.

Printed in the United States of America

CONTENTS

DEDICATION

I dedicate this book to my parents (Figure 1) and grandparents (Figure 2) for their affection, kindness, and generosity in supporting me throughout my childhood, adolescence and young adulthood.

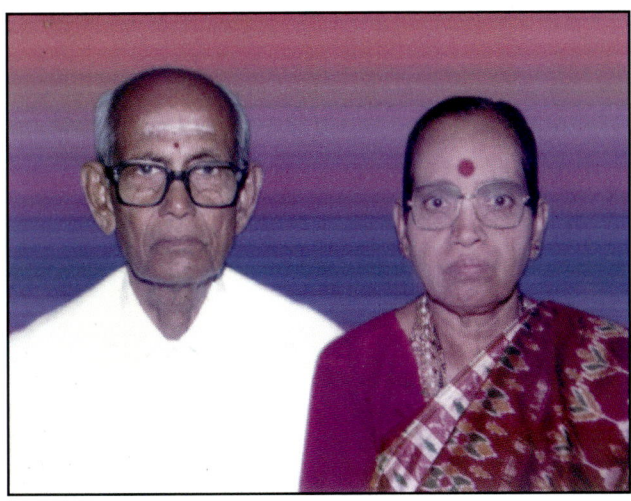

Figure 1. Late Sri P. V. B. Krishna Rao, BE (Hon) and Late Srimathi
Patnana Savithramma

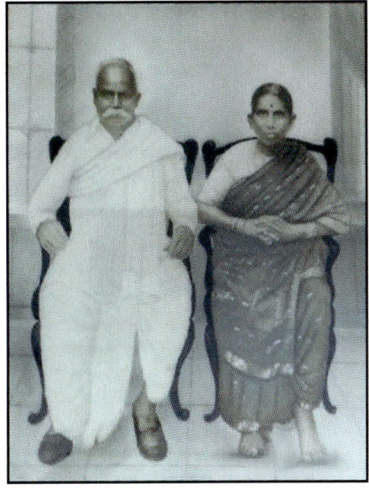

Figure 2. Late Sri Patnana Swamy Chetty and Late Srimathi
Patnana Rathnalamma

They were instrumental in me becoming a physician and have always encouraged me in pursuing my dreams. My gratitude and thanks are indebted to them forever, but unfortunately never expressed to them when they were alive.

P. Syamasundar Rao, MD

PREFACE

I was encouraged by my friends and classmates to write a memoir reviewing my scientific accomplishments, particularly by my college (Mrs. A.V.N. College, Visakhapatnam, Andhra Pradesh, India) and medical school (Andhra Medical College, Visakhapatnam) classmate, Dr. Gopalrao Nemana, a retired cardiologist from Sacramento, California. But I did not want to undertake such a task, given my health and other academic commitments. Suddenly, Dr. K.C. Chaudhuri Foundation/Indian Journal of Pediatrics bestowed upon me the honor of the Lifetime Achievement Award in 2017; the award required that I present an "Oration" outlining my lifetime accomplishments at the All India Institute of Medical Sciences (AIMS), New Delhi in September 2017. It was also required that the oration is published in the Indian Journal of Pediatrics. The published oration (Rao P.S., The Journey of an Indian Pediatric Cardiologist: Dr. K.C. Chaudhuri Lifetime Achievement Award, Oration at AIIMS, New Delhi, September 2017. Indian J Pediat 2017; 84:848-58) rekindled the thought of writing the memoir and forms the outline for this book.

The field of Pediatric Cardiology was in early development when I began my career in the mid 1960s. I had the opportunity to witness first-hand the stepwise evolution of Pediatric Cardiology over the last fifty years. Therefore, a unique historical perspective can be provided. I have bestowed considerable attention to the development of new knowledge, while providing care to patients with heart disease over a fifty-year period. These developments along with my contributions to Pediatric Cardiology were included in a companion book titled "Pediatric Cardiology: How It Has Evolved Over the last 50 Years." In this memoir, I will portray my journey and include subjects that are not in the purview of the evolution of Pediatric Cardiology. Along the way, art and science of interventional pediatric cardiology will be presented, as applicable to each chapter in both books.

Developments such as early detection of the neonates with serious heart disease and their rapid transport to tertiary care centers, availability of highly sensitive non-invasive diagnostic tools, advances in neonatal care and anesthesia, progress in trans-catheter interventional procedures and extension of complicated surgical procedures to the neonate and infant have advanced to such a degree that almost all congenital cardiac defects can be diagnosed and "corrected". The defects that could not be corrected could be effectively palliated. Cardiac defects that were once fatal in infancy are now treatable. These principles will be incorporated into the respective chapters, as applicable. Although every attempt was made to minimize repetition, there was some degree of replication, which was unavoidable to preserve the continuity of thought and discussion.

P. Syamasundar Rao, MD

A C K N O W L E D G E M E N T

Apart from my parents and grandparents mentioned in the dedication, I desire to thank my teachers and mentors, Dr. (Mrs.) Lavanya Mukherjee, Dr. Herman W. Lipow, Dr. Norman J. Sissman, Dr. Jerome Liebman, and Dr. Leonard M. Linde, for imparting the knowledge that is useful for the rest of my career, and my wife, Hymavathi, and children, Dr. Vijay K. Patnana, Dr. Madhavi Patnana, and Ms. Radhika N. Patnana for their love, encouragement and support.

I also wish to acknowledge the courage and wisdom of the patients and their parents who kindheartedly participated as volunteer research subjects in numerous clinical trials quoted in this book. An equal credit goes to the physicians, nurses and cardiologists of these subjects who convinced their patients/parents of children to participate in these clinical studies. These folks, through their kind efforts, advanced and created a knowledge base that is likely to form a foundation of immense implication for future generations of patients to come.

I also thank several societies and institutions who have, over the years, conferred distinction and/or recognized my clinical, teaching, and research contributions and these include: Telugu Association of North America (Award for Outstanding Contribution to Pediatric Cardiology, 1989); Swedish Pediatric Association, Gothenburg, Sweden (John Lind's Lecture, 1992); Wisconsin Nicaragua Partners of the Americas, Madison, Wisconsin (Meritorious Service Award, 1993); Healing the Children of Wisconsin, Madison (Outstanding Service Award, 1993); American Association of Cardiologists of Indian Origin (Outstanding Scientist Award, 1996); Tufts University, New England Medical Center, Boston, Massachusetts (Kreidberg's Lecture, 2005); North American Telugu Association (Outstanding Scientist Award, 2012); American Telugu Association (Outstanding Scientist Award, 2012); University of Texas, McGovern Medical School (Dean's Teaching Excellence Award, 2014); and most recently, the trustees of the Dr. K. C. Chaudhuri Foundation and Dr. I. C. Verma (Dr. K. C. Chaudhuri Lifetime Achievement Award, September 2017) and the Executive Committee and Trustees of the Telugu Cultural Association of Houston (Life Time Achievement Award, March 2018).

During the multitude of academic endeavors over the last fifty years, I collaborated with a number of my teachers and colleagues, post-doctoral fellows, resident physicians, medical students, nurses/nurse practitioners, electrocardiography, echocardiography, and cardiac catheterization technologists, and statisticians; these are too numerous to list, but are included in references throughout the book. While the contributions of these individuals were partly acknowledged at the time of respective publications by their inclusion in the list of authors, it is prudent to thank them again in this book for their contribution, counsel and cooperation.

Finally, I thank Dr. William B. Strong, my senior associate when I was at the Medical College of Georgia, for his continued support even after I left the institution by the way of continued encouragement of my professional and academic activities.

P. Syamasundar Rao, MD

THE JOURNEY BEGINS

INTRODUCTION

When my last book, "Perinatal Cardiology: A Multidisciplinary Approach" was published in 2015,[1] I thought that would be the last book that I would work on and stated so to several of my friends and colleagues. Then, in 2017, I was conferred a Lifetime Achievement Award by Dr. K. C. Chaudhuri Foundation/Indian Journal of Pediatrics/All India Institute of Medical Sciences, New Delhi. The conditions of the award were that I make a presentation at the award ceremony in New Delhi and that the award acceptance oration is published in the Indian Journal of Pediatrics. When this publication came out,[2] again several friends, including those that I mentioned in the Acknowledgement section, enticed me to publish a memoir including my contributions to the medical literature. After a long thought, I have decided to accept this challenge. This book is a product of such considerations.

A large volume of my contributions to the literature is concurrently published in a book titled "Pediatric Cardiology: How It Has Evolved Over the Last 50 Years," which is a companion to this book. This book focuses on my memoir and other contributions that could not be included in the book on Pediatric Cardiology evolution.

In this chapter, the beginnings of the journey will be presented and I and my family will be introduced.

THE BEGINNING

I was born on September 21, 1941, to Sri Patnana Venkata Bala Krishna Rao and Srimathi Savithramma in the village of Ullibhadra, which is located four miles from the town of Parvathipuram. Parvathipuram was in the district of Srikakulam, state of Madras in the pre-independent India. Over the last nearly eight decades, several political changes have occurred so that the village is now in the district of Vijayanagaram, state of Andhra Pradesh in the independent India.

CHILDHOOD AND EARLY EDUCATION

My childhood was generally unremarkable, although the remembrances of these events are vague. Getting involved in an accident in which my finger got caught in a folding chair while caring for my younger sister, going to the hospital, and coming back with bandages are definite remembrances. This accident resulted in shortening of the ring finger of my right hand which is still obvious (Figure 1). I also recall going to school (third grade) in Mambalam in the city of Madras (now Chennai) and going to fourth grade in Parvathipuram, where I stood first in the class are definitive recollections of my early years. Because of this exceptional school performance, my parents decided that I skip fifth grade and had me take an entrance test and admitted me into sixth grade in high school in Ananthapuram where my father was working at that time. My only recollection of that year was participating in football (soccer) in the school team; indeed, I served as a team captain. In the middle of that year, my father was transferred away from Ananthapuram and my parents decided that I should stay with my grandparents in Parvathipuram so that I have an undisturbed education.

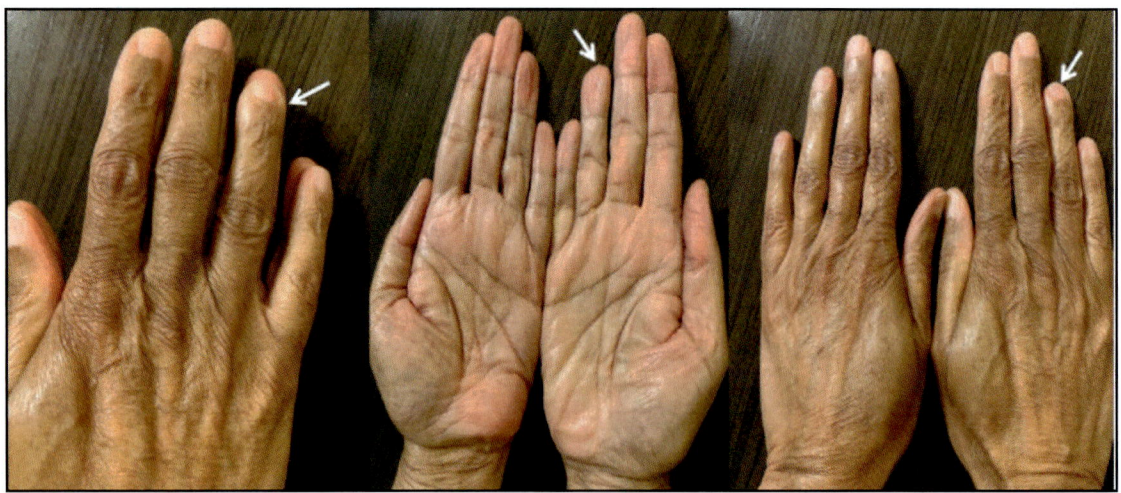

Figure 1. Photographs of my hands illustrating short ring finger (arrows) of my right hand.

Because I left in the middle of the school year, I again had to take another entrance test to get admission to the seventh grade in the Board High School, Parvathipuram where my grandparents live. Luckily, I passed the test again. The education continued with an interruption to go to Vijayawada for tenth grade because I was unhappy at Parvathipuram. During that year, I went to school at S. K. P. V. V. Hindu High School in Gandhinagar, a suburb of Vijayawada. As I finished the tenth grade, my father was again transferred, resulting in me returning to

Parvathipuram to finish eleventh grade and I graduated in 1956 achieving certification of Secondary School Leaving Certificate (SSLC) (Figure 2). Taking pictures was not in vogue in those days and after an extensive look at what could be found, I could only locate one picture taken (Figure 3) during my high school years.

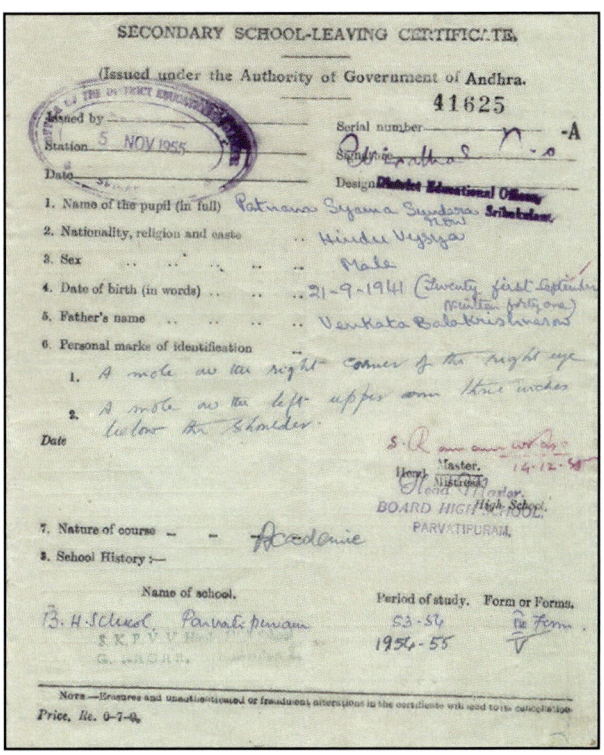

Figure 2. My Secondary School Leaving Certificate (SSLC).

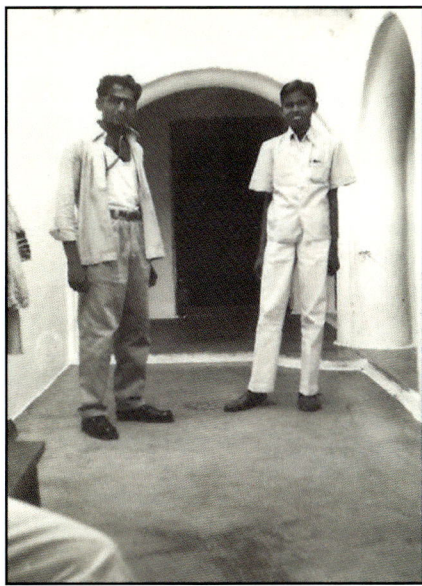

Figure 3. My photograph (right) with a family friend, a homeopathic doctor, during high school years.

GRANDPARENTS AND PARENTS

A few words about my grandparents and parents are in order at this time. My paternal grandfather, Patnana Swamy Chetty (Figure 4) is considered to be the first person to go to college from our Kalinga Vysya community; in those days, most people in our community went into business without going to studies beyond high school. My grandmother (Patnana Ratnalamma - Figure 4) was a homemaker and took care of the children. My grandfather's college consisted of two years of college and he graduated FA (Fellow of Arts). Following graduation, he joined the Revenue Department and rose in ranks to become a Tahasildar, a prestigious position. He was briefly promoted to a Deputy Collector, but was demoted shortly thereafter and he retired as a Tahasildar. His wish, as I was told, was to make one of his sons a Deputy Collector. Though he did not see that while he was alive, his second son did indeed achieve such a distinction by becoming a Deputy Collector in the Revenue Department. Following retirement from the Revenue Department, my grandfather served as a Dewan (Chief Minister) of Bobbili Raja before complete retirement and return to Parvathipuram, our native place.

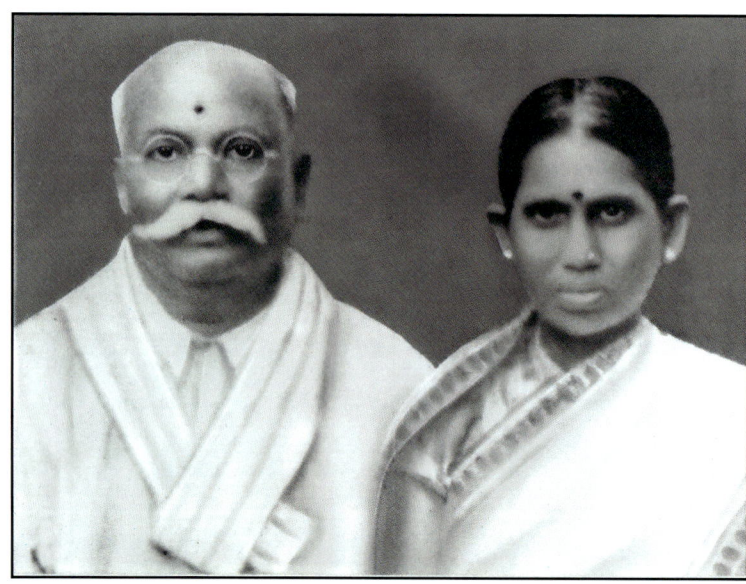

Figure 4. My paternal grandparents.

My maternal grandfather, Podugu Satyanarayana was a businessman in Ullibhadra and passed away before I was born and therefore, I do not know much about him with the exception that he was a very successful businessman. My maternal grandmother (Podugu Manikyalamma) was also a homemaker and took care of the children.

As mentioned, my paternal grandfather was very much interested in education. Because of this reason, education was considered very important in our family and indeed, seven of the eight sons of my grandfather pursued higher education (and became engineers, accountants or lawyers) and only one went into business. None of them were interested in becoming doctors and therefore, my grandparents were set out to make me, their eldest grandson, a physician. They encouraged, rather, indoctrinated me to become a doctor. This was an easy task for them since I was living with them during most of my high school studies. My grandfather did not live to see me as a doctor, but knew that I will be a doctor since he passed away when I was in the fourth year of medical school. My grandmother, however, lived longer and saw me not only becoming a doctor, but also achieving distinction in a foreign land, the USA.

My father (Patnana Venkata Bala Krishna Rao - Figure 5) was a very bright student and stood first in his class all through elementary school, high school and college and was able to secure a seat at the prestigious Gundy Engineering College, the only engineering college in the state of Madras (now Tamil Nadu) at that time. He continued his brilliance in studies and graduated with honors (BE Hon). He joined the state Electricity Department as a Junior Engineer and rose to the rank of Deputy Chief Engineer and Superintending Engineer. He was the first electrical engineer in our Vysya community and he was also the first to achieve distinction as Superintending Engineer. He was sent to England on a fellowship to learn about the Electrical Engineering in Briton and following his return, he submitted a report of how the Department of Electricity should modernize, but he was very disappointed that none of the recommendations were implemented by the government. Nevertheless, he enjoyed the distinction of "foreign-returned;" this was considered an accomplishment in those days. He is an avid fan of exercise and this is prior to the fad of exercise that developed years later in the medical community and among the public. He did not take (nor require) any medication until his death at age ninety-two because of sepsis related to a large boil in his thigh. He, like his father, was also very much interested in education and encouraged all his children to study so that three of us became doctors, two accountants and only one went into business, that too managing a wholesale medical store.

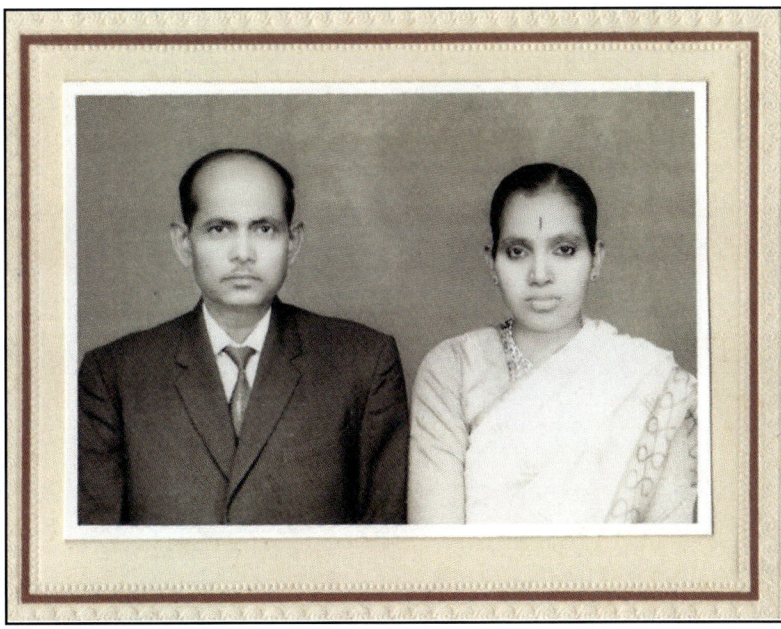

Figure 5. My parents.

My mother (Patnana Savithramma - Figure 5) was a homemaker and took care of the children. The family photo (Figure 6) shows my parents and siblings. She was very much interested in seeing Telugu movies, which is in contradistinction to my dad who did not want to go see any movies. She was also very much into gold jewelry. Because of these two reasons, each time I went to India (almost once every year), I made it a point to take her to as many movies as possible and either buy gold jewelry for her and if that is not possible, have a local jeweler make some jewel for her during each of my visits. She passed away at age eighty-five; shortly after a new set of gold bangles were gifted to her by me and my wife.

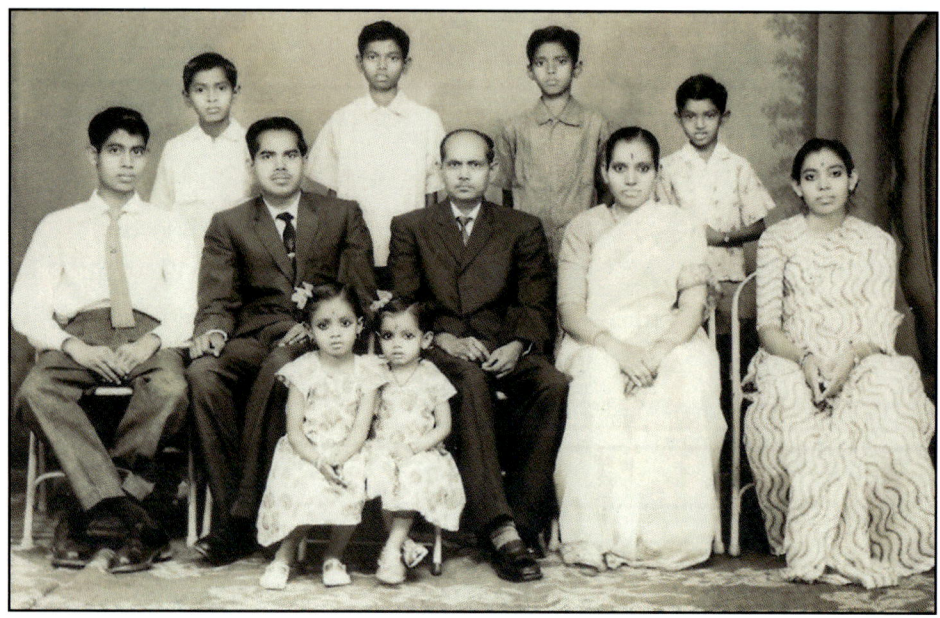

Figure 6. My parents and siblings. Standing, Muralidhar, Jayakeerti, Dr. Ratna Someswara Rao, and Bhaskar Rao; Middle row, Dr. Sambasiva Rao, me, my dad, PVB Krishna Rao, my mother, Savithramma, Kalyani; front row, Uma Devi and Anuradha.

COLLEGE, MEDICAL SCHOOL, AND DCH

Following graduation from high school as described in the section on "Childhood and Early Education," I went on to college studies; joined intermediate in Art and Science (IASc) at Mrs. A.V.N. College, Visakhapatnam, Andhra Pradesh. This was the last intermediate batch and subsequently a new system of education with introduction of PUC (Pre-University Course) started in Andhra University. Photographs taken during college, solo (Figure 7) and a with friend (Figure 8), are shown in figures 7 and 8. Following graduation in 1958 (Figure 9), I joined medical school.

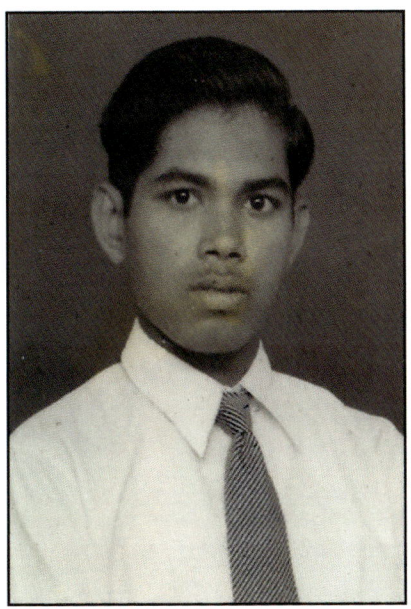 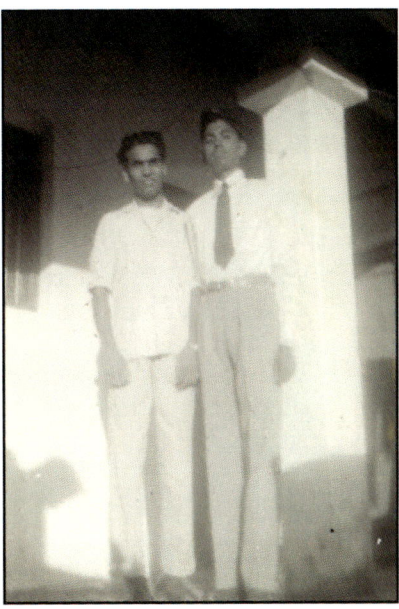

Figure 7. My photograph during college. **Figure 8.** My (right) photograph with a friend during college.

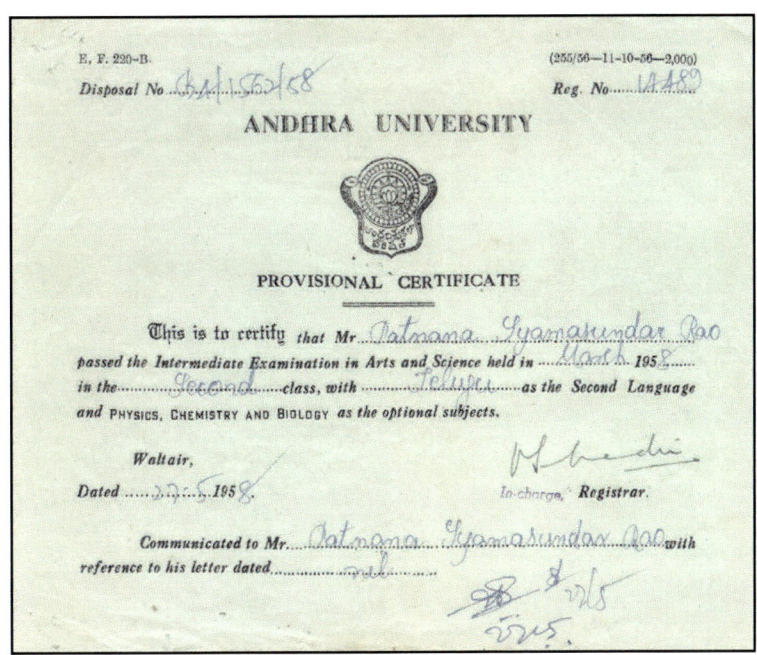

Figure 9. My Intermediate in Arts & Science Certificate of Graduation.

Medical school was a joyful experience for the most part. There was some ragging at the time of entry into the medical school, but fortunately it was not too bad for me since I did not live in the hostel. I stayed in a private housing and lodge in the first couple of years and moved to an Industrial Estate complex during the third year, since my dad was posted as an Industrial Estate Engineer overseeing that complex. When he went to England, I and the rest of the family moved into a private residence in Daba Gardens, a suburb of Visakhapatnam. When my father returned from England, he was posted away from Visakhapatnam. So, I moved into the Medical College Men's Hostel for the last couple of years of medical school. Some photographs taken during the medical school years are shown in figures 10, 11, 12 and 13.

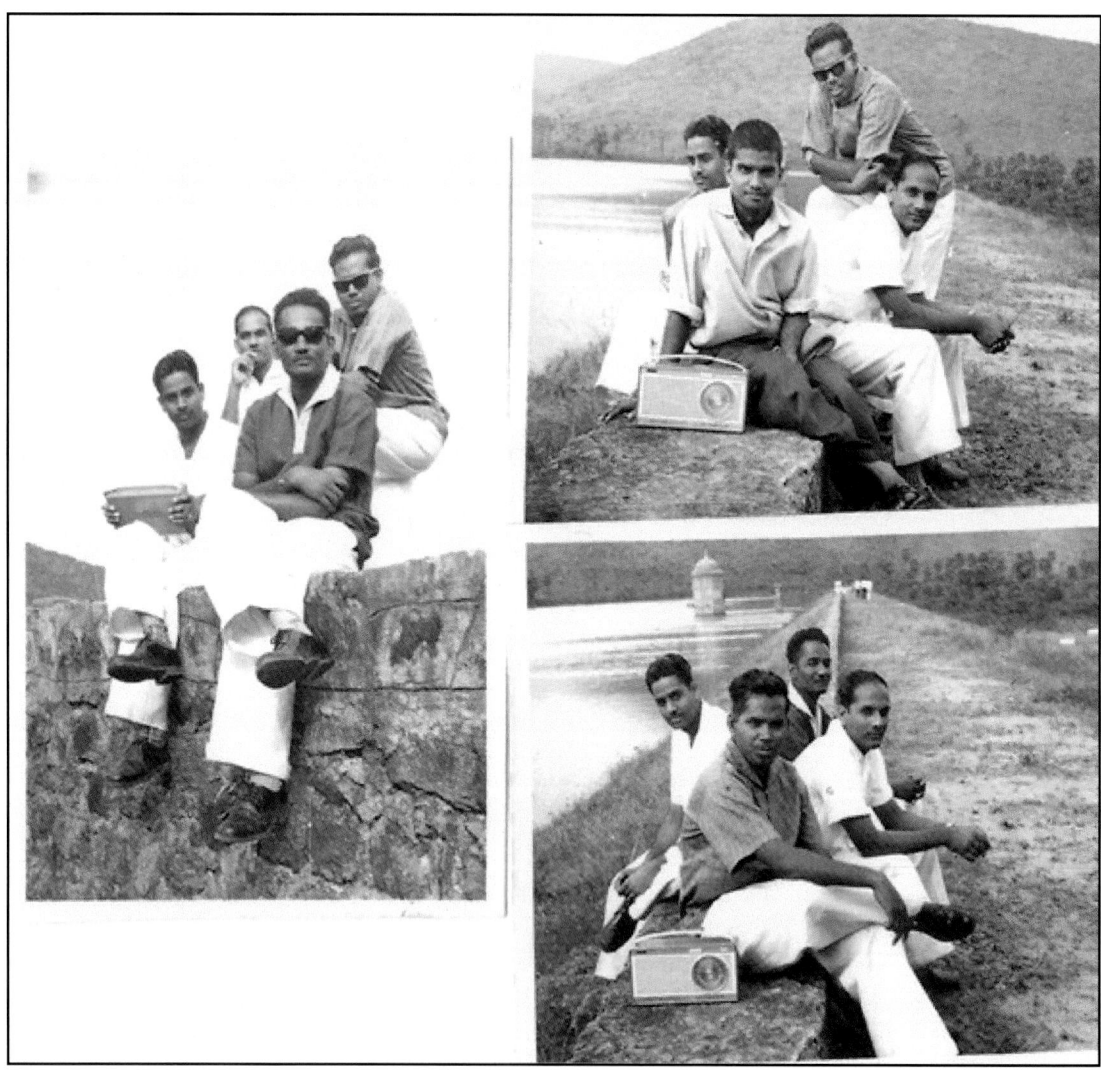

Figures 10. Me along with medical school classmates during a picnic at Aruku Valley.

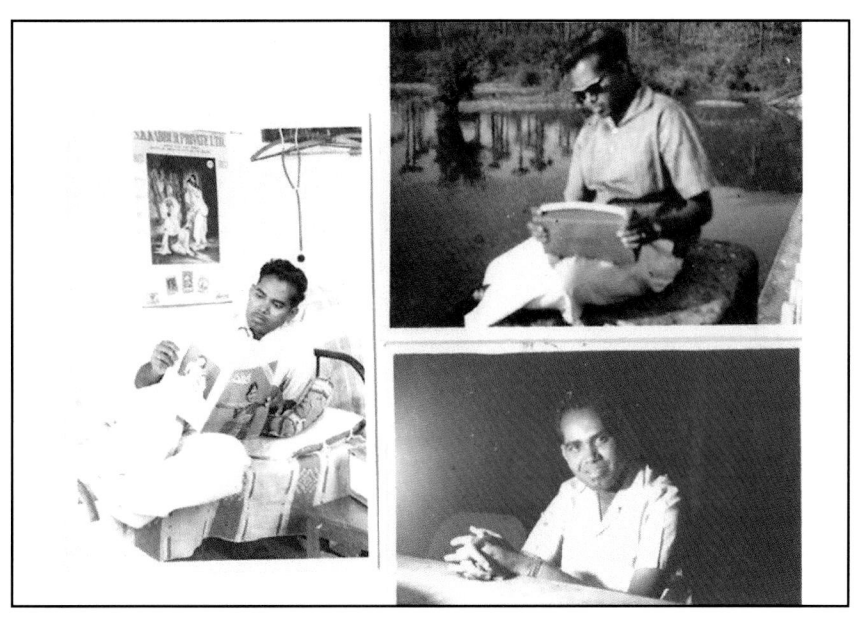

Figures 11. Photograph of myself during medical school.

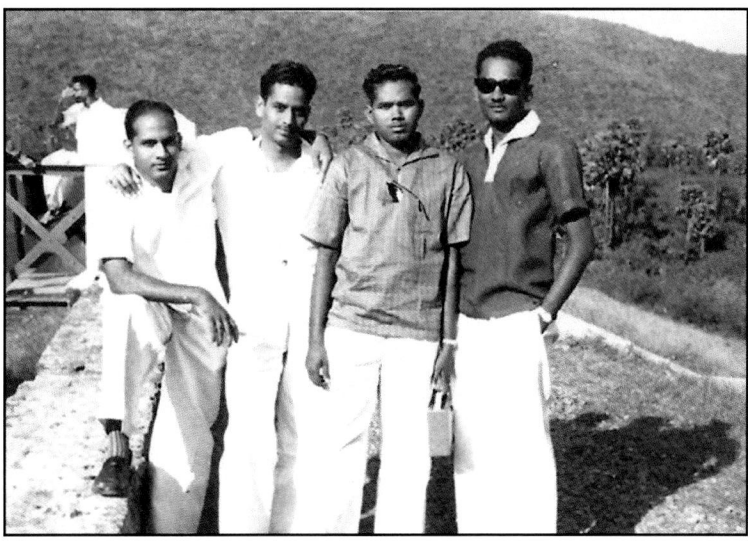

Figures 12. Photograph of me along with medical school classmates.

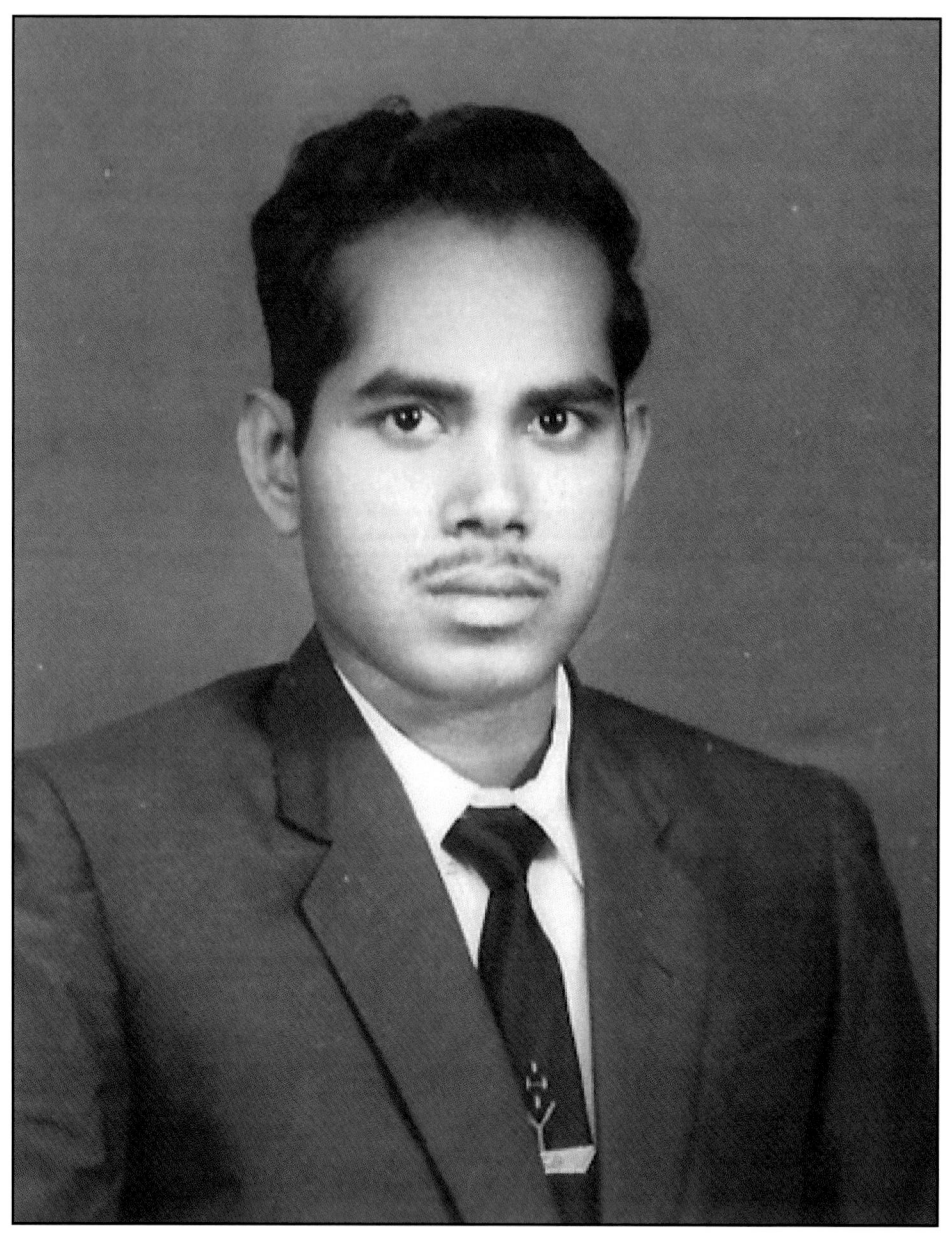

Figure 13. My photograph during medical college.

There was nothing remarkable about the studies and I progressed in a normal fashion and graduated in 1964 (Figures 14 and 15). However, there were disappointments because I failed to get elected as the class representative to which I contested. However, when I was a house surgeon, I was elected as the President of the House Surgeon's Association. During that period, I was instrumental in creating a state-wide House Surgeon's Association and became the President of the association. The association under my leadership organized and pleaded with the Health Minister to increase the stipend for the house surgeons, which was only ninety rupees per month at that time. The government refused; then, the association gave a strike notice. The government caved in and increased the stipend to 120 rupees before the strike started. This was considered an accomplishment.

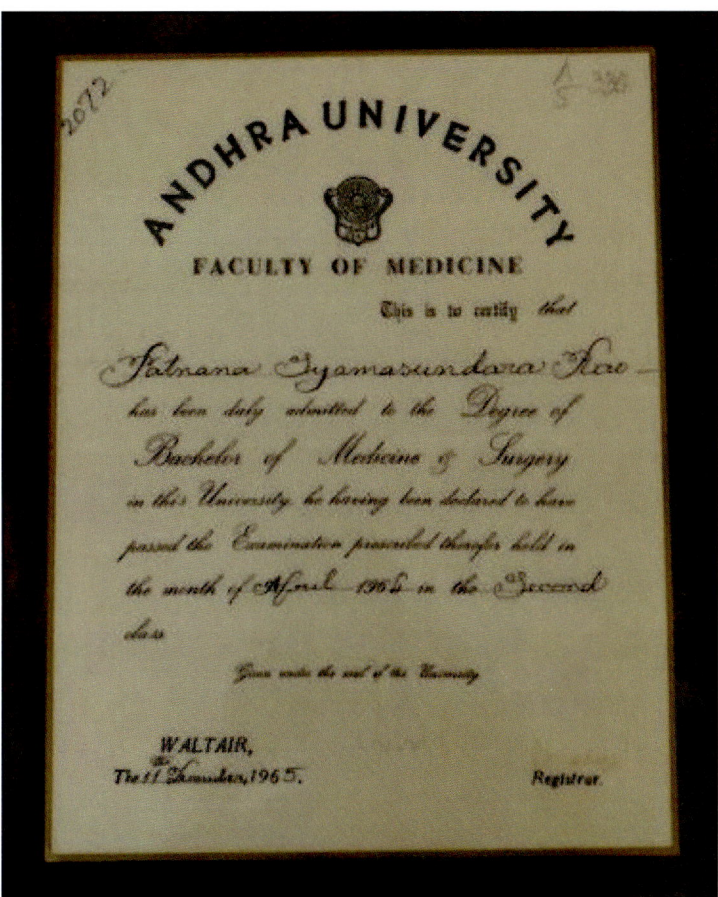

Figure 14. My medical school graduation Diploma.

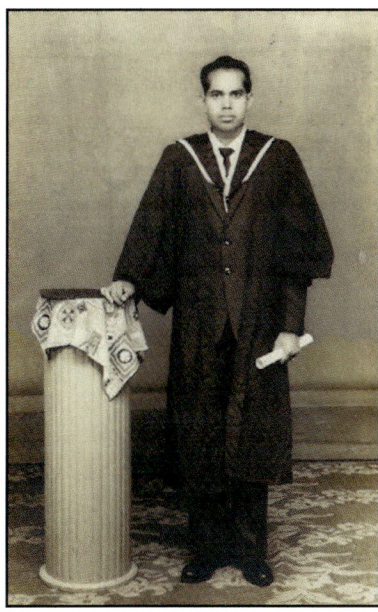

Figure 15. My medical school graduation photograph.

While I was a house surgeon, we were required to rotate through multiple specialties (Figure 16); this gave a wide range of experience. After completion of my house surgeon training, I secured a license to practice medicine, which was issued by the Andhra Medical Council (Figure 17).

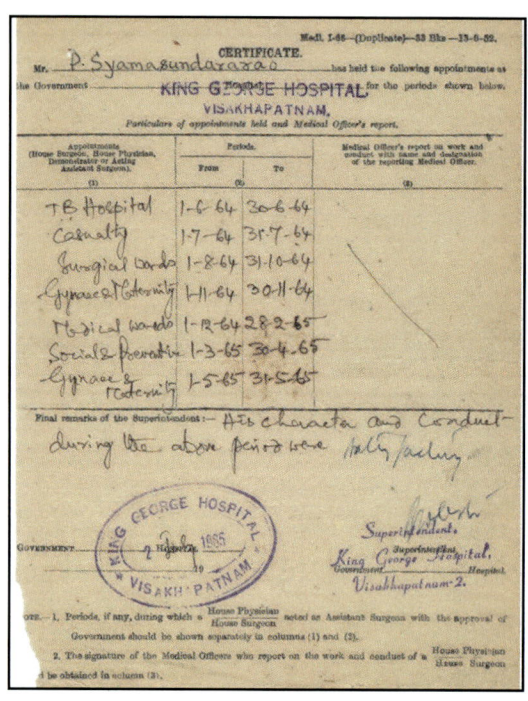

Figure 16. My specialty rotations during house surgeoncy at the King George Hospital.

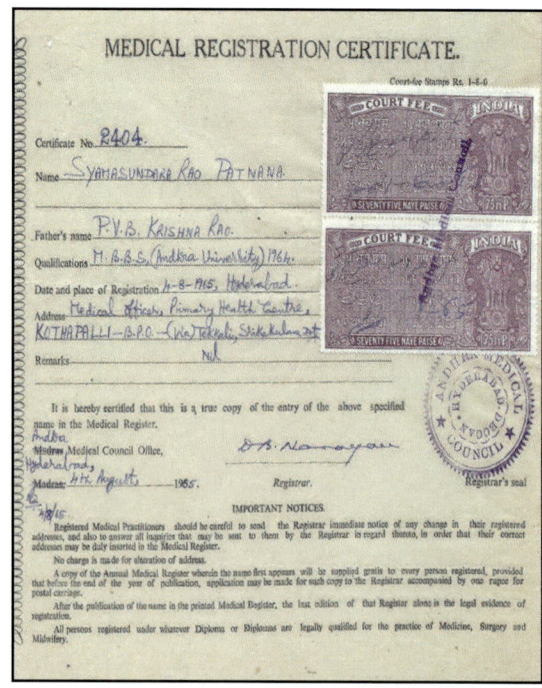

Figure 17. My license to practice medicine issued by the Andhra Medical Council.

Following the completion of my house surgeon training, I joined Diploma in Child Health (DCH) after a short detour as a medical officer, which will be described in the chapter on "The Journey to USA." This was a concentrated learning of diseases of childhood and formed the basis of my pediatric experience for the rest of my career. Some photographs with the other postgraduate students are shown in figure 18. I was conferred the Diploma in Child Health (DCH) in June 1966 (Figure 19), shortly before leaving for USA. To my surprise, I achieved distinction by being first in the university DCH examination that year (Figure 20).

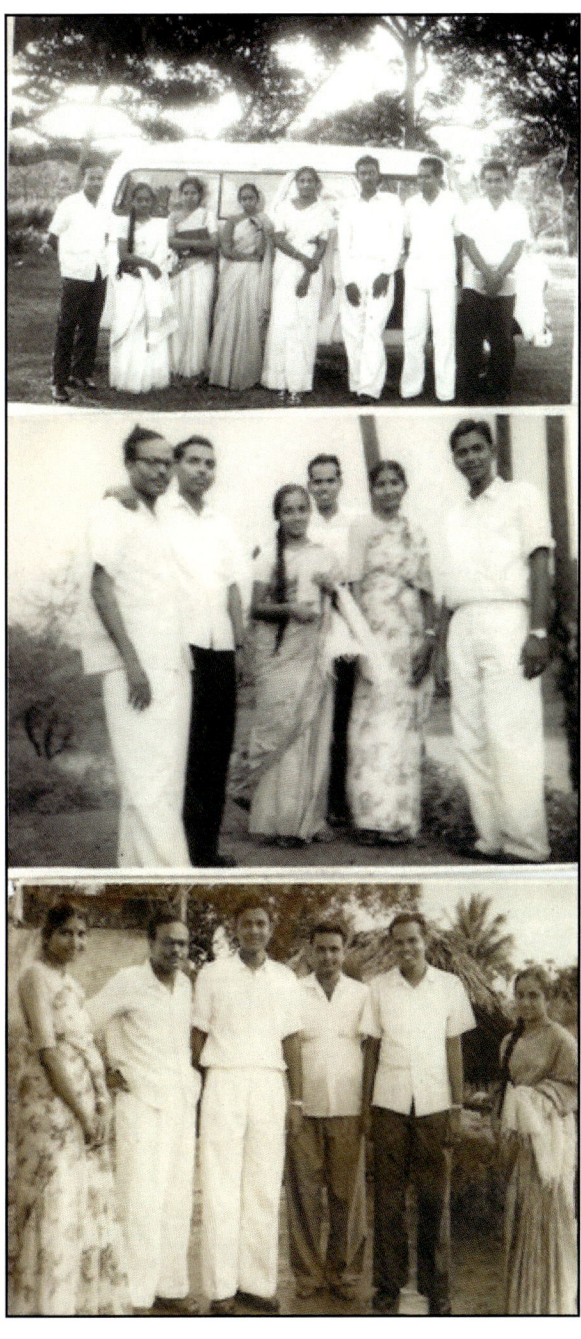

Figure 18. My photographs with the other postgraduate students during DCH studies.

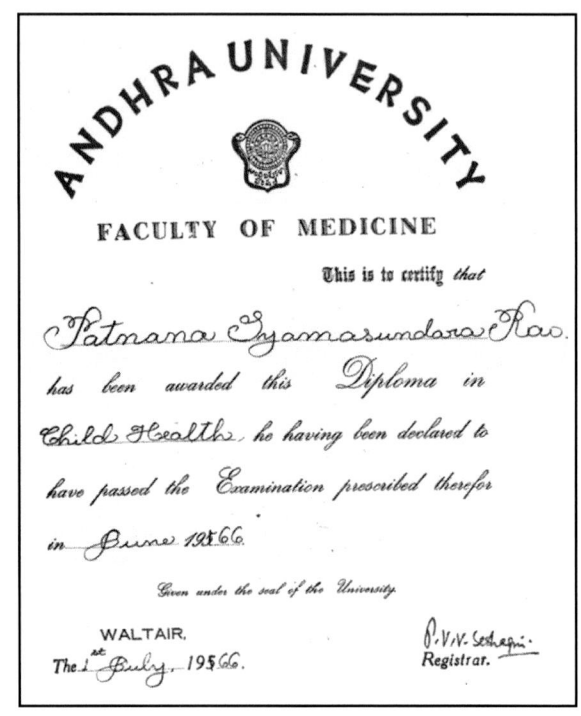

Figure 19. My DCH Graduation Diploma.

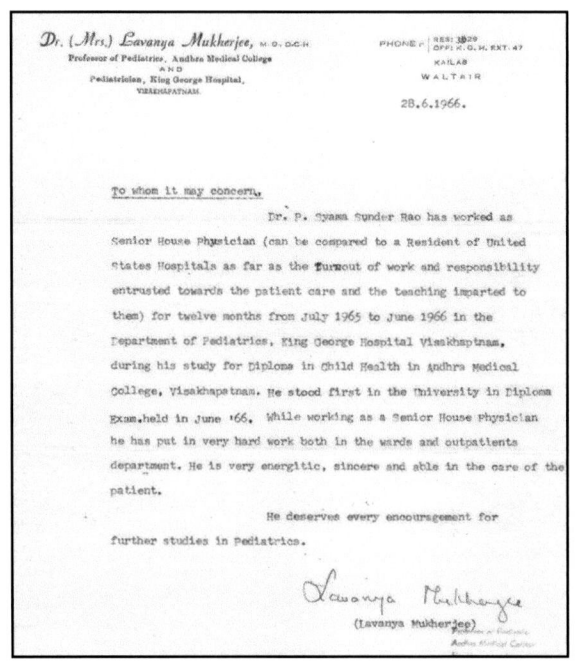

Figure 20. Letter from the professor stating that I achieved distinction by being first in the university DCH examination.

MARRIAGE AND FAMILY

Shortly before I came to USA, I married Doki Hymavathi, the youngest daughter of Sri Doki Lakshmana Murty and Srimathi Ammadamma (Figure 21) of Harischandrapuram, a village near Srikakulam in Andhra Pradesh.

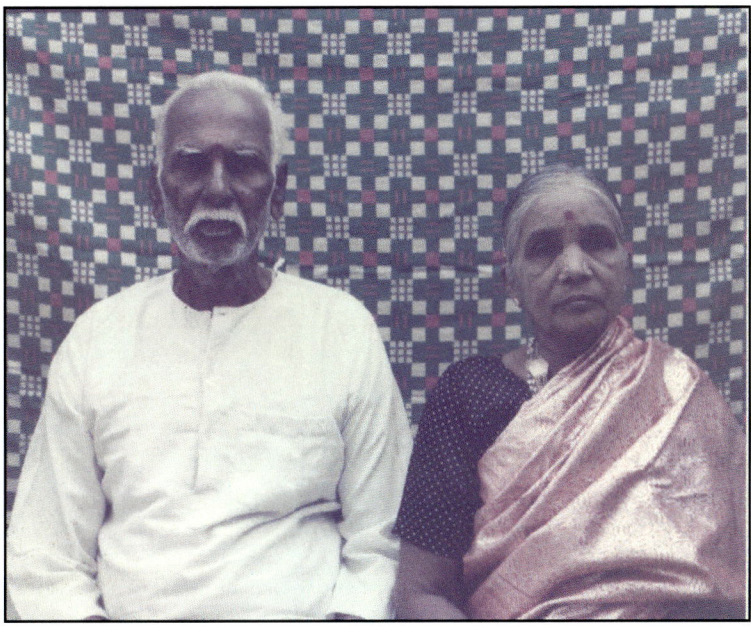

Figure 21. My wife's parents.

The marriage took place at Harischandrapuram with invitations printed in our native language, Telugu (Figure 22) and English (Figure 23).

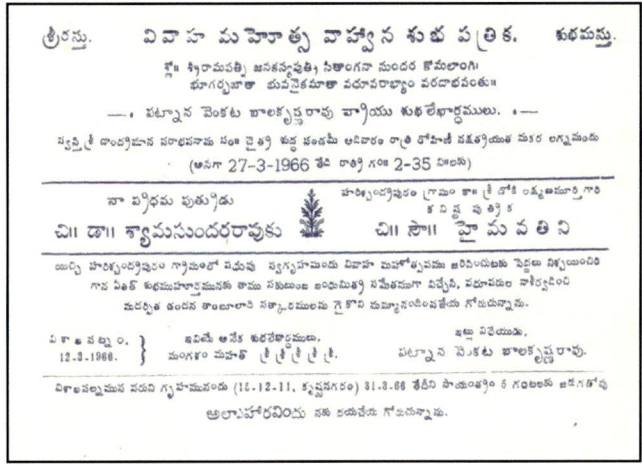

Figure 22. My marriage invitation in Telugu.

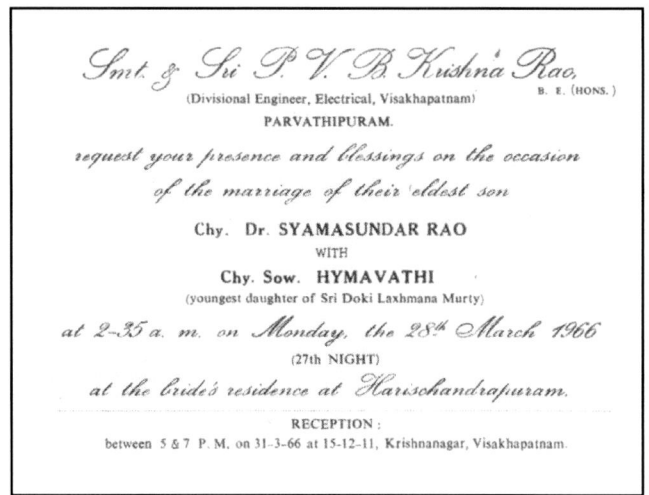

Figure 23. My marriage invitation in English.

The marriage was performed in a Hindu tradition (Figures 24 through 27) on the night of March 27, 1966.

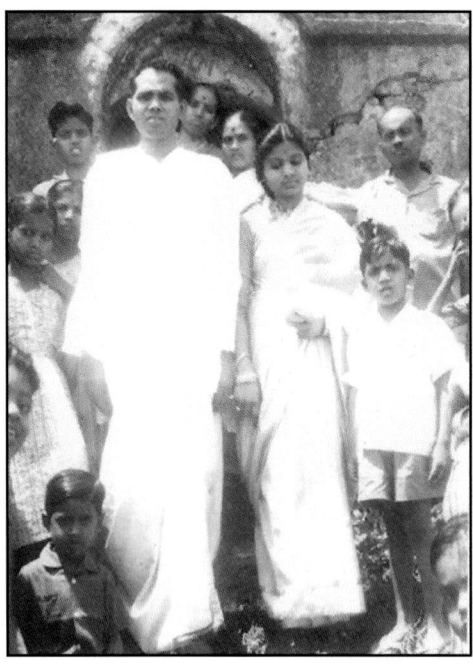

Figure 24. Photograph during morning ceremony of the wedding.

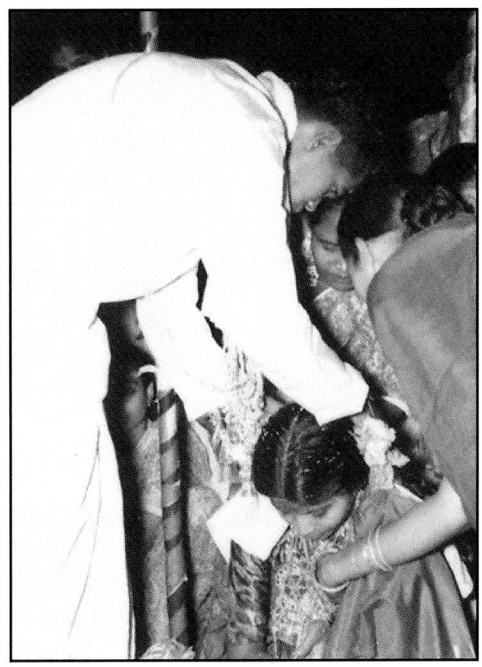

Figure 25. Tying mangalasutra, the most important part of the Hindu wedding ceremony, consummating the marriage.

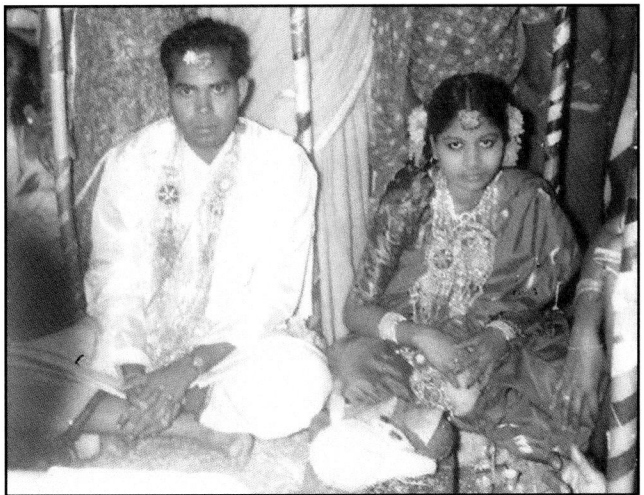

Figure 26. Photograph with the new bride soon after the formalities of the wedding.

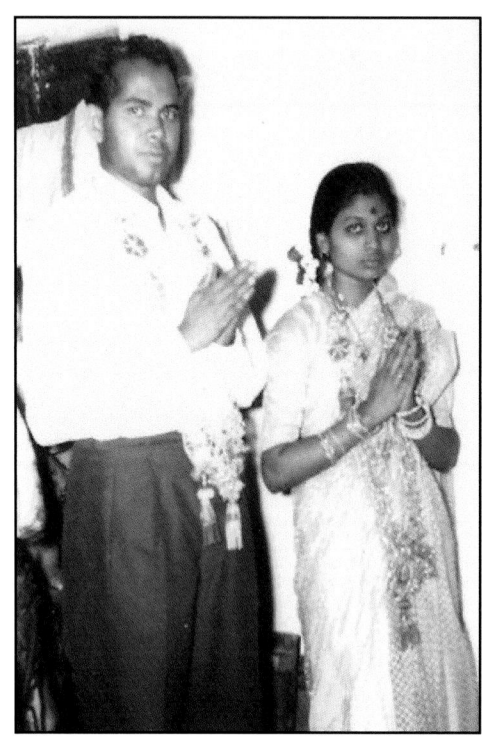

Figure 27. Photograph of the new couple praying to God immediately after returning to my parent's home following the wedding.

Some of the other marriage related photos are shown in figures 28 through 33.

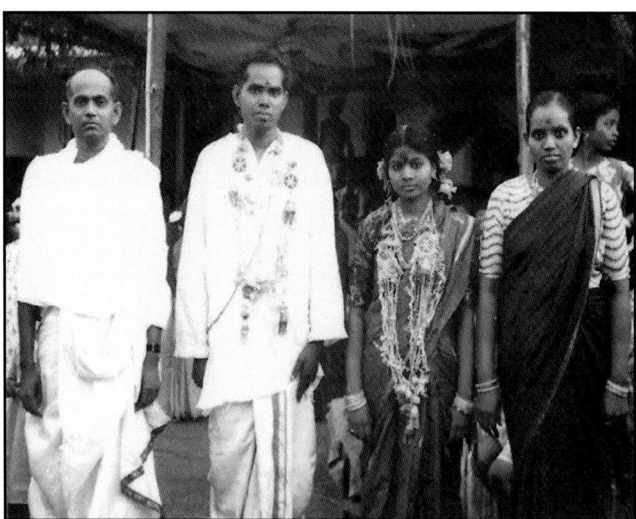

Figure 28. Photograph of the newly wedded couple with my parents.

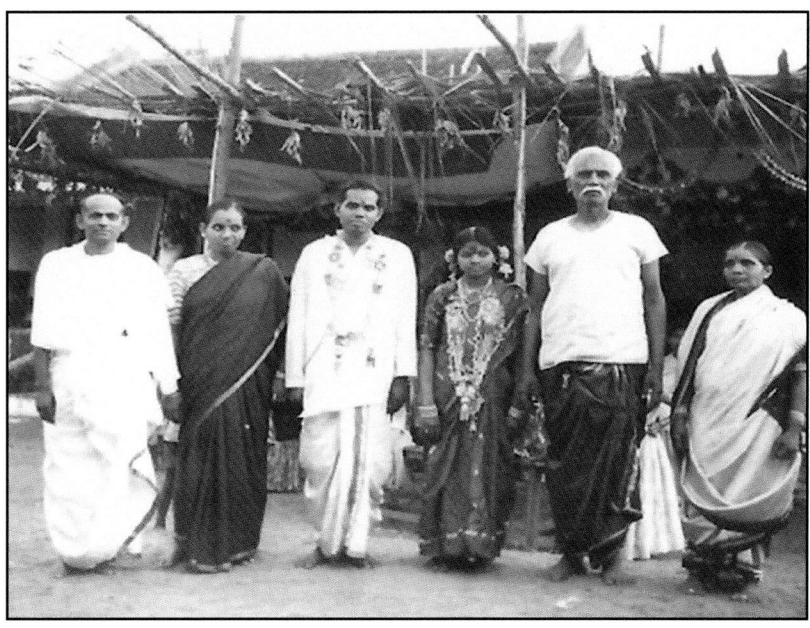

Figure 29. Photograph of the newly wedded couple with my parents (left) and the bride's parents (right).

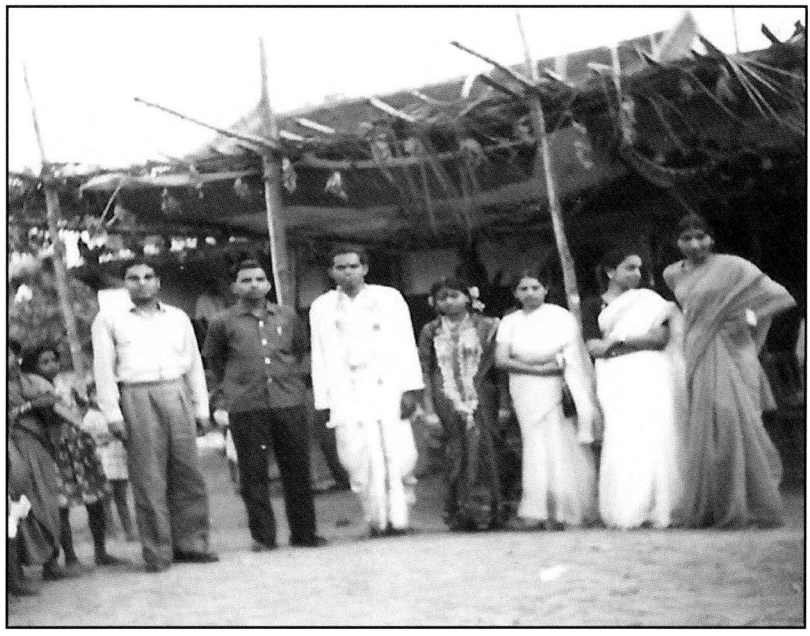

Figure 30. Photograph of the newly wedded couple with my colleague postgraduate students.

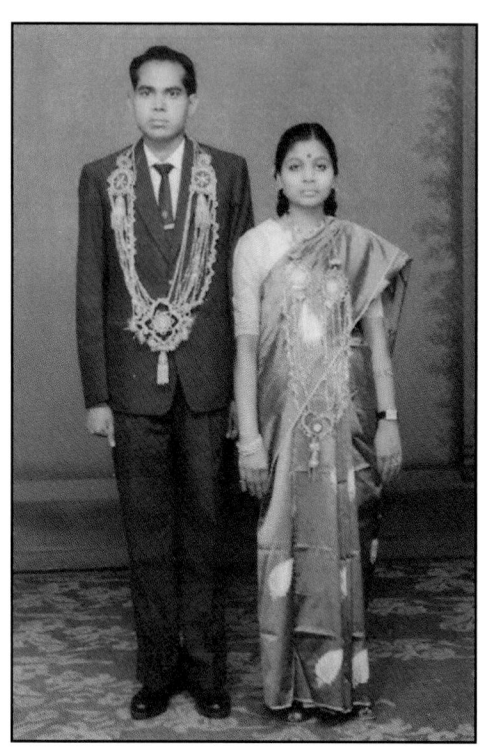

Figure 31. Photograph of the newly wedded couple in a photo studio setting.

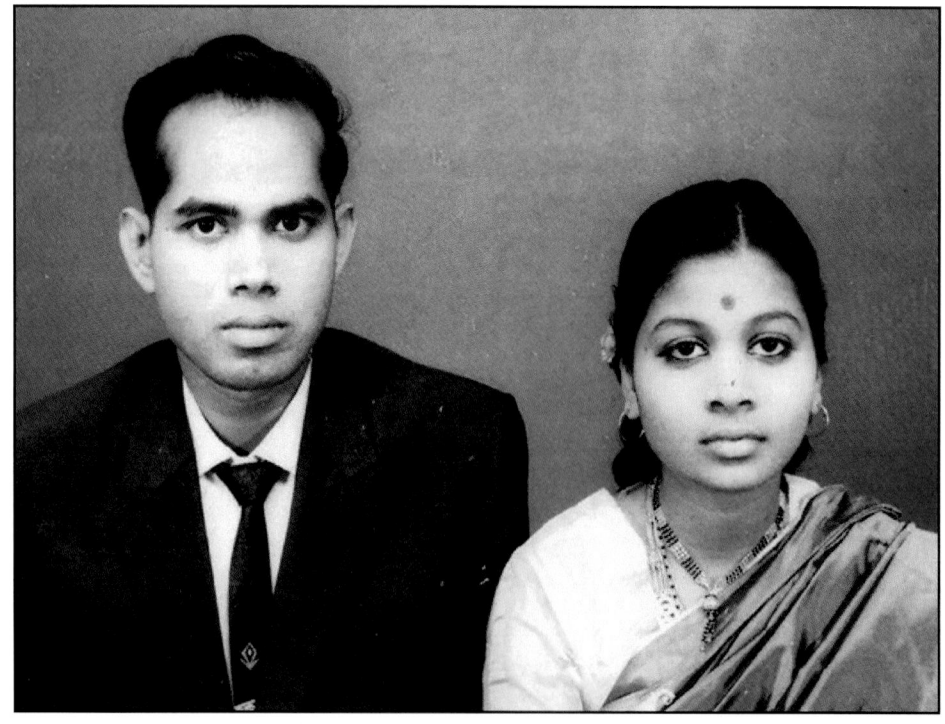

Figure 32. Photograph of the newly wedded couple in a photo studio setting, close-up view.

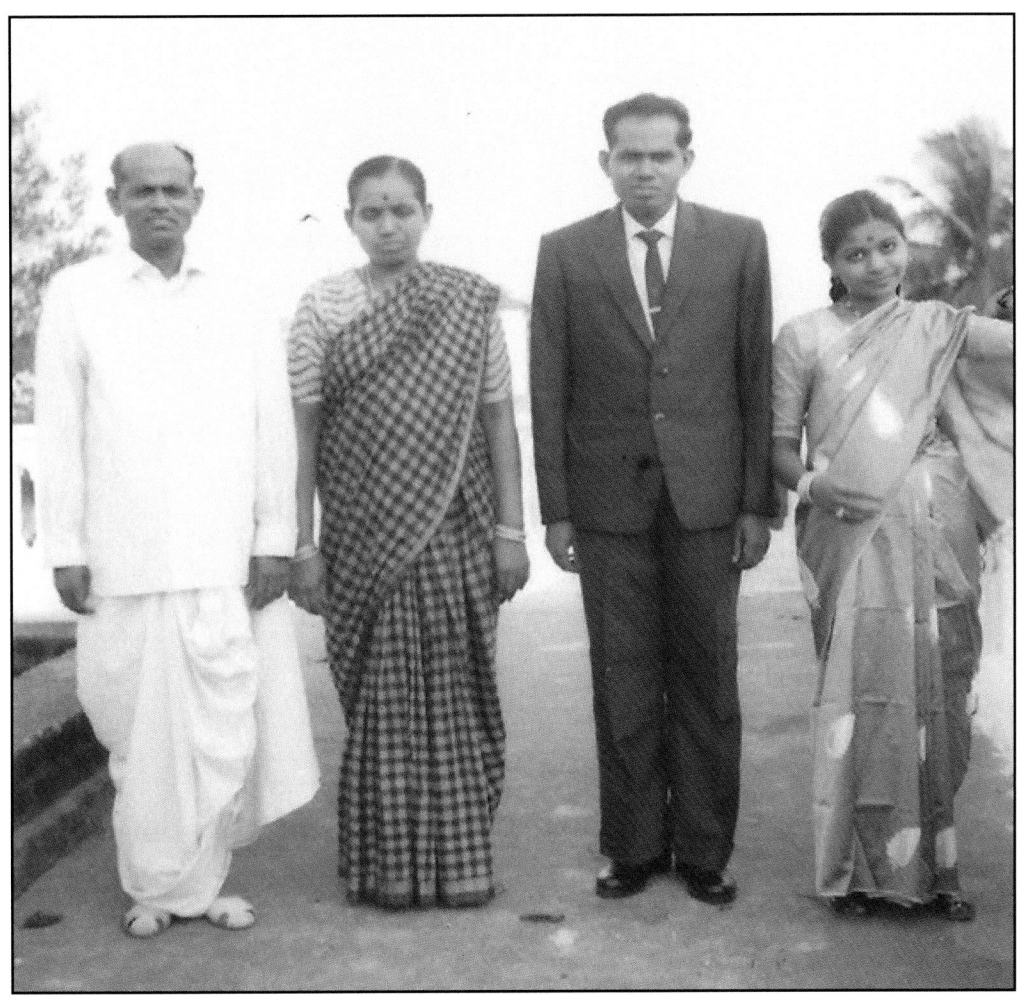

Figure 33. Photograph of the newly wedded couple with my parents shortly before the wedding reception.

My wife came along with me in my journey to USA as will be described in Chapter 2 on "The Journey to USA." We had three beautiful children (Figures 34 through 46). The oldest is a son who became a physician (Dr. Vijay K. Patnana) and Vijay practices Anesthesiology in St. Louis, Missouri. The second is a daughter who also became a physician (Dr. Madhavi Patnana) and Madhavi is currently the Professor of Radiology at the University of Texas, MD Anderson Cancer Center in Houston, Texas. The third is also a daughter (Ms. Radhika N. Patnana) who dabbles in fashion and marketing. Photographs of the children as they grew up (Figures 34 through 38) and them with me and my wife (Figures 39 through 46) are shown in figures 34 through 46.

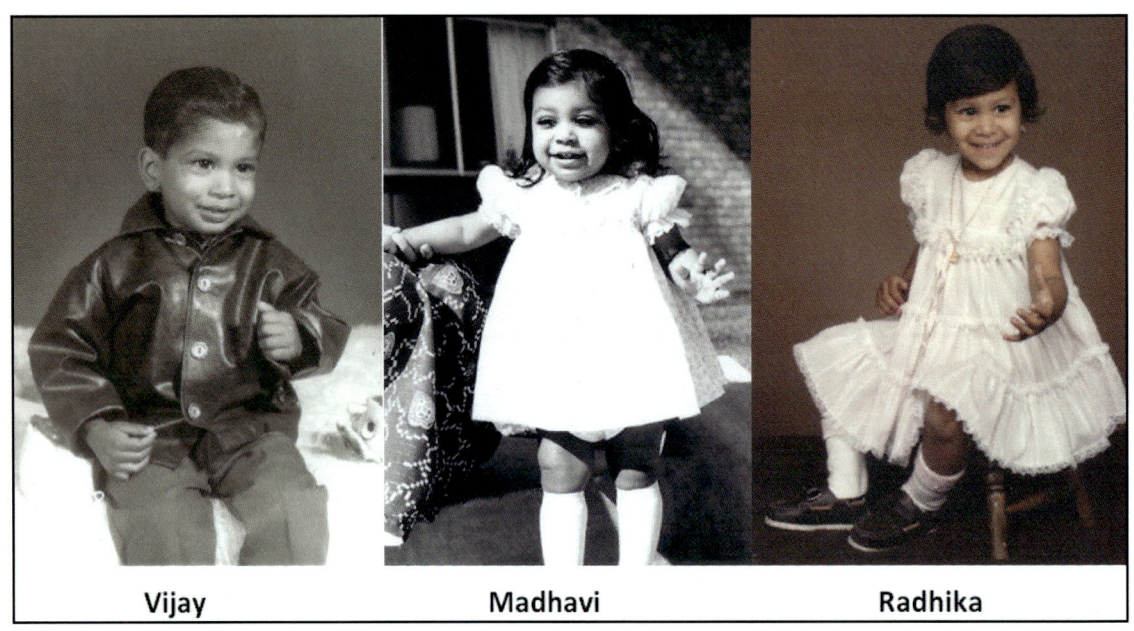

Figure 34. Our son and daughters at a young age.

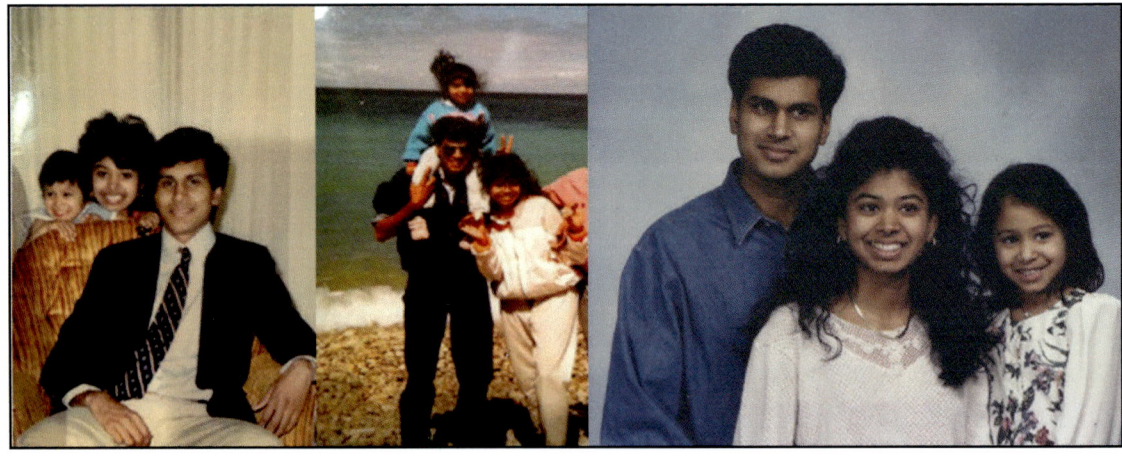

Figure 35. Our son and daughters as they grew up.

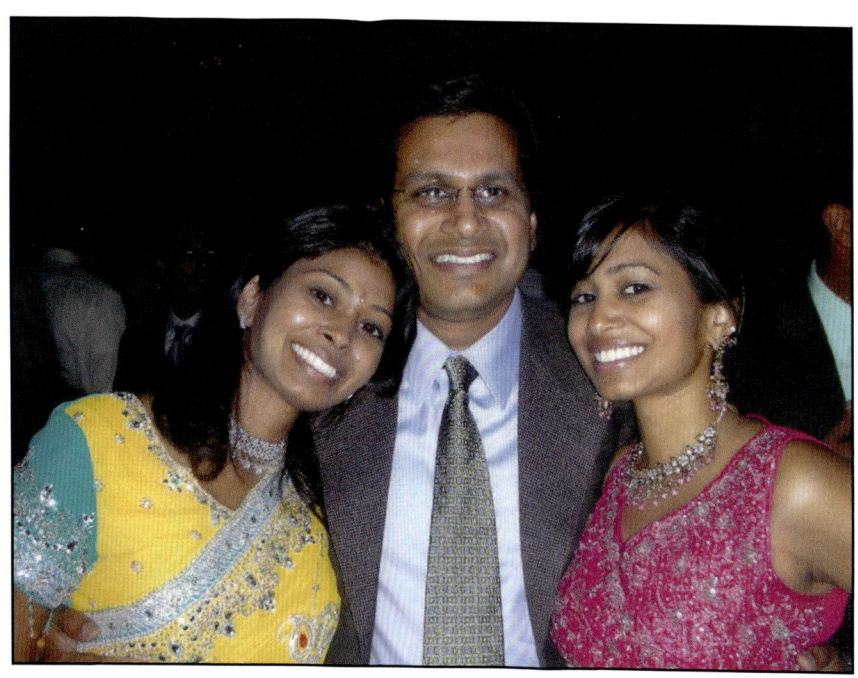

Figure 36. Our son and daughters in early 2000s, Madhavi, Vijay and Radhika.

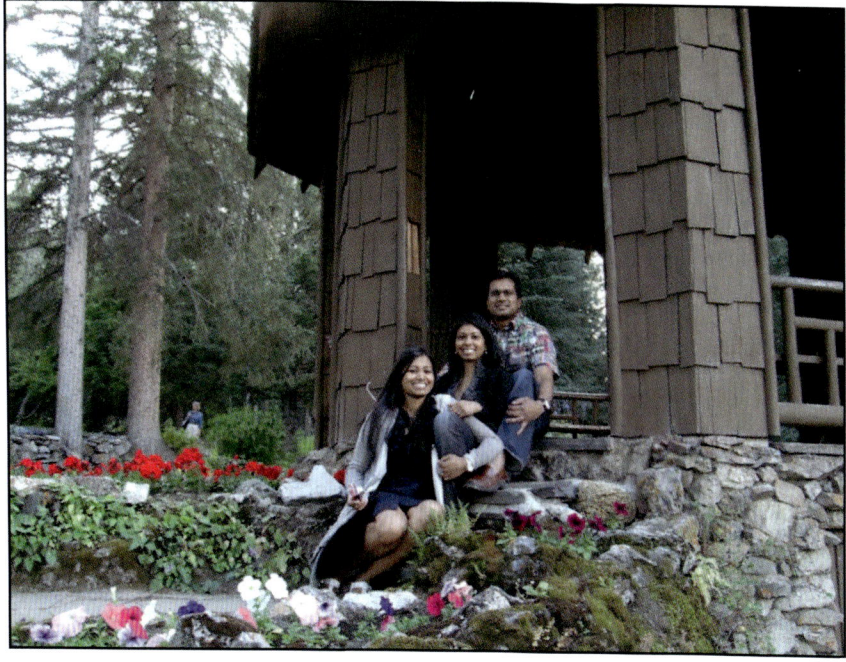

Figure 37. Our son and daughters at a Canadian Resort in 2011. Top to bottom, Vijay, Madhavi, and Radhika.

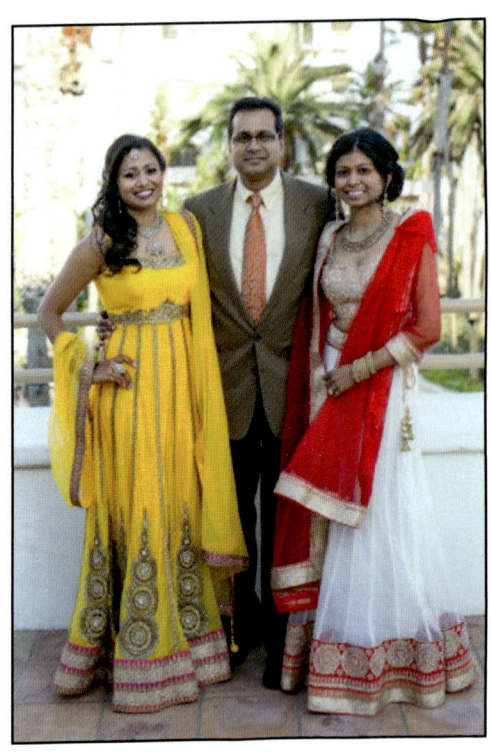

Figure 38. Our son and daughters in 2016, Radhika, Vijay, and Madhavi.

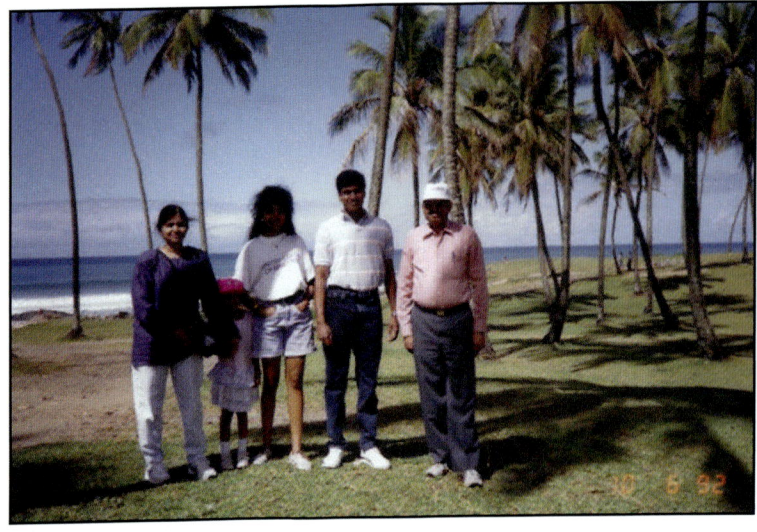

Figure 39. Me with my wife, son and daughters. Hymavathi, Radhika, Madhavi,

Vijay, and me.

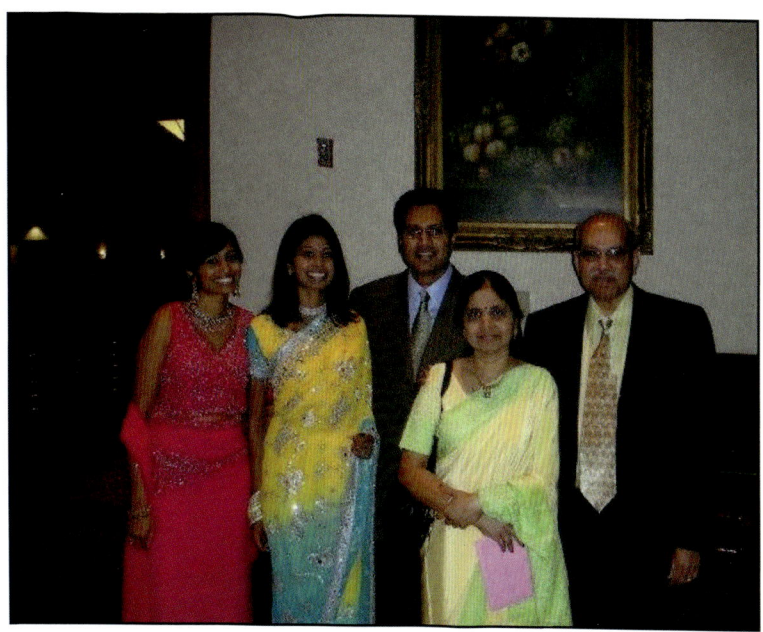

Figure 40. Me with my wife, son and daughters. Radhika. Madhavi, Vijay, Hymavathi, and me.

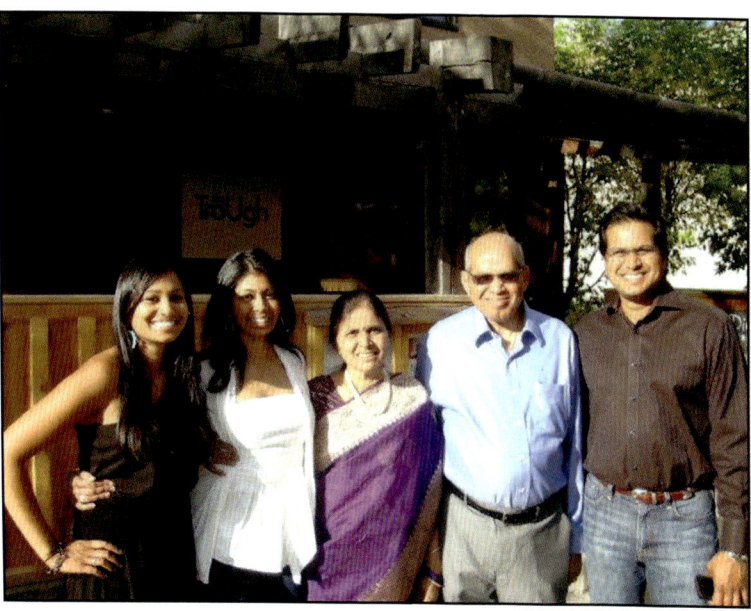

Figure 41. Me with my wife, son and daughters. Radhika, Madhavi, Hymavathi, me, and Vijay.

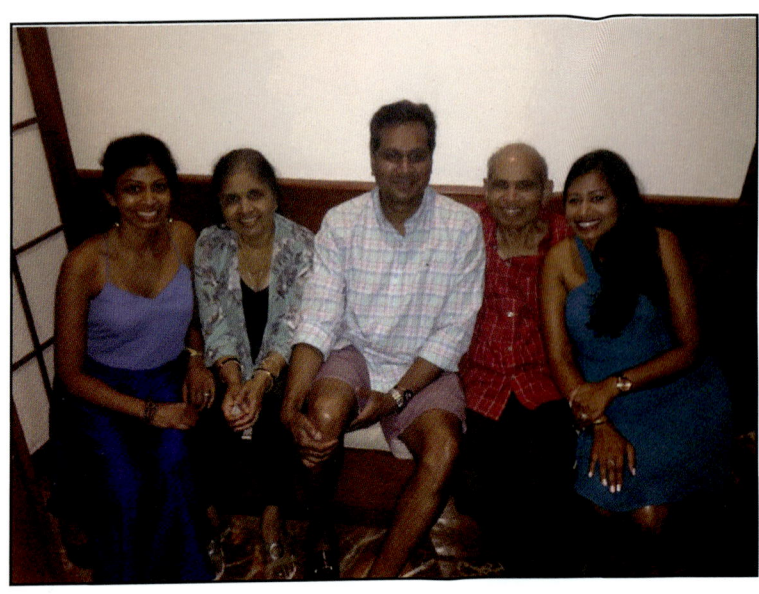

Figure 42. Me with my wife, son and daughters. Madhavi, Hymavathi, Vijay, me, and Radhika.

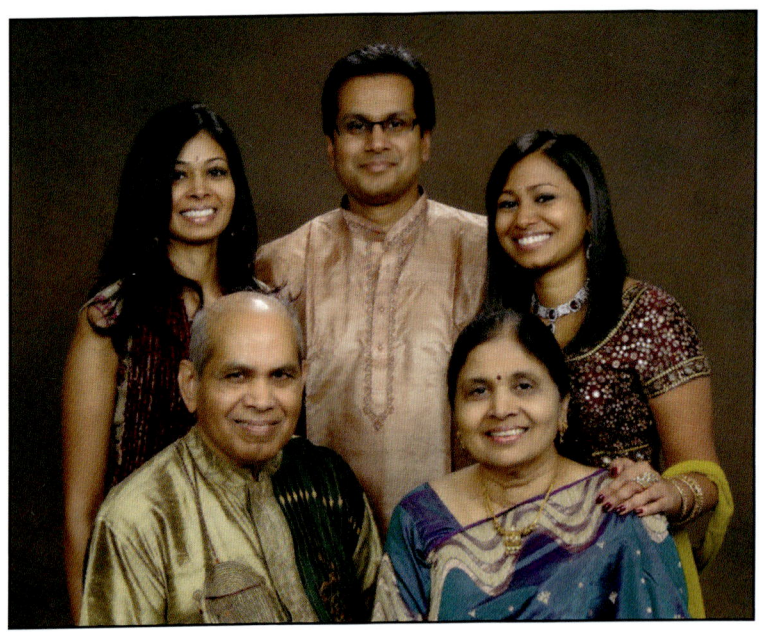

Figure 43. Me with my wife, son and daughters in 2014. Top row, Madhavi, Vijay and Radhika. Bottom row, me and Hymavathi.

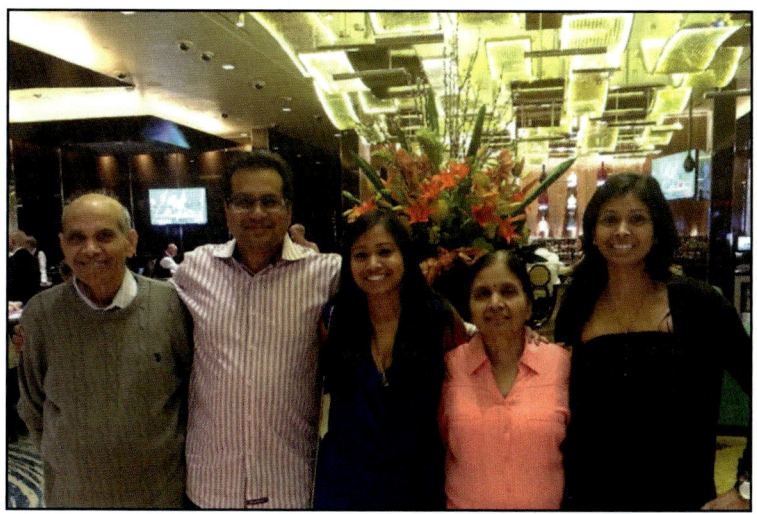

Figure 44. Me with my wife, son and daughters in 2016. Me, Vijay, Radhika, Hymavathi and Madhavi.

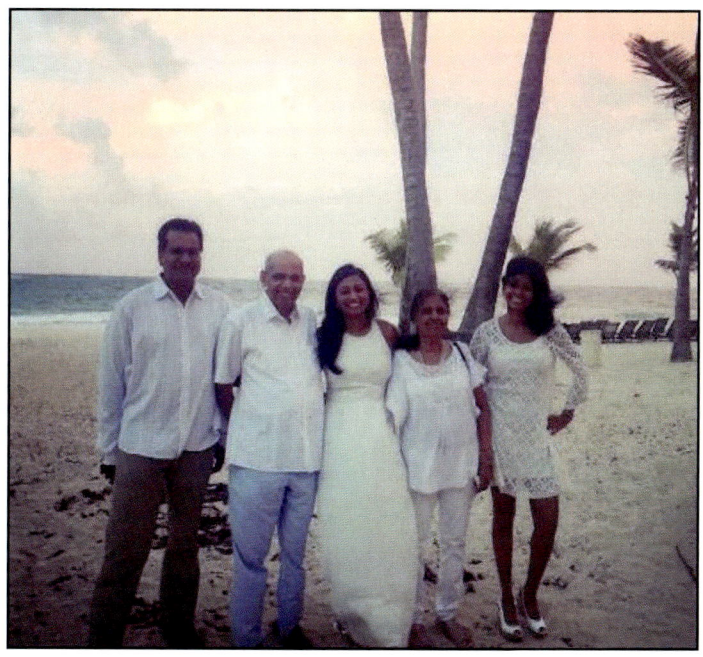

Figure 45. Me with my wife, son and daughters in 2017 at a resort. Vijay, me, Radhika, Hymavathi, and Madhavi.

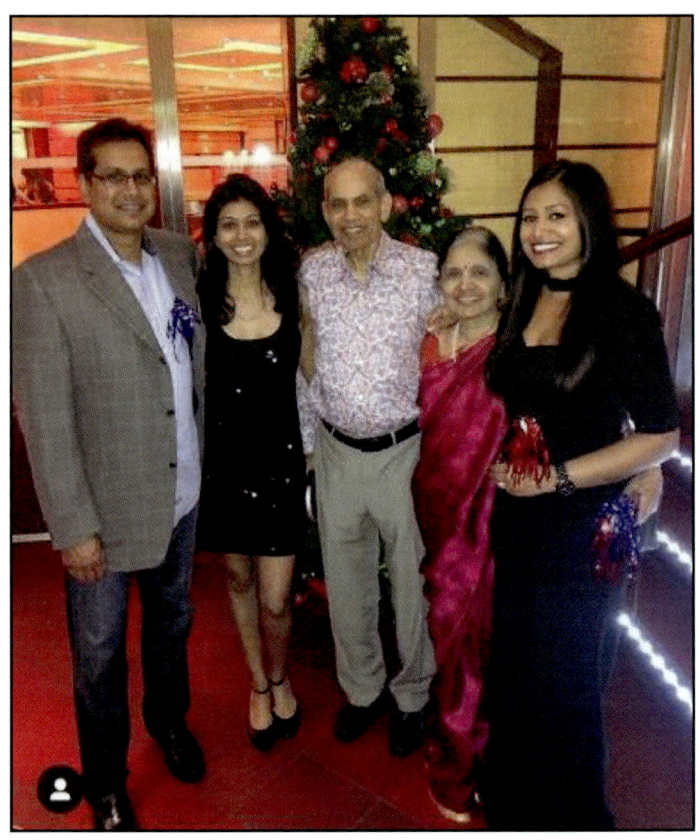

Figure 46. Me with my wife, son and daughters at a Thanksgiving get-together. Vijay, Madhavi, me, Hymavathi, and Radhika.

Photographs of daughters with me and my wife are shown in figures 47 through 49.

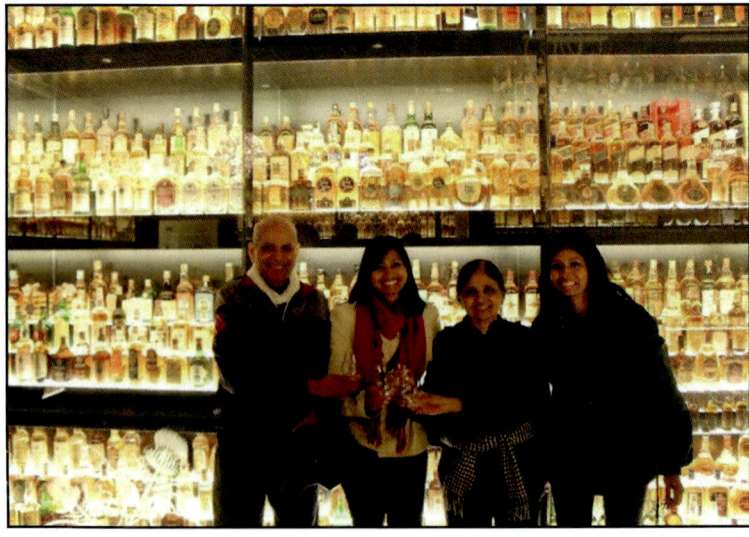

Figure 47. Me with my wife and daughters while in Iceland. Me, Radhika Hymavathi, and Madhavi.

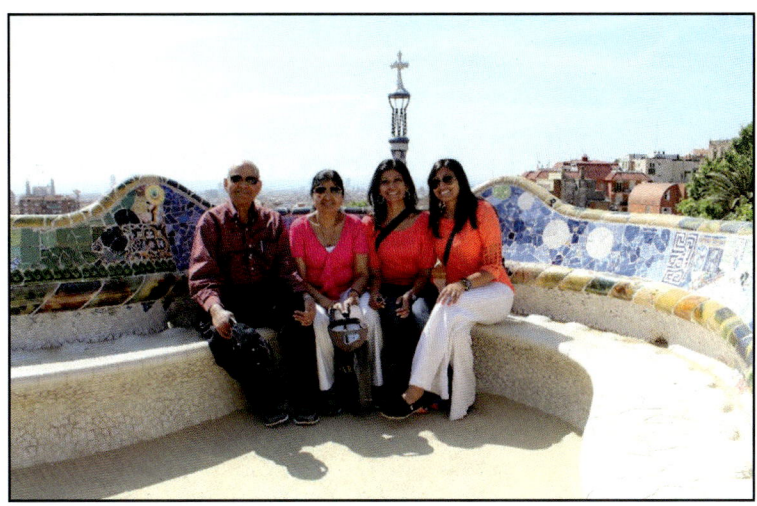

Figure 48. Me with my wife and daughters while in New Orleans. Me, Hymavathi, Madhavi, and Radhika.

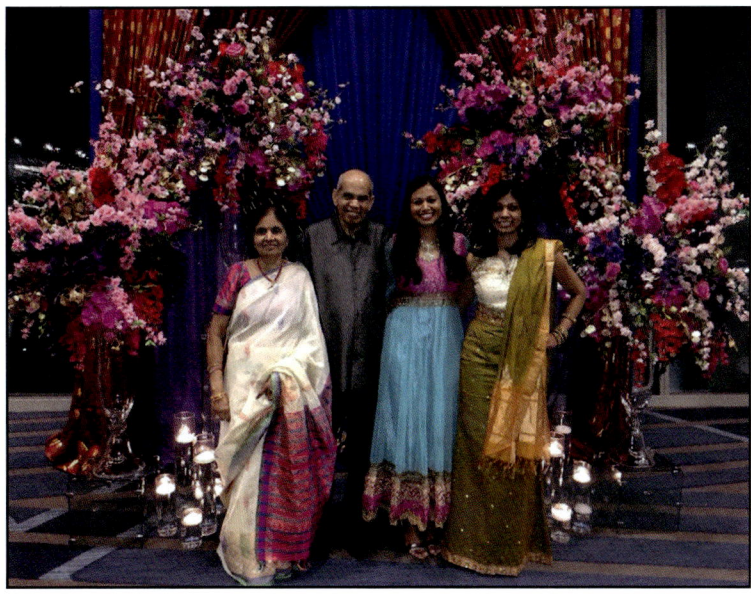

Figure 49. Me with my wife and daughters. Hymavathi, me, Radhika, and Madhavi.

We are blessed with three granddaughters and their photographs by themselves (Figures 50 & 51) as well as with me and my wife (Figure 52) are shown as follows.

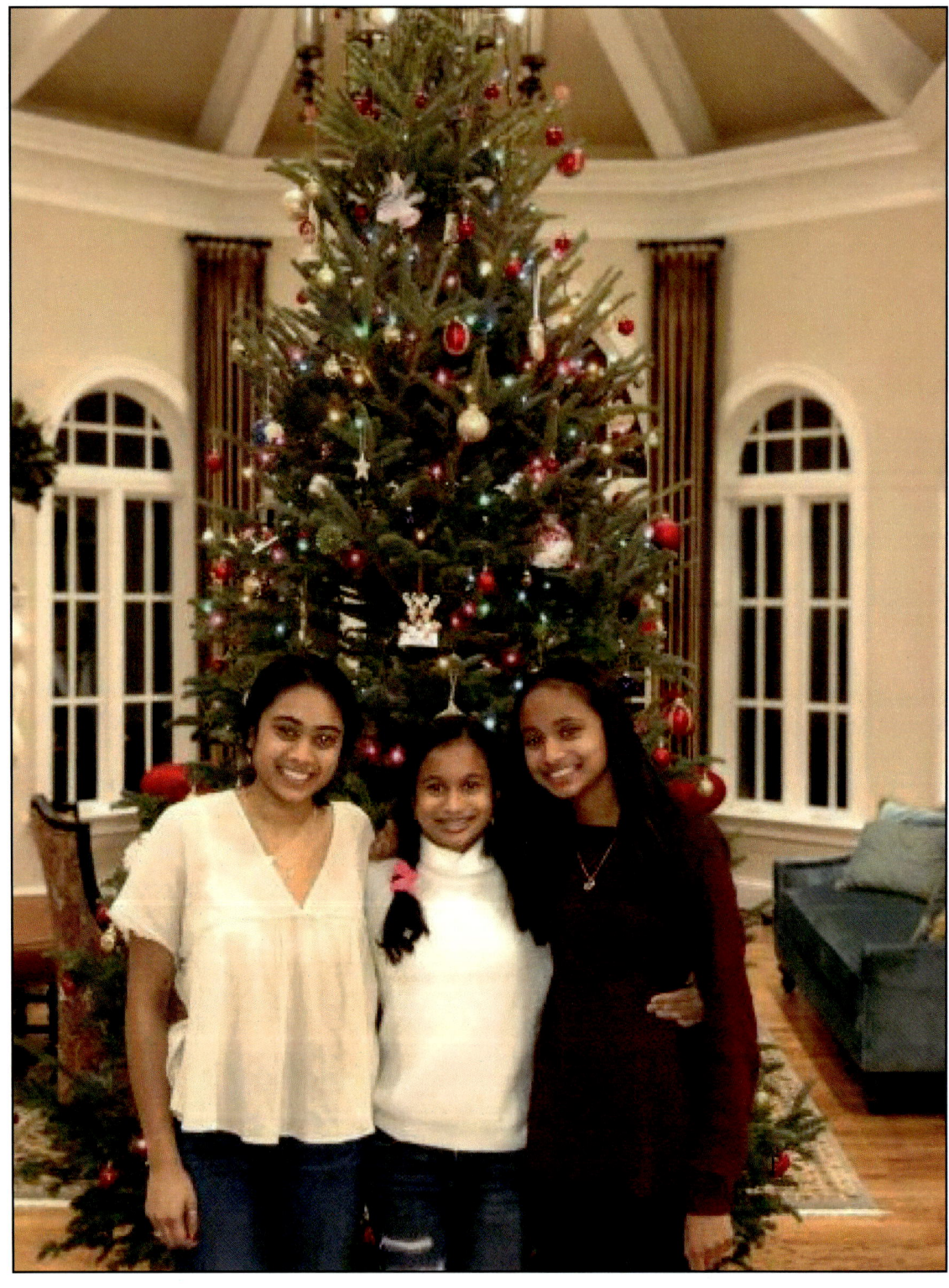

Figure 50. Our granddaughters, Meghana, Anjali, and Rhea.

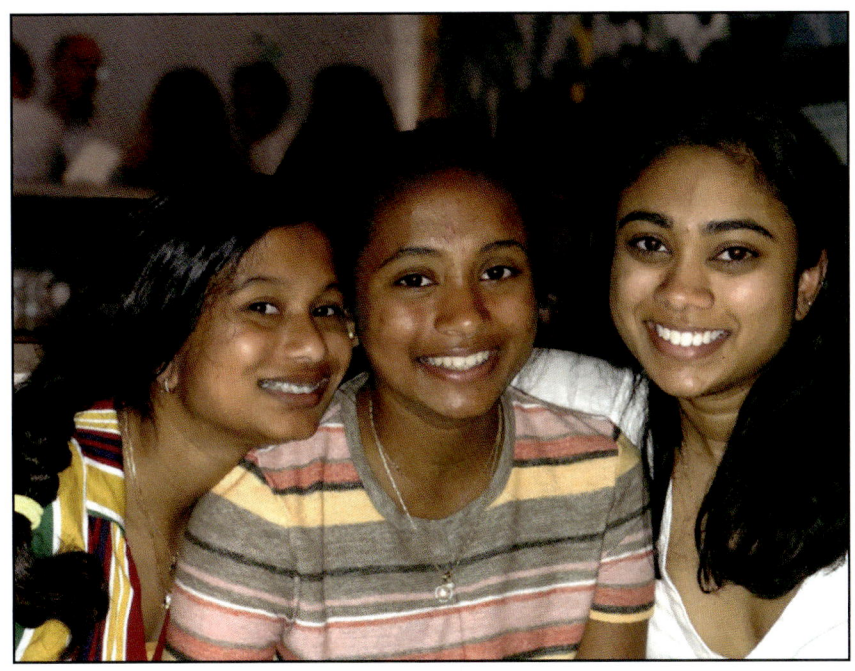

Figure 51. Our granddaughters, Anjali, Rhea, and Meghana.

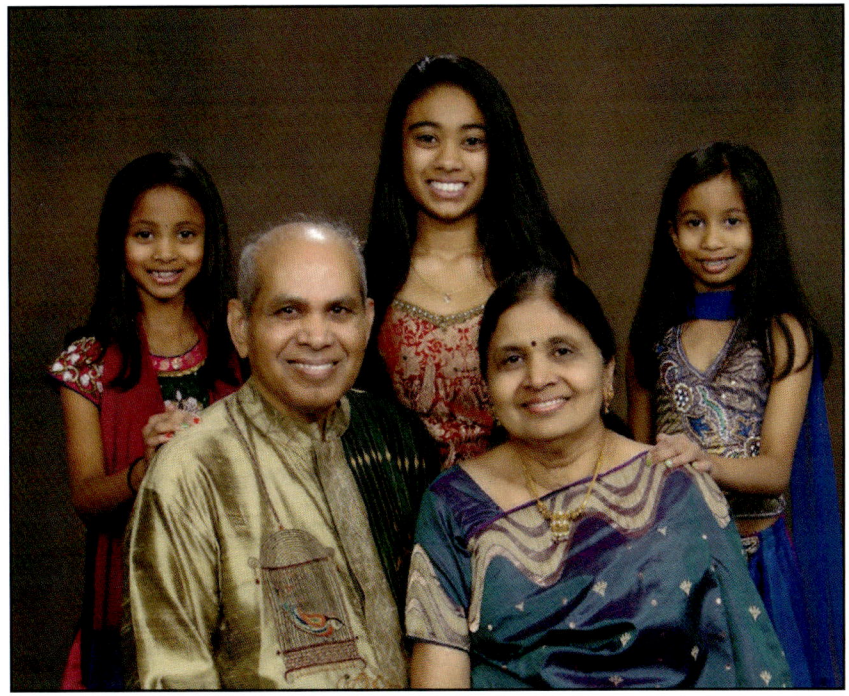

Figure 52. Me with my wife and granddaughters in 2014. Top row, Rhea, Meghana and Anjali. Bottom row, me, and Hymavathi.

My wife has always been a helpful companion, supporting me to prepare for multiple examinations that I had to take during my training, raise our children, take care of my parents during their old age, and take care of me when I was sick with a severe heart attack in 2015. Most importantly, she was very supportive of me in providing financial support to my father in educating four of my brothers and performing marriages of three sisters since my dad retired shortly after my next brother's graduation from medical school.

A pictorial presentation of some of the events during the journey will be presented in figures 53 through 82.

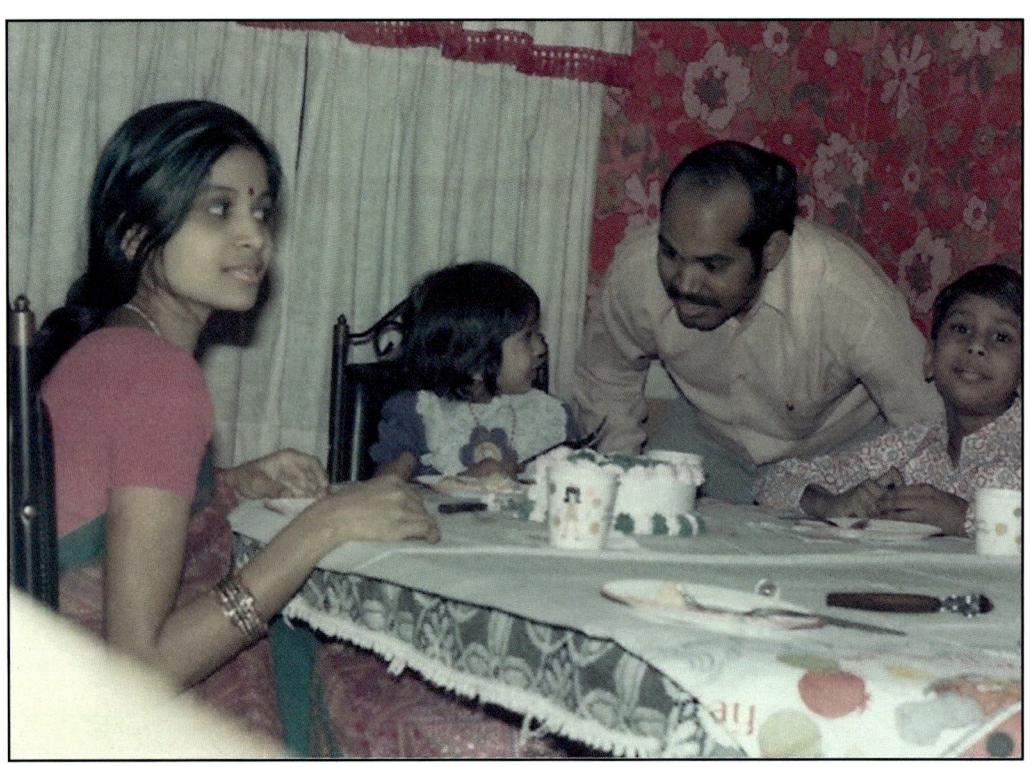

Figure 53. Celebrating daughter, Madhavi's birthday in mid 1970s with Vijay, on-looking. Hymavathi, Madhavi, me, and Vijay.

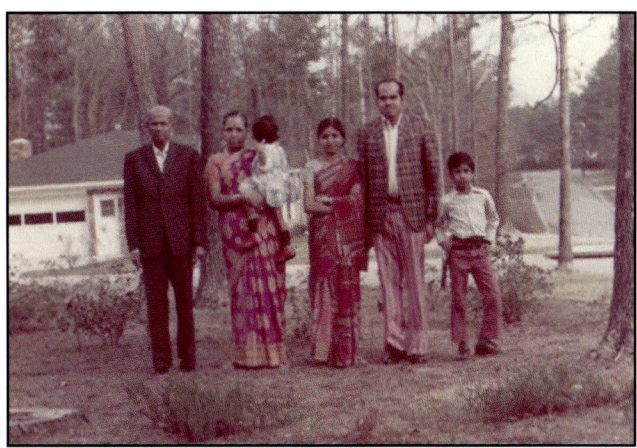

Figure 54. Our family photo when my parents were visiting with us while we were in Augusta, Georgia in mid 1970s. My dad, my mom, Madhavi, Hymavathi, me, and Vijay.

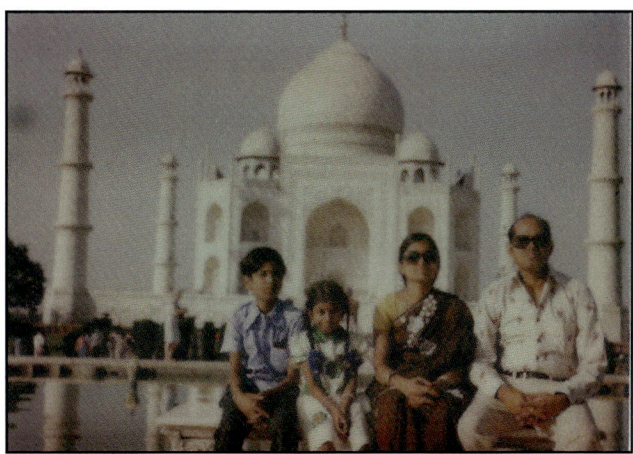

Figure 55. Photograph during a visit to the Taj Mahal in mid 1970s. Vijay, Madhavi, Hymavathi, and me.

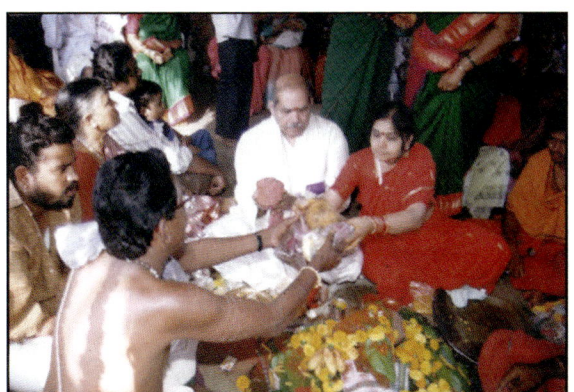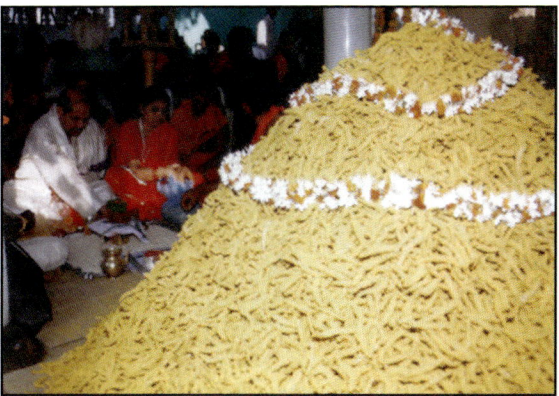

Figure 56. Photograph taken during the performance of Lakshapasupu Vratham in India in 1980s.

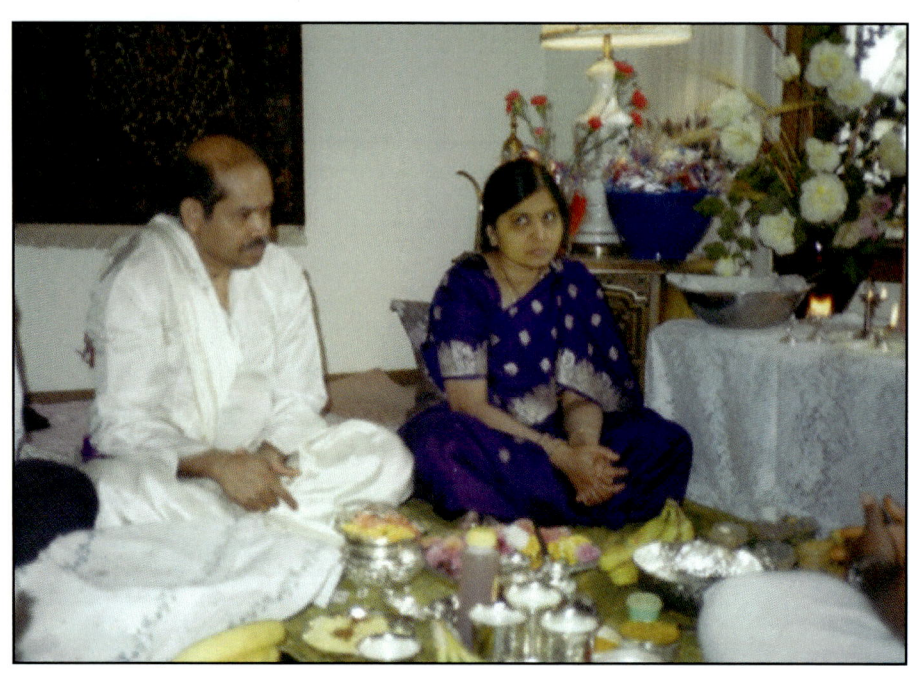

Figures 57. Photograph while performing Sri Satyanarayana Vratham in late 1980s in USA.

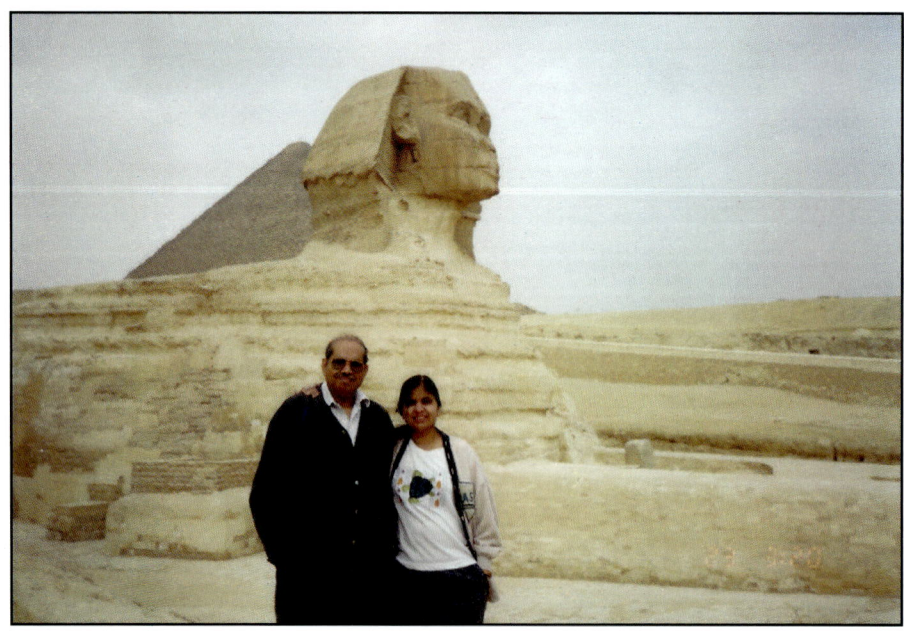

Figure 58. Hymavathi and I during a visit to Sphinx on the west bank of the Nile in Giza, Egypt.

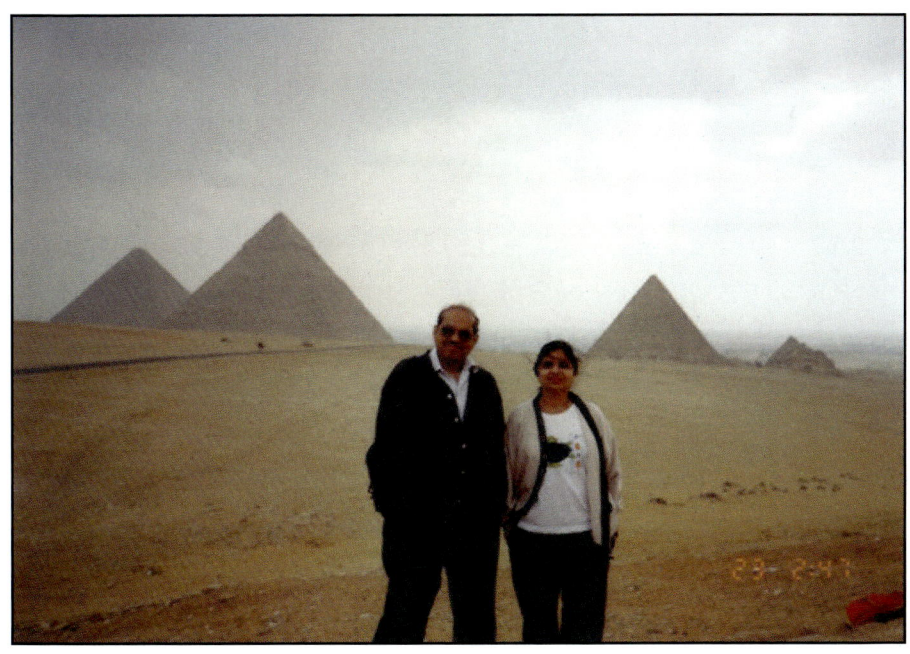

Figure 59. Hymavathi and I during a visit to the Pyramids in Egypt.

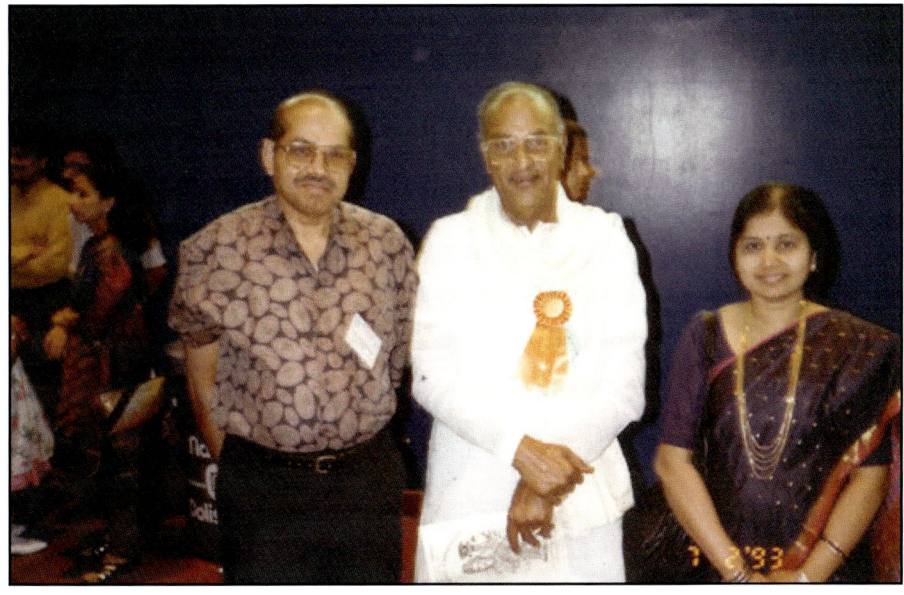

Figure 60. Photograph with a famous cine actor, Gummadi. Me, Gummadi,
and Hymavathi.

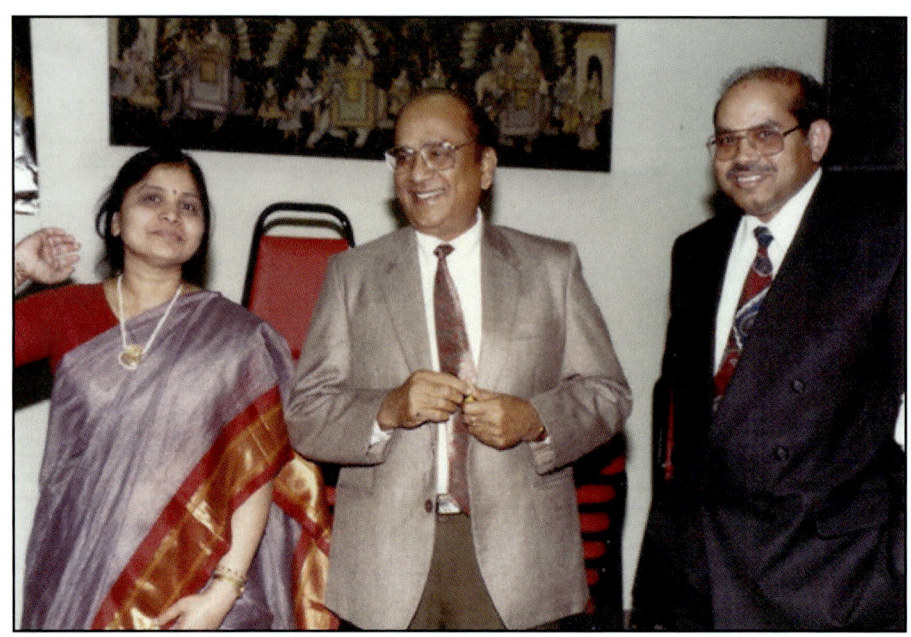

Figure 61. Photograph with another famous cine actor, Akkineni. Hymavathi, Akkineni, and me.

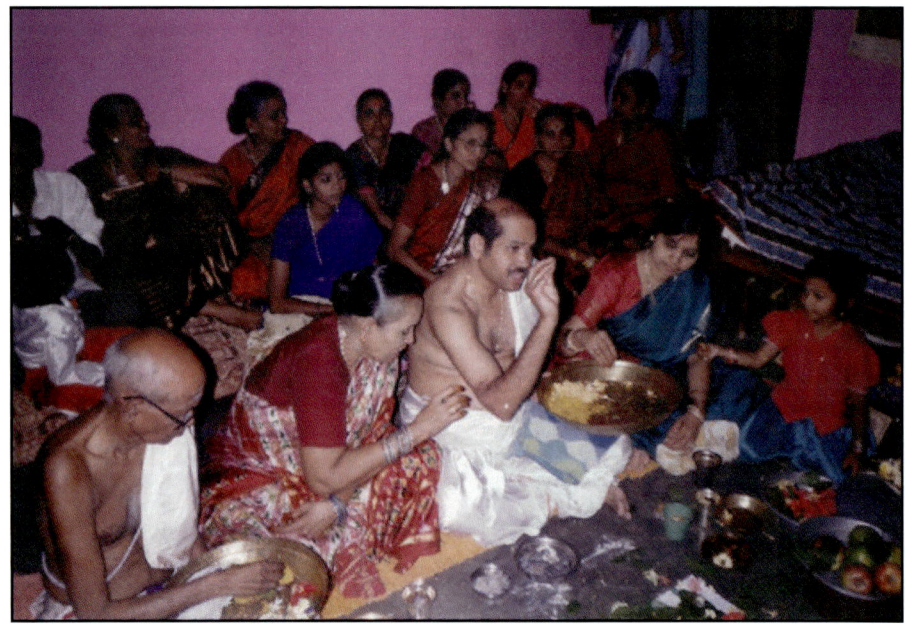

Figures 62. Photograph while performing Sri Satyanarayana Vratham in late 1980s in India. My dad, my mom, me, Hymavathi, and Radhika. On the back rows, relatives attending the ceremony.

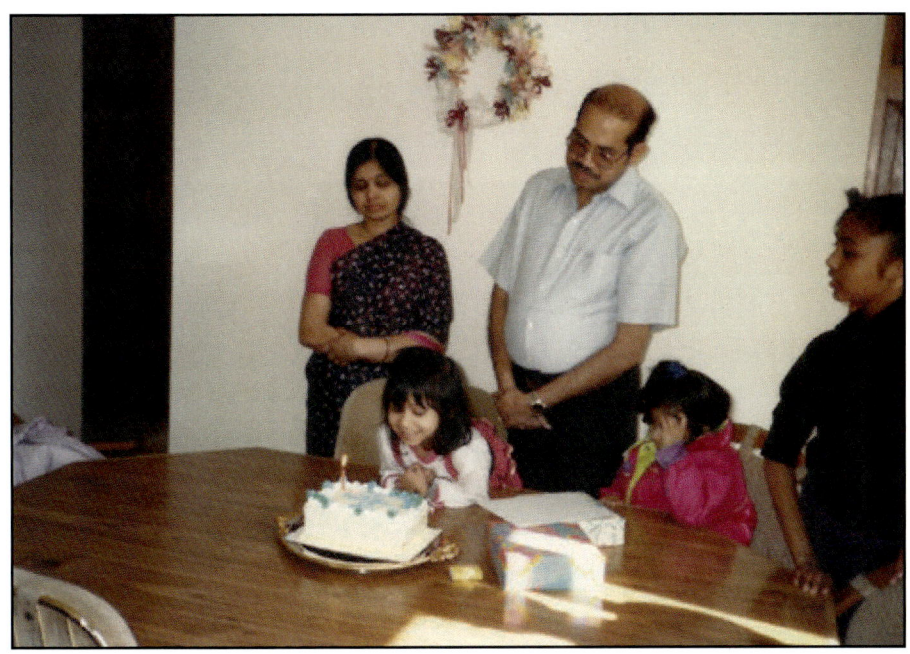

Figure 63. Celebrating daughter, Radhika's birthday in late 1980s.

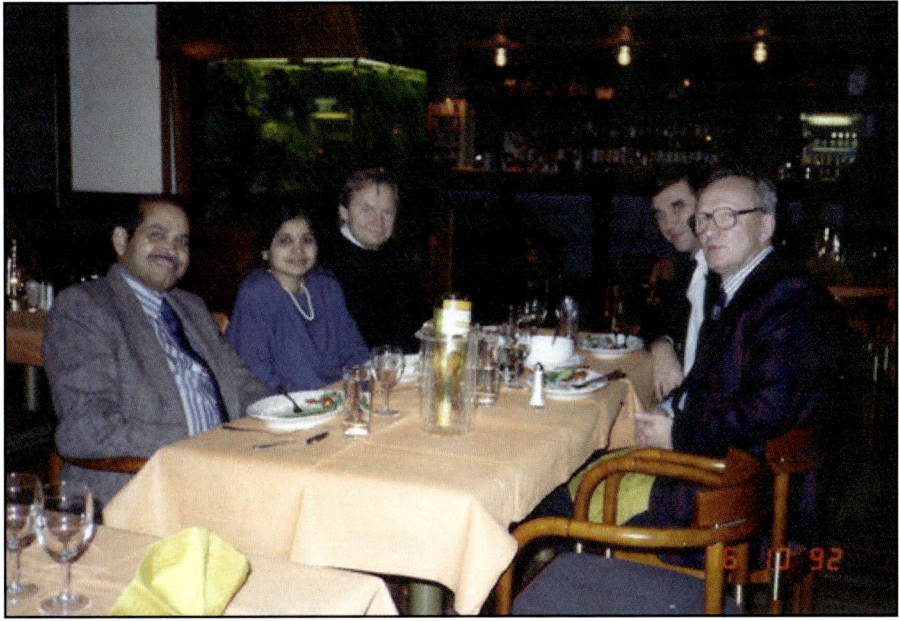

Figure 64. Photograph taken in Sweden when I was invited to deliver John Lind's lecture at the Swedish Pediatric Association Meeting in late 1992.

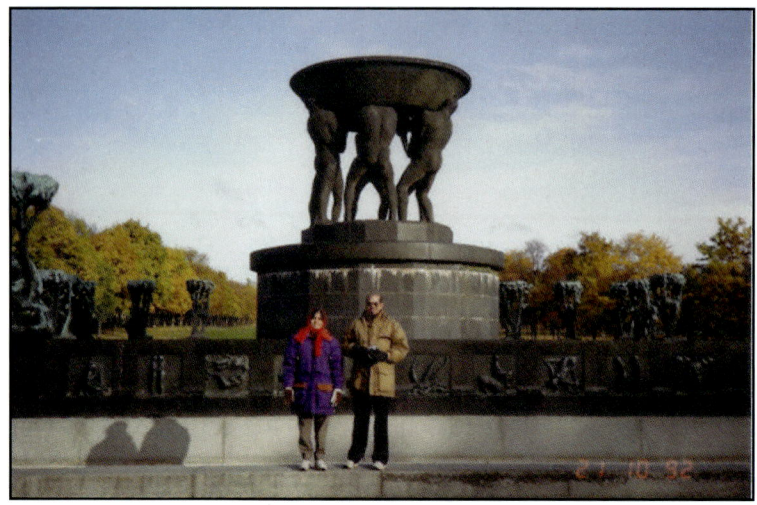

Figure 65. Photograph taken in Norway following the delivery of John Lind's lecture in Sweden in late 1992.

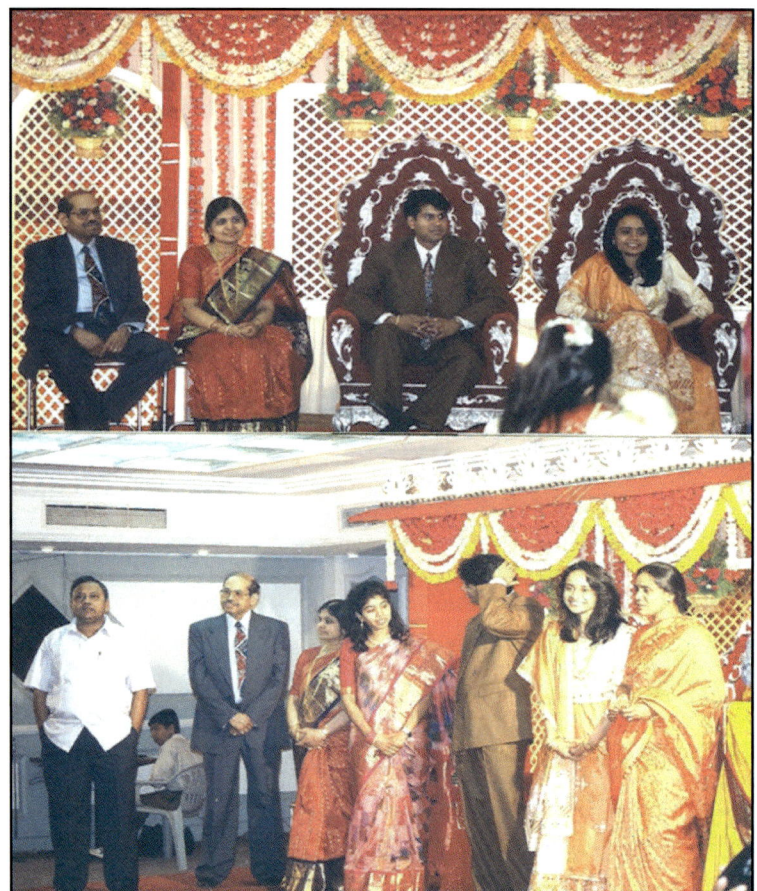

Figure 66. Photographs during our son's wedding reception in India. Top, me, Hymavathi, Vijay and my son's new bride, Radha. Bottom, Nageswararao (Radha's dad), me, Hymavathi, Madhavi, Vijay, Radha, and Sujatha (Radha's mom).

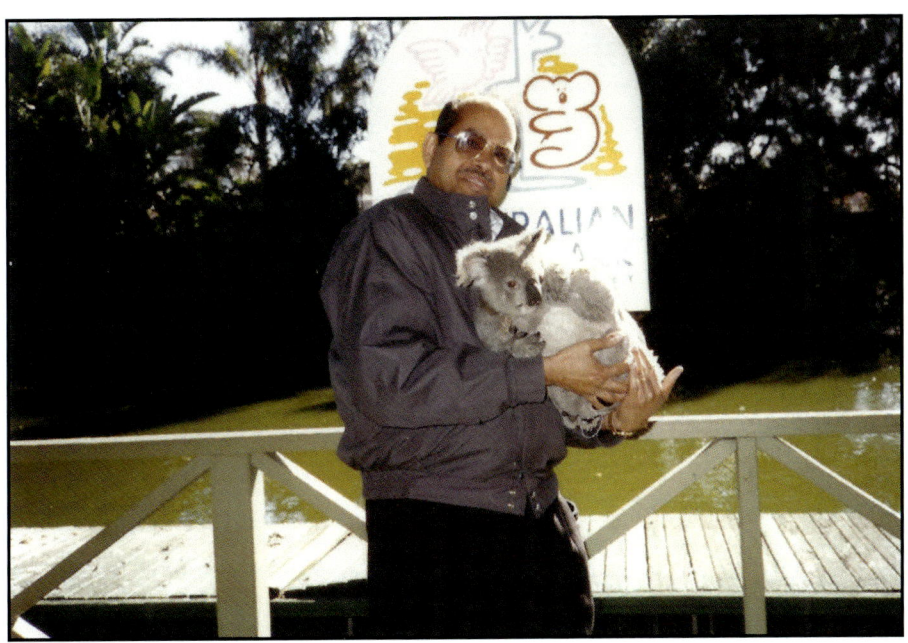

Figure 67. With a Koala bear in Australia

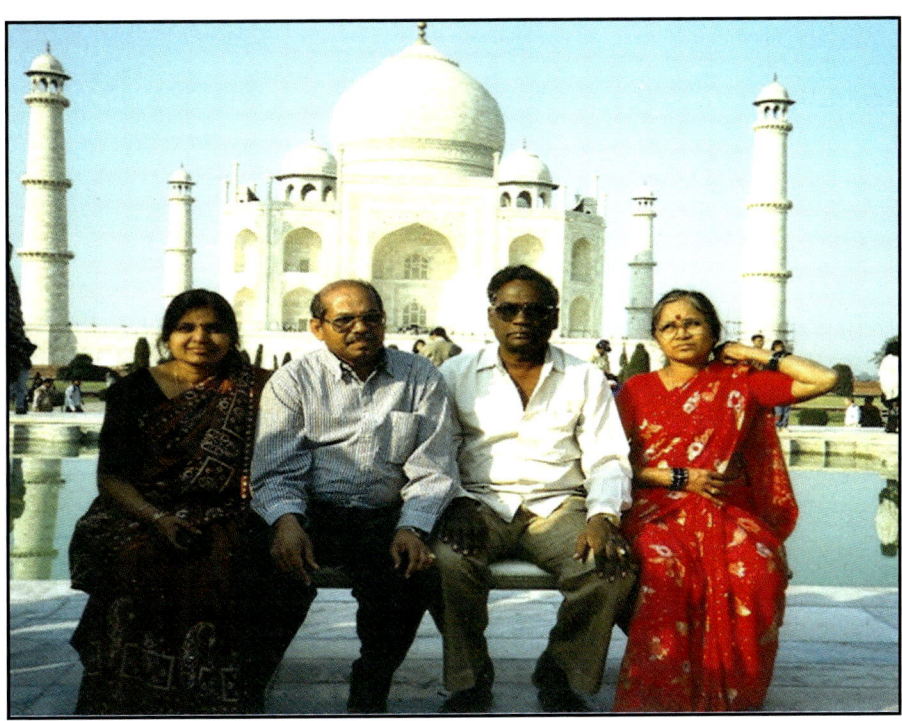

Figure 68. Photograph with my wife, my wife's sister (Prema Kumari) and her husband (T. Narasimha Murty), while touring the Taj Mahal.

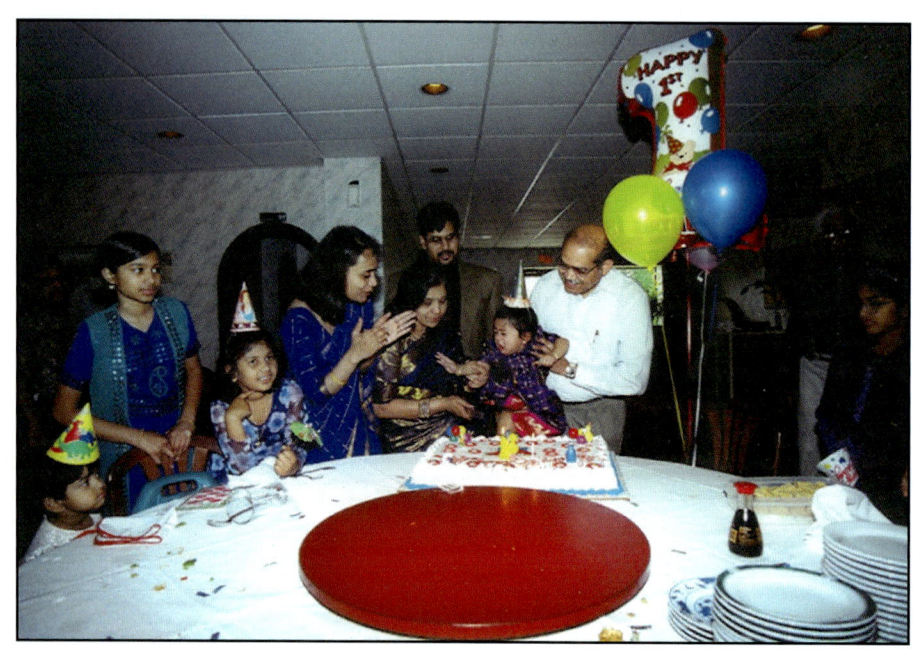

Figure 69. Celebrating granddaughter, Meghana's first birthday.

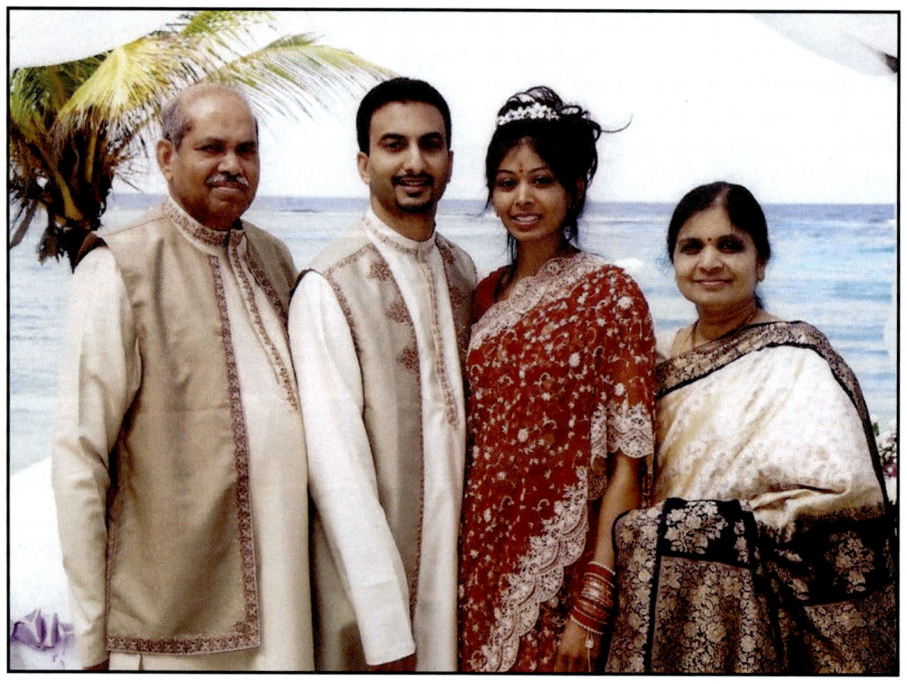

Figure 70. Photographs during our daughter, Madhavi's wedding. Me, Ravi Krishna, Madhavi, and Hymavathi.

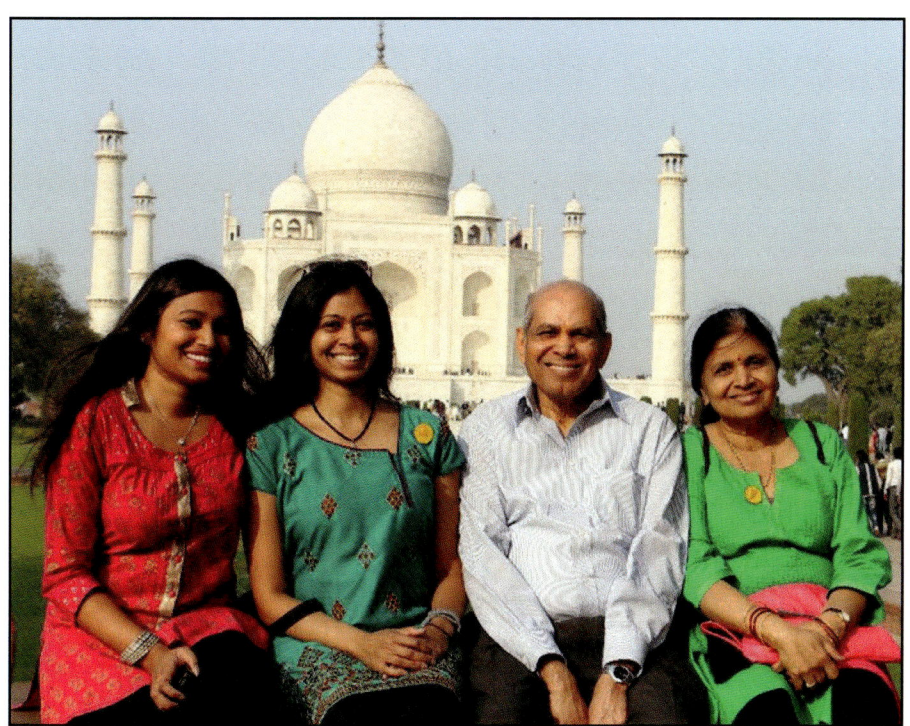

Figure 71. Photograph with my wife and daughters during a visit to the Taj Mahal. Radhika, Madhavi, me, and Hymavathi.

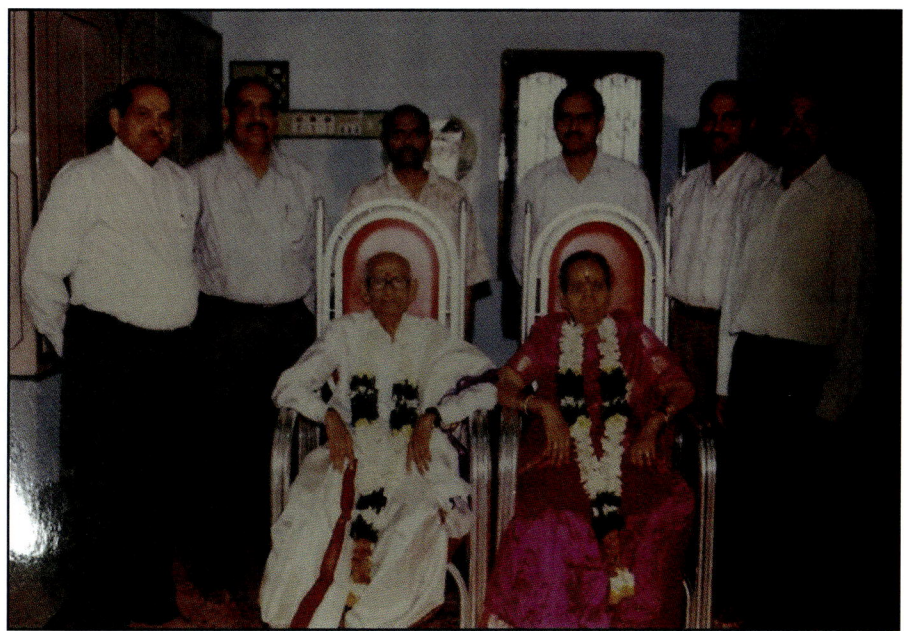

Figure 72. Photograph taken during a ceremony called "Pada Puja" of our parents, performed in India. Standing - Me and my brothers, Sambasiva Rao, Jayakeerti, Ratna Someswara Rao, Muralidhar, and Bhaskar Rao. Sitting - My dad, PVB Krishna Rao, and my mom, Savithramma.

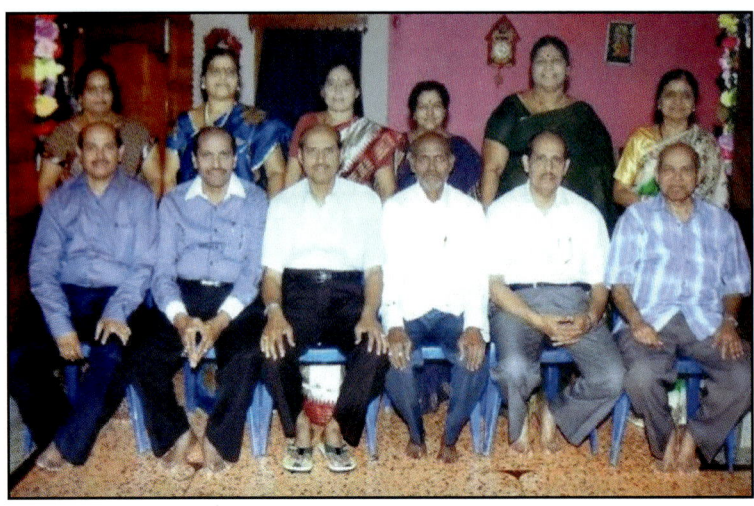

Figure 73. Photograph taken while in India with all my brothers and their wives. Standing - Jayasree, Geetha, Lakshmi Kumari, Saraswathi, Vidyavathi and Hymavathi. Sitting - Bhaskar Rao, Muralidhar, Ratna Someswara Rao, Jayakeerti, Sambasiva Rao, and me.

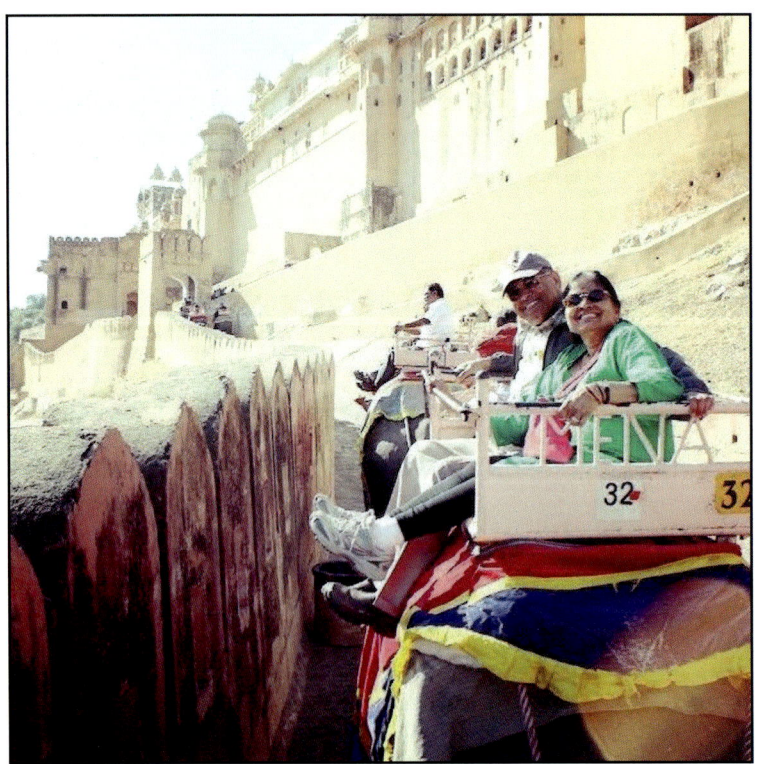

Figure 74. Elephant ride while in Rajasthan during "Palace on the Wheels" tour in India.

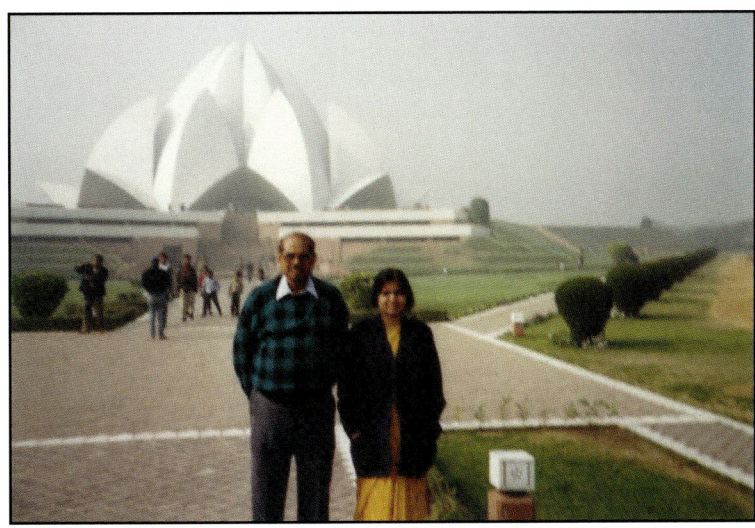

Figure 75. Photograph during a visit to the Lotus Temple in New Delhi.

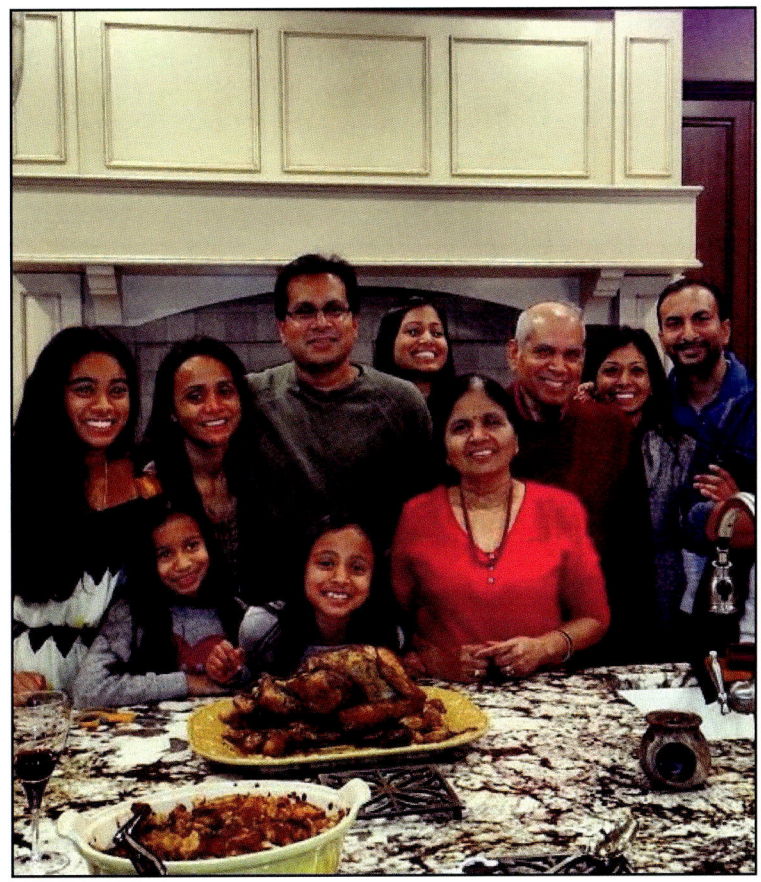

Figure 76. Photograph taken while in St. Louis at my son's home during a Thanksgiving dinner. Back Row - Maghana, Radha, Vijay, Radhika, me, Madhavi and Ravi. Front Row - Anjali, Rhea, and Hymavathi.

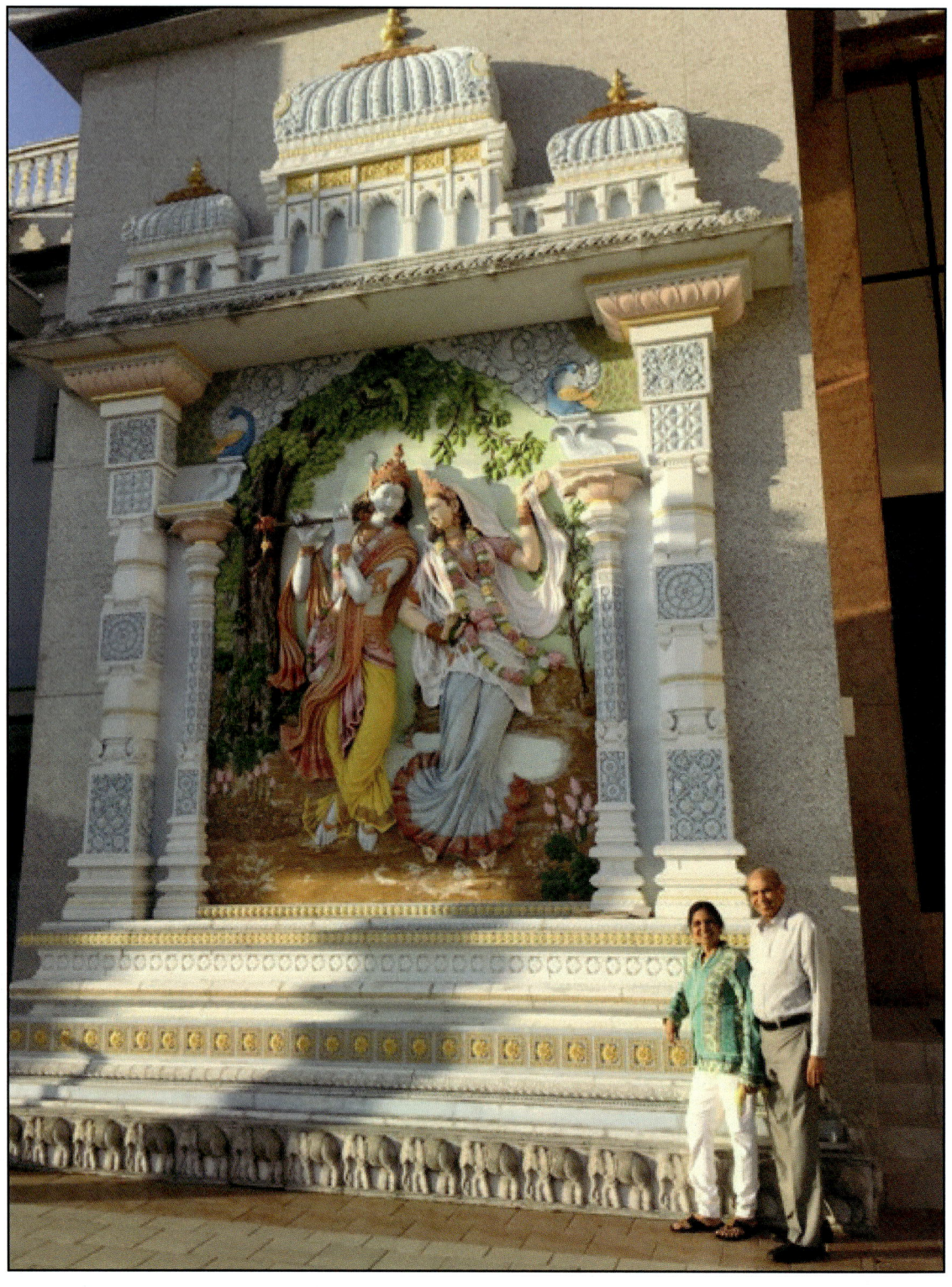

Figure 77. Photograph taken during a visit to Radhakrishna Temple in Austin.
Me and Hymavathi standing at the right lower corner.

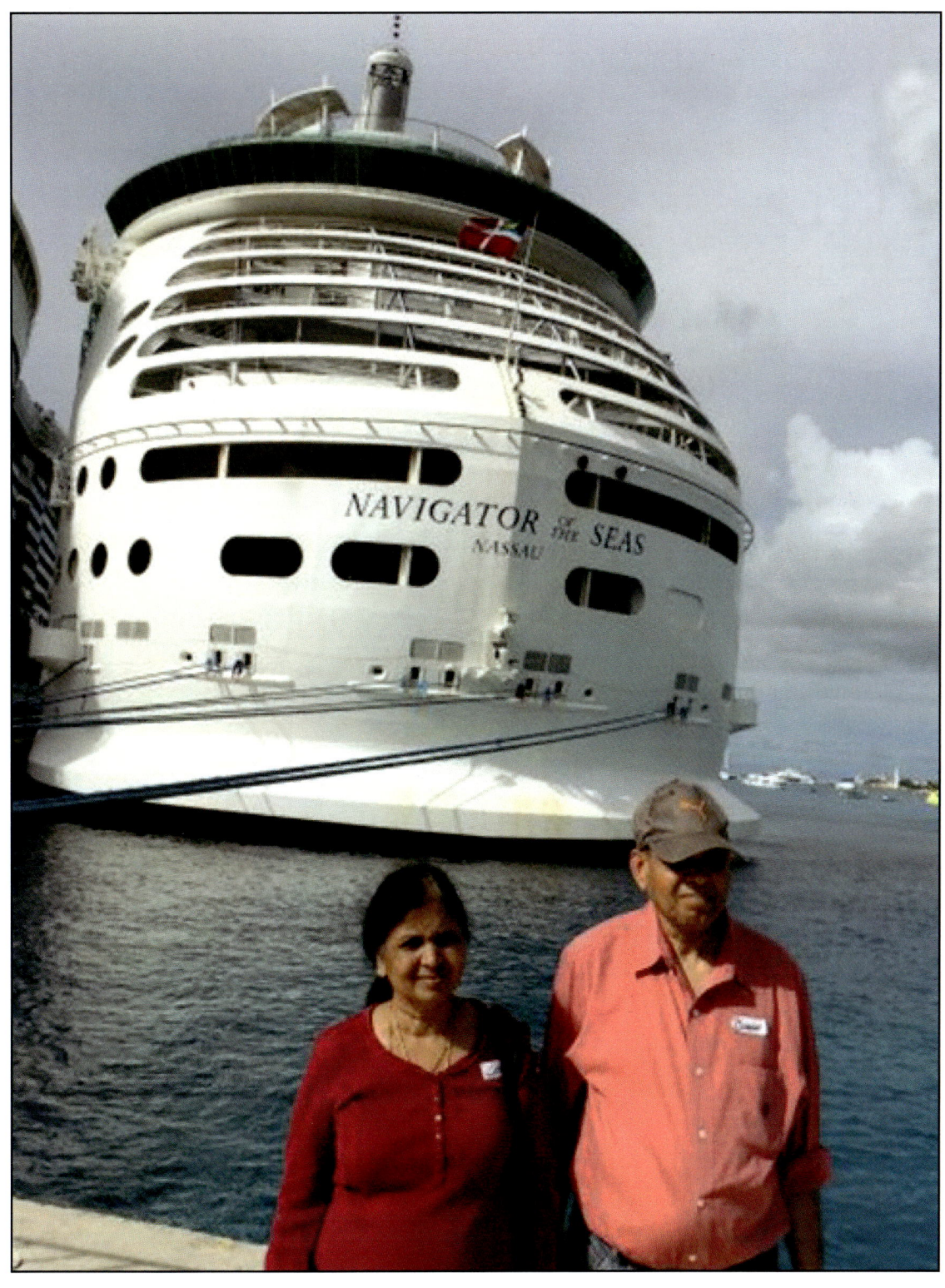

Figure 78. Photograph taken during Caribbean cruise.

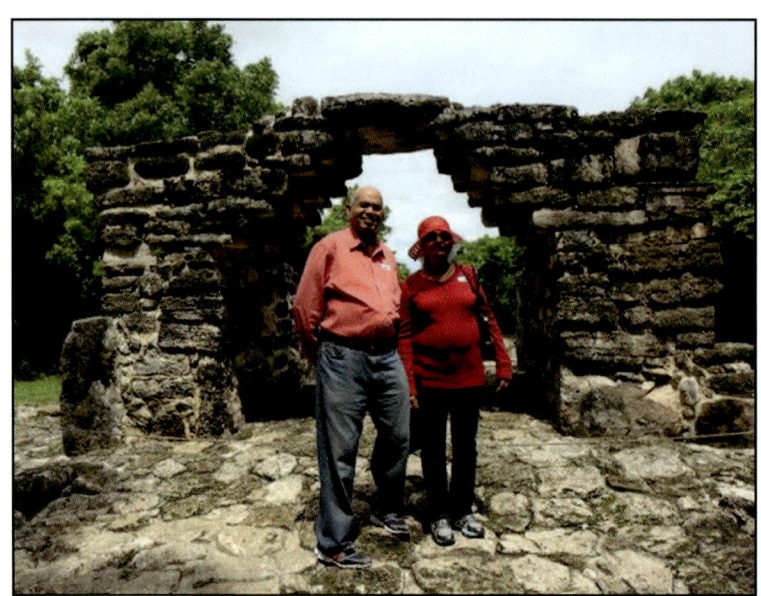

Figure 79. Photograph taken during Caribbean cruise.

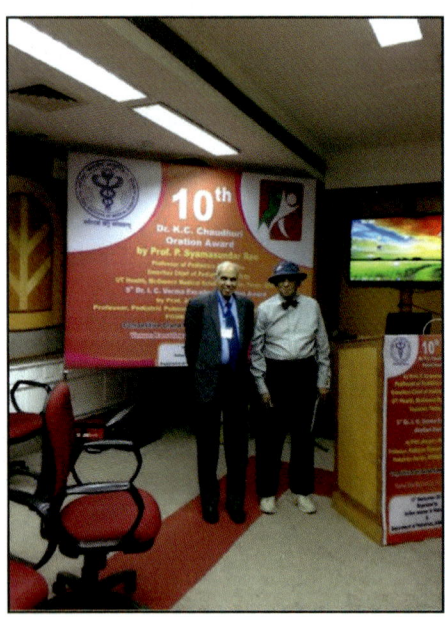
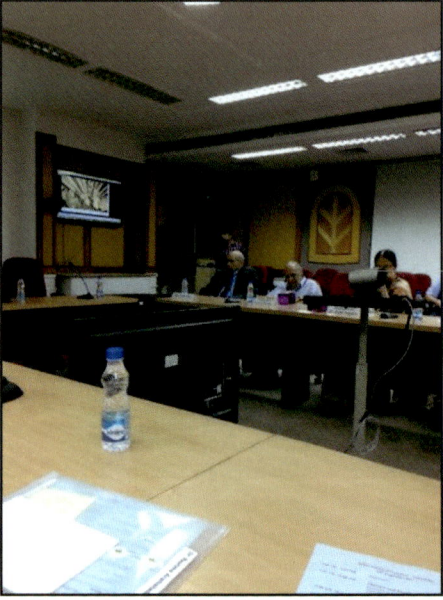

Figure 80. Photographs taken during Lifetime Achievement Award presentation
in New Delhi in September 2017.

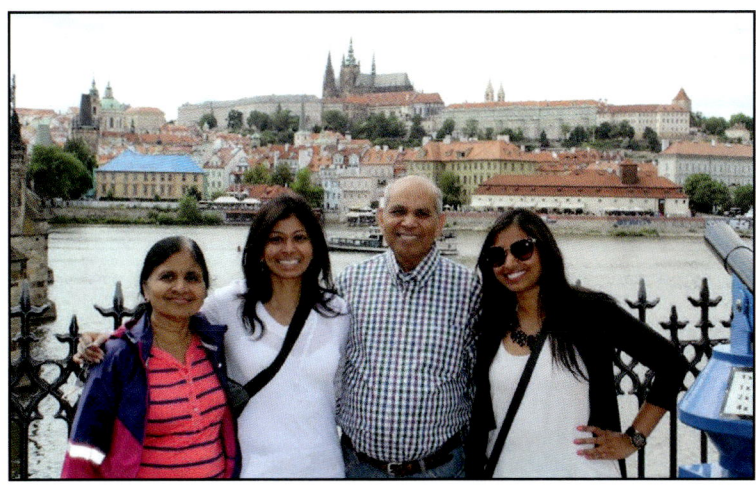

Figure 81. Photograph taken during Viking River Cruise in Europe. Hyamvathi, Madhavi, me, and Radhika.

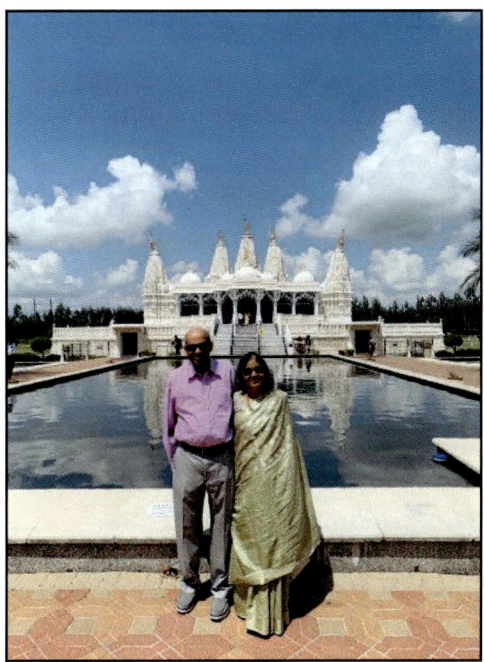

Figure 82. Photograph taken during a visit to the Swamy Narayan Temple in Houston in August 2019.

Sixtieth (Figures 83 and 84), seventieth (Figures 85 through 88) and seventy-fifth (Figures 89 through 94) birthday celebration photographs and fiftieth marriage anniversary pictures (Figures 95 through 108) are presented in that order.

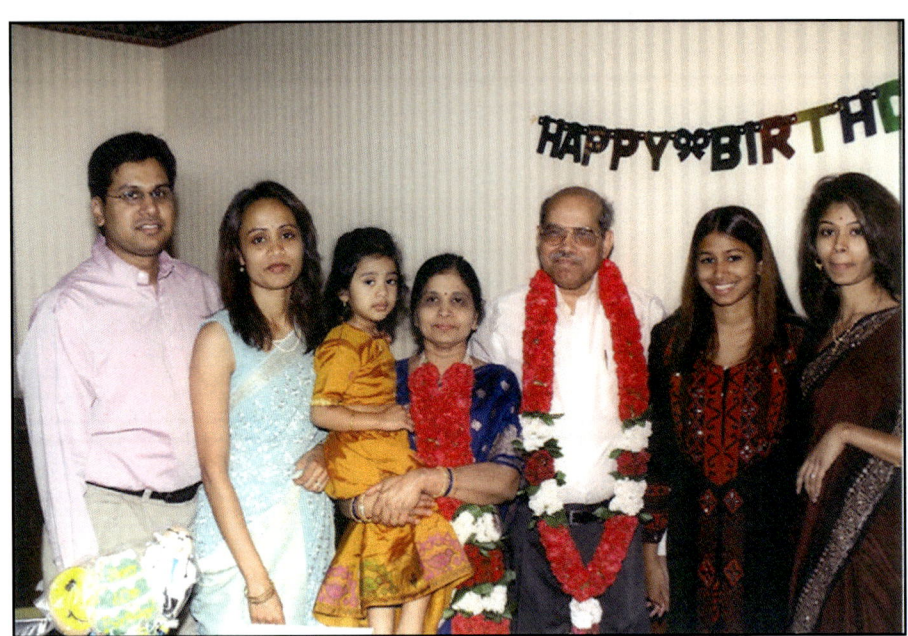

Figure 83. Celebrating my sixtieth birthday with the rest of the family. Left to right, Vijay, Radha, Meghana, Hymavathi, me, Radhika, and Madhavi.

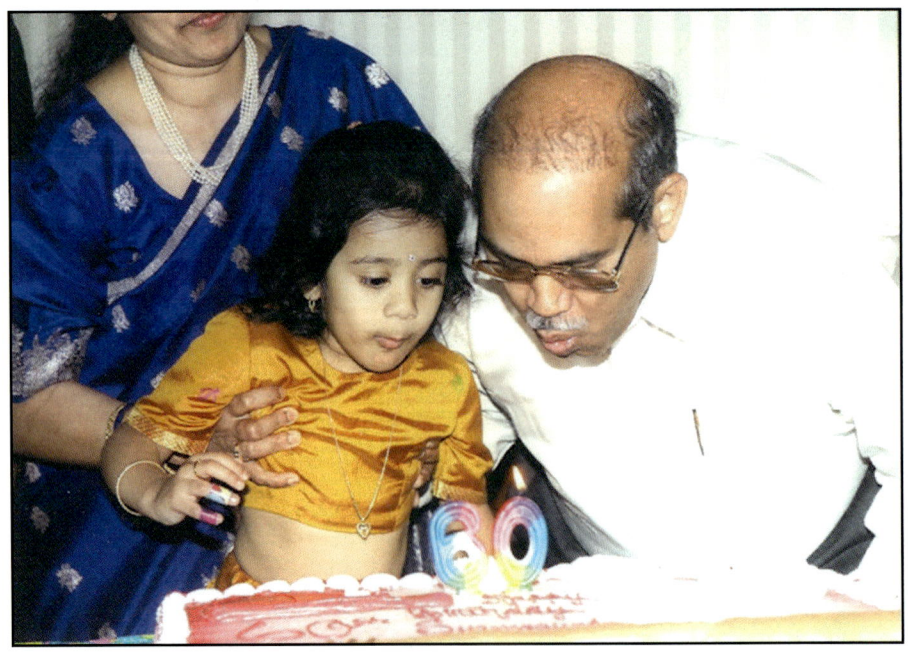

Figure 84. Granddaughter, Meghana, helping to blow my sixtieth birthday candle

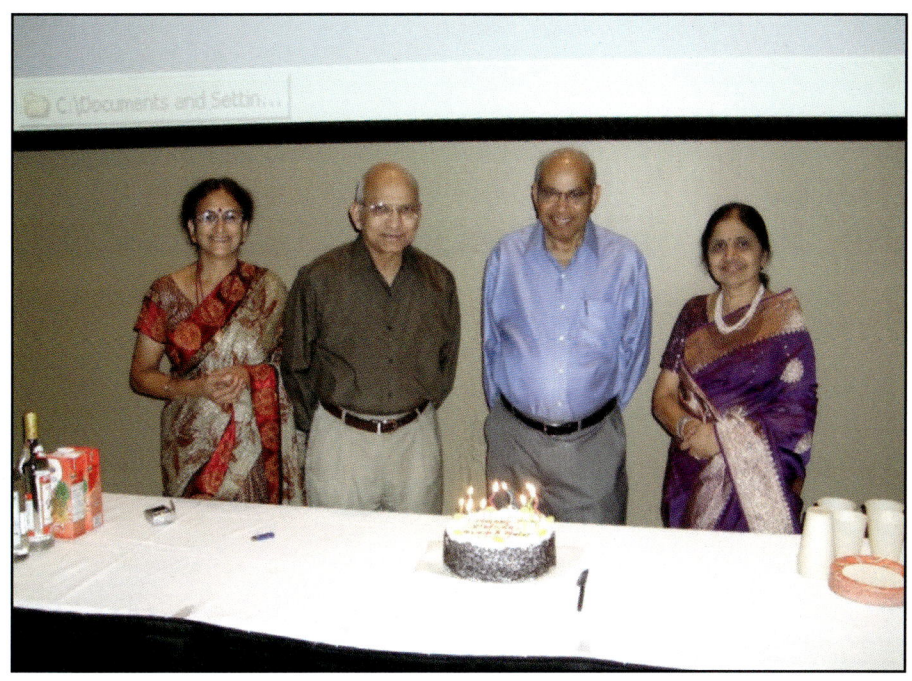

Figure 85. Photograph taken during my seventieth birthday celebration at a Canadian resort along with my daughter's in-laws. Mrs. Satyavathi, Mr. Pratap Chundru, me, and my wife, Hymavathi.

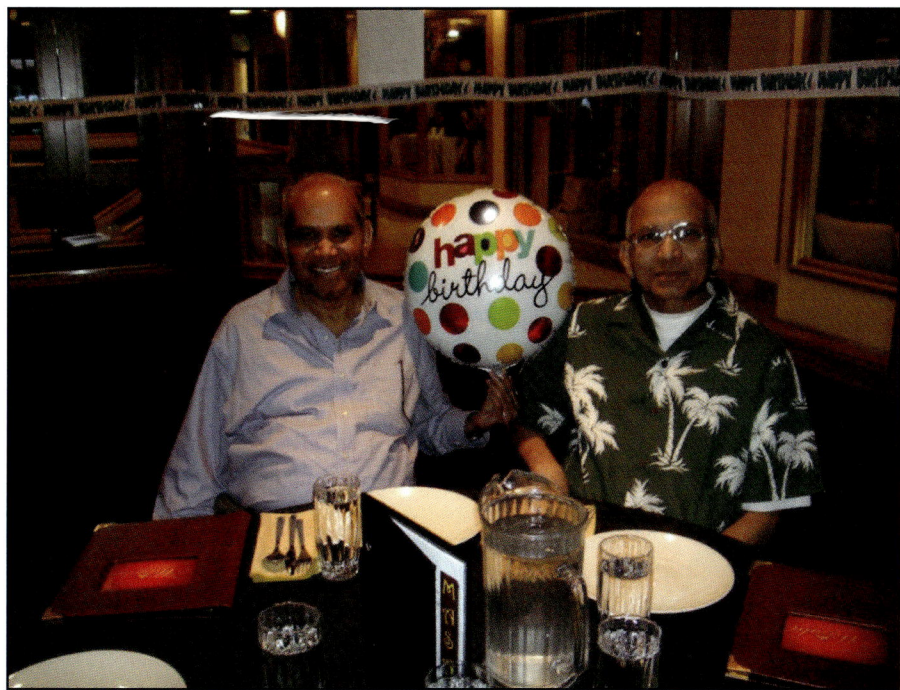

Figure 86. Photograph taken during my seventieth birthday celebration at a Canadian resort along with Mr. Pratap Chundru whose birthday is on the same day as that of mine.

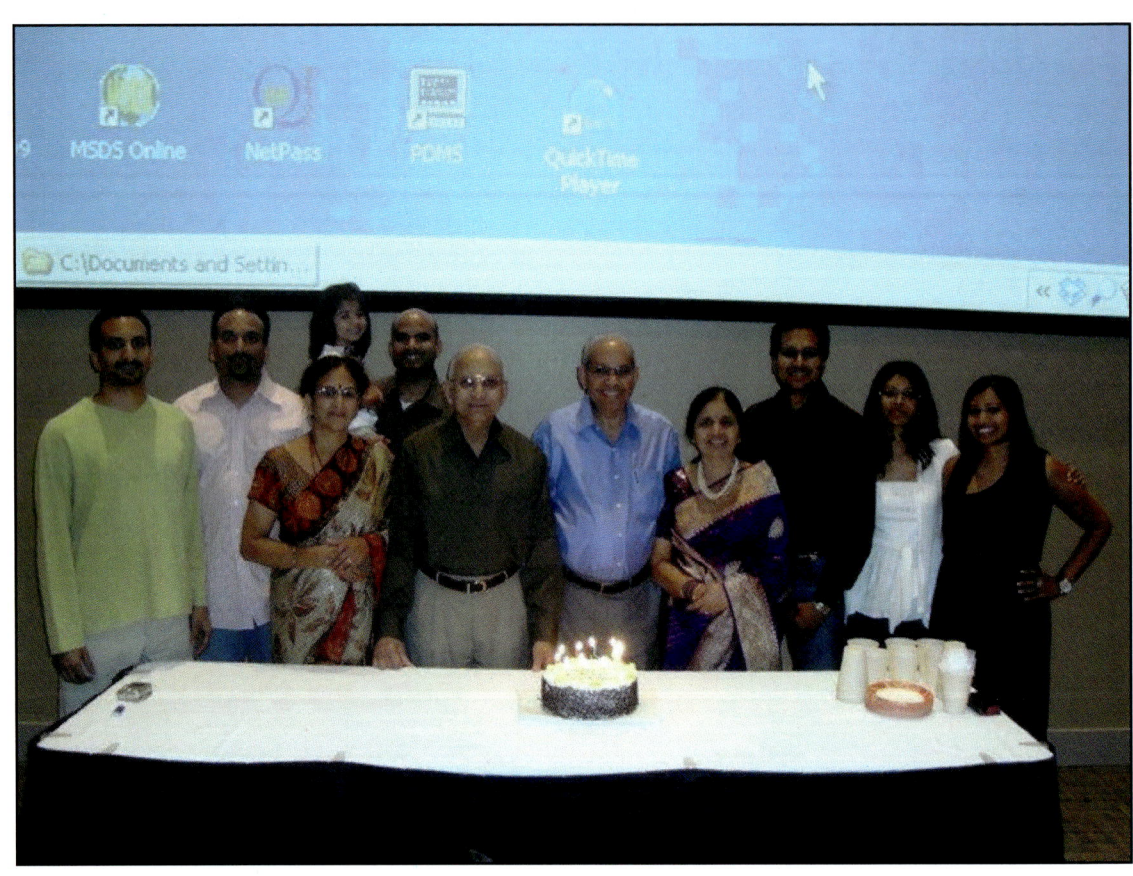

Figure 87. Photograph taken during my seventieth birthday celebration at a Canadian resort along with my and Mr. Pratap Chundrus' families.

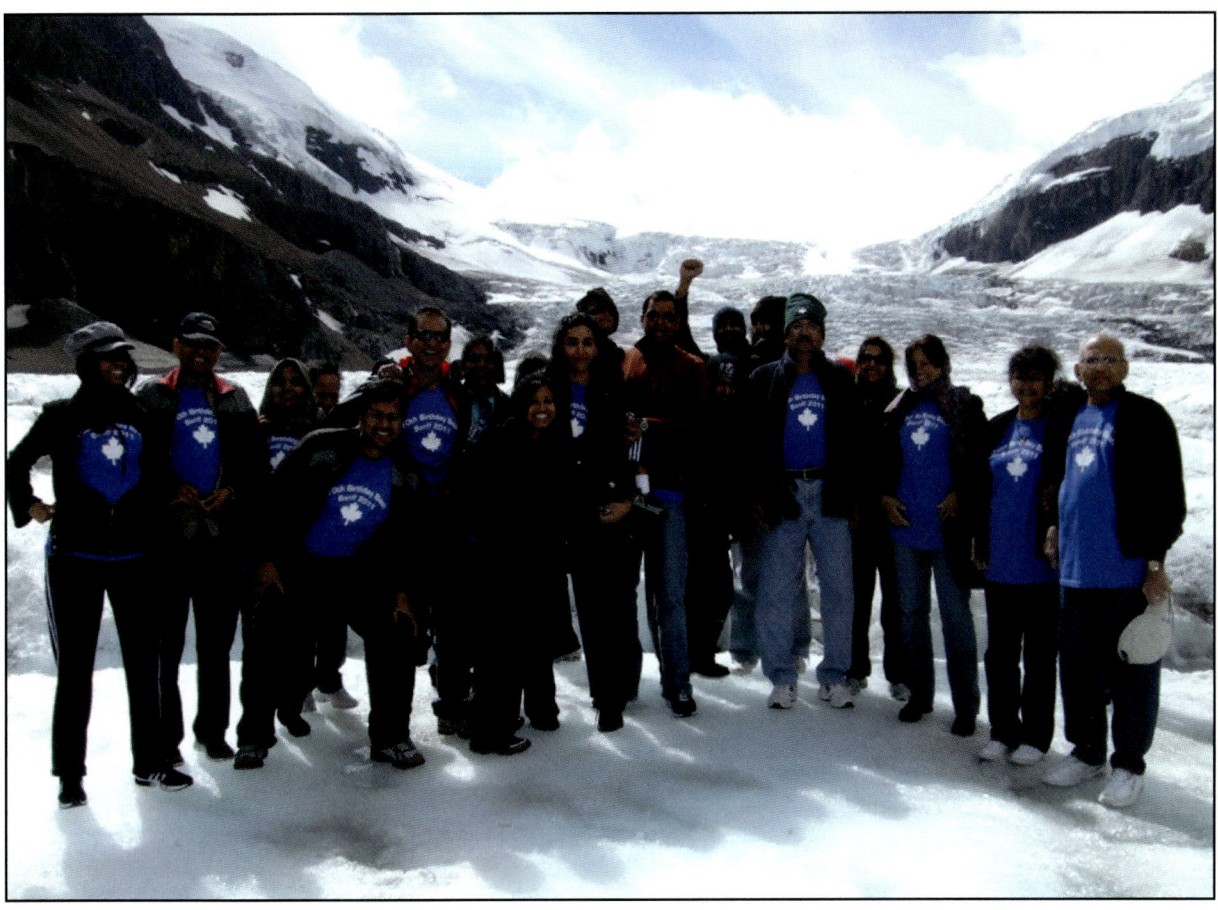

Figure 88. Photograph taken during my seventieth birthday celebration at a Canadian resort along with family and friends of myself and Mr. Pratap Chundru.

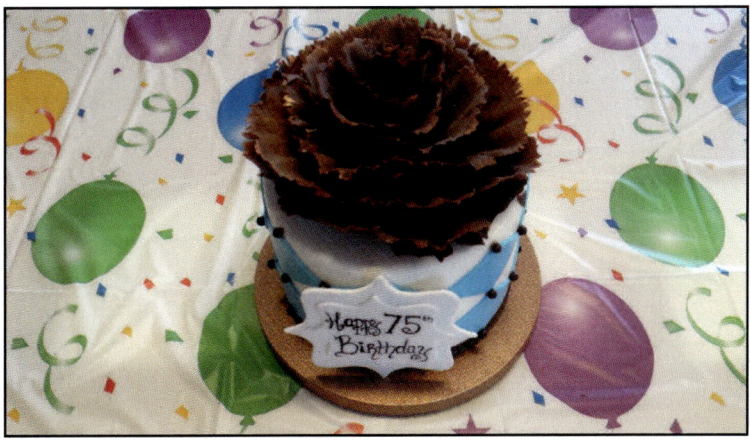

Figure 89. Photograph taken during my seventy-fifth birthday celebration in Las Vegas.

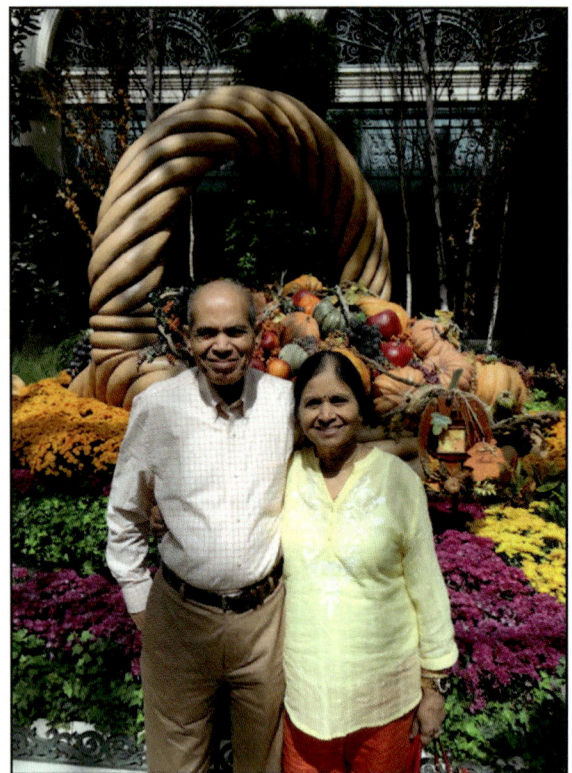
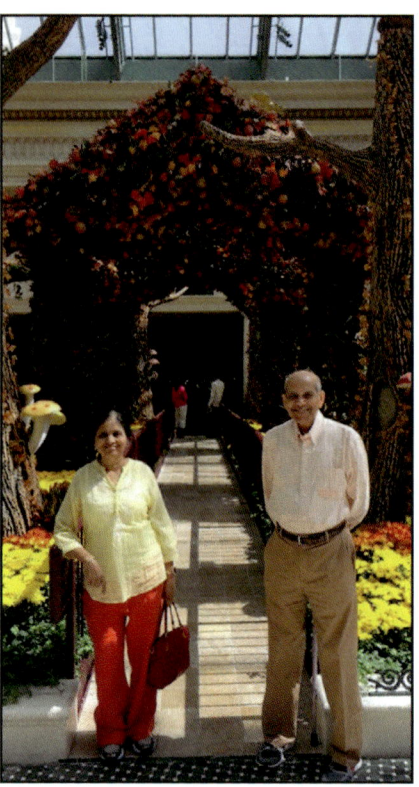

Figures 90 & 91. Photographs with my wife taken during my seventy-fifth birthday celebration in Las Vegas.

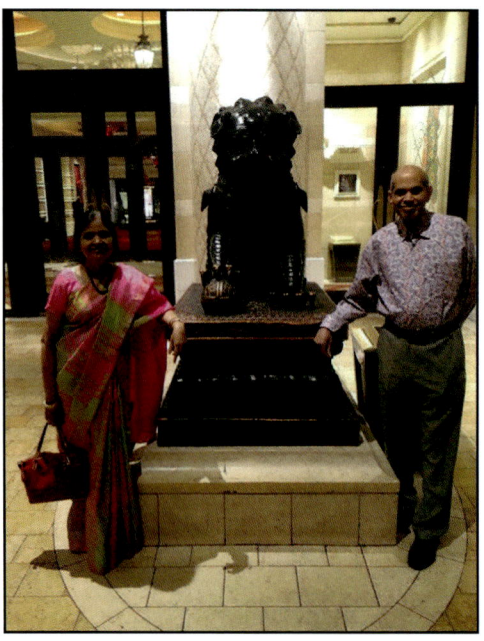

Figure 92. Photograph with my wife taken during my seventy-fifth birthday celebration in Las Vegas.

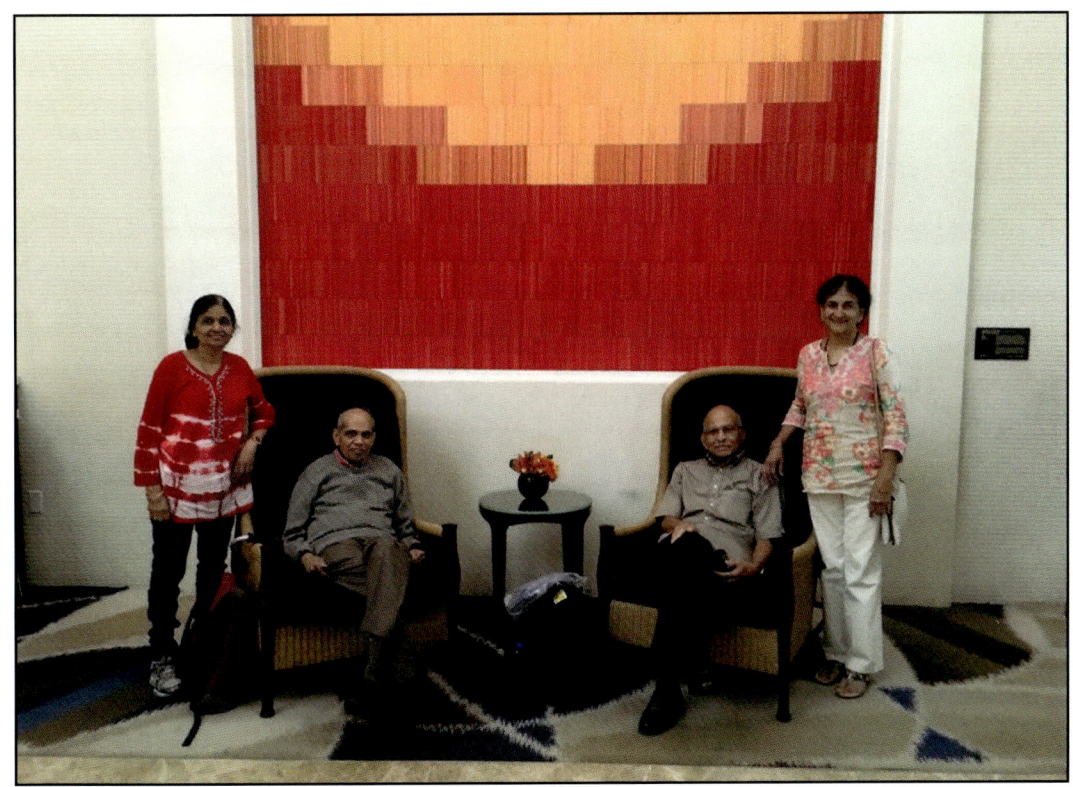

Figure 93. Photograph taken during my seventy-fifth birthday celebration in
Las Vegas with my daughter's in-laws (Hymavathi, me, Mr. Pratap Chundru, and
Mrs. Satyavathi).

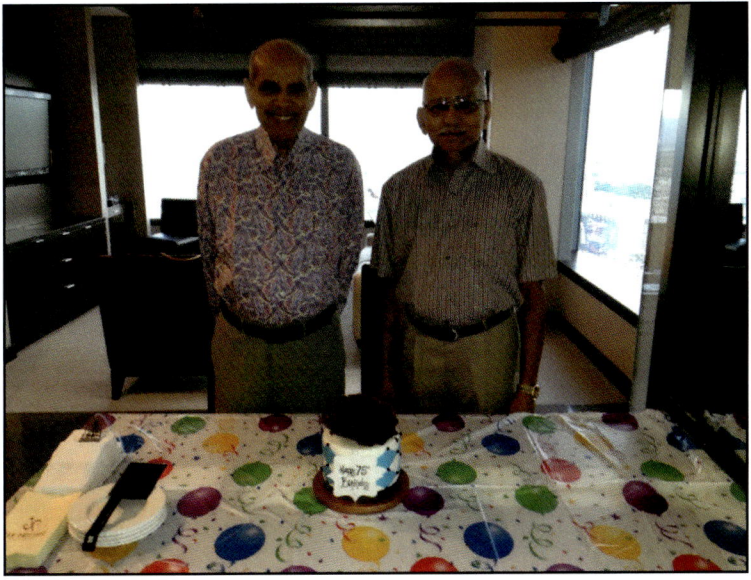

Figure 94. Photograph taken during my seventy-fifth birthday celebration in
Las Vegas along with Mr. Pratap Chundru whose birthday, as mentioned above,
is on the same day as that of mine.

My wife and I celebrated our fiftieth marriage anniversary three year ago and some of the pictures are shown in Figures 95 through 108.

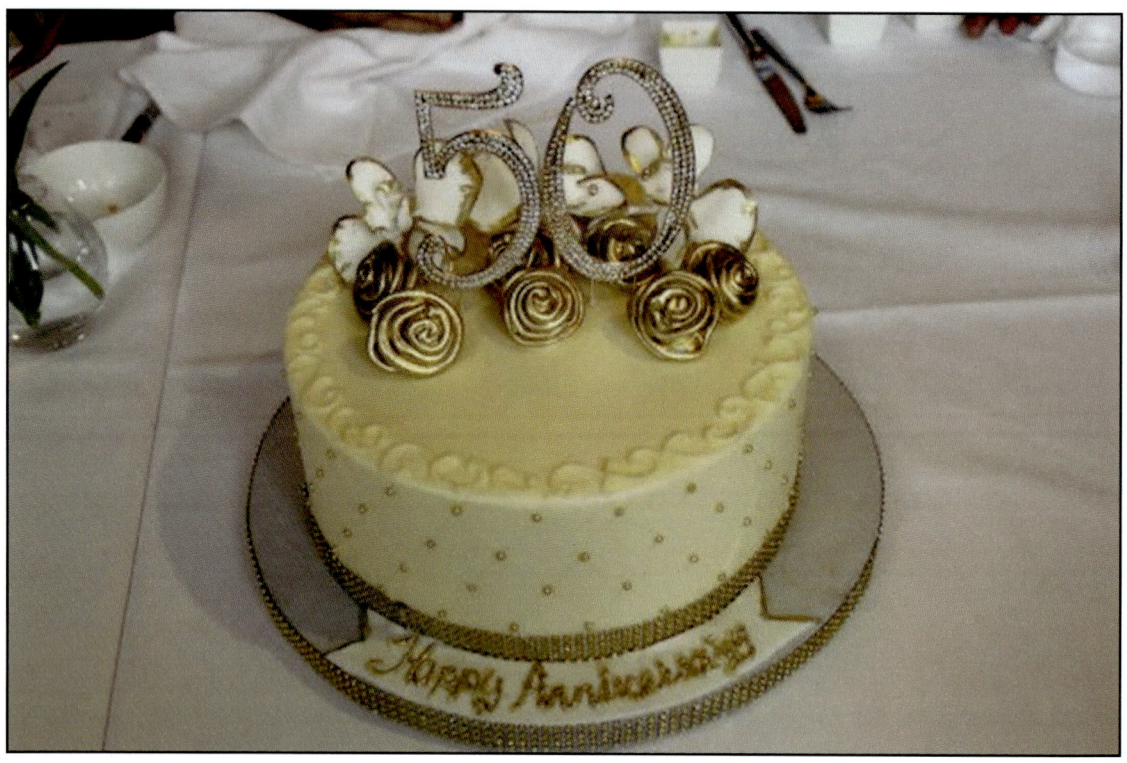

Figure 95. Photograph taken during our fiftieth marriage anniversary celebrations.

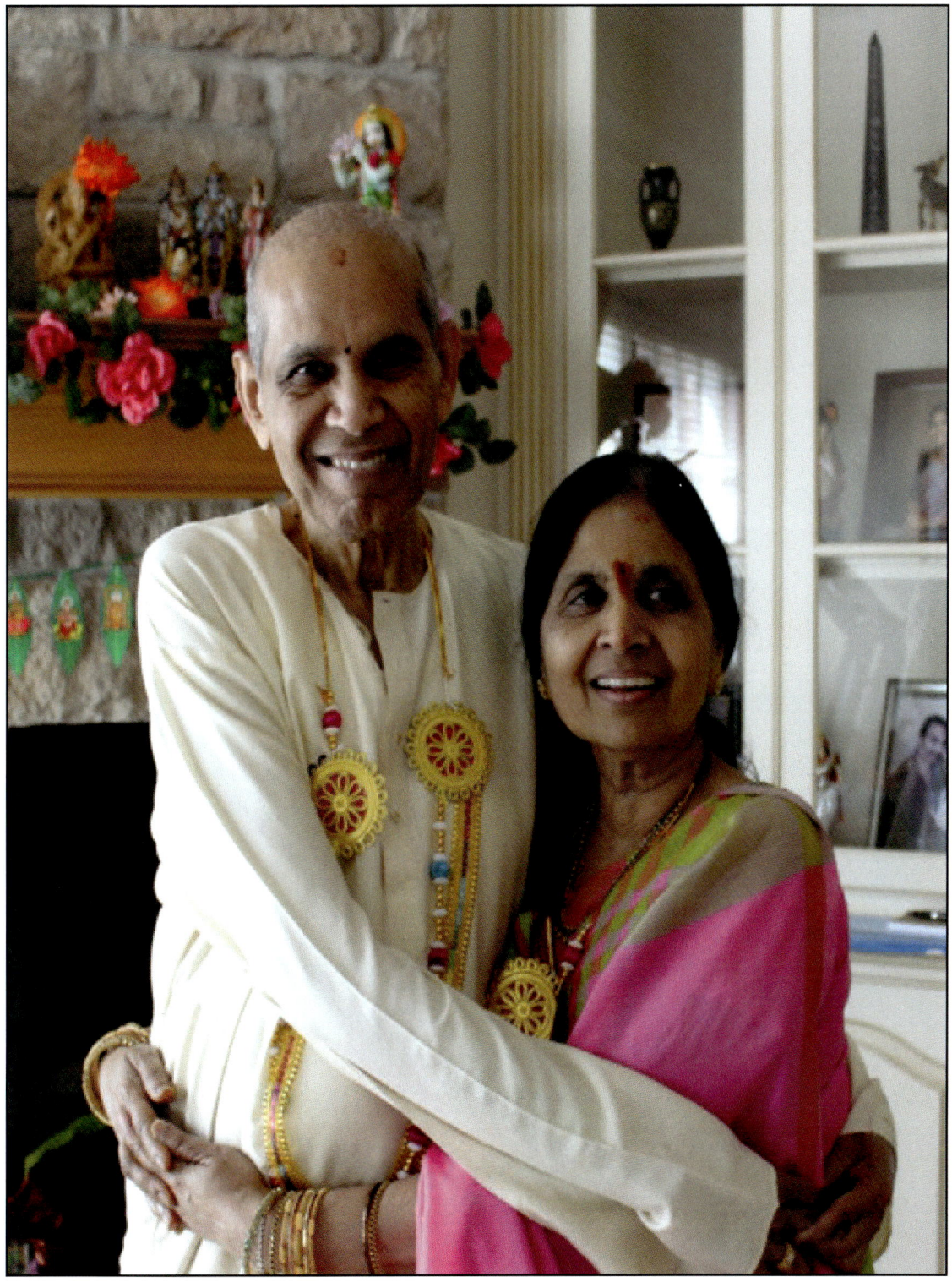

Figure 96. Photograph taken during our fiftieth marriage anniversary celebrations.

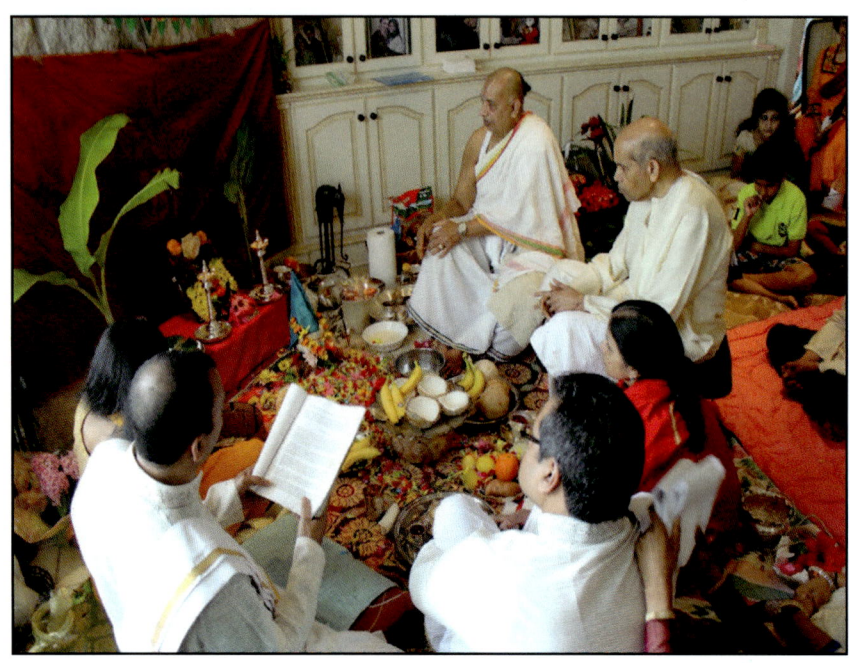

Figure 97. Photograph taken during Sri Satyanarayana Vratham on the occasion of our fiftieth marriage anniversary.

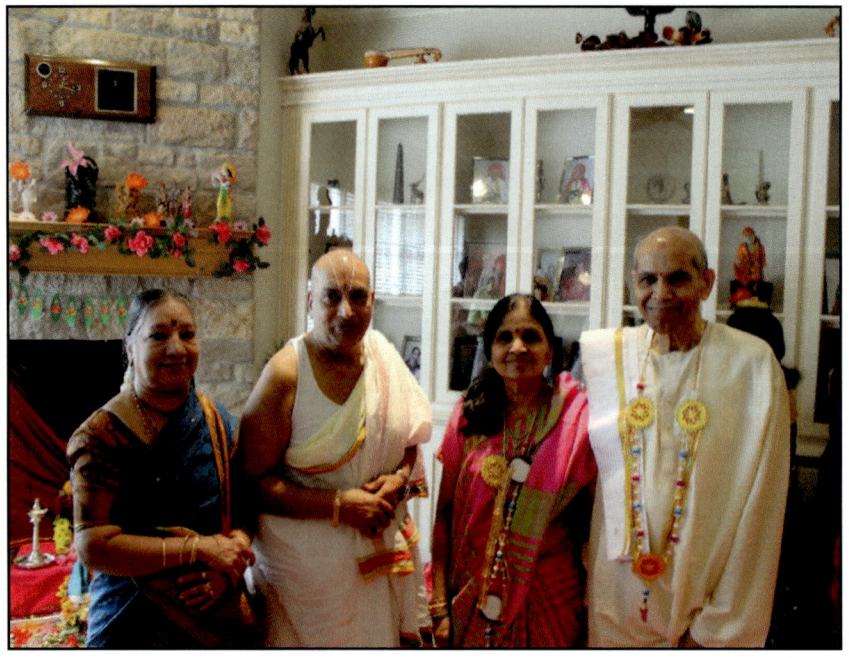

Figure 98. Photograph with my wife, pourohith (priest) who performed Sri Satyanarayana Vratham and his wife on the occasion of our fiftieth marriage anniversary.

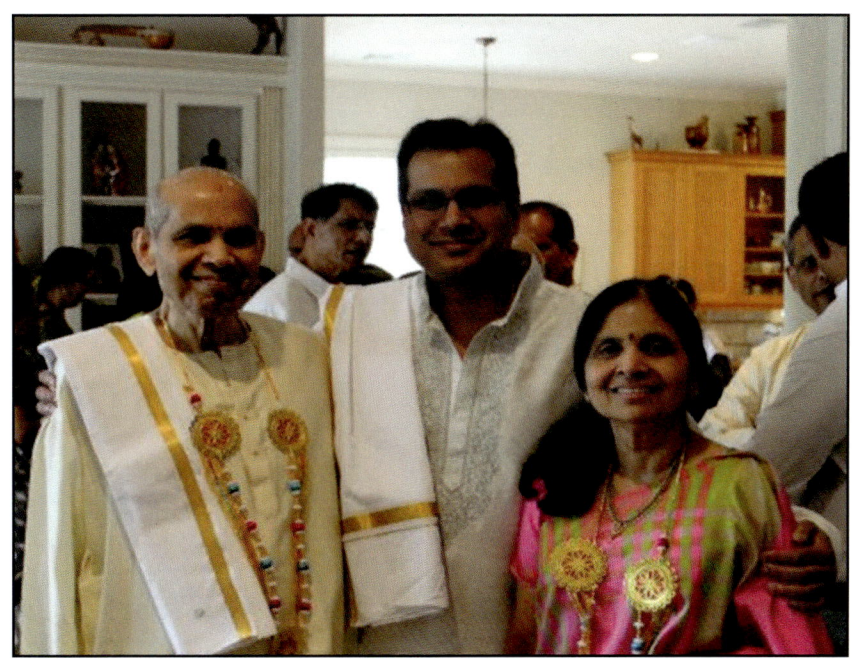

Figure 99. Photograph with my wife and son, Dr. Vijay K. Patnana, taken during our fiftieth marriage anniversary celebrations.

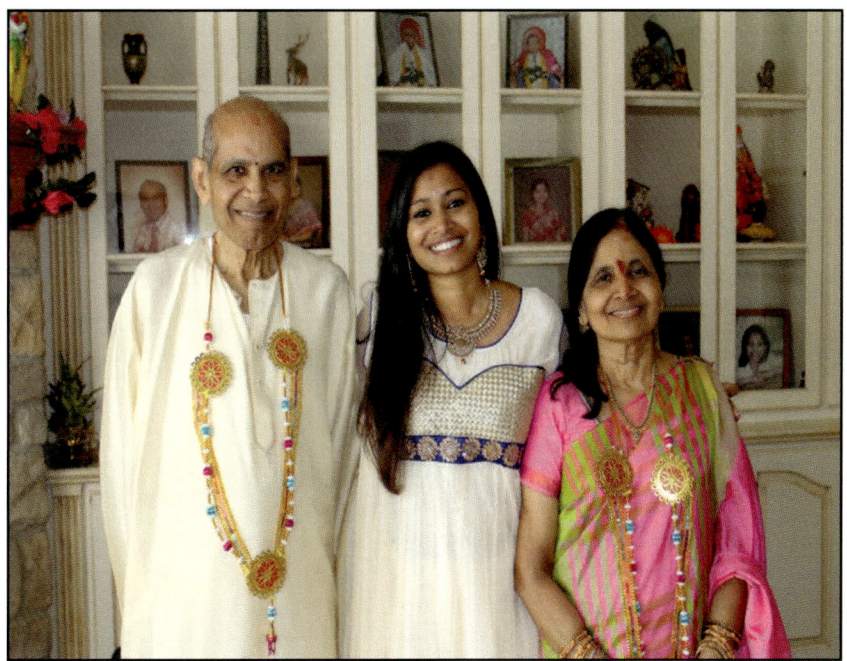

Figure 100. Photograph with my wife and daughter, Ms. Radhika N. Patnana, taken during our fiftieth marriage anniversary celebrations.

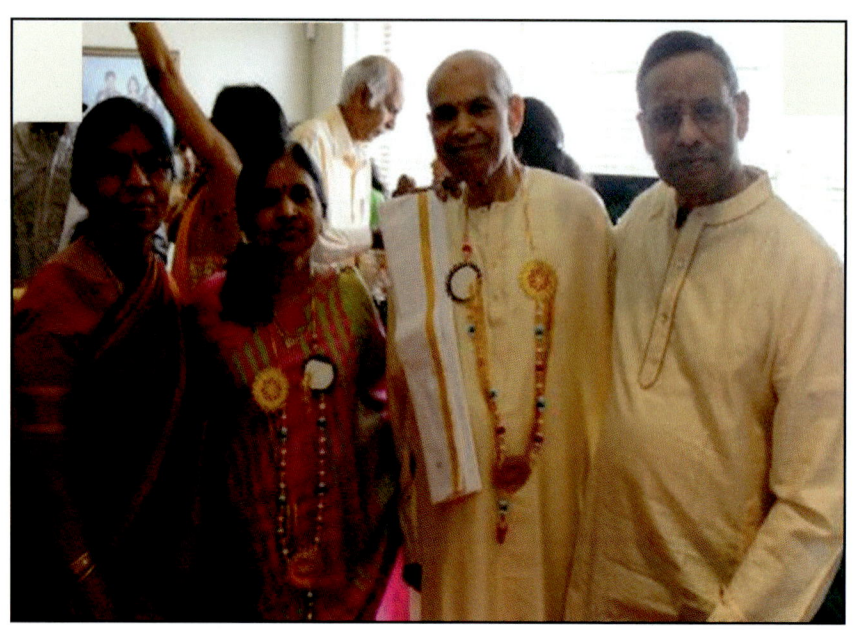

Figure 101. Photograph with my wife and my medical school classmate and friend, Dr. Sambasiva Rao, and his wife, Girija, taken during our fiftieth marriage anniversary celebrations.

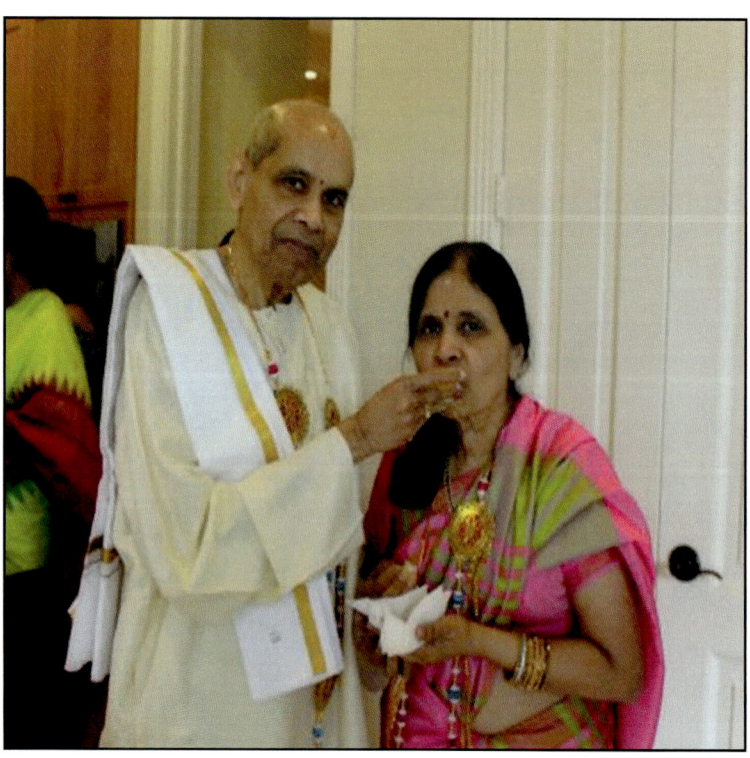

Figure 102. Photograph taken during our fiftieth marriage anniversary celebrations.

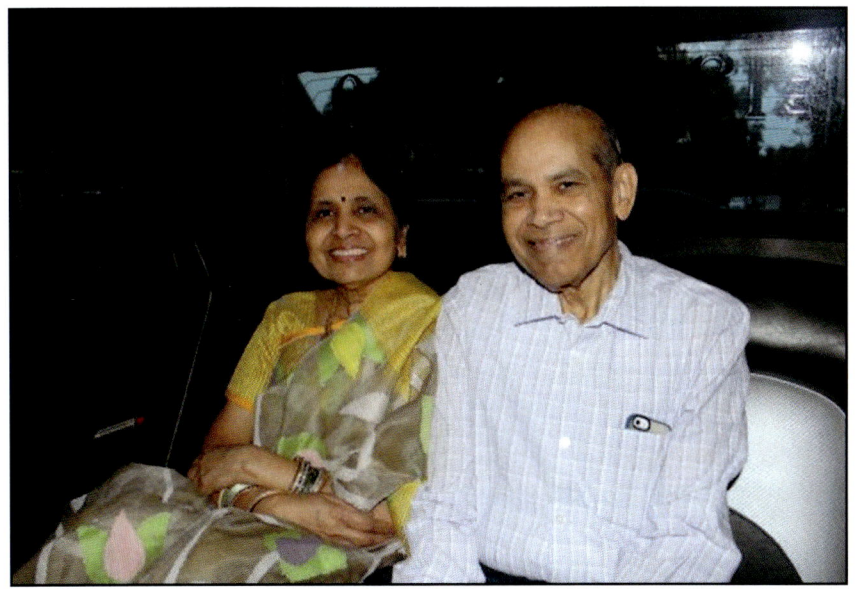

Figure 103. Photograph taken during our fiftieth marriage anniversary celebrations.

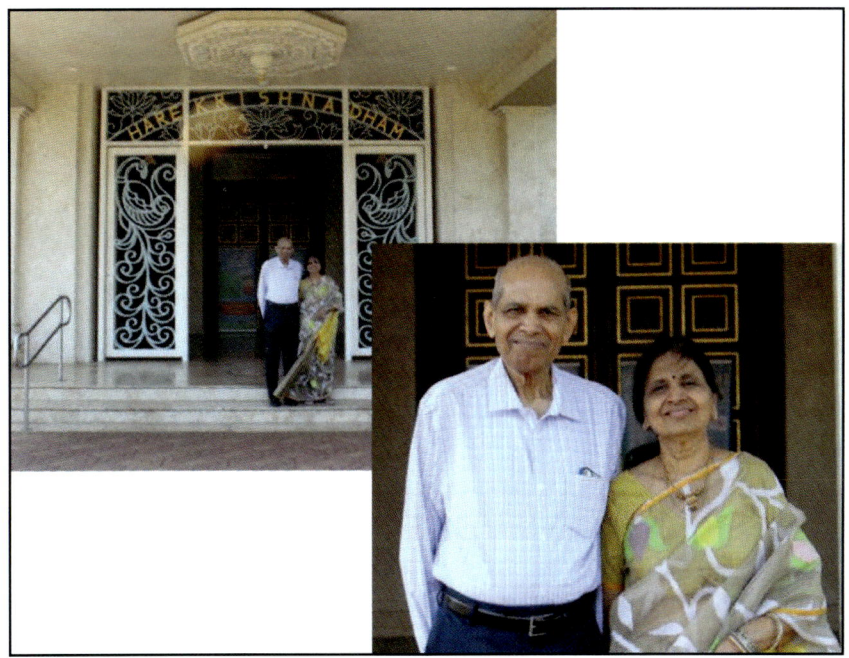

Figure 104. Photograph taken at the Hare Krishna Temple during our fiftieth marriage anniversary celebrations.

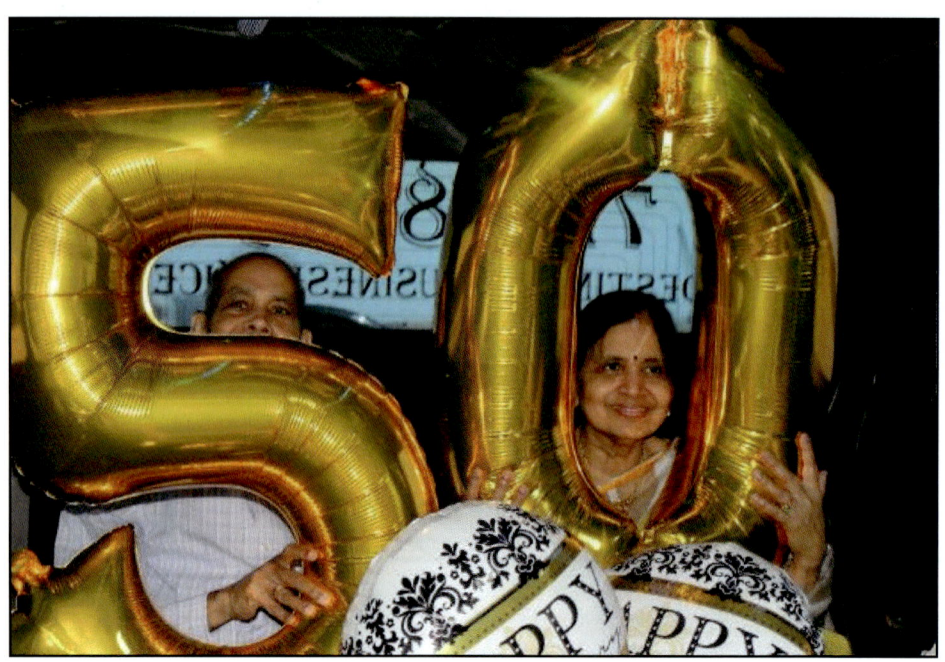

Figure 105. Photograph taken during our fiftieth marriage anniversary celebrations.

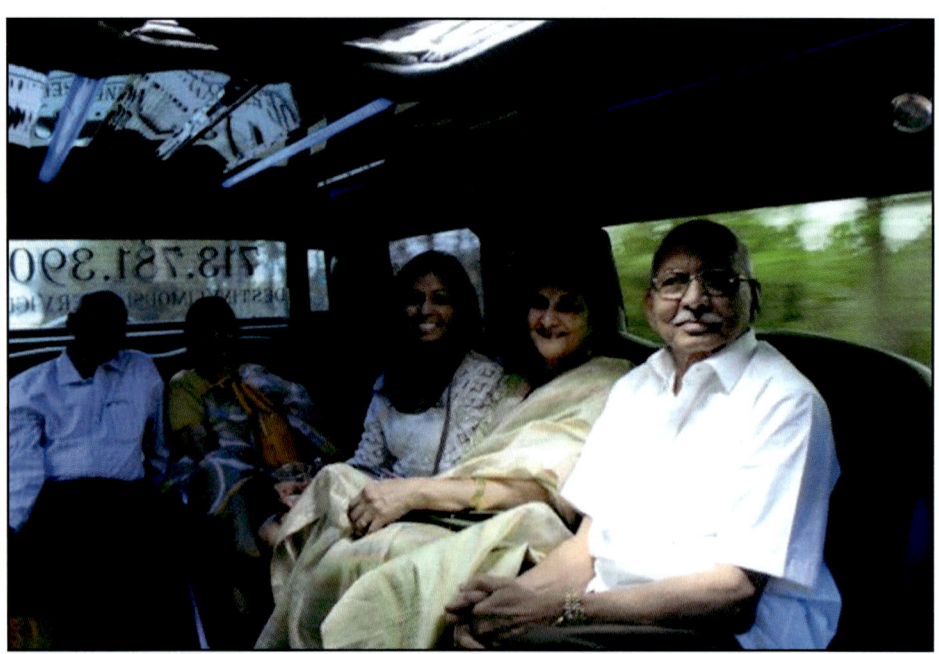

Figure 106. Photograph taken during our fiftieth marriage anniversary celebrations along with daughter, Dr. Madhavi Patnana, and her in-laws (Mrs. Satyavathi and Mr. Pratap Chundru).

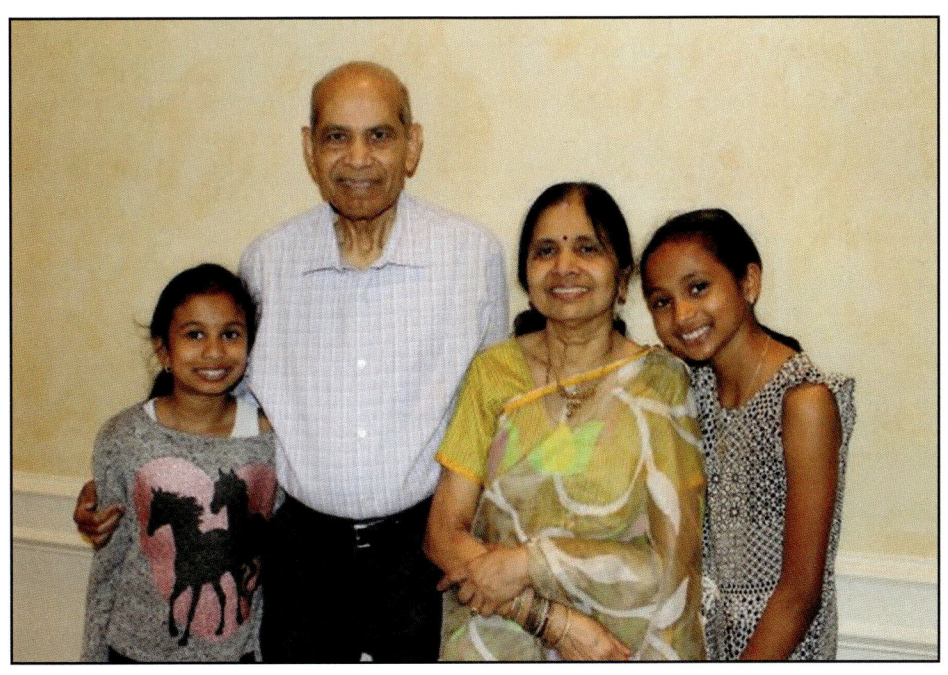

Figure 107. Photograph taken during our fiftieth marriage anniversary celebrations along with granddaughters, Anjali and Rhea.

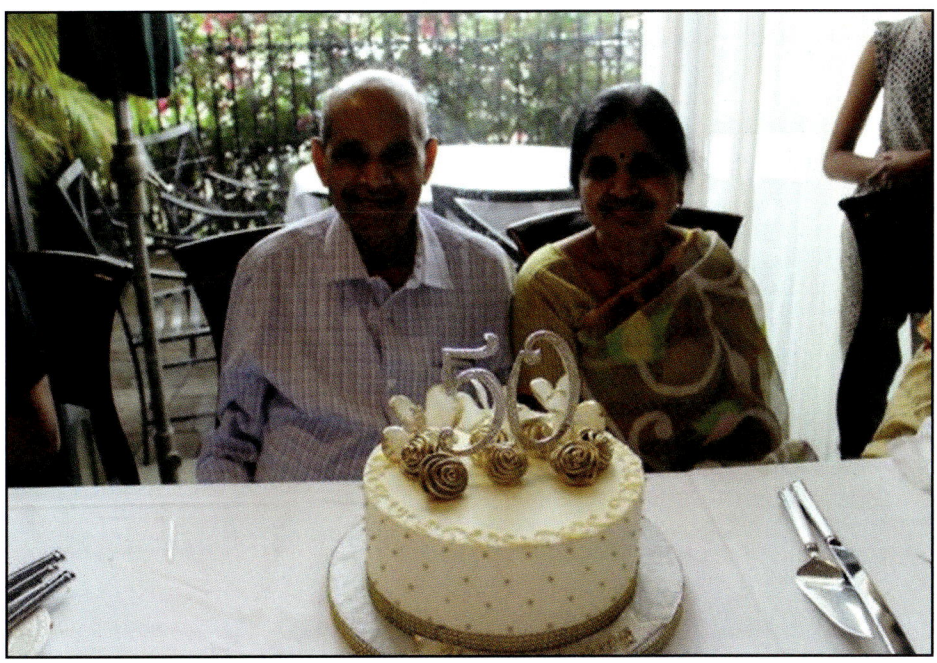

Figure 108. Photograph taken during our fiftieth marriage anniversary celebrations.

Following our trip to New Delhi to receive the Life Achievement Award on September 10, 2017, we visited my wife's native place, Harischandrapuram, where all her brothers and their children reside. Hymavathi's nephew, Doki Ravi Kumar, arranged a birthday party to celebrate both our birthdays (Hymavathi's birthday was on September 12 and my birthday was on September 21); the party was scheduled on a Sunday between both our birthdays. Nearly 500 people attended the party and some of the photographs taken during the function are shown in figures 109 through 123.

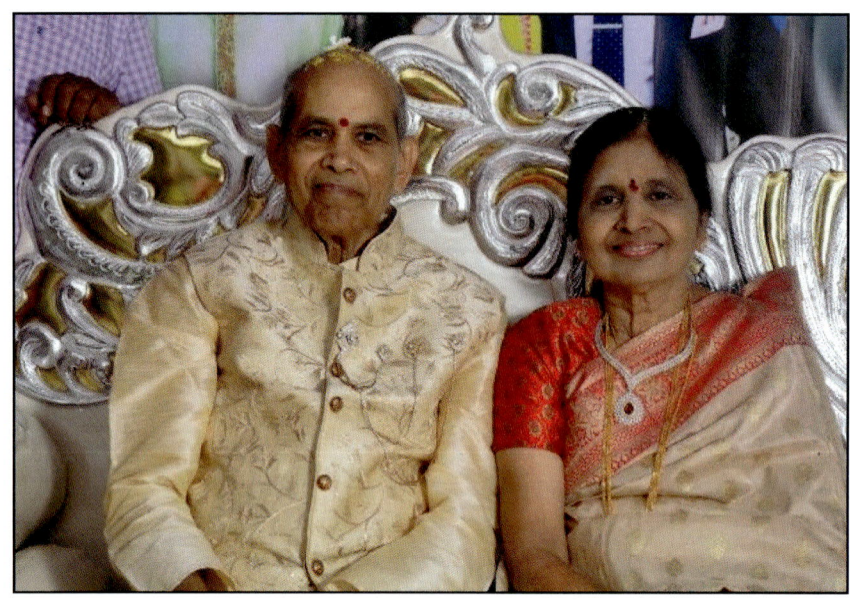

Figure 109.

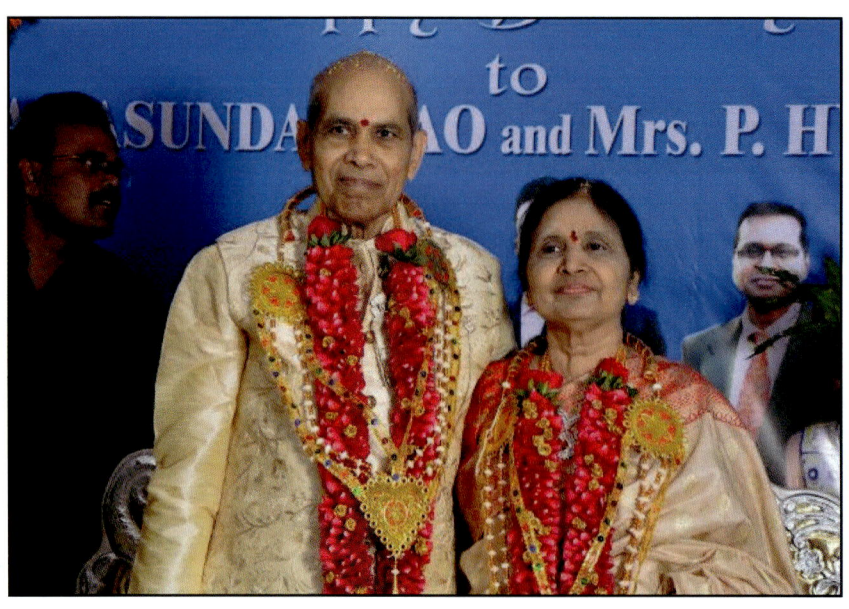

Figure 110.

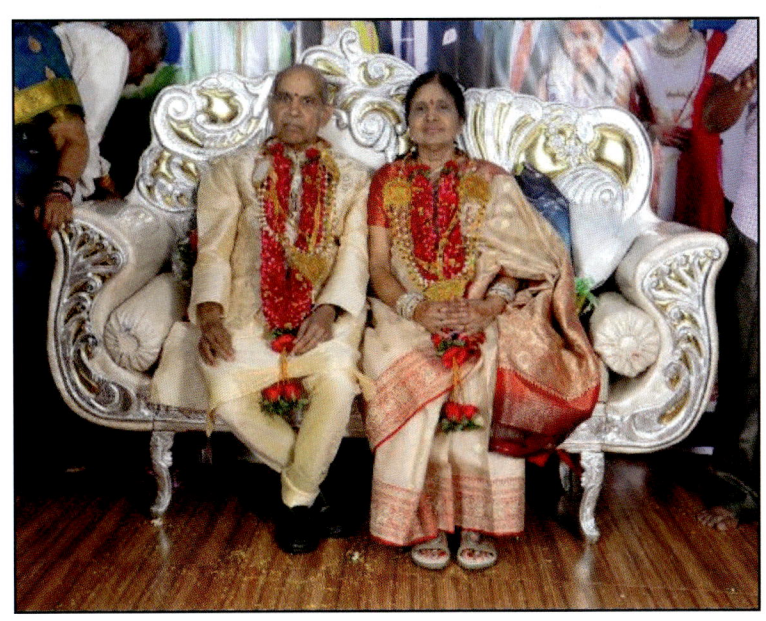

Figure 111.

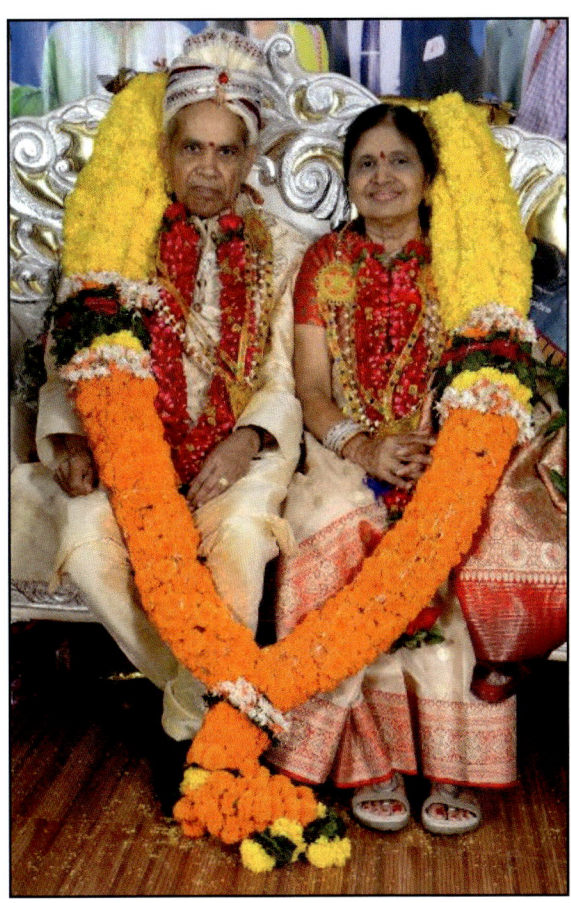

Figure 112.

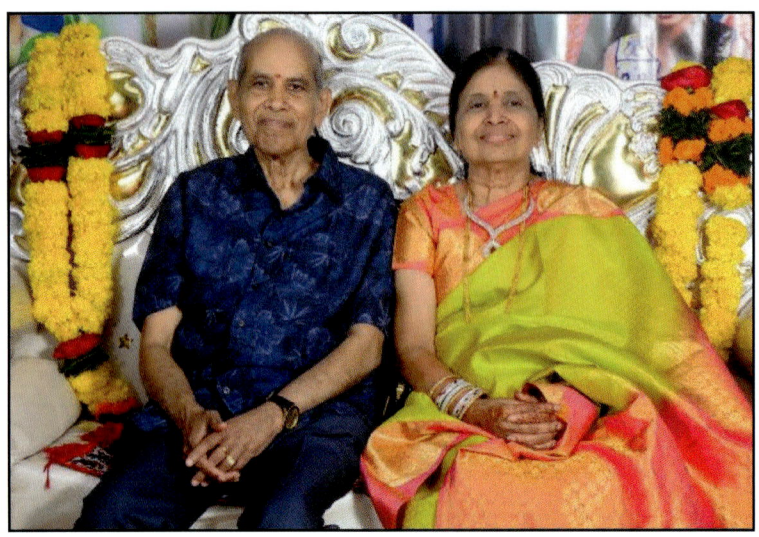

Figure 113.

Figures 109 through 113. Photographs of Hymavathi and me taken during our birthday celebrations.

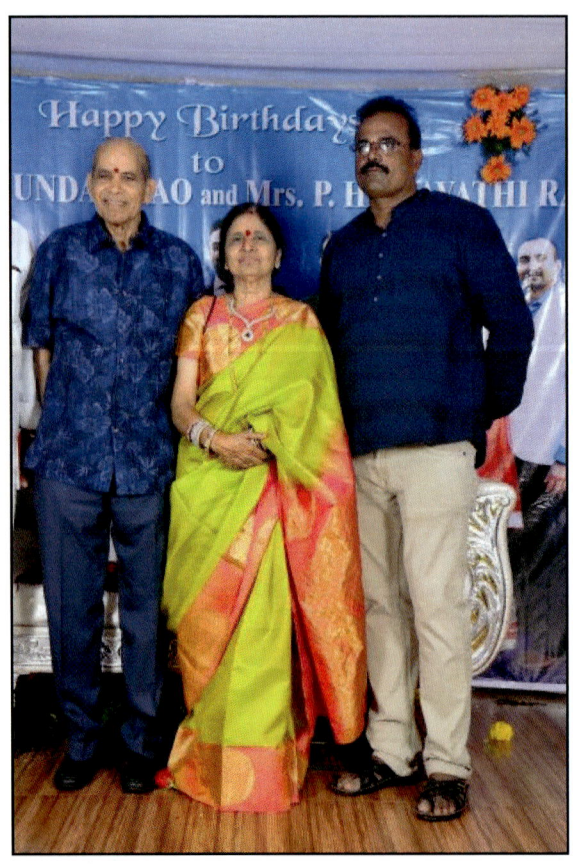

Figure 114. Photograph of Hymavathi and I along with Ravi Kumar, Hymavathi's nephew, who organized the birthday celebration.

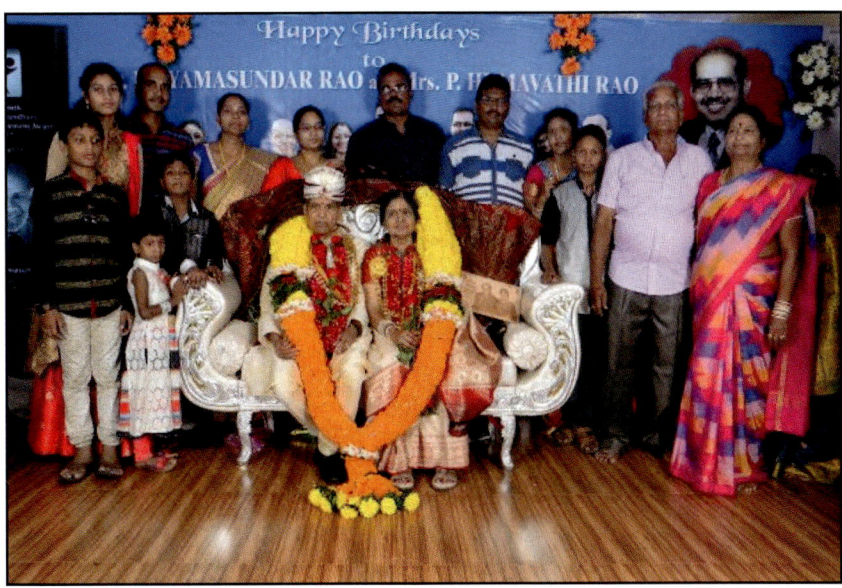

Figure 115. Photograph of Hymavathi and I along with Hymavathi's brother, Doki Bhaskararao, and his entire family taken during our birthday celebrations.

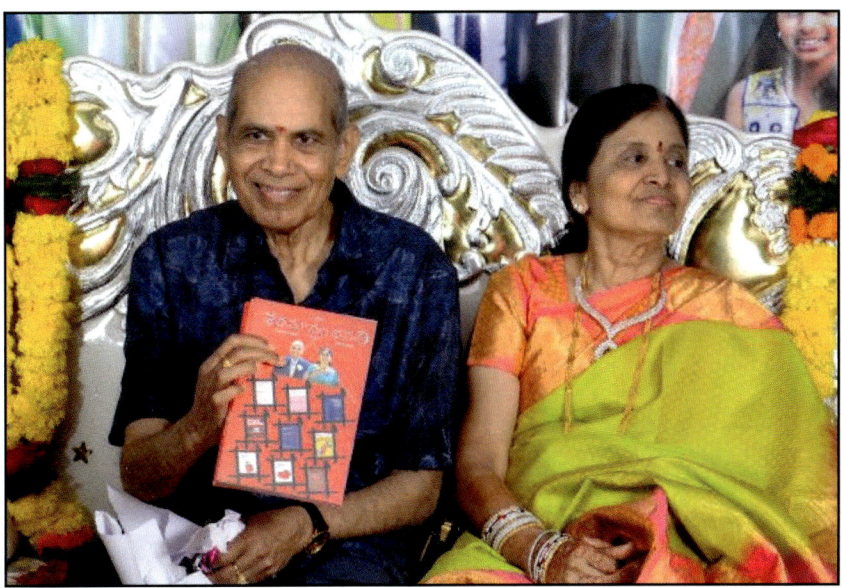

Figure 116. Photograph of Hymavathi and I with me showing the booklet published for distribution during our birthday celebrations.

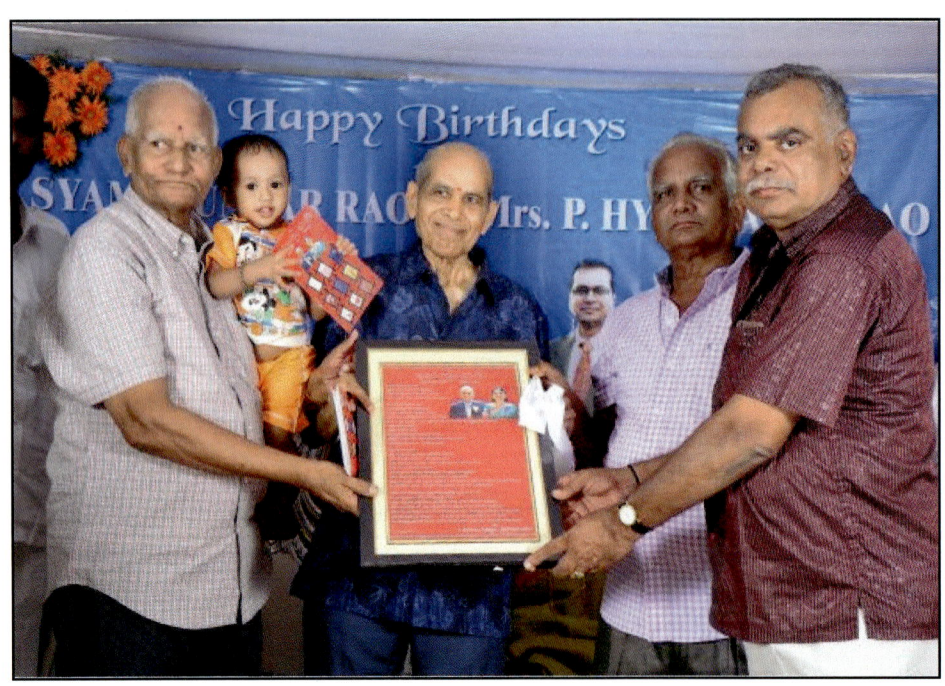

Figure 117. Photograph showing the presentation of a plaque by Hyamvathi's brothers and nephew during our birthday celebrations.

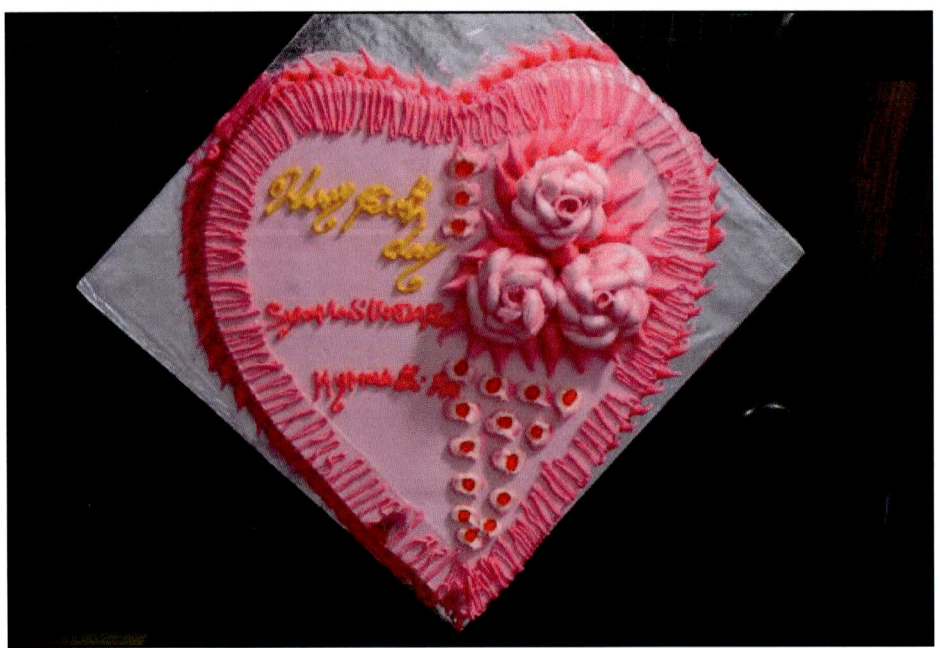

Figure 118. Photograph of the birthday cake.

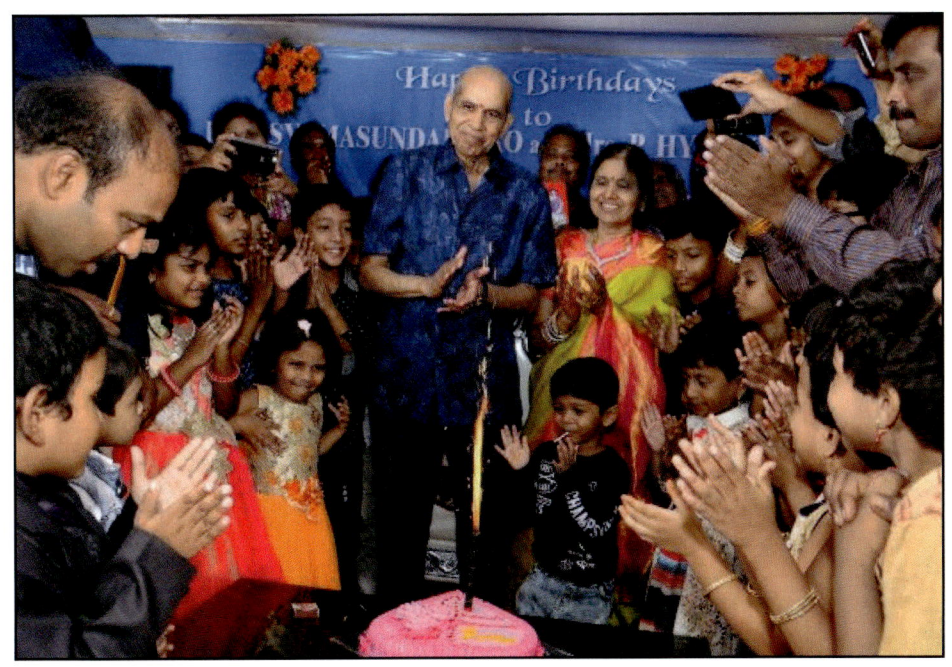

Figure 119. Lighting the birthday candle.

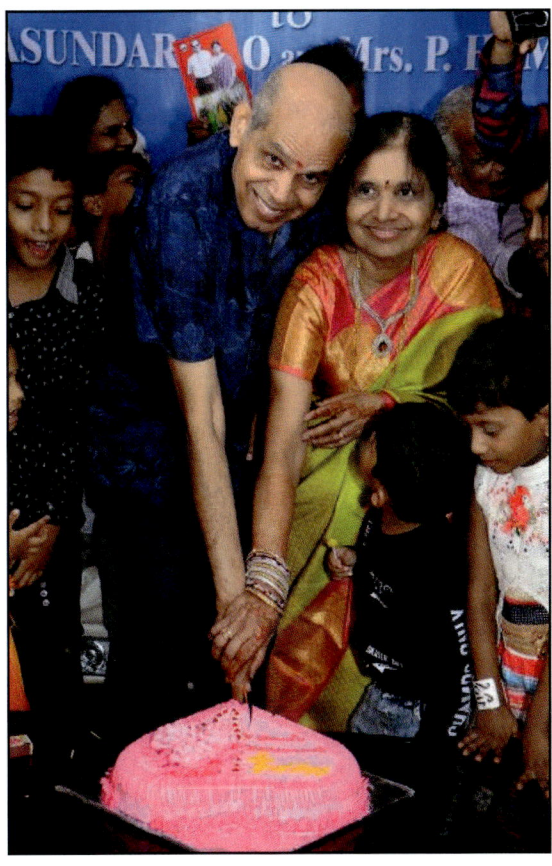

Figure 120. Cutting the birthday cake.

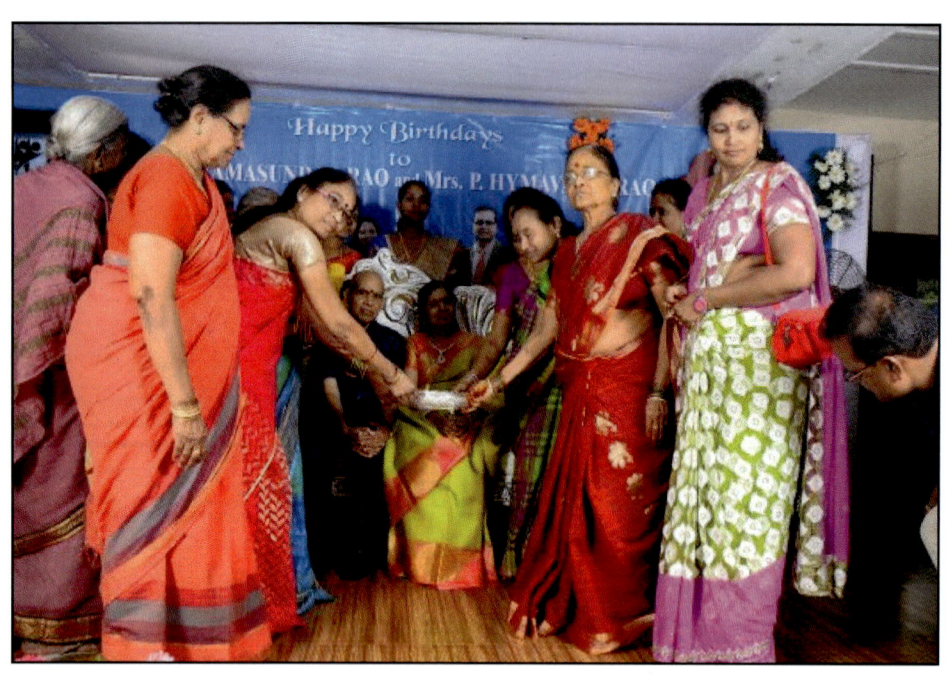

Figure 121. Harathi to the birthday couple.

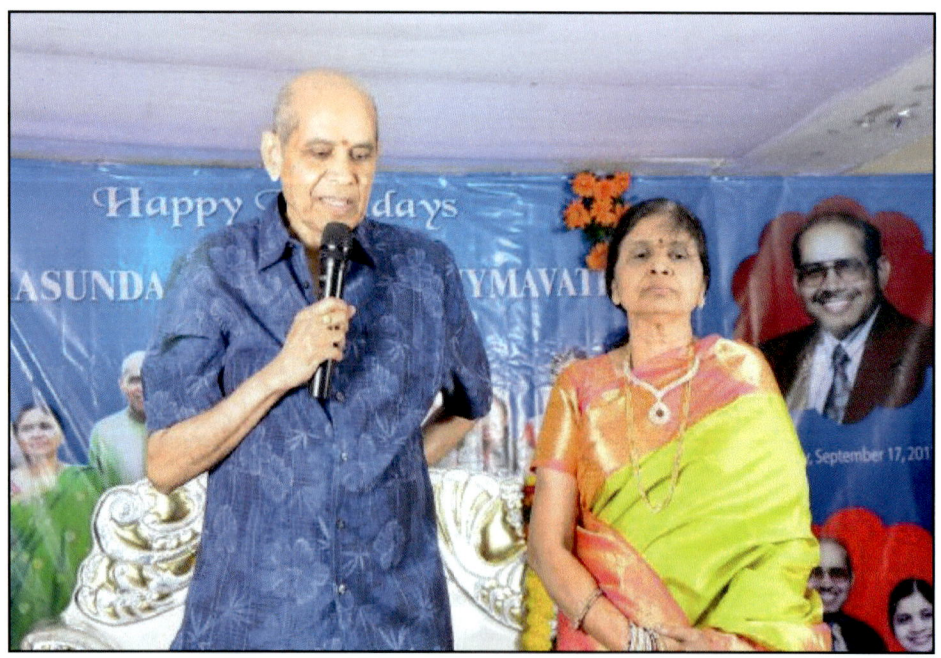

Figure 122.

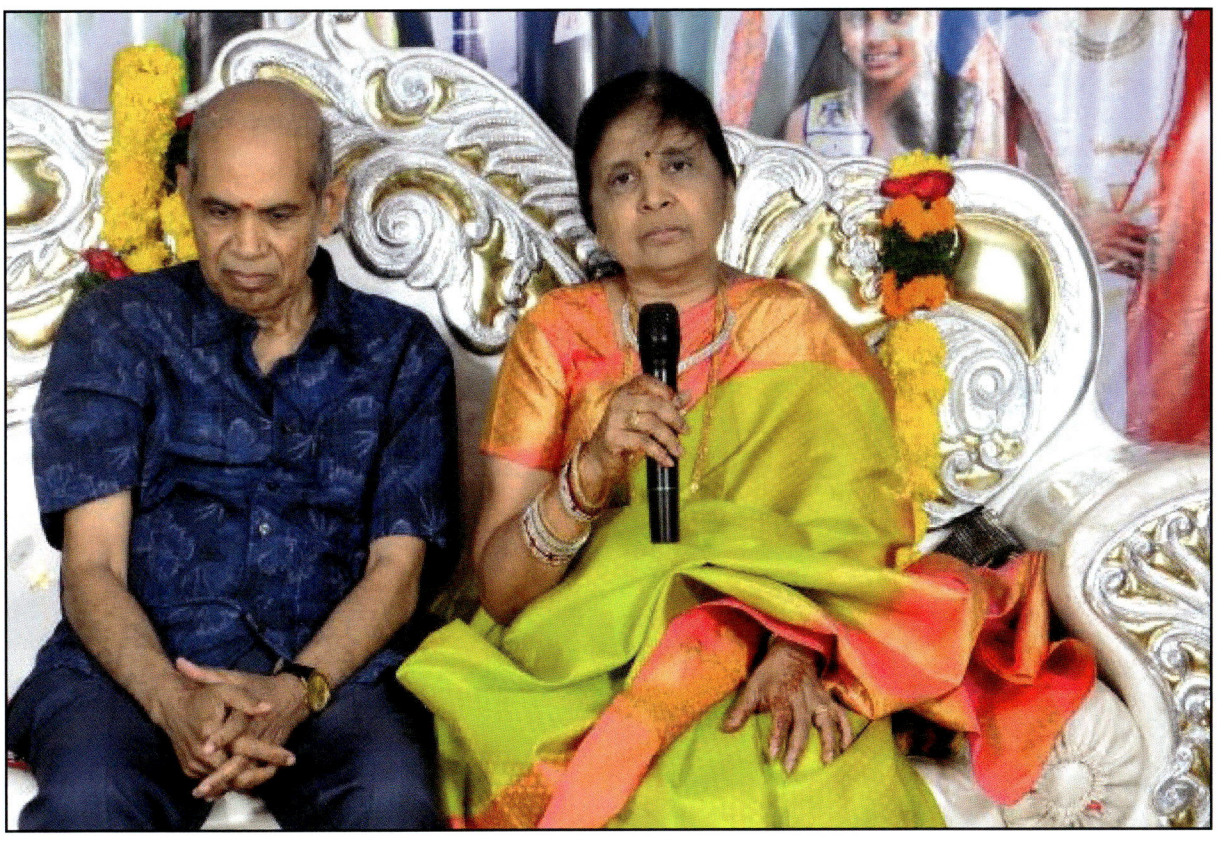

Figure 123.

Figures 122 and 123. Speeches conveying thanks immediately following our birthday celebrations.

With time, we grew in age and the family grew in numbers. A pictorial presentation of our couple through the years (Figures 124 through 136) and of the family (Figures 137 through 141) is made in figures 124 through 141. The next two figures (Figure 142 and 143) are portraits of the entire family, both in Indian traditional (Figure 142) and in American casual (Figure 143) clothes. The final four pictures of this chapter introduce the newest member of our family, my daughter Radhika's puppy, Mango (Figures 144 through 147).

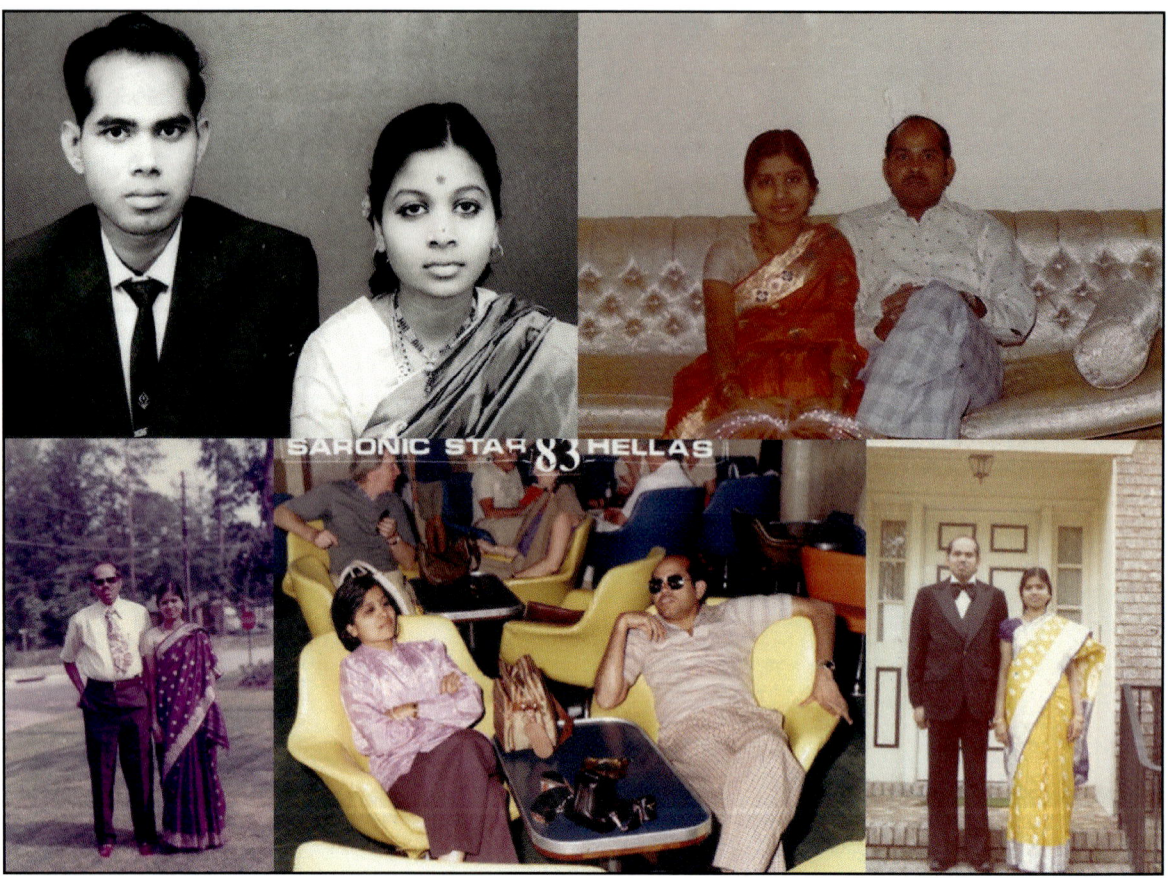

Figure 124.

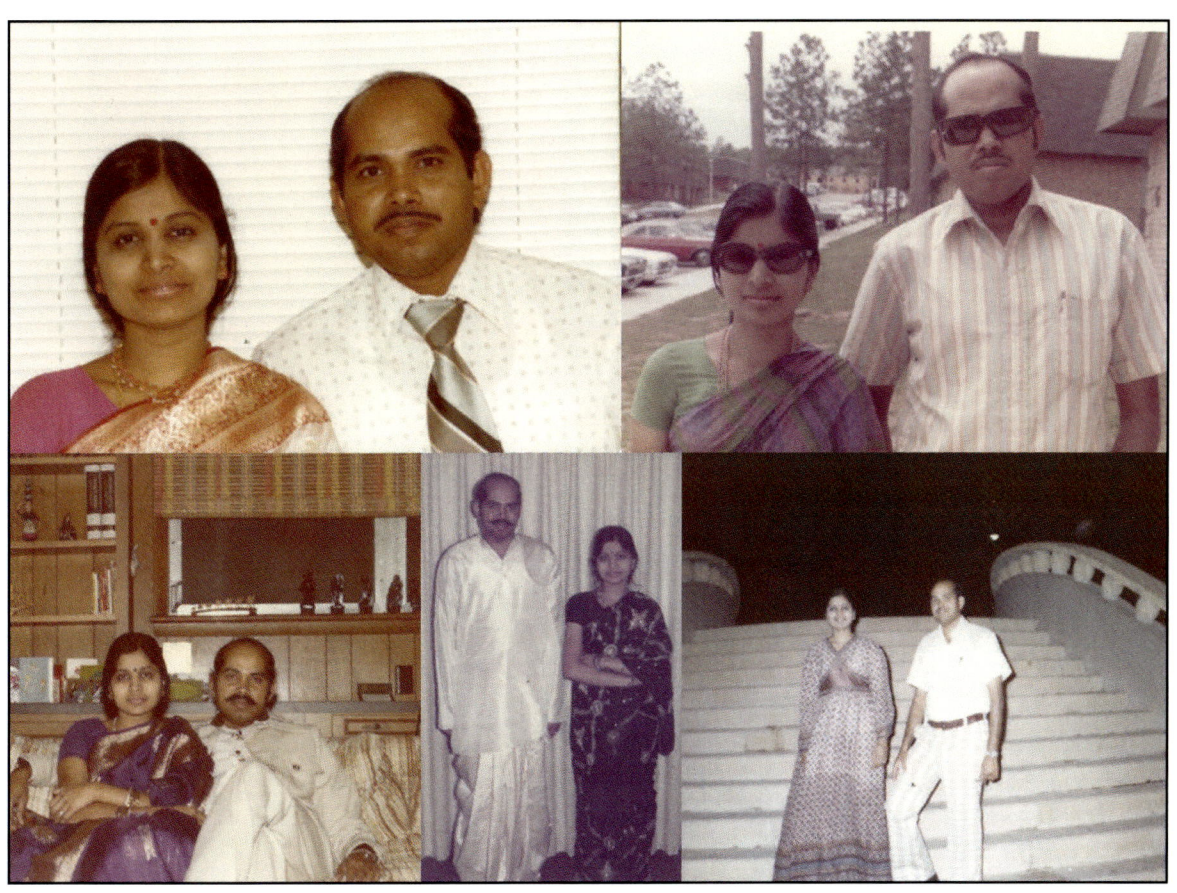

Figure 125.

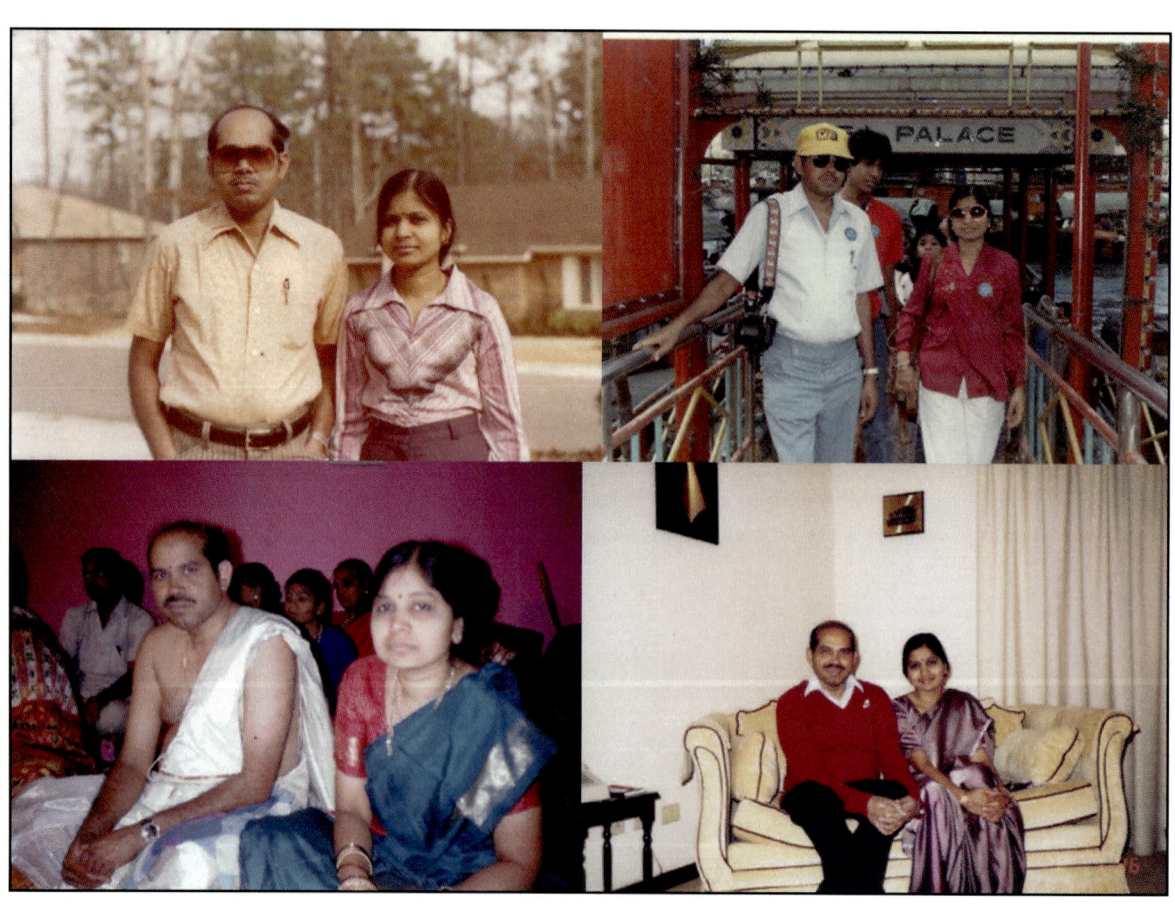

Figure 126.

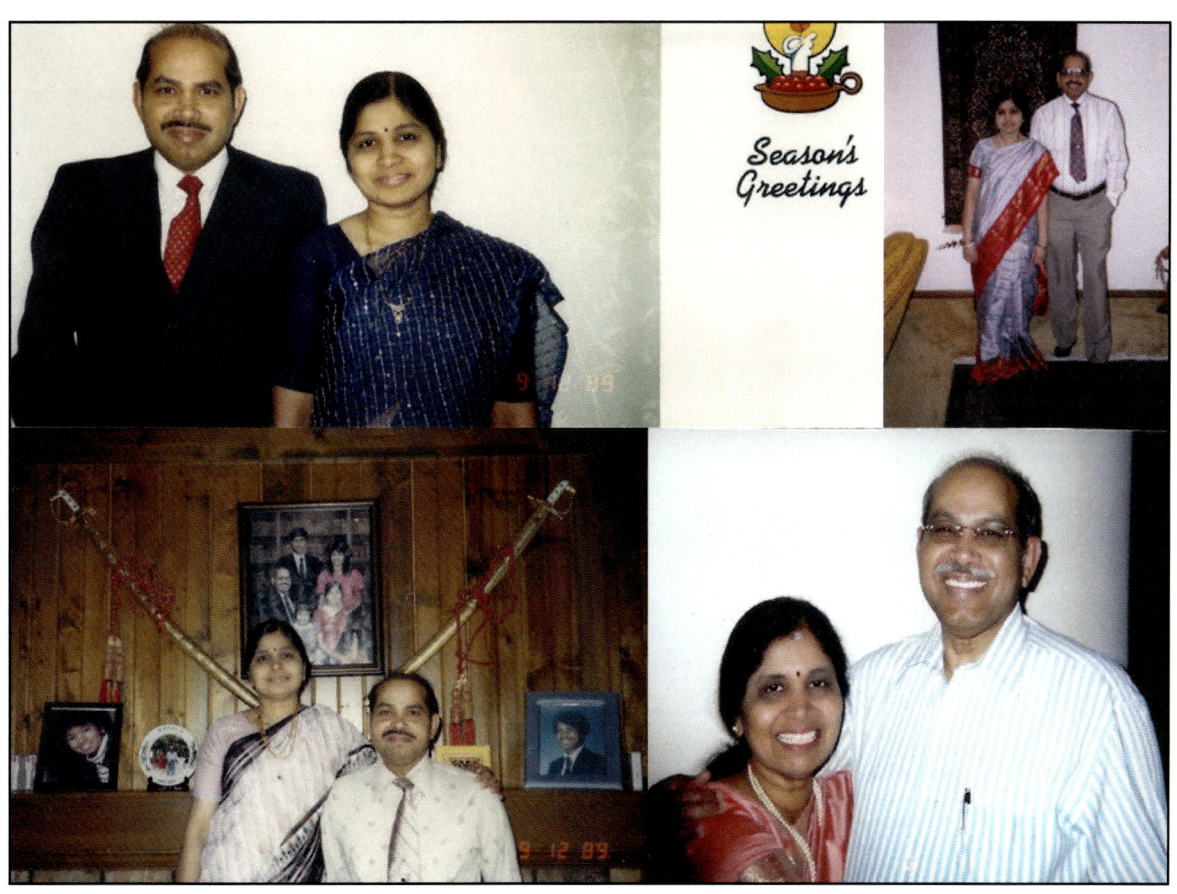

Figure 127.

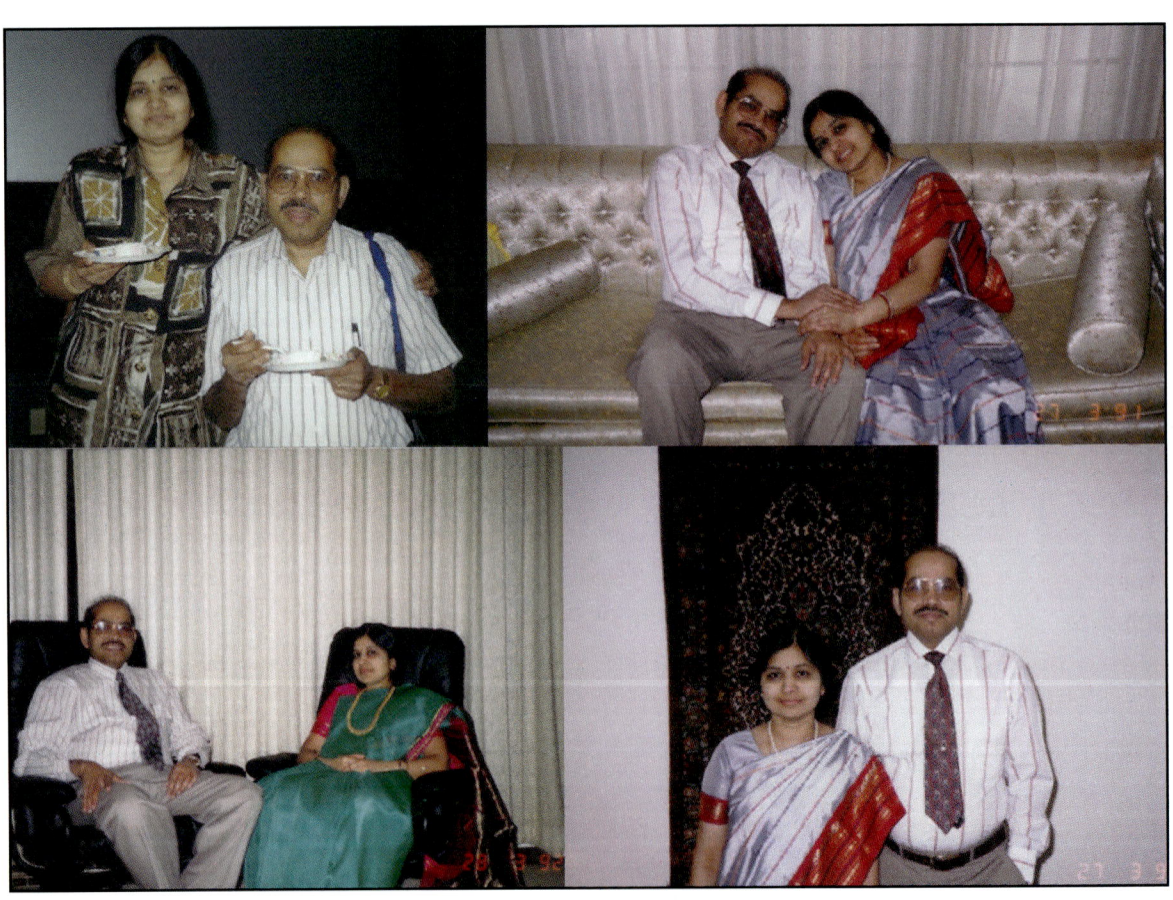

Figure 128.

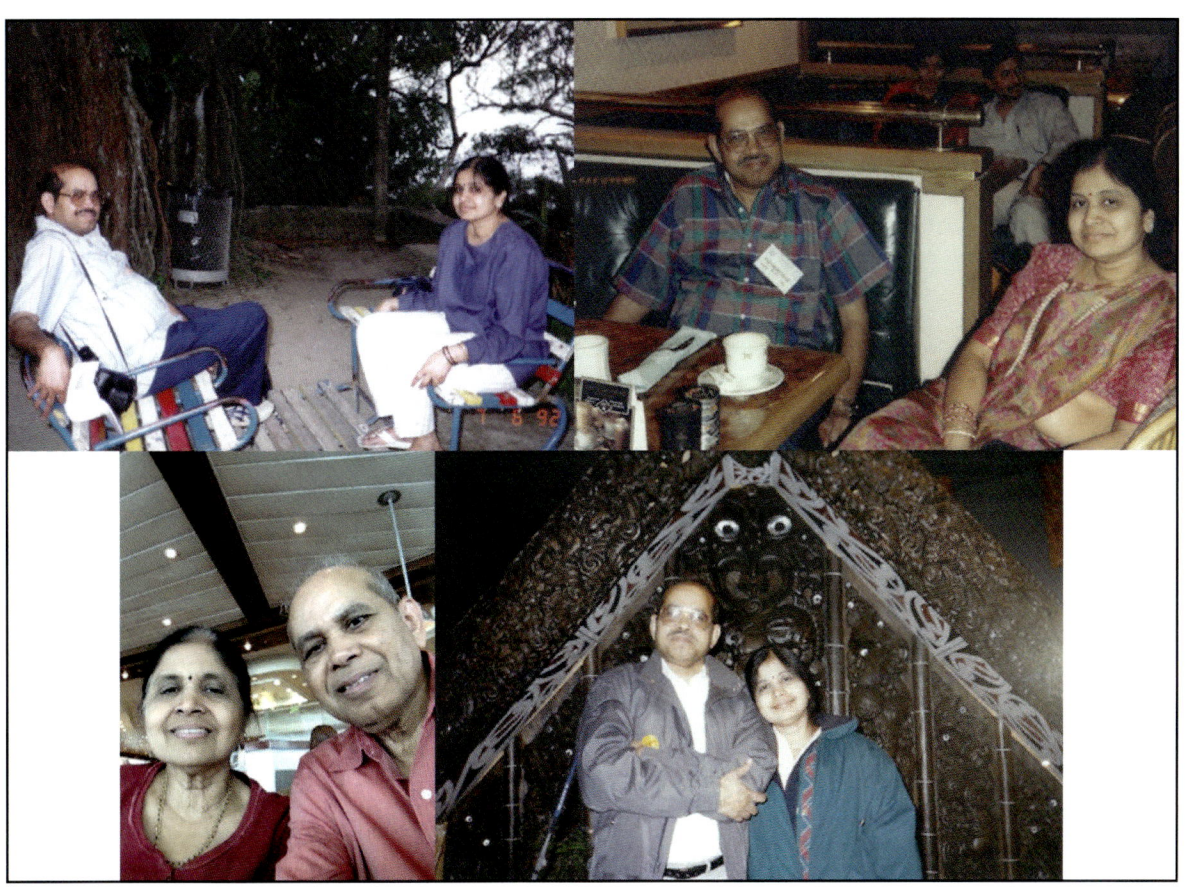

Figure 129.

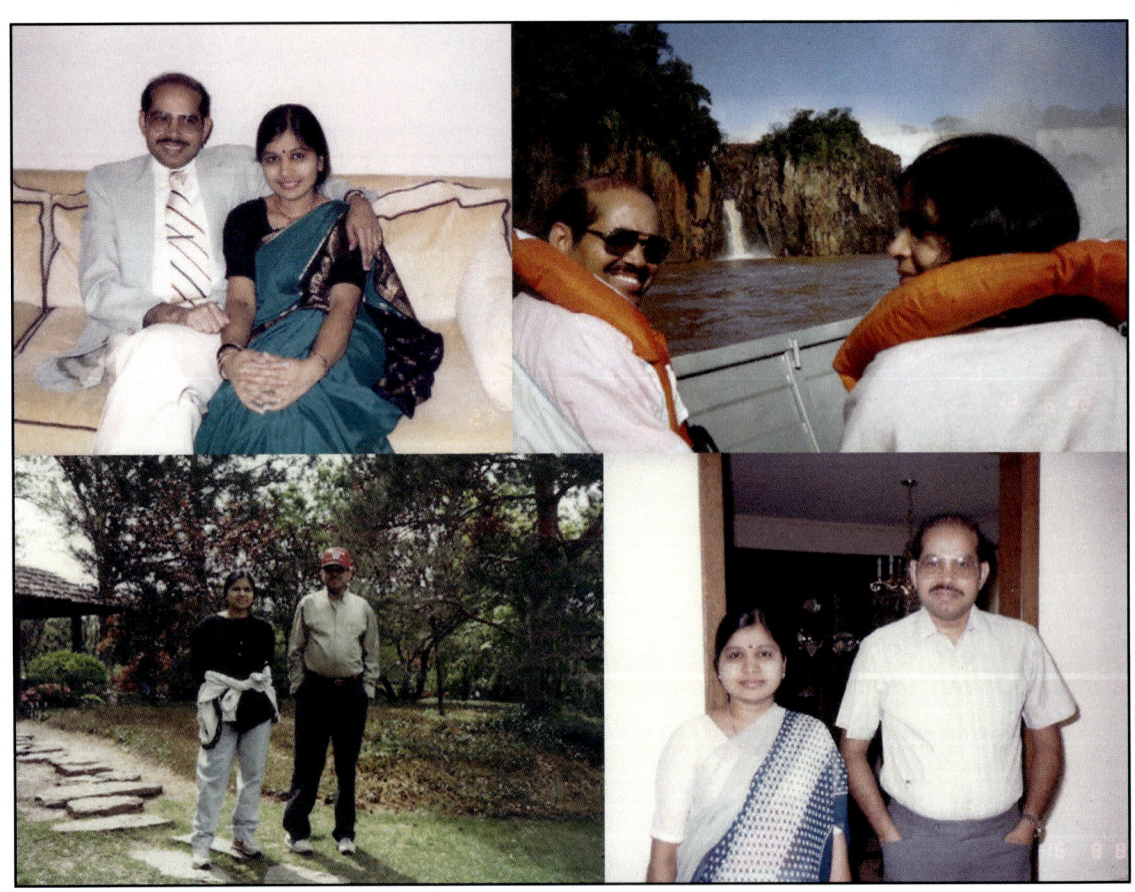

Figure 130.

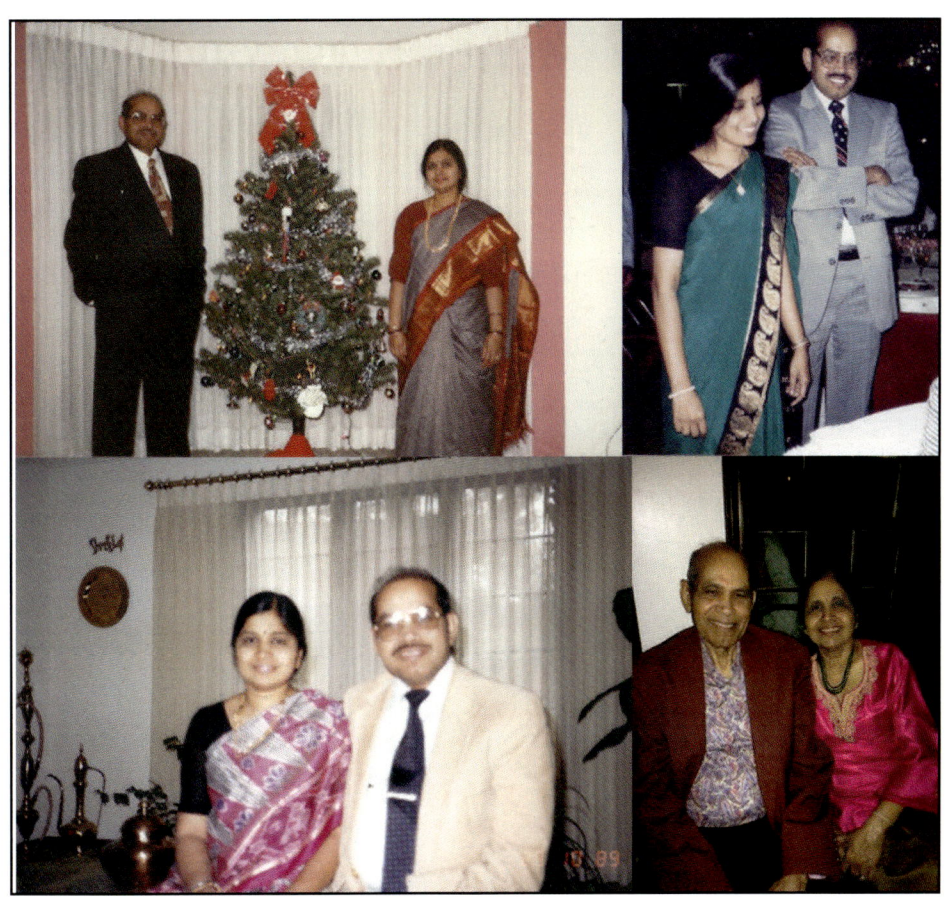

Figure 131.

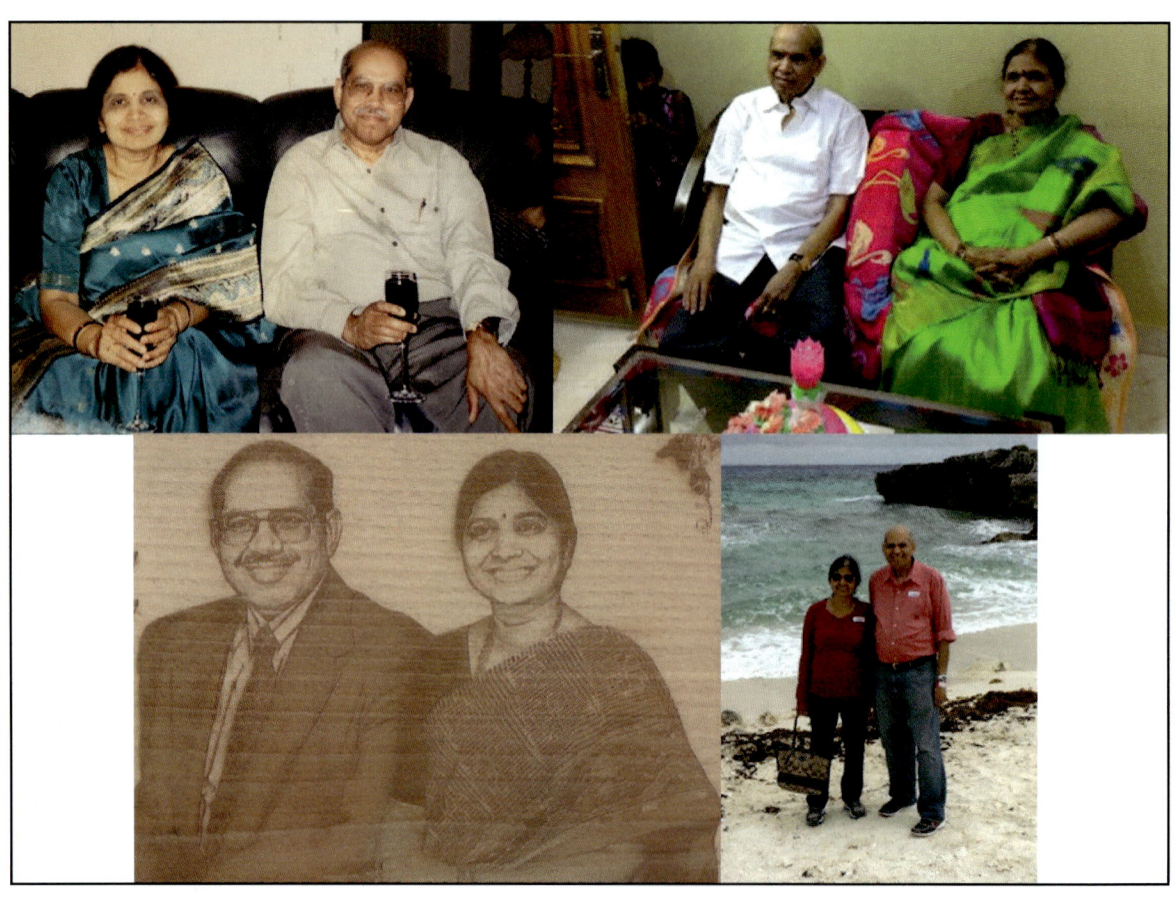

Figure 132.

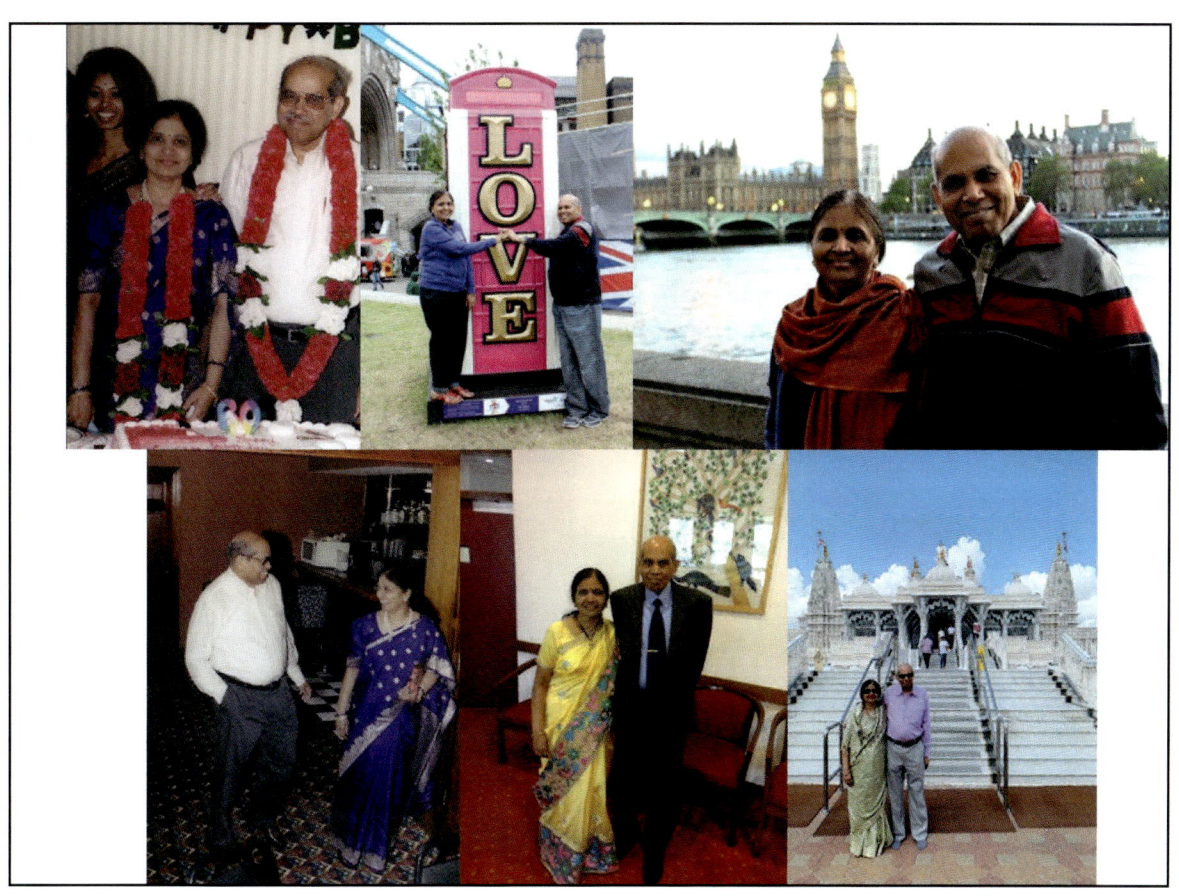

Figure 133.

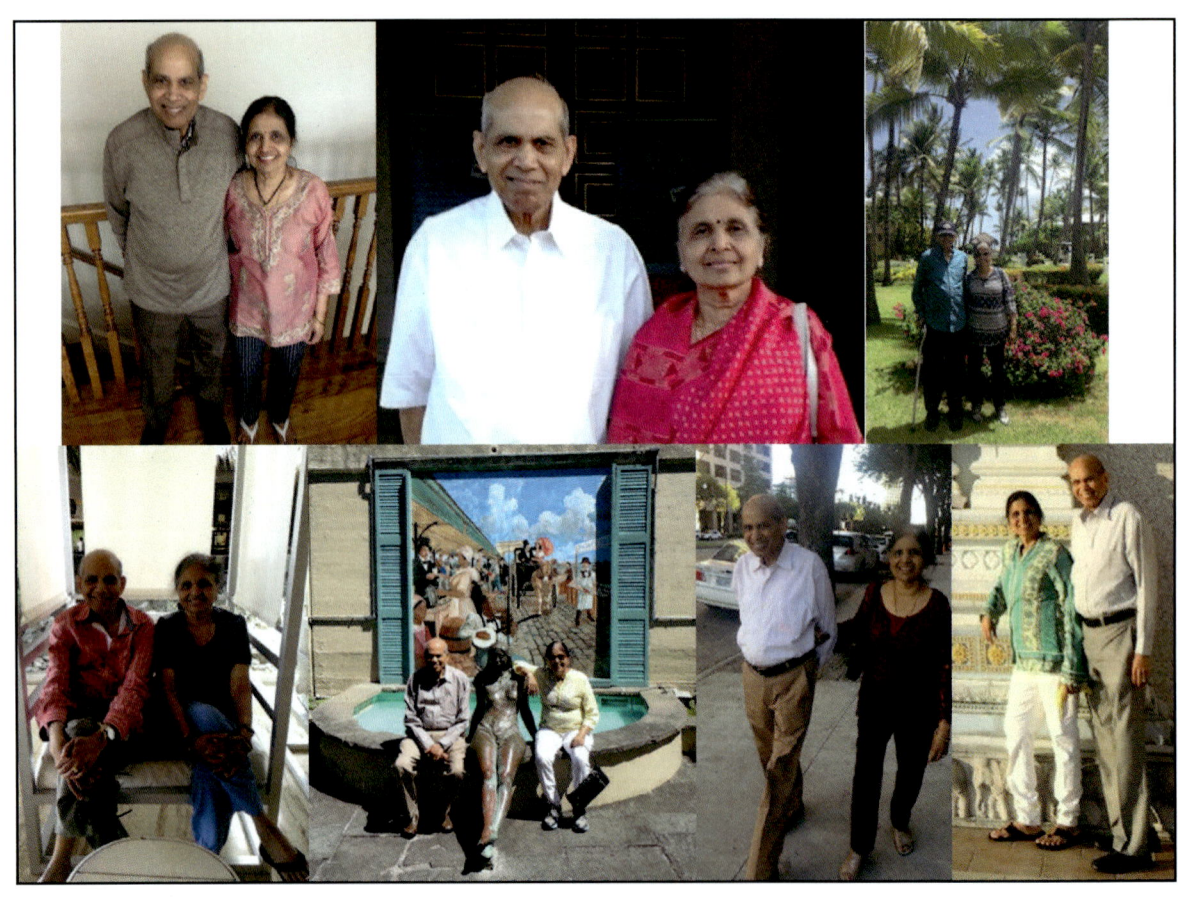

Figure 134.

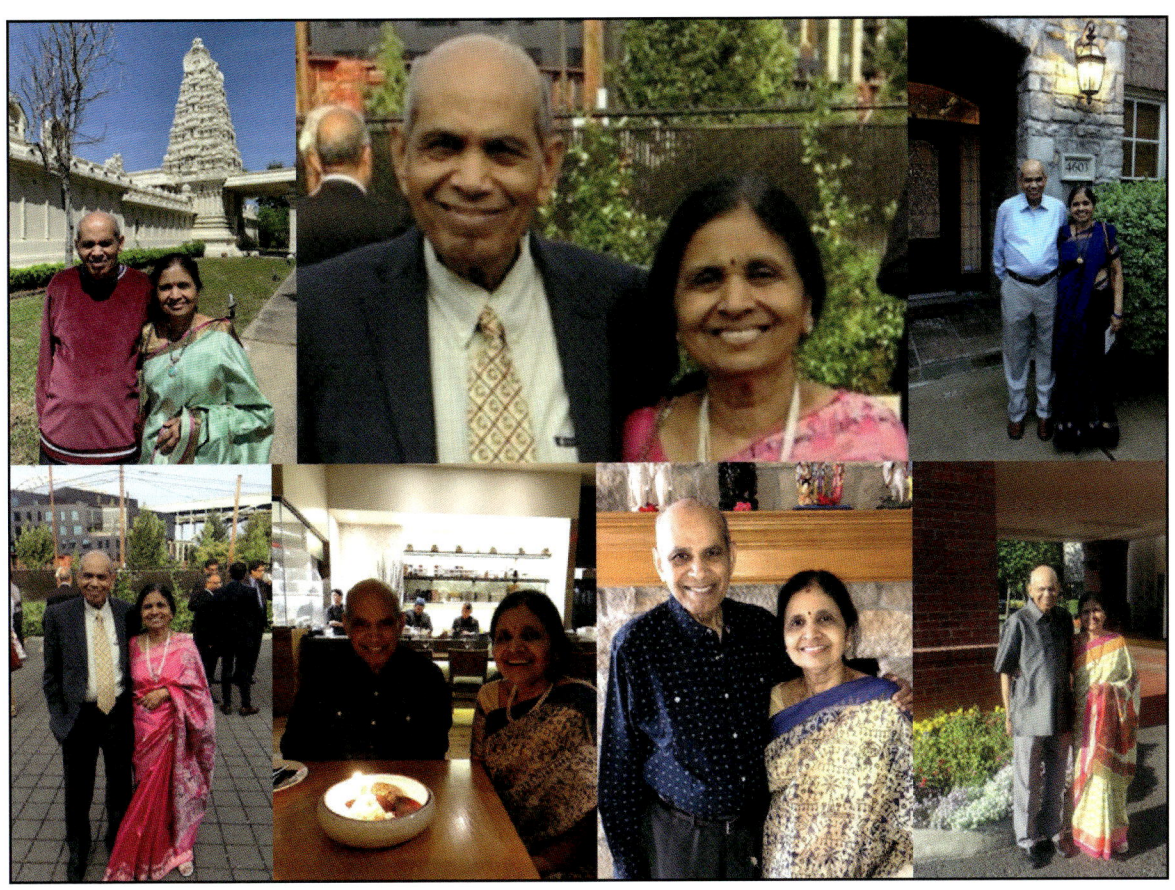

Figure 135.

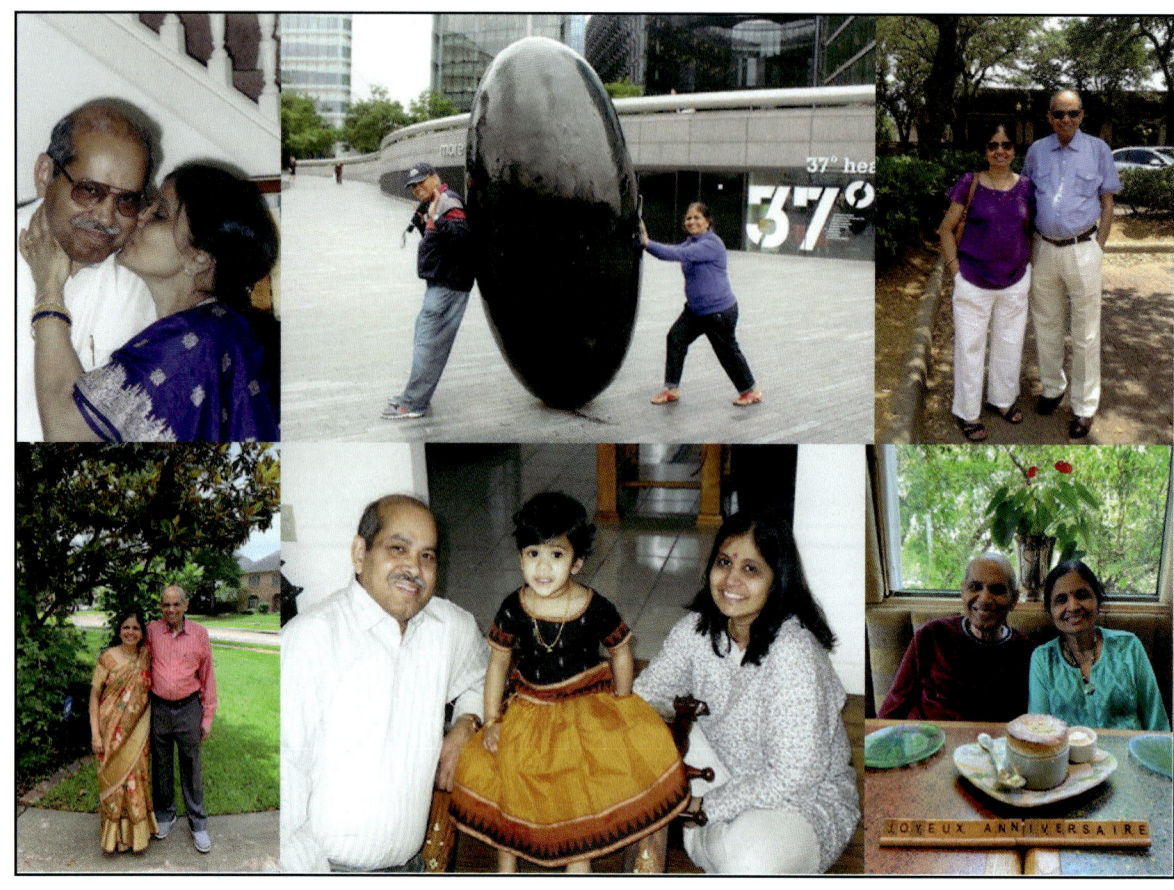

Figure 136.

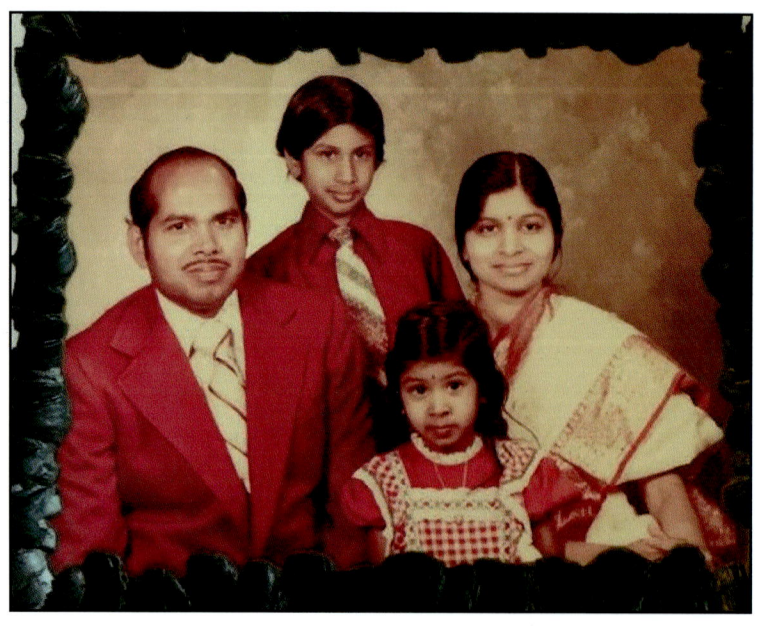

Figure 137. Family portrait taken in mid 1970s. Me, Vijay, Madhavi.
and Hymavathi.

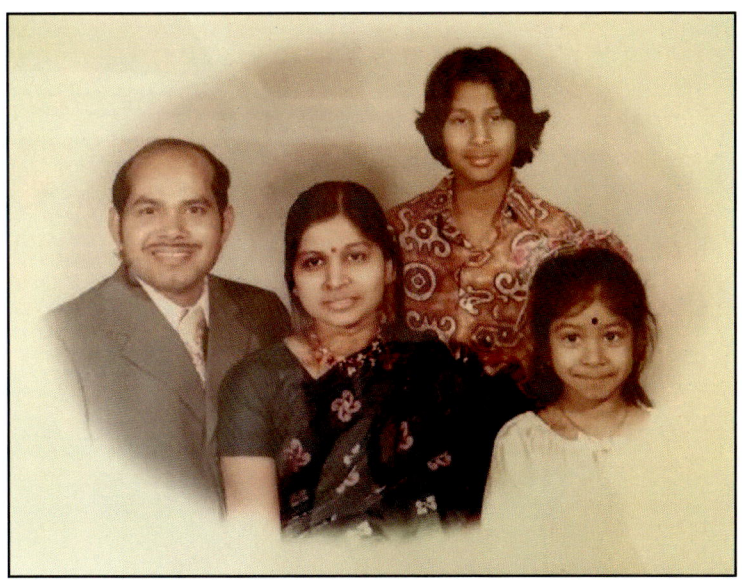

Figure 138. Family portrait taken in late 1970s. Me, Hymavathi, Vijay, and Madhavi.

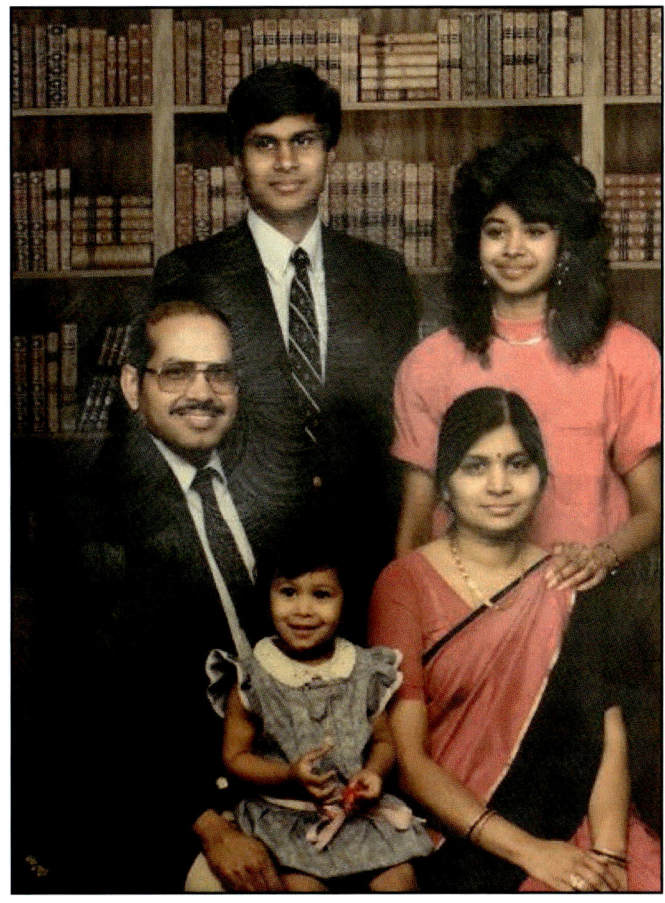

Figure 139. Family portrait taken in late 1980s. Vijay, Madhavi, me, Radhika, and Hymavathi.

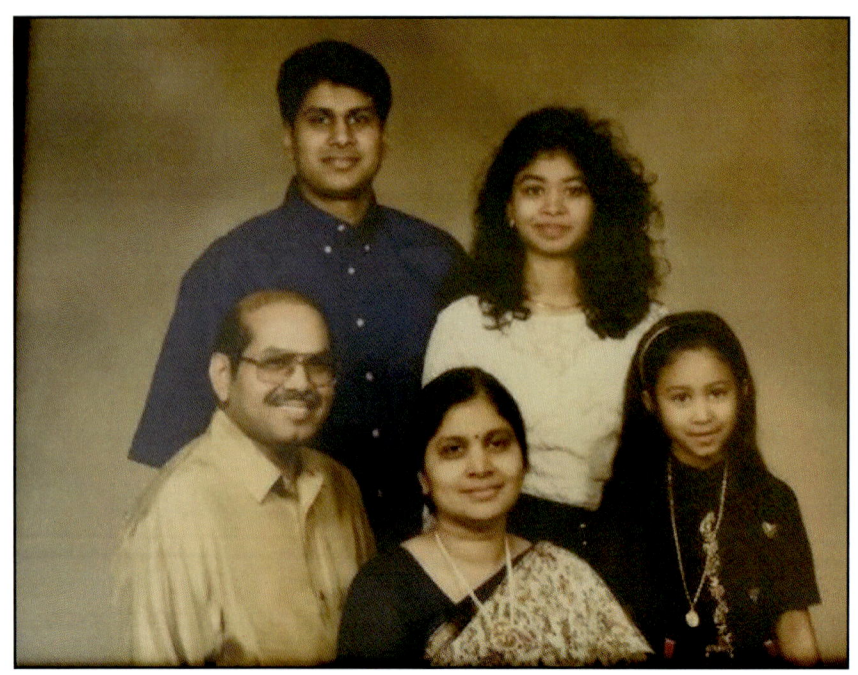

Figure 140. Family portrait taken in early 1990s. Vijay, Madhavi, me, Hymavathi, and Radhika.

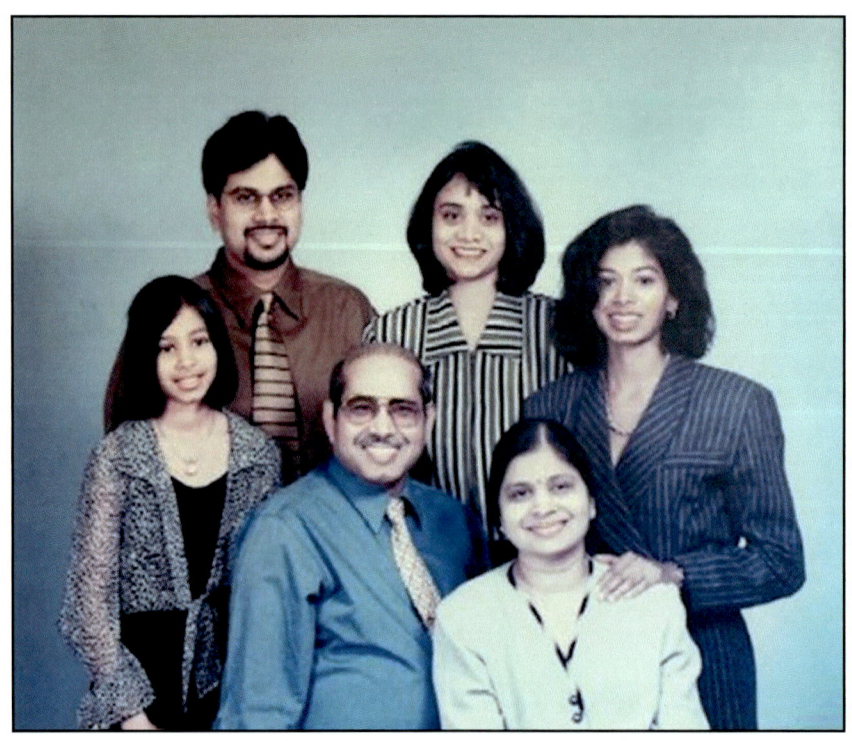

Figure 141. Family portrait taken in mid 1990s. Vijay, Radha, Madhavi, Radhika, me, and Hymavathi.

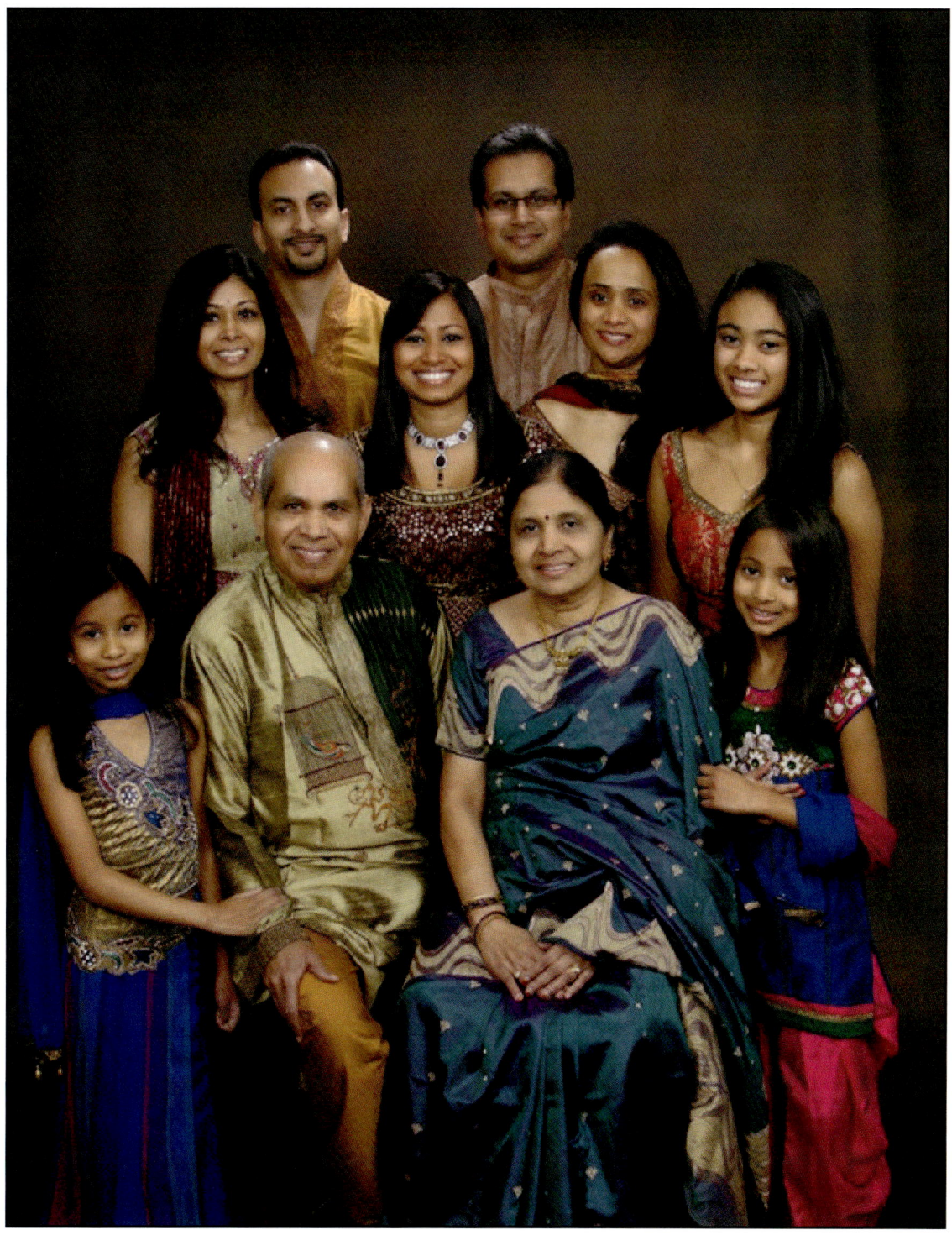

Figure 142. Family portrait in Indian traditional dresses. Top row - Ravi (Madhavi's husband) and Vijay; middle row - Madhavi, Radhika, Radha, and Meghana; bottom row - Anjali, me, Hymavathi, and Rhea.

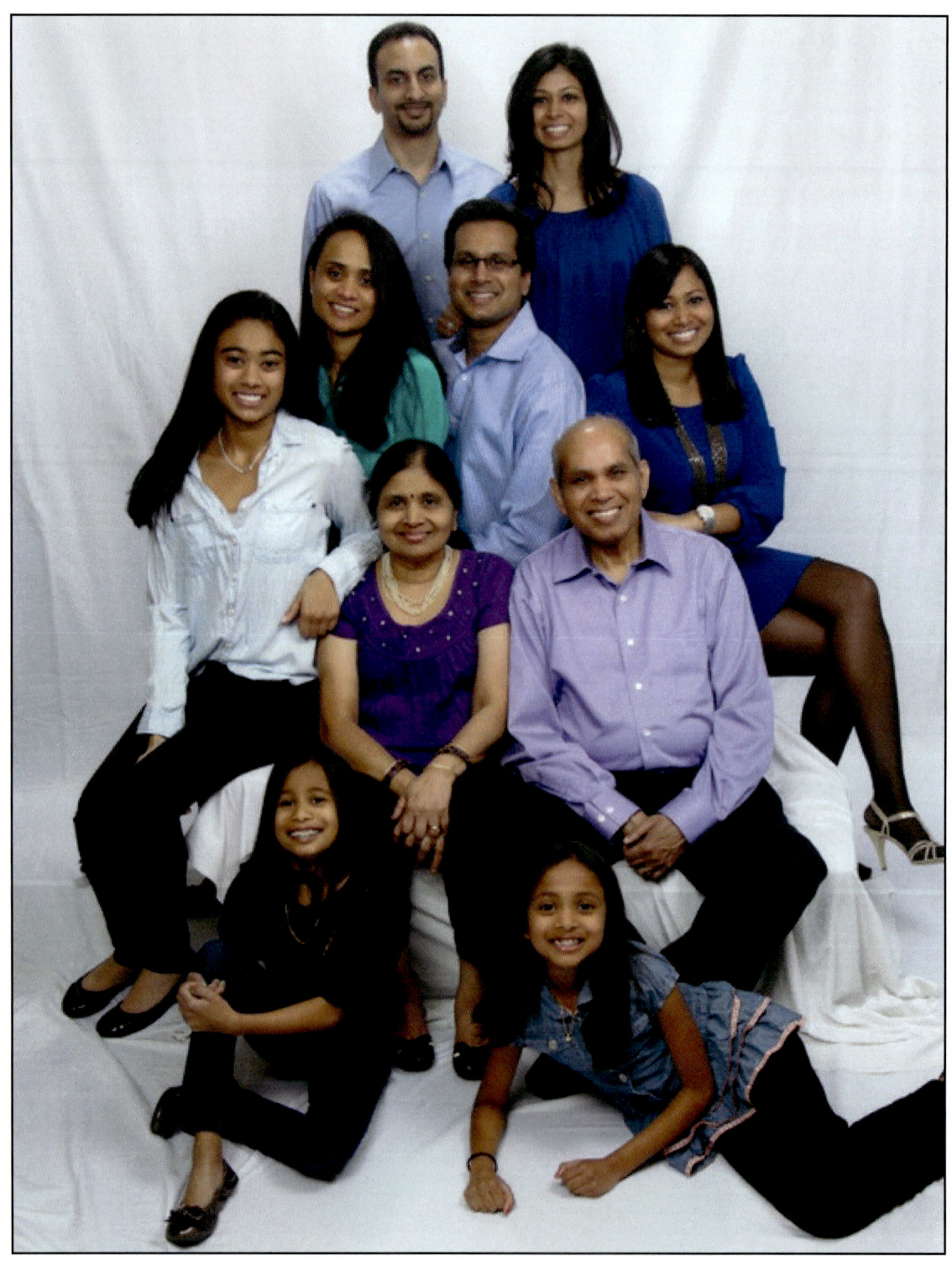

Figure 143. Family portrait in American casual dresses. Top row - Ravi and Madhavi; middle row - Meghana, Radha, Vijay, and Radhika; next row - Hymavathi and me; on the floor - Anjali and Rhea.

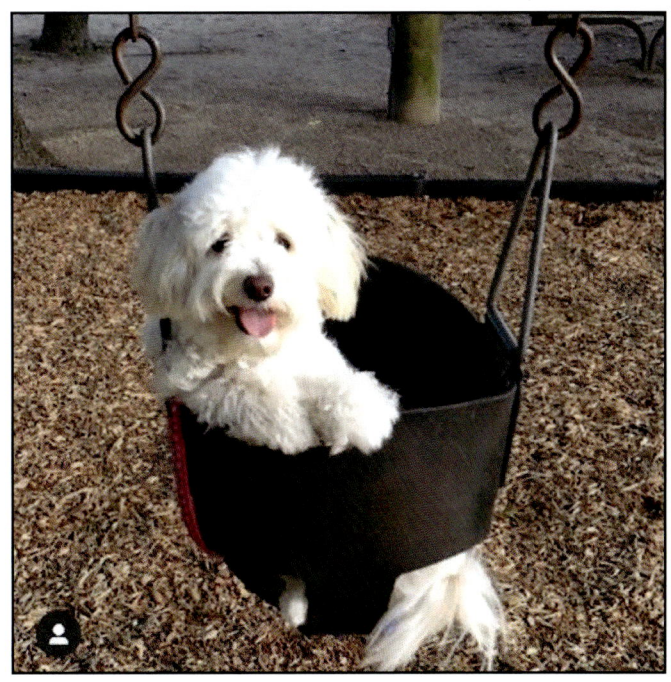

Figure 144. Photograph of Mango.

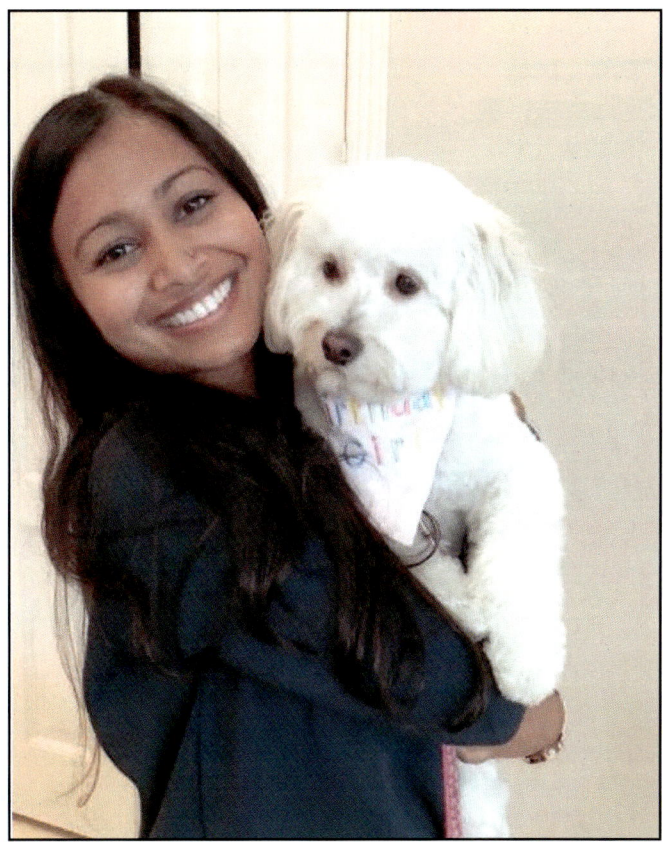

Figure 145. Photograph of Mango with Radhika.

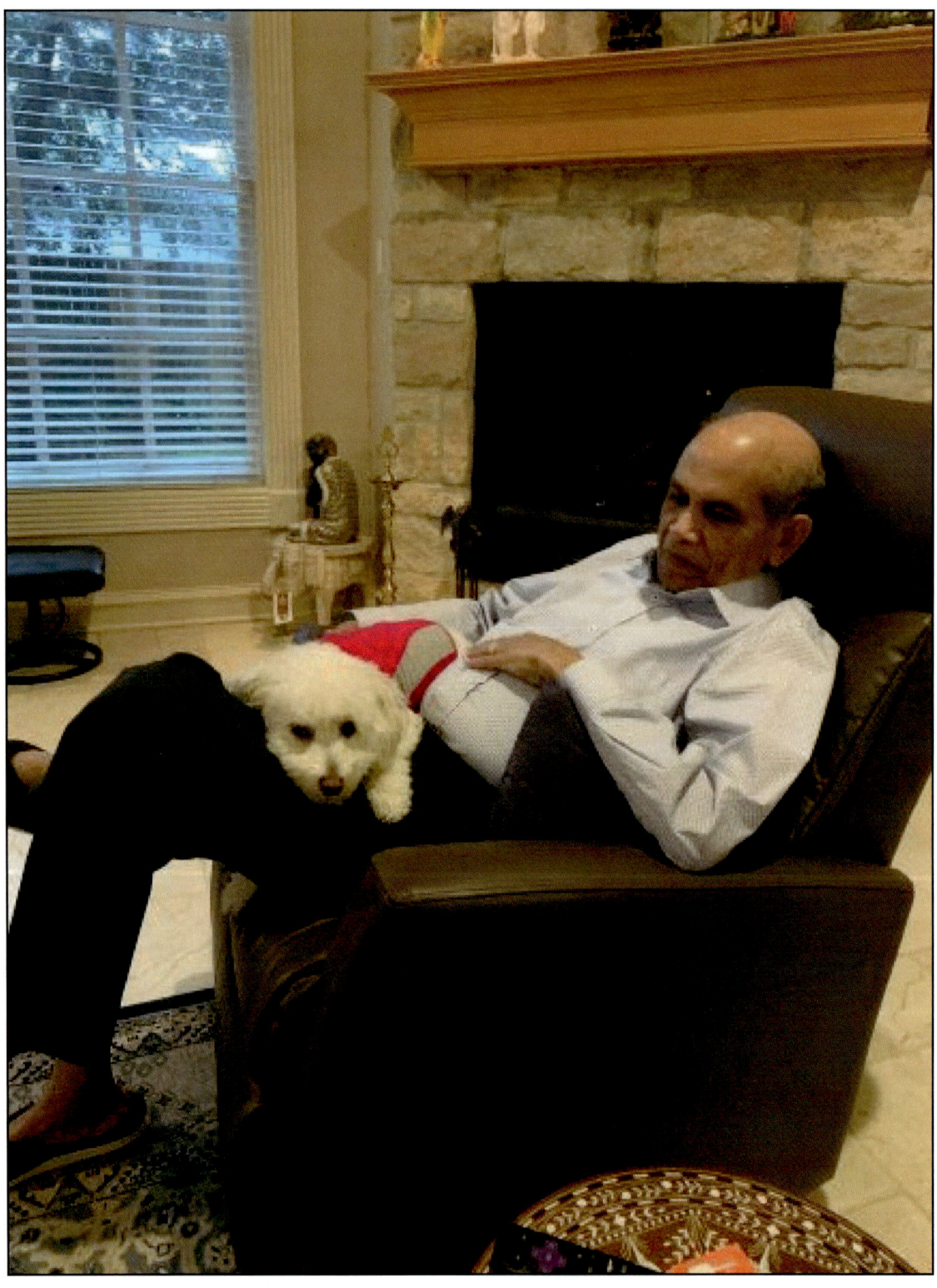

Figure 146. Mango with me.

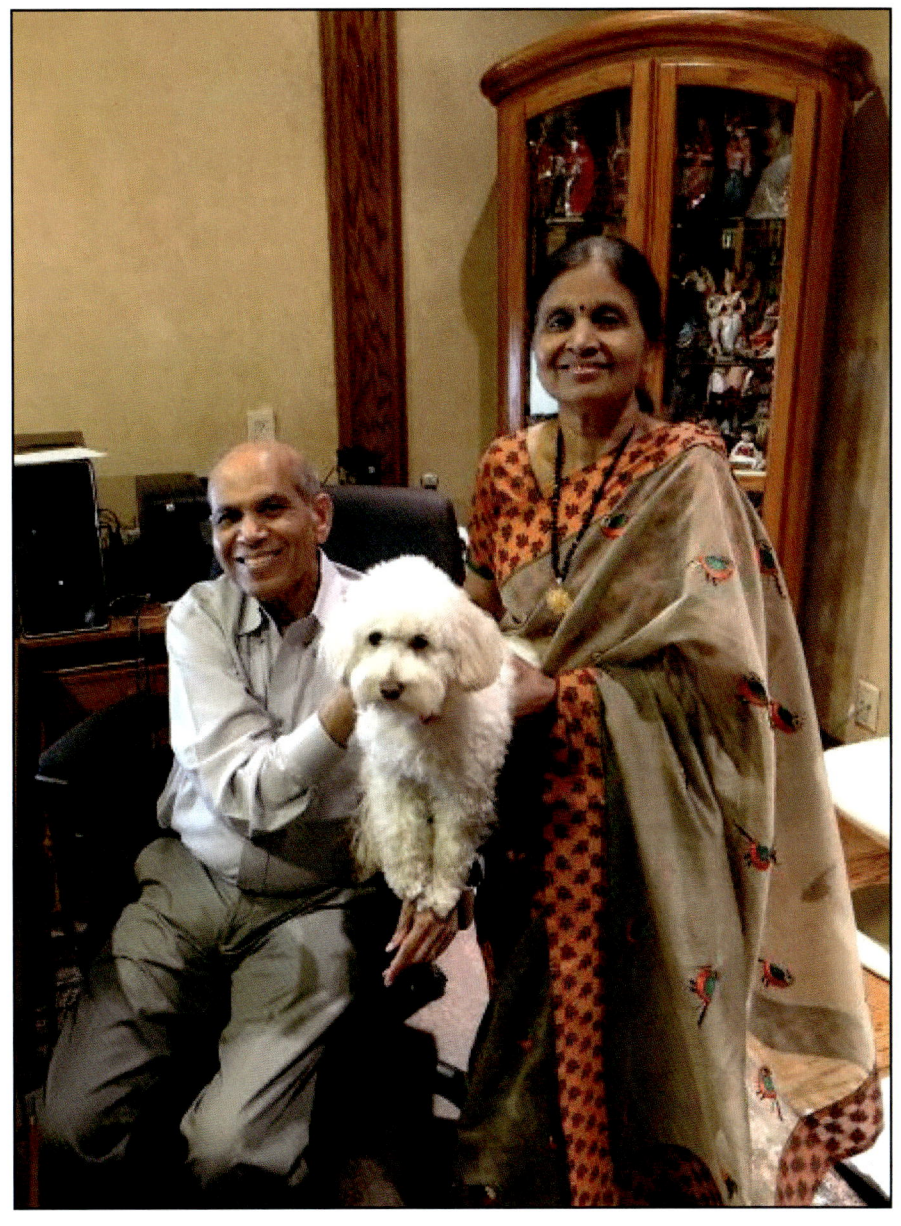

Figure 147. Mango with me and Hymavathi.

REFERENCES

1. Rao PS, Vidyasagar D. (editors), *Perinatal Cardiology: A Multidisciplinary Approach*, Minneapolis, MN, Cardiotext Publishing, 2015.

2. Rao PS, *The Journey of an Indian Pediatric Cardiologist, Dr. K. C. Chaudhuri Lifetime Achievement Award/Oration at AIIMS, New Delhi, September 2017* (Indian J Pediat 2017; 84:848-58).

CHAPTER 2

THE JOURNEY TO USA

INTRODUCTION

In this chapter, the reasons for why and how I became a pediatric cardiologist and how the journey to USA took place will be reviewed.

WHY AND HOW I BECAME A PEDIATRIC CARDIOLOGIST

While I was a student at the Andhra Medical College, Visakhapatnam (one of the ten medical schools in India at the time of the Indian independence), I was entertaining a career choice of either going into surgery or pediatrics. Suddenly, during house surgeoncy, I was involved in taking care of two cyanotic infants to whom only blow-by oxygen could be administered; unfortunately, both babies died. These infants turned out to have severe congenital heart defects, namely, transposition of the great arteries and tricuspid atresia, respectively. These incidents prompted the thought that I should go to USA, get training to turn into a pediatric cardiologist and return to India to serve the people in India. This contemplation may probably have dwindled away, but for the fact that one of my professors, Dr. Laxhmana Rao, who just then returned from USA after a sabbatical at Johns Hopkins University, Baltimore, Maryland, invited Dr. Helen B. Taussig (considered the mother of Pediatric Cardiology) to come to our medical school as a visiting professor. The faculty and staff of the Department of Pediatrics, Andhra Medical College/King George Hospital, Visakhapatnam, gathered a large number of patients with heart disease and presented to Dr. Taussig during a three-day period. Dr. Taussig reviewed the clinical, chest X-ray, electrocardiogram (ECG) and the blood work findings of each these children in detail and discussed each case with a focus on diagnosis and management. I was privileged to be present at these deliberations, which further strengthened my desire to become a pediatric cardiologist.

Less than two years later, I departed to USA (see the next section), fulfilled pediatric training requirements to join pediatric cardiology fellowship program with the intent to go to Johns Hopkins University Hospital in Baltimore, Maryland. Unfortunately, however, this was not feasible since the funding for pediatric cardiology fellowship at Johns Hopkins at that time required immigrant or citizenship status (I was on J-1visa), a requirement imposed by the National Institute of Health, the agency that funded fellowship programs in those days. Fortunately, I was able to secure pediatric cardiology training at Stanford University, Palo Alto, California, Case-Western Reserve University, Cleveland, Ohio and University of California at Los Angeles, California.

My unsuccessful attempts to return to India after completion of pediatric cardiology training and career in pediatric cardiology will be reviewed in the subsequent chapters.

THE JOURNEY TO USA

Most physicians from my prior generations have opted to go to England, mostly related to the fact that India was ruled by British prior to independence. On the basis of exposure to, and to some degree, indoctrination from elders, teachers and history learned, from the beginning I was against going to Briton, and instead, toying with the idea of going to USA as an alternative to conventional postgraduate education in India itself. As these ideas were developing in my mind, suddenly, my attention was drawn to a poster exhibited at the entrance of the Andhra Medical College Library during the final year of the medical school. The poster was an advertisement from the Mercy Hospital in Des Moines, Iowa, USA. The poster was advertising that they are seeking to recruit interns and a photograph of the hospital along with their address was boldly displayed on the poster. I immediately sent a letter to the Mercy Hospital, seeking for a formal application form. The Medical Director of the hospital promptly responded; not only did he send an application form, but also included a booklet and application form for applying for certification by the Educational Council for Foreign Medical Graduates (ECFMG) and stated that the certification by the ECFMG is a prerequisite for acceptance as an intern at their, and at any other institution in the USA. I promptly filled the ECFMG application and took it to Dr. V. S. Raghunadhan, Principal of Andhra Medical College, for his signature to certify that I am indeed a student/graduate of the Andhra Medical College. He discouraged me to take this type of detour in my career and encouraged me to do MD or MS in India. I persisted and persuaded and Dr. Raghunadhan finally signed the application form. The duly filled application form, along with the required attachments, was sent by airmail to the ECFMG office in Evanston, Illinois. The ECFMG scheduled me for the ECFMG examination in March 1965 in Madras (now Chennai). I was happy with these developments.

Suddenly, news broke out that the Government of India issued a GO (Government Order) that physicians should serve for at least seven years in Primary Health Care Centers (PHCs) prior to being granted permission to go abroad. Given this development, I felt that there is no point in going to Madras to take ECFMG examination since one can't leave the county even after passing ECFMG and dropped this idea altogether. Shortly before March 1965 ECFMG examination, when I was a house surgeon rotating in the Department of Pediatrics, one of the postgraduate students in Pediatrics, Dr. Subba Rao, enticed me to go ahead and take the ECFMG examination and mentioned the benefit of going to Tirupathi to perform Dharsan of Lord Venkateswara on the way back from the ECFMG examination. It should be mentioned that it was a ritual for almost every medical graduate to visit Tirupathi for Dharsan of Lord Venkateswara in those days and neither I nor Dr. Subba Rao had done this following our graduation from medical school. Based on these considerations, I decided to travel to Madras to take the ECFMG examination and Dharsan of Lord Venkateswara. As Dr. Subba Rao and I entered the train compartment, to our surprise, we found a bunch of doctors who were travelling to Madras to take the ECFMG examination. They were all carrying multiple choice question booklets helping to prepare for the ECFMG examination. Dr. Subba Rao and I had not prepared for the examination because it was a sudden decision to take the ECFMG examination, but took the opportunity to review the questions with the others in the train compartment. This was the only ECFMG examination preparation for me and Dr. Subba Rao. The trip to Madras was uneventful and we took the examination and then travelled to Tirupathi for a successful Dharsan of Lord Venkateswara. A few weeks later, the results came out, and both Dr. Subba Rao and I (Figure 1) passed the ECFMG examination. While I was able to utilize the ECFMG certification, to the best of my knowledge, Dr. Subba Rao did not go to USA, but, I was given to the understanding that he had a successful pediatric practice in his native town.

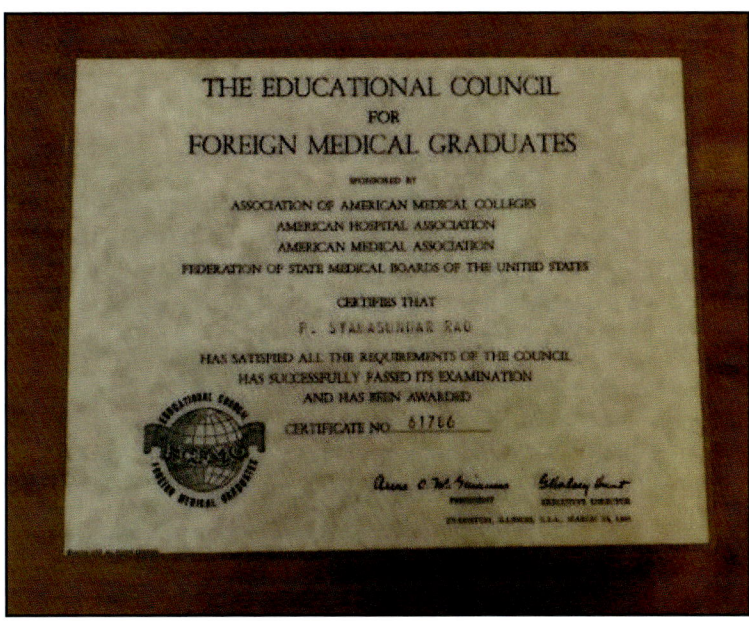

Figure 1. My ECFMG Certificate.

The GO that was mentioned above is still in force, but it became known that a physician in the state of Kerala filed a court case challenging that the GO is unconstitutional. Therefore, there was some hope that the courts might overrule the GO. Having this faith, I thought that some service to the country by serving in PHC may be in order and accordingly applied for a position as a medical officer to the Director of Medical Services (DMS) of Andhra Pradesh following completion of house surgeoncy. I was posted to a PHC at a village by the name of Kothapalli, a remote village in the district of Srikakulam in Andhra Pradesh. Since the intent was to perform service while waiting to go to USA, I did not protest and went to Kothapalli.

The village of Kothapalli is approximately four to five miles away from either the nearest bus or railway stations and I had to walk this distance to reach the destination. Since that was a rainy season, the roads were filled with mud, making travel somewhat difficult. Despite this inconvenience, I opted to fulfill the duties of medical officer since the intent was to provide service "en-route" to USA.

The PHC was located in a small building at the outskirts of Kothapalli and I was able to secure accommodation in the village. Since my predecessor did not regularly go to the PHC, as I was told, my daily attendance at the PHC resulted in a large number of patients coming to PHC to seek medical attention. With this volume of patients, the medical supplies rapidly dwindled. In those days, there was really no value to prescriptions written by the doctor;

it is the medicines that are given by doctor that are of any value. To replenish the medical supplies, I travelled to a medical store in Tekkali, a nearby town, with the PHC's compounder (pharmacist) and purchased medicines to the tune of 150 rupees. This is the maximum amount authorized to procure medicines by a medical officer by the government. Given the high volume of patients visiting the PHC, these medicines exhausted in a few days. I then sent the compounder to the same medical store in Tekkali to procure more medicines. The proprietor of the medical store denied supplying additional medicines since the initial 150 rupees had not been paid by the office of Block Development Officer (BDO); the proprietor indicated to the compounder that some money has to be paid to the staff in the BDO's office to complete the necessary paperwork to get paid. The proprietor of the medical store in Tekkali was unwilling to go through these hoops, especially since his medical store is striving well with local people buying the medicines from his store. Then, I travelled to the BDO's office and discussed with the BDO to help expedite paying the medical store owner so that medicines will be available to serve the patients coming to PHC. The BDO told me not to interfere with administrative matters and that things will happen in due course.

As this was going on, I was posted as a medical officer with additional charge for the Government Dispensary in a nearby village by the name of Pathapatnam, since that physician was leaving to Visakhapatnam for postgraduate studies. I took charge of the new posting and decided to go to the Pathapatnam medical dispensary one day a week.

Suddenly, I received a letter from the Andhra Medical College that I was accepted for postgraduate studies in Diploma in Child Health (DCH). Largely related to lack of medicines at the PHC, I accepted to join in the DCH course in Andhra Medical College. Then I travelled to Srikakulam to meet the District Medical Officer (DMO) and with great difficulty convinced the DMO to relieve me from the medical officer duties from Kothapalli and Pathapatnam.

I returned to Visakhapatnam after forty days of service at Kothapalli and Pathapatnam and joined the DCH course. Since I was hoping for a favorable outcome of the writ petition filed by the Kerala physician, a formal application for internship at Mercy Hospital in Des Moines, Iowa, along with all the required documents was sent and in a few weeks, a letter came from the Mercy Hospital giving me an appointment as an intern at the Mercy Hospital. I wrote a letter to Mercy Hospital's medical director seeking for postponement of joining their program by six months along with the reason for such a request, which was the GO from the Indian government. This request for extension to join the internship was accepted by the Mercy Hospital. By the end of December 1965, the Kerala physician's writ petition was still not concluded and rumors were circulated that the case is on the way to Supreme Court of India in New Delhi. I again wrote to the Mercy Hospital requesting extension for three more months; this request was again granted by the Mercy Hospital. In February 1966, the Supreme Court of India decreed that the GO is unconstitutional; the government can restrict its citizens to go abroad, but can't specifically deny a class of people (for example, physicians, lawyers or accounts). The GO was thus invalidated by the Supreme Court of India. The passports held by the office of DMS, including that of mine were released. By that time, my marriage date was fixed in March 1966 and the DCH examinations were scheduled for April 1966. I promptly wrote to the Mercy Hospital administration, seeking for another extension and clearly indicated that the GO was struck down by the Supreme Court of India and that I was free to go to USA to join their program. I stated reason for this extension was marriage and DCH exam dates. The Mercy Hospital responded by saying that they wanted me to join the internship in July 1966 and that no further extensions will be granted.

THE SAGA OF PASSPORTS

A few words about securing passports are in order at this juncture. I applied for a passport while still in Kothapalli. All the paper work for the passport was smooth and orderly through the Collector's office in Srikakulam, presumably because I was a medical officer. Indeed, it was very strange that the constable assigned to verify my credentials came to my office in PHC and saluted, saying with a smile that he is the one that will be reporting on my credentials. I thanked him and eventually the passport was issued, but was confiscated by the government pursuing to GO discussed above and was kept in the office of DMS in Hyderabad and, as mentioned above, the passport was released after the Supreme Court declared the GO is null and void. My wife's passport was different matter. Immediately following the marriage, I filled the appropriate passport application for my wife, had her sign it, and submitted it to the Collector's office in Visakhapatnam. Assuming that it will be processed in a manner similar to that of my passport application, a few weeks later I contacted the passport office in Madras and was told that the passport application from Visakhapatnam has not arrived. I took this issue to my dad who was Divisional Engineer in Visakhapatnam and he contacted the District Collector who advised that I should meet with the Collector in his office. The Collector called the clerical staff in-charge of processing the passport applications, ordered him to bring the application and asked why it was not forwarded to the passport office in Madras. The staff had no explanation and the Collector ordered the staff to immediately process the application. I later learned that the clerical staff expected a mammul (a form of payment for services to be performed). A few weeks later, the passport office in Madras notified me that the passport is ready.

Since the marriage and DCH examinations were completed and my wife's passport was ready, travel to Madras to pick up the passport and secure visas to go to USA was undertaken. On the way to Madras, a short visit to Bangalore and Mysore for a short honeymoon was planned. The trip to Bangalore and Mysore (Figure 2) was enjoyable, especially in view of visit with a friend who has the same name as mine (Dr. Pullela Syamasundar Rao - Figure 3) and who also got recently married. The parents of my friend's wife were very hospitable and treated us as their own. Securing my wife's passport was uneventful, but getting the visas to go to USA was somewhat laborious and involved getting medical examination, chest x-ray and laboratory tests. Luckily, both my wife and I were successful in passing these hurdles and returned to Visakhapatnam, ready to pack for the USA trip.

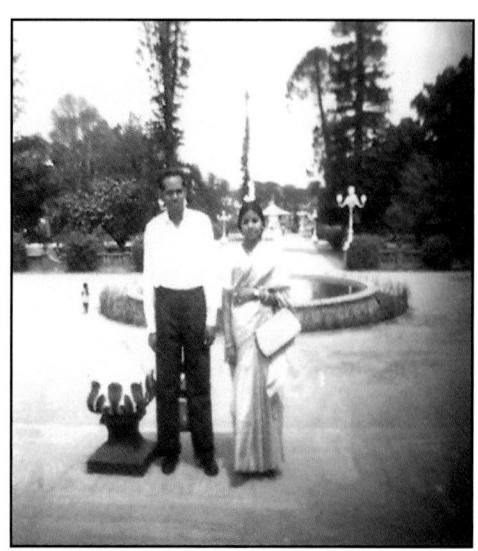

Figure 2. My wife and I in Brindavan Gardens in Mysore.

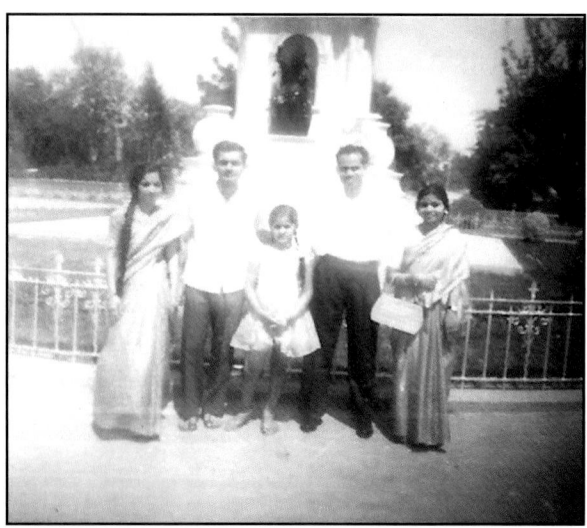

Figure 3. Photograph of me with my wife and the other Syamasundar Rao and
his new bride (and her sister) in Brindavan Gardens in Mysore.

It is worthwhile mentioning the generosity of the Mercy Hospital at this juncture. When the internship position was initially offered by the Mercy Hospital, I requested for assistance for airline ticket to USA since I did not want to burden my dad with the expense associated with the travel. The Mercy Hospital agreed to send a pre-paid ticket, but stated that they would deduct the amount from my paycheck. When my wife was also coming to USA, a similar request for her ticket was also made; again, the Mercy Hospital agreed with the provision that her ticket amount will also be deducted from my bi-weekly salary.

With the passports in hand and pre-paid tickets from the Mercy Hospital just arrived, we began packing for the trip. Since my dad returned from England a few years earlier, his experience in what to take, etc., the packing became easy. We packed all that we thought that we would need in four small suitcases.

Since this was the first trip of this sort in our region, save my dad's trip to England a few years earlier, a lot of relatives and friends, numbering in nearly hundred people came to the airport to give the new couple a sendoff. It was a mixed feeling for me and my wife, excited to see and experience the new country and sad to leave parents, brothers, sisters, other relatives and friends.

This was a long journey requiring seven different flights. We both first got up in a very small, old plane called Dakota for the first flight from Visakhapatnam to Hyderabad. At Hyderabad, we enplaned on a more modern plane by the name of Viscount, which took us to Bombay. In Bombay, we boarded a jet, Boeing; this flight took us to Cairo, Egypt, where we were required to deplane for a short while. Then we re-boarded the same flight to London. After a few hours of stay in the London airport, we flew to New York City. From New York to Chicago and from there to Des Moines. It was fortunate that all the flights were on time and we did not miss any connection. As we landed in Des Moines on July 4 (not knowing that it is the US Independence Day), we were received by a person familiar to me. This gentleman was several years senior to me who had completed MS in Ophthalmology, but because of his frequent stopovers at Osler's Lodge to visit his friend where I was also residing during some of the medical school years. His name is Dr. Rajeswara Rao; since the last parts our names are same, the secretary to the Medical Director at the Mercy Hospital actually thought that we are related to each other and enticed Dr. Rajeswara Rao to receive us at the Des Moines airport. To find a familiar face in an unfamiliar land was a great relief.

Since Dr. Rajeswara Rao did not drive at that time, he sought the help of a friend of his, Mr. Raman Nayer, who had a car and drove. They took both of us to the already allotted (by the hospital) apartment. Fortunately, the apartment was fully furnished and equipped with central air and heat and was located just behind the hospital. We had a long nice sleep after more than two days of international travel, apart from the twelve hours of time difference.

Next morning, I went to the hospital and met with the Medical Director (Dr. Howard G. Ellis) and his secretary. Since we only had ten US dollars in our possession,* the hospital administration was generous in loaning me US $100 with the provision that this amount along with travel expenses already paid will be deducted from the bi-weekly paychecks. Later that day, Mr. Nayer and Dr. Rajeswara Rao took us to a departmental store by the name of Arden where we could buy all household stuff including groceries. That weekend they took us to the city of Ames, Iowa, and introduced us to two Telugu families (Dr. and Mrs. Avula and Dr. and Mrs. Sriharsha) who were at the University of Iowa in Ames. These generous efforts by Mr. Nayer and Dr. Rajeswara Rao made our young family settle in the new land for which we are ever grateful to them. Subsequent journey will be described in sections on postgraduate education and academic career of the Chapter 3 titled, "The Journey Continues."

*The Government of India in those days only granted foreign exchange to the tune of five US dollars per each traveler going abroad. Since I felt that this was insufficient money to get by prior to the first paycheck, I sought Reserve Bank of India's approval for an additional US $100. I was informed that this exchange can be undertaken at the Bombay airport prior to departure abroad. Accordingly, I carried the required amount in rupees, but could not exchange for dollars because the bank at the airport was closed for such a transaction, although the five US dollars per each traveler was provided. This is the reason for having only ten US dollars on arrival in Des Moines.

CHAPTER 3

THE JOURNEY CONTINUES

INTRODUCTION

In this chapter, my postgraduate education and academic career along with my extracurricular activities will be reviewed. My attempts to return to India as well as my contributions to education of physicians in India will also be reviewed.

POSTGRADUATE EDUCATION

My postgraduate education began soon after graduation from medical school in 1964 and indeed, this training as a house surgeon is a requirement for graduation from medical school in India. The clinical training while a house surgeon and during Diploma in Child Health (DCH) were reviewed in the Chapter 1 on "The Journey Begins." As mentioned in the Chapter 2 on "The Journey to USA," I (along with my wife) arrived in Des Moines, Iowa, in July 1966 to begin the internship. Although, similar training (house surgeon at the King George Hospital in Visakhapatnam) was received in the past, this internship was considered as an entry point to US medical system and as such, accomplished that purpose. I was introduced to the US system of medical practice and rotated through multiple specialties including pediatrics with eventual successful completion of the internship (Figure 1). Rotation in pediatric service with two pediatricians, Dr. M.E. Alberts and Dr. J.J. Polish has exposed me to US pediatrics. In addition, the opportunity to attend pediatric grand rounds every Friday noon at the Raymond Blank Children's Hospital was provided, broadening my knowledge in pediatrics.

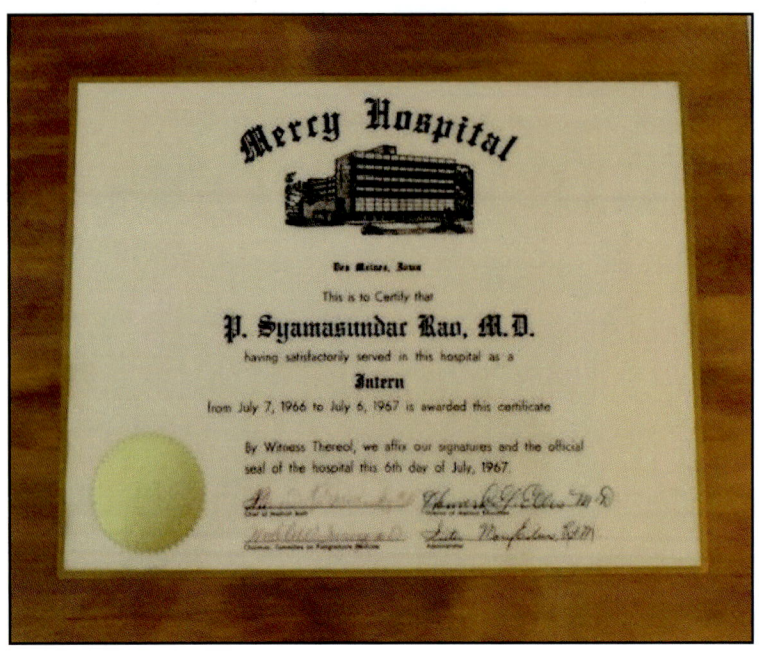

Figure 1. Certificate of completion of internship at the Mercy Hospital, Des Moines, Iowa.

While undergoing the internship, I applied to multiple pediatric training programs in Iowa City, Iowa; Flint, Michigan; Chicago, Illinois; Cincinnati, Ohio; Phoenix, Arizona; among others. When interviewed in Phoenix in January 1967, the weather in Phoenix was a lot warmer than that in Des Moines. Since I was not used to the cold weather of Des Moines, Phoenix weather was a welcoming attraction. Furthermore, the Good Samaritan Hospital in Phoenix, AZ, was unique in those days because its medical staff included multiple pediatric subspecialists, which is unusual in those days at institutions outside University Hospital setting. It should be noted that there were no medical schools in Arizona at that time and the Good Samaritan Hospital served as a referral hospital for pediatric subspecialty issues for the entire state. Furthermore, the Good Samaritan Hospital had an active approved pediatric cardiology fellowship program, another attraction for me. This turned out to be an excellent opportunity in advancing my goals to become a pediatric cardiologist. Apart from general pediatric and pediatric subspecialty exposure, I was given the opportunity to rotate through pediatric cardiology service for a period of six months under the direction of Dr. Marian Molthan, a pediatric cardiologist trained at the Children's Memorial Hospital/North-Western University in Chicago, IL. There was also encouragement for academic activities with resultant publication of multiple papers.[1-8] Another important factor that was recognized later was that formal letters of recommendation by Dr. Herman W. Lipow, Director of the Pediatric Residency Program and Dr. Belton Meyer, Director of Neonatology who were both trained at Stanford University in Palo Alto, California, were very helpful in securing a fellowship in pediatric cardiology for me at Stanford University. The resident staff of the Good Samaritan Hospital consisted of both American-trained and foreign-trained physicians (Figure 2) and as such helped me to get adjusted to the local circumstances. Following completion of this training (Figure 3), I was certified by the American Board of Pediatrics (Figure 4).

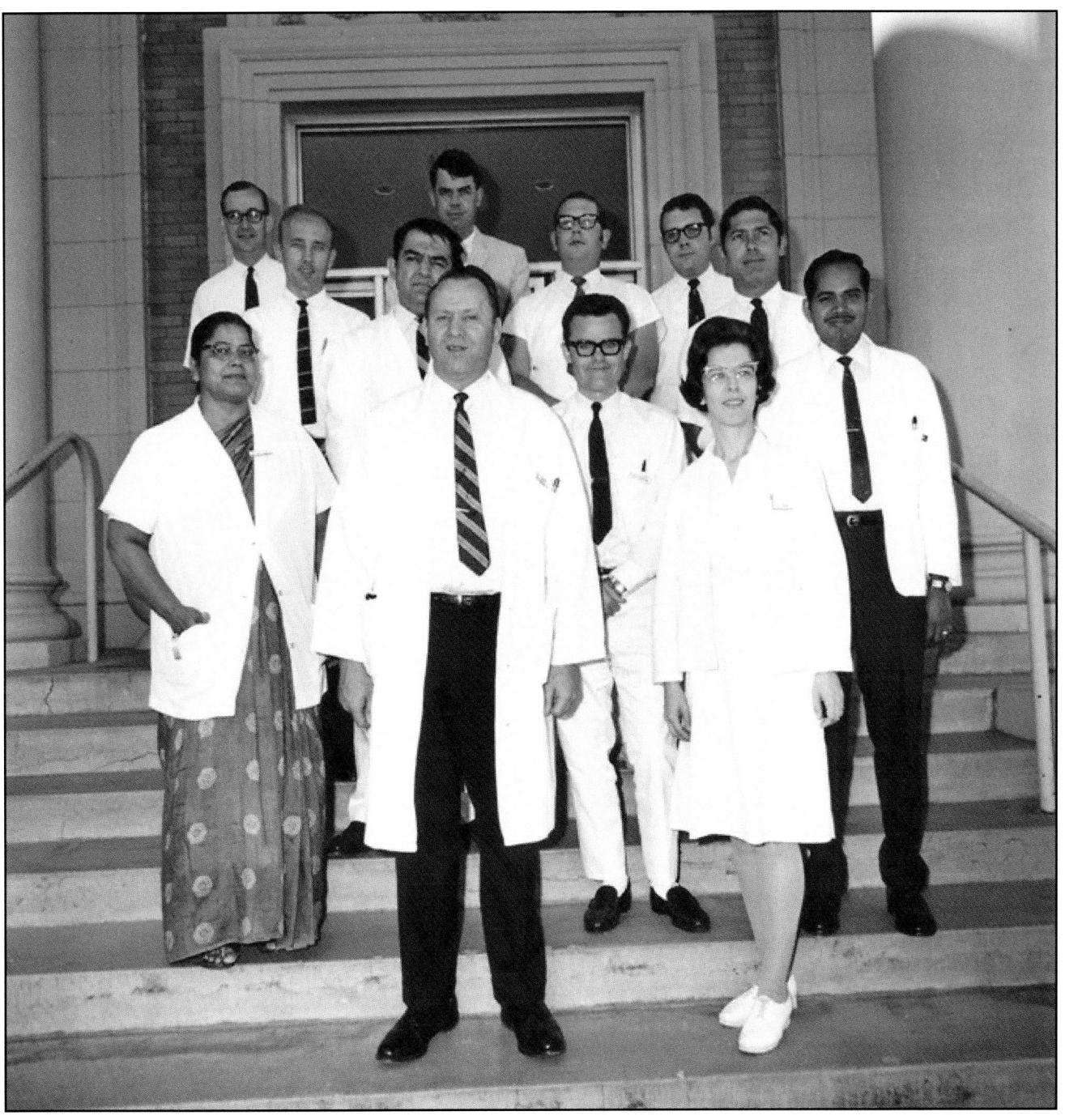

Figure 2. Photograph of myself with Dr. Herman Lipow, Pediatric Program Director (in the center), teaching staff and the other pediatric residents at the Good Samaritan Hospital in Phoenix, AZ, 1969.

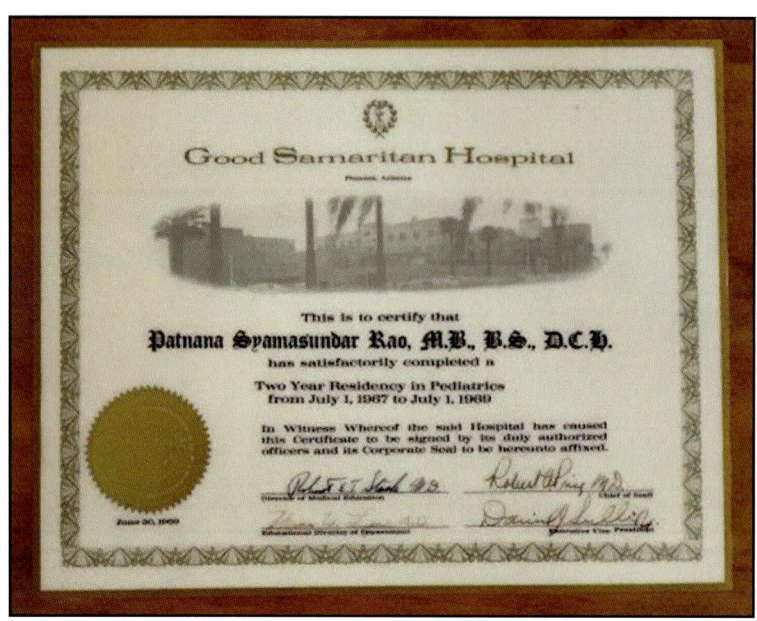

Figure 3. Certificate of Completion of Pediatric Residency at the Good Samaritan Hospital, Phoenix, AZ.

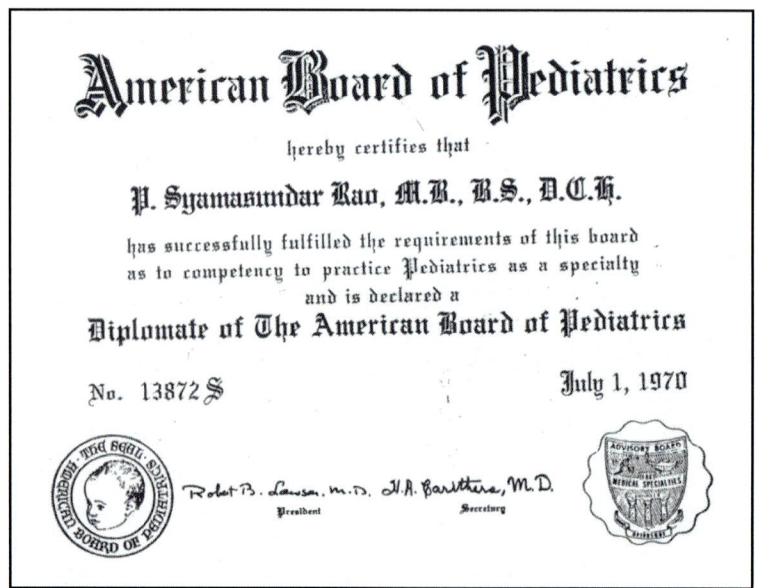

Figure 4. Certification by the American Board of Pediatrics.

As alluded to in the Chapter 2 on "The Journey to USA," my intent was to get pediatric cardiology training at the Johns Hopkins Hospital and that it was not possible to do so because of fellowship funding issues. Following successful completion (Figure 3) of pediatric training at the Good Samaritan Hospital, I joined the pediatric cardiology fellowship program at Stanford University; thanks to Evelyn L. Nizer Foundation, which supported my fellowship. The pediatric cardiology knowledge gained at the Good Samaritan Hospital in Phoenix, AZ, under the tutelage of Dr. Marian Molthan was very helpful to me during the initial phases of my fellowship at Stanford. The pediatric cardiology mentors at Stanford, Dr. Norman J. Sissman and Dr. Emmanuel Mesel and at its affiliated Santa Clara Valley Medical Center, Dr. Philip Bernaren were great teachers and advanced my pediatric cardiology knowledge. In addition, there was opportunity for clinical research resulting in multiple publications[9-13] and presentations at international scientific socities.[14,15] The fellowship programs were of two years' duration in those days and my intent was to complete the fellowship program at Stanford. But unfortunately, both the mentors at Stanford were planning to leave Stanford the following year. Therefore, I sought to find a second-year spot elsewhere and was offered positions at University of Kansas in Kansas City, Kansas, and Babies and Children's Hospital of Cleveland/ University Hospitals of Cleveland/Case-Western Reserve University, Cleveland, Ohio. I selected the Cleveland program because of the reputation of the program director, Dr. Jerome Liebman as a great teacher. Following successful completion of the first-year fellowship at Stanford (Figure 5), I moved to Cleveland.

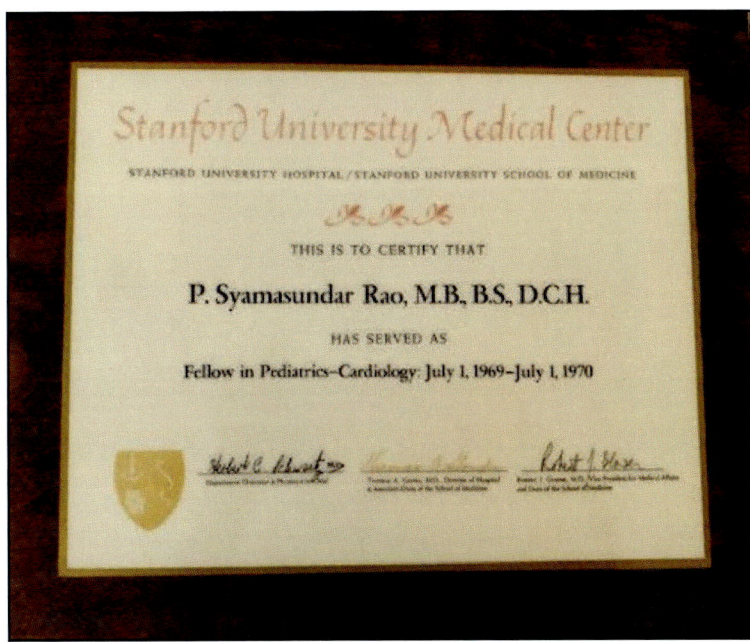

Figure 5. Certificate of completion of one year of Pediatric Cardiology Fellowship at Stanford University Medical Center.

Second-year fellowship under the tutelage of Dr. Jerome Liebman and Dr. Daniel Silbert was gratifying, confirmed the known reputation of Dr. Liebman as a great teacher, and provided further refinement of my pediatric cardiology skills acquired at the Good Samaritan Hospital and Stanford University. In addition, the opportunity to participate in clinical studies, resulting in several publications,[16-19] was provided to me. Furthermore, I was offered with a chance to train for a month in congenital heart disease pathology with Dr. Maurice Lev, Congenital Heart Disease Research and Training Center, Hektoen Institute for Medical Research, Chicago, Illinois. This training was undertaken during the month of February 1971 during which time literally hundreds of hearts were examined under the direction of Dr. Lev, an expert in congenital heart disease pathology and I accompanied Dr. Lev to multiple clinical-pathological conferences at several University Medical Centers in Chicago. These experiences were very useful for the reminder of my career in interpretation of pathologic, angiographic and echocardiographic anatomy of the heart. Following the successful completion of the second-year fellowship at the University Hospitals of Cleveland/

Case-Western Reserve (Figure 6) and certification by the Sub-board of Pediatric Cardiology (Figure 7), my intension was to return to India as will be detailed in the section on "Attempts to Return to India."

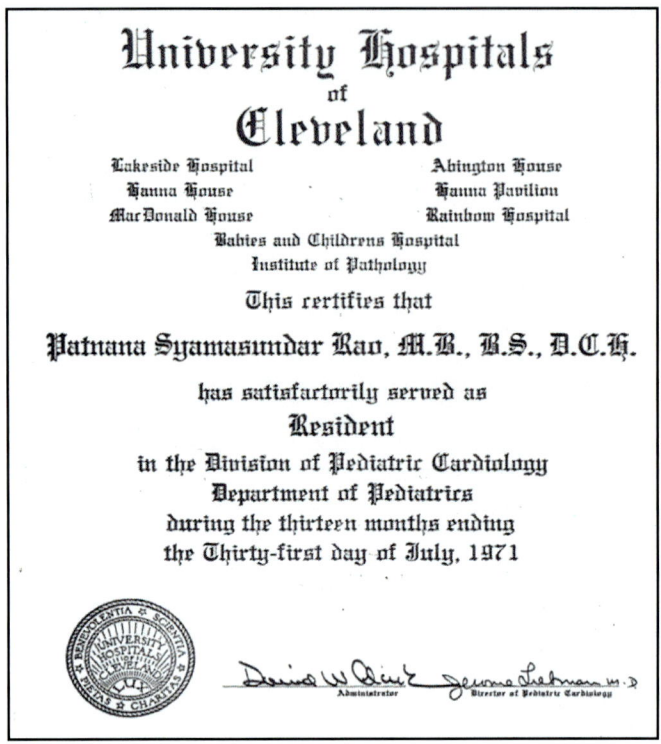

Figure 6. Certificate of completion of second year of the Pediatric Cardiology Fellowship (Residency) at the University Hospitals of Cleveland.

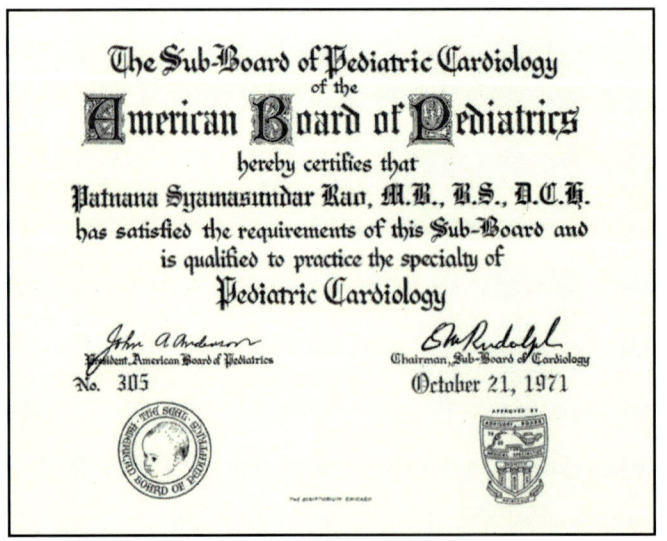

Figure 7. Certification by the Sub-Board of Pediatric Cardiology of the American Board of Pediatrics.

But, returning to India did not happen. Consequently, I sought for a third-year research fellowship at University of California at Los Angeles (UCLA) preparatory to an academic career in pediatric cardiology. This was a cardiovascular research fellowship under the direction of Dr. Leonard M. Linde (Figure 8).

UNIVERSITY OF CALIFORNIA
GRADUATE DIVISION · LOS ANGELES

CERTIFICATE OF POSTDOCTORAL STUDY

P. SYAMASUNDAR RAO, M. D.

HAS SATISFACTORILY ENGAGED IN POSTDOCTORAL STUDIES
IN THE FIELD(S) OF
PEDIATRIC CARDIOLOGY
ON THE LOS ANGELES CAMPUS OF THE UNIVERSITY
COVERING A PERIOD OF TWELVE MONTHS
BETWEEN THE DATES OF JULY 1, 1971 AND JUNE 30, 1972

JULY 1, 1971
DATED

CHANCELLOR

DEAN, GRADUATE DIVISION
pro tem

DEPARTMENT CHAIRMAN

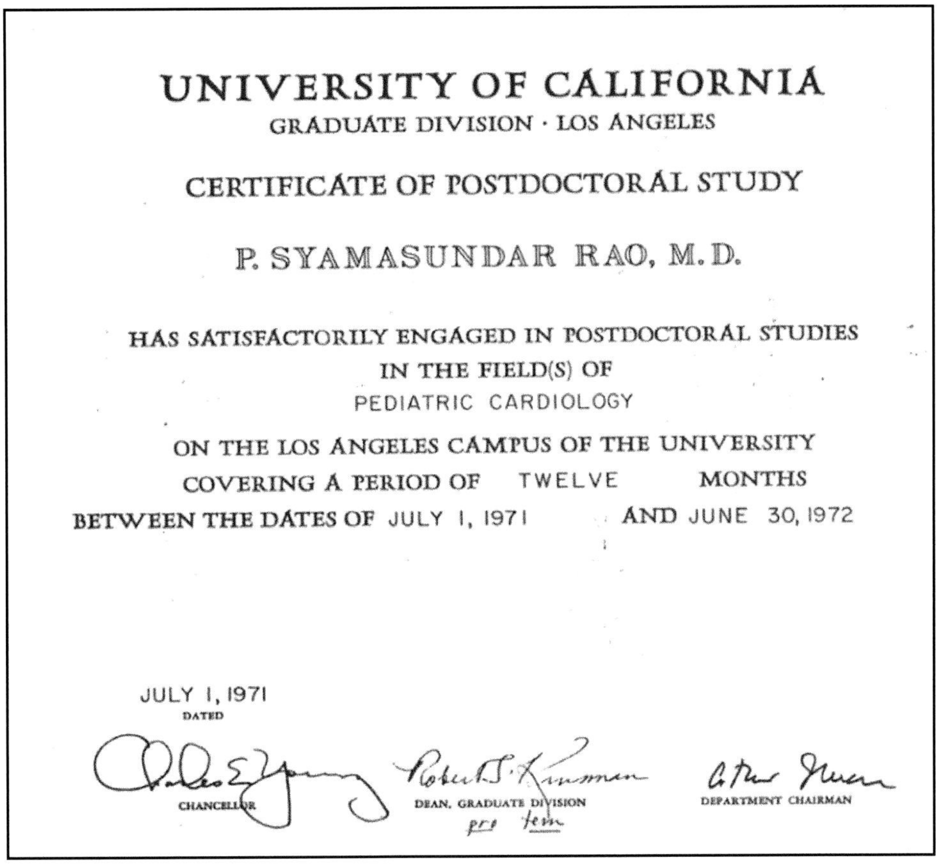

Figure 8. Certificate of Completion of post-doctoral study at the University of California at Los Angeles, CA.

Apart from participating in the experiments in the cardiovascular physiology laboratory, I also participated in clinical activities including cardiac catheterization laboratory and clinical research. A photograph with the faculty and other fellows is shown in figure 9, although my research mentor, Dr. Leonard M. Linde, was absent when this picture was taken. The activities at UCLA resulted in publication of a number of papers[20-25] and presentations at regional,[26,27] national[28] and international[29] scientific societies.

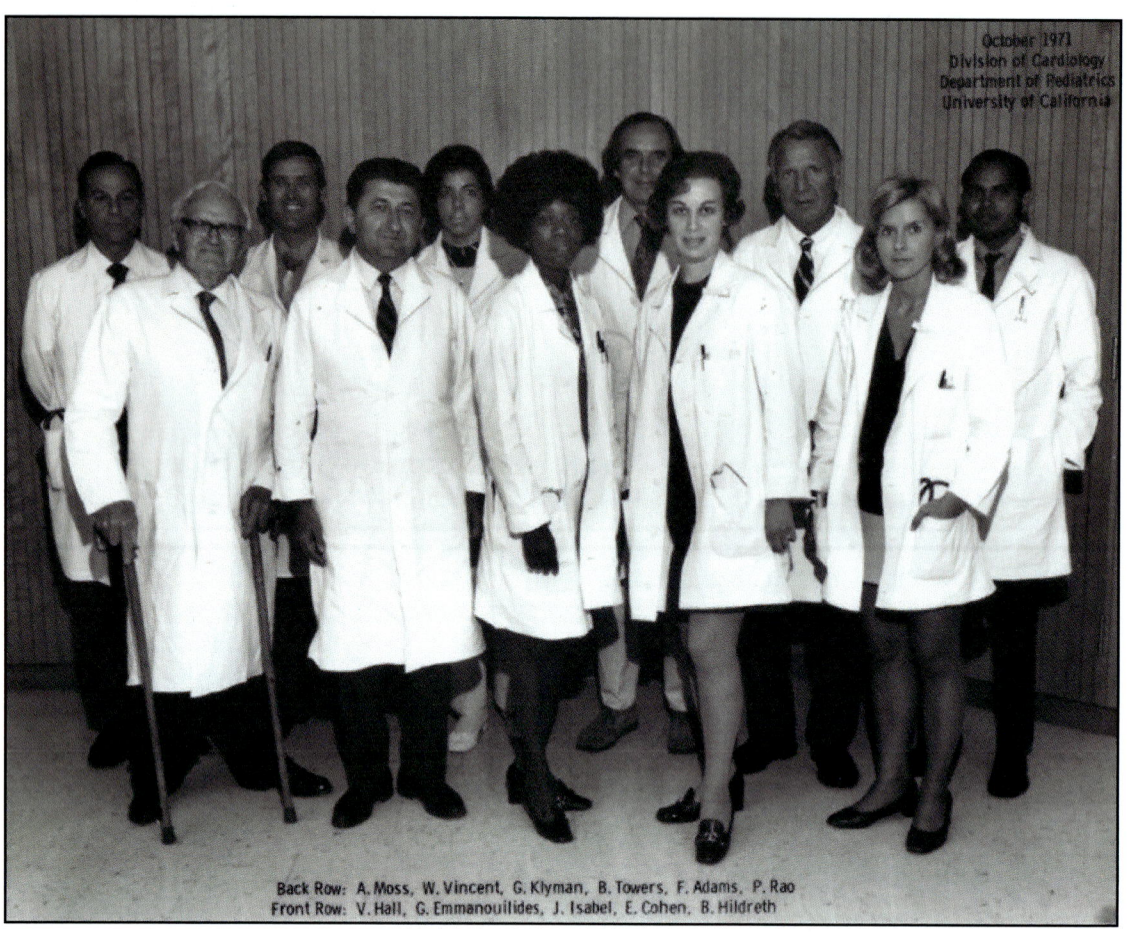

Back Row: A. Moss, W. Vincent, G. Klyman, B. Towers, F. Adams, P. Rao
Front Row: V. Hall, G. Emmanouilides, J. Isabel, E. Cohen, B. Hildreth

Figure 9. Photograph of myself with faculty and other Pediatric Cardiology fellows at UCLA, 1971-72.

ACADEMIC CAREER

As will be reviewed below in the section on "Attempts to Return to India," my attempts to go back to India immediately after training were unsuccessful and therefore, I took additional research training, as reviewed in the preceding section and subsequent to that I accepted a faculty position (Assistant Professor) in 1972 at the Medical College of Georgia, Augusta, Georgia (Figure 10). I was promoted to the rank of Associate Professor in 1975 (Figure 11) and to full Professor in 1979 (Figure 12). I also served as Assistant Professor of Physiology because of my interest in research related to cardiovascular physiology. During my tenure at the Medical College of Georgia, I not only participated in clinical care of the patients, but also initiated experimental studies in pulmonary vascular impedance[30] and organized and conducted multiple clinical studies, which will be reviewed in the companion book, "Pediatric Cardiology: How It Has Evolved Over the last 50 Years" and in the forthcoming chapters.

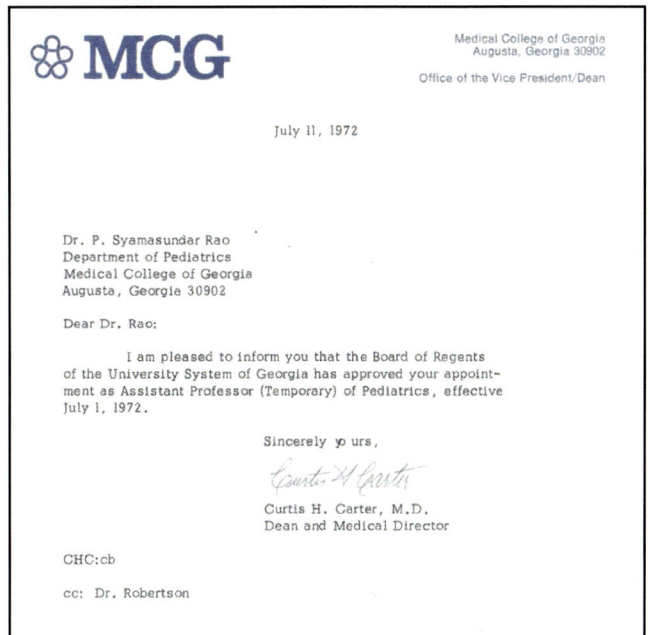

Figure 10. Letter of appointment as Assistant Professor of Pediatrics at the Medical College of Georgia.

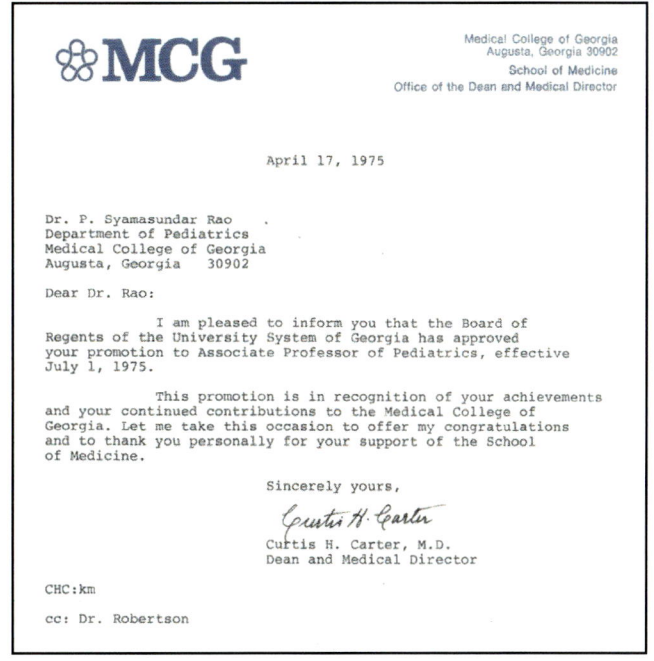

Figure 11. Letter from the Dean informing me of my promotion to Associate Professor of Pediatrics.

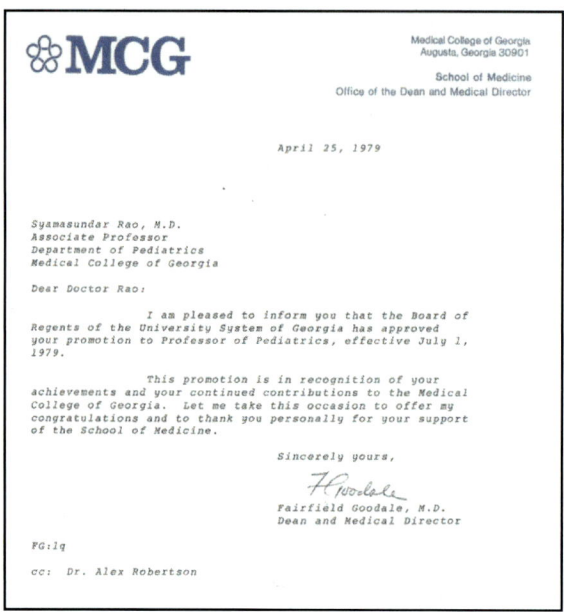

Figure 12. Letter from the Dean informing me of my promotion to Professor of Pediatrics.

I also served on multiple committees, the notable of which is: Chairman of Faculty Appointments, Promotions and Tenure Committee of School of Medicine of the Medical College of Georgia (Figure 13). In June 1976, I took a mini-sabbatical with Dr. William B. Rashkind at Children's Hospital of Philadelphia, PA, at the conclusion of which, I became one of the few in the world that could trans-catheter occlude atrial septal defects as will be detailed in the chapter on "Atrial Septal Defects" in the book titled, "Pediatric Cardiology: How It Has Evolved Over the last 50 Years."

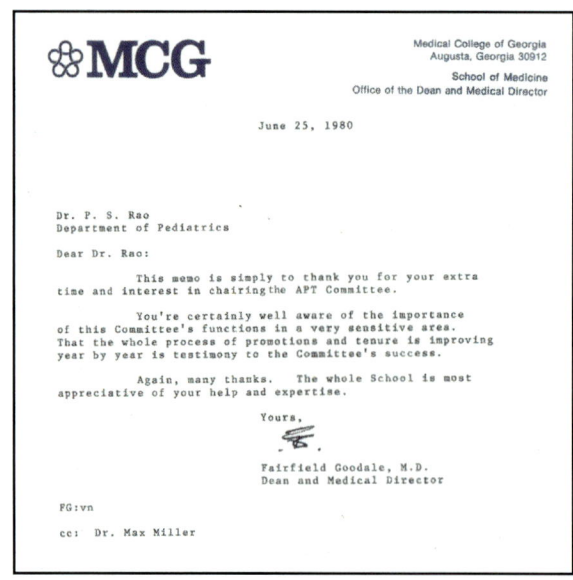

Figure 13. Letter from the Dean thanking me for chairing Appointments, Promotions and Tenure committee of the School of Medicine.

I was also appointed as Associate Director of Pediatric Cardiology and Director of Pediatric Cardiac Catheterization Laboratory (Figures 14 and 15) during my tenure at the Medical College of Georgia. Some photographs while at the Medical College of Georgia are shown in figures 16 and 17.

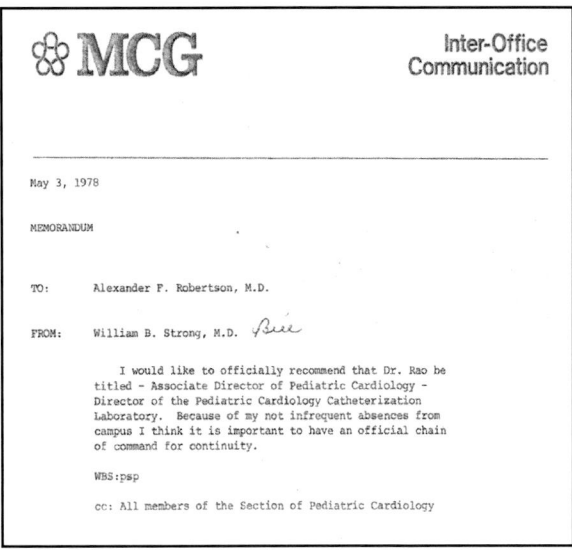

Figure 14. Letter from the Section Director recommending that I be appointed as the Associate Director of Pediatric Cardiology and Director of Pediatric Cardiac Catheterization Laboratory.

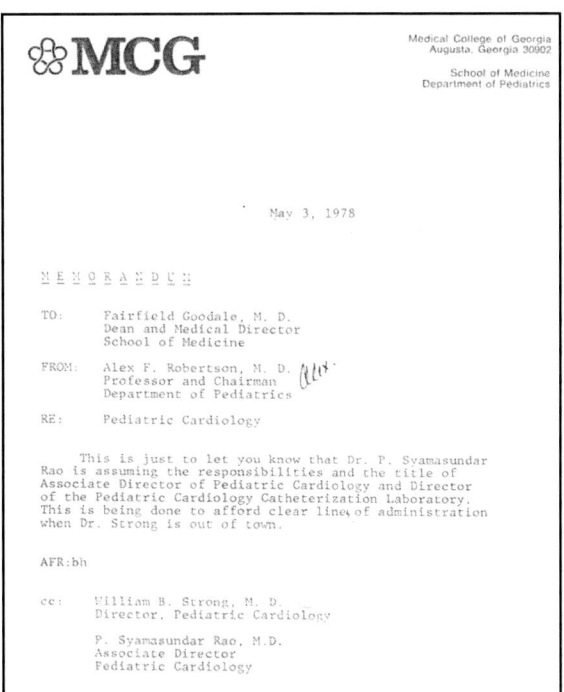

Figure 15. Letter from the Chairman of the Department of Pediatrics appointing me as the Associate Director of Pediatric Cardiology and Director of Pediatric Cardiac Catheterization Laboratory.

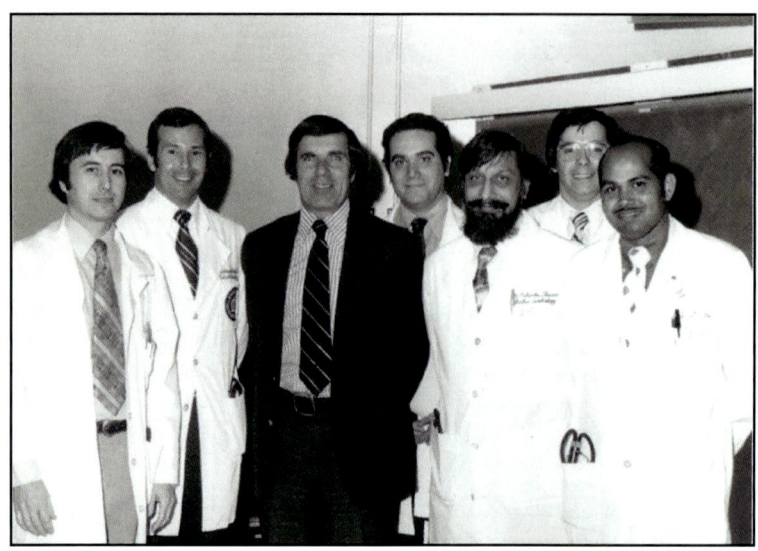

Figure 16. Photograph of myself with the faculty and other Pediatric Cardiology fellows at the Medical College of Georgia during a visiting professor's (Dr. Norman S. Talner) visit.

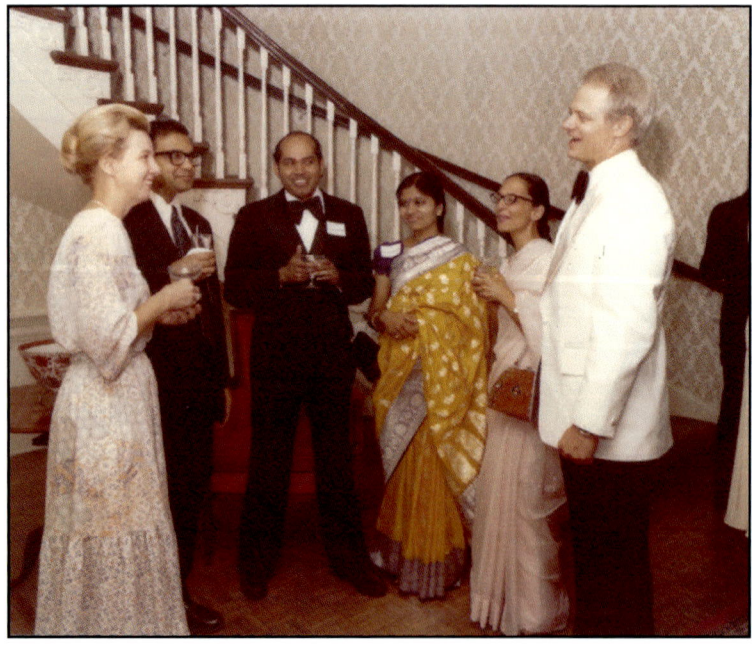

Figure 17. Photograph with wife (middle) during a reception at the Medical College of Georgia.

After unsuccessful attempts to go to India on a sabbatical, as will be reviewed in the section on "Attempts to Return to India," I moved to the King Faisal Specialist Hospital & Research Center, Riyadh, Saudi Arabia, in 1981 as a Consultant Pediatric Cardiologist. In addition to taking care of children with heart disease and establishing satellite clinics in Dammam, Dhahran and Al-Khobar, I undertook multiple administrative and committee responsibilities including: Associate Chief of Staff for Inpatient Affairs; Chairman, Ad Hoc Committee on Medical Education; Chairman, Pediatric Symposium Committee; Chairman, Pediatric Cardiology Symposium Committee; Research Advisory Committee; Medical Council; Research Council; Chairman, Quality Assurance Committee, Research Center Bylaws Committee; Medical Staff Bylaws Committee; among others. I was appointed as the Chairman of the Department of Pediatrics in 1986. Photograph of the medical staff of the Department of Pediatrics at the King Faisal Specialist Hospital & Research Center are shown in figure 18 with me in the center. Most importantly, I initiated catheter based interventional pediatric cardiology during my tenure at the King Faisal Specialist Hospital & Research Center, resulting in multiple publications which will be reviewed in the forthcoming chapters and in the book titled, "Pediatric Cardiology: How It Has Evolved Over the last 50 Years." Most important, however, was the advancement of trans-catheter therapy for heart defects in children.[31-33]

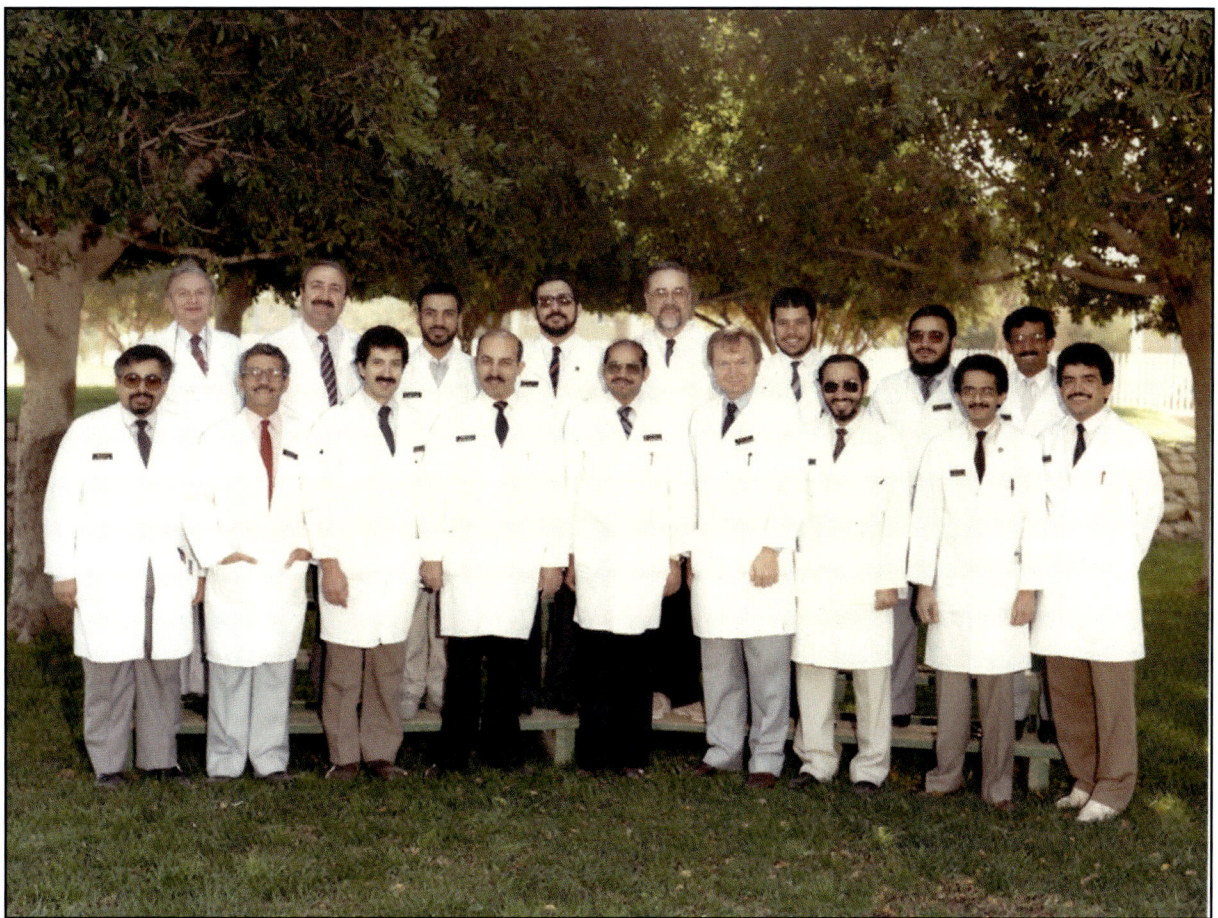

Figure 18. Photograph of the medical staff of the Department of Pediatrics at the King Faisal Specialist Hospital and Research Center with me in the center.

Following the tenure at the King Faisal Specialist Hospital & Research Center (Figures 19, 20 and 21), I moved to Madison, Wisconsin as a Professor of Pediatrics and Director of Pediatric Cardiology at the University of Wisconsin Medical School, Madison, WI.

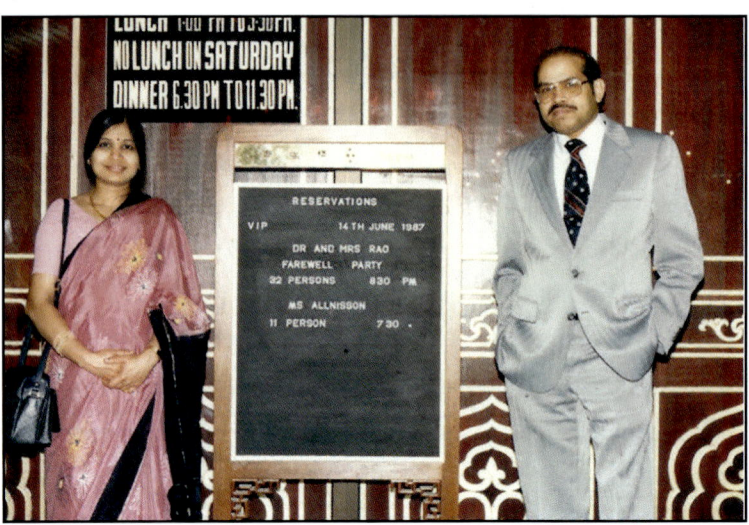

Figure 19. Photograph 1 during send-off from the King Faisal Specialist Hospital.

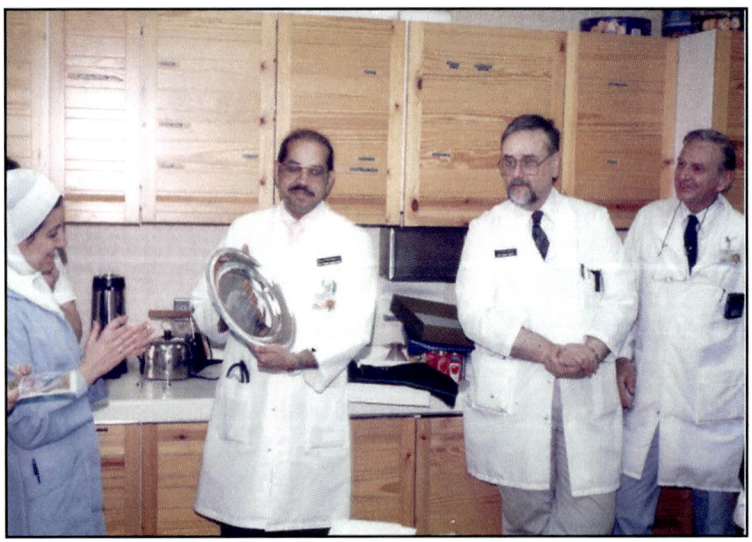

Figure 20. Photograph 2 during send-off from the King Faisal Specialist Hospital.

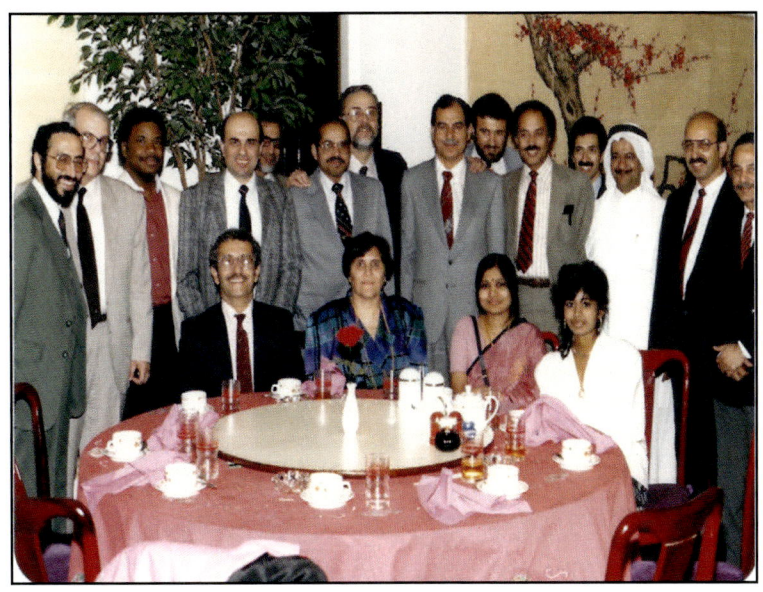

Figure 21. Photograph 3 during send-off from the King Faisal
Specialist Hospital.

At the University of Wisconsin, apart from directing and developing the Division of Pediatric Cardiology, I attempted to advance the application of balloon valvuloplasty/angioplasty techniques[34-41] to treat children with heart disease and initiated local, national and international clinical trials of buttoned device occlusion of atrial septal defects[42-46] and patent ductus arteriosus,[47-49] which will also be reviewed in the forthcoming chapters and in the book titled, "Pediatric Cardiology: How It Has Evolved Over the last 50 Years" and will not be repeated here. Our photograph with the Chairman of Pediatrics, Dr. Philip Ferrel and his wife is shown in figure 22.

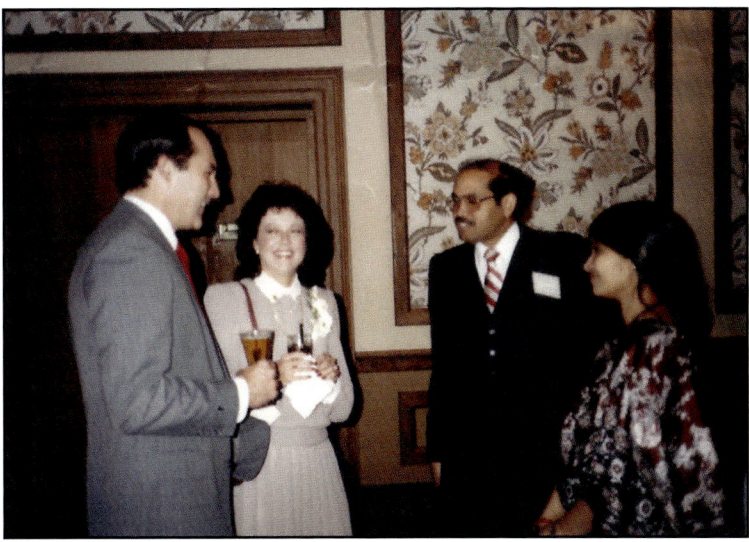

Figure 22. Our photograph with Chairman of Pediatrics at University of
Wisconsin and his wife.

Then, I moved to the St. Louis University School of Medicine/Cardinal Glennon Children's Hospital, St. Louis, Missouri, in 1994 as Professor of Pediatrics and Director of Pediatric Cardiology and continued the research on trans-catheter interventions in children and adults[50,51] and again, these will be reviewed in multiple chapters to follow and in the book titled, "Pediatric Cardiology: How It Has Evolved Over the last 50 Years." As noted in the "Disappointments" section of the next chapter, I relocated to the University of Texas McGovern Medical School/ Children's Memorial Hermann Hospital, Houston, Texas in 2002 as the Professor of Pediatrics and Director of Pediatric Cardiology. Here, apart from continuing the work on interventional pediatric cardiology, I spent considerable amount of time to establish new pediatric cardiac and pediatric cardiovascular surgery programs, ACGME-approved pediatric cardiology fellowship program, and Texas State Medical Board-approved interventional pediatric cardiology fellowship program.

During more than fifty years of pediatric cardiology practice, in addition to taking care of patients with heart disease, I showed substantial interest in the development of new knowledge and training and teaching physicians around the world. These endeavors resulted in travel to a number of countries including India, Argentina, Australia, Egypt, Finland, France, Jordan, Nicaragua, Sweden, Germany, New Zealand, Brazil, and Japan and several cities in USA, to deliver scientific presentations and/or to demonstrate catheter interventional techniques. Some of the pictures of these presentations are shown in figures 23 through 29.

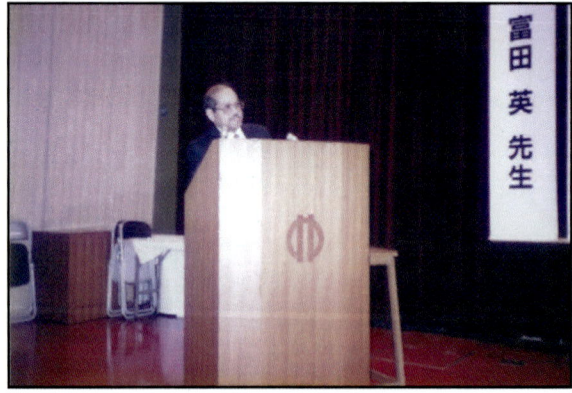
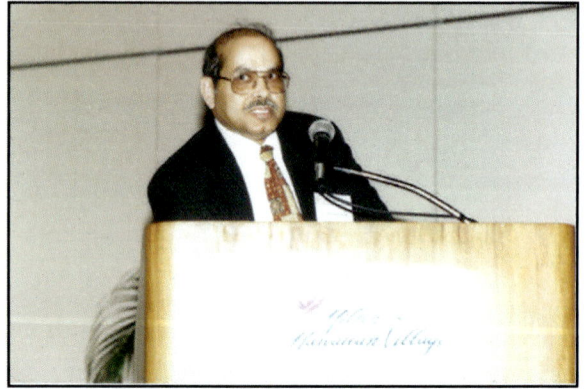
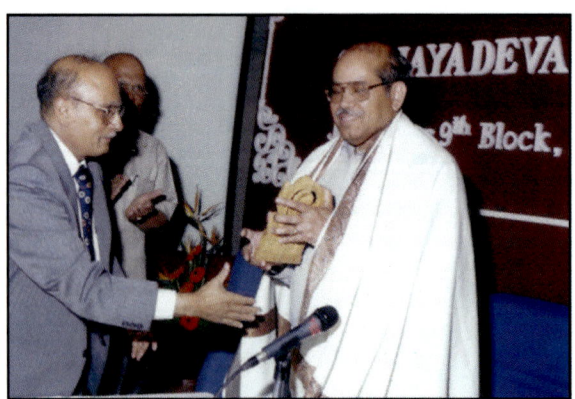
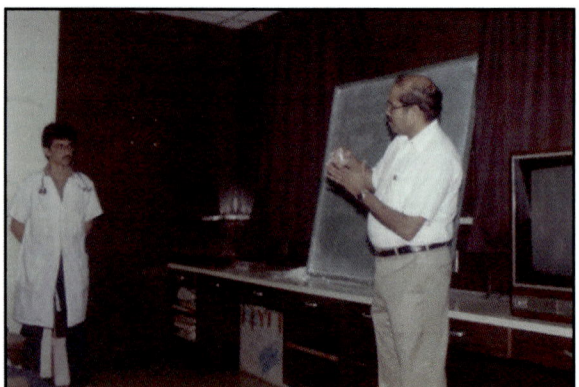

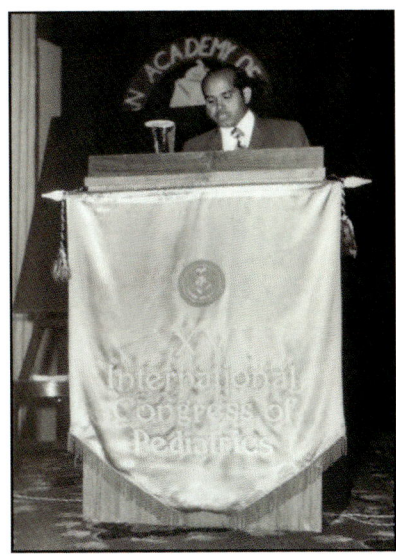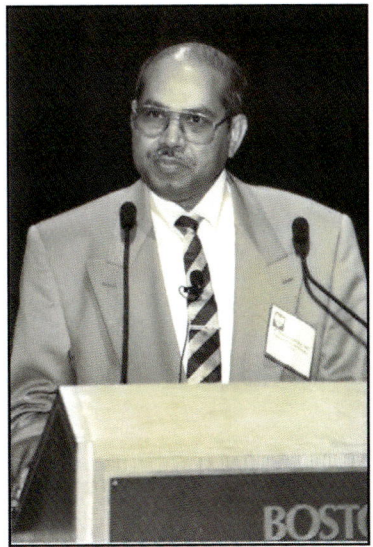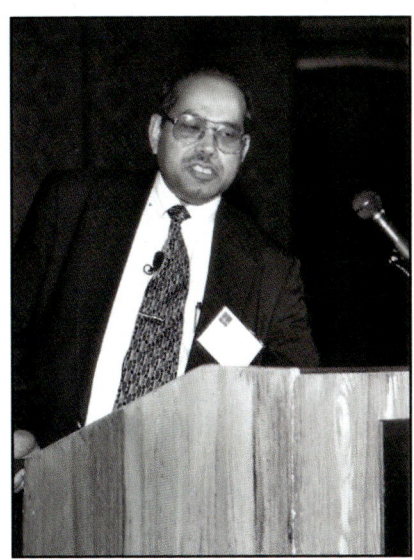

Figures 23 through 29. Photographs of lecture presentations/receipt of facilitations at multiple locations.

The interest in clinical research resulted in publication of 390 papers in journals (as first or senior author), 230 abstract presentations, 14 monographs and books and 150 book chapters as well as 160 invited presentations and lectureships.

EXTRACURRICULAR ACTIVITIES

My participation in extracurricular activities will be reviewed in this section; the material will be separately presented for each stage of my career.

High School and College

My involvement in soccer in the early years of high school was mentioned in the first chapter. As I arrived in Parvathipuram for the seventh grade, the rules by my grandparents were different. I had to return home from school soon after the classes were finished and no post-school sports were allowed with their philosophy that education is important at that stage and not play. However, they allowed me to join Auxiliary Cadet Corps (ACC) and participate in the drills, etc. associated with the ACC at the behest of my uncles who argued that ACC participation might be considered as an extracurricular activity that may be counted favorably towards medical school admission.

With a similar philosophy, I joined in the National Cadet Corps (NCC) soon after admission to intermediate in Arts and Science (IASc) at Mrs. A. V. N. College, Visakhapatnam (Figure 30). With the previous experience in ACC in high school, I easily earned a 'B' certificate in infantry (Figure 31).

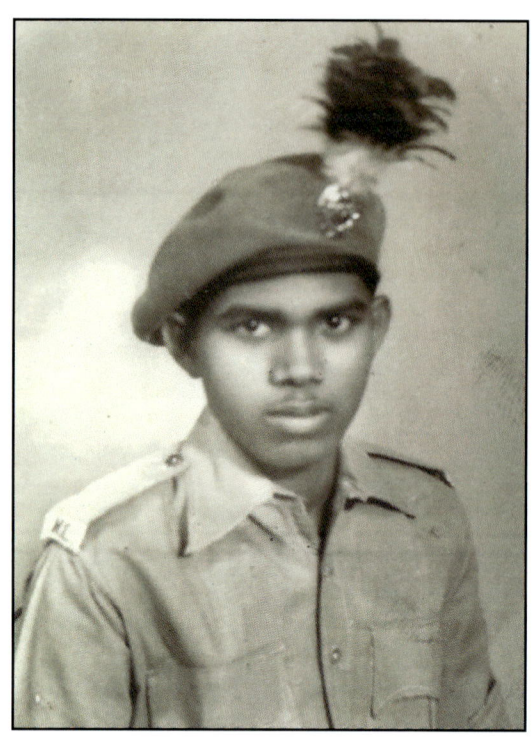

Figure 30. My photograph while a NCC cadet at Mrs. AVN College in Visakhapatnam in 1957.

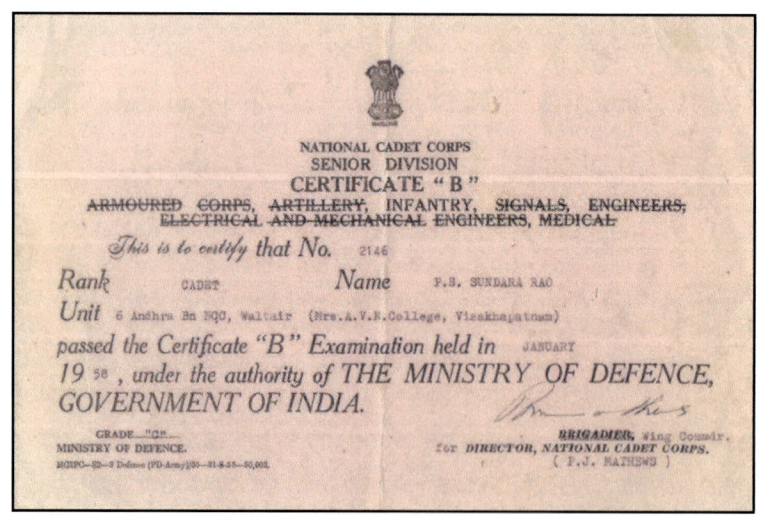

Figure 31. Infantry 'B' Certificate.

While I did secure reasonably good scores in Science subjects in the IASc examination, it is generally thought that the NCC experience along with other sports and social service participation (Figures 32 and 33) has helped me in securing medical school admission.

DEPARTMENT OF PHYSICAL EDUCATION,
MRS. A. V. N. COLLEGE, VISAKHAPATNAM.

Name of the Student: P. Syam Sundar Rao.

Class: Intermediate.

Period of Study: 1956-1958

Games and sports participated: Foot-Ball, Hockey, Basket-Ball and Badminton.

Tournaments participated: nil.

General remarks: nil.

Date 20.7.1958

20.7.58
Physical Director.

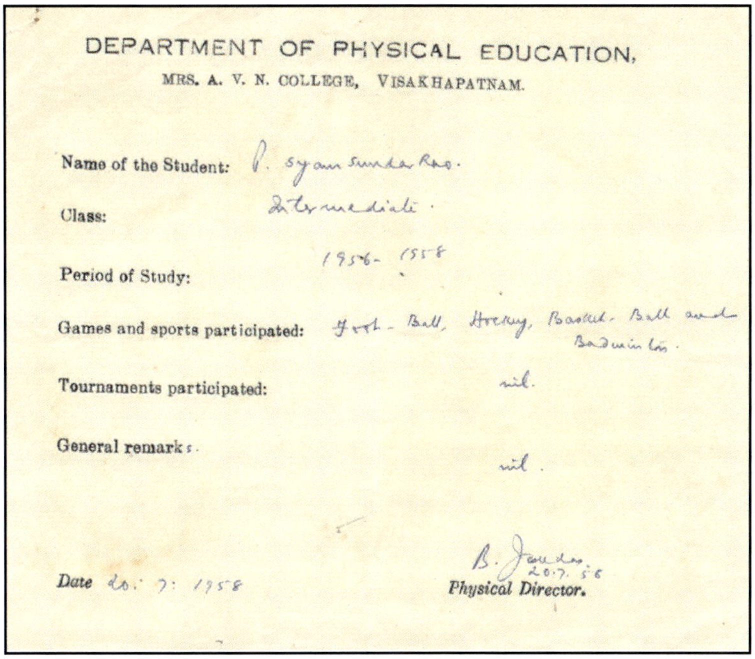

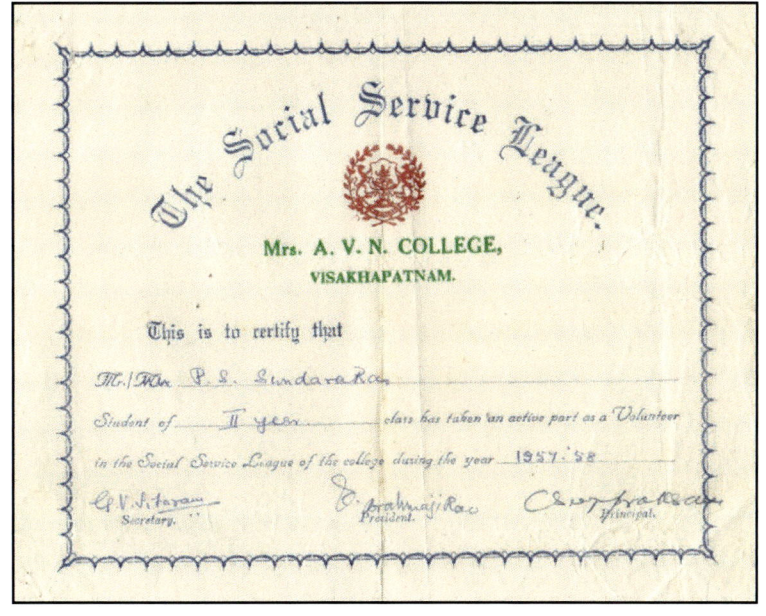

Figure 32. Certificate of my participation in sports while at Mrs. AVN College in Visakhapatnam (1956-58).

The Social Service League

Mrs. A. V. N. COLLEGE,
VISAKHAPATNAM.

This is to certify that

Mr./Miss P. S. Sundara Rao

Student of II year class has taken an active part as a Volunteer in the Social Service League of the college during the year 1957-58

G. V. Sitaram
Secretary.

President.

Principal.

Figure 33. Certificate of my participation in The Social Service League while at Mrs. AVN College in Visakhapatnam (1957-58).

Medical School

While the NCC was no longer required for the purpose of securing educational advantage, I had by this time developed an affinity with the NCC and therefore, joined the Army Medical NCC unit in Andhra Medical College. A few months passed by with regular attendance in the NCC activities along with medical school classes. The final examination for Chemistry was scheduled for late December 1959, but all the NCC cadets were required to attend the NCC camp planned for mid-December 1959. I sought for exemption from attending the camp because of closeness to the public examination, but the NCC officials denied such request prompting me to resign from the NCC. A few months later, a new Navy Medical NCC unit was established in the Andhra Medical College. Because of past NCC experience including 'B' certification, I was invited to join the new Navy Medical unit with a promise for rapid promotion. I accepted the invitation, joined the Navy Medical unit, and was given the Leading Cadet rank upon joining. I participated in all the activities of the Navy Medical unit and passed the Navy Medical 'B' certificate (Figure 34) with a resultant promotion to Cadet Captain (Figure 35).

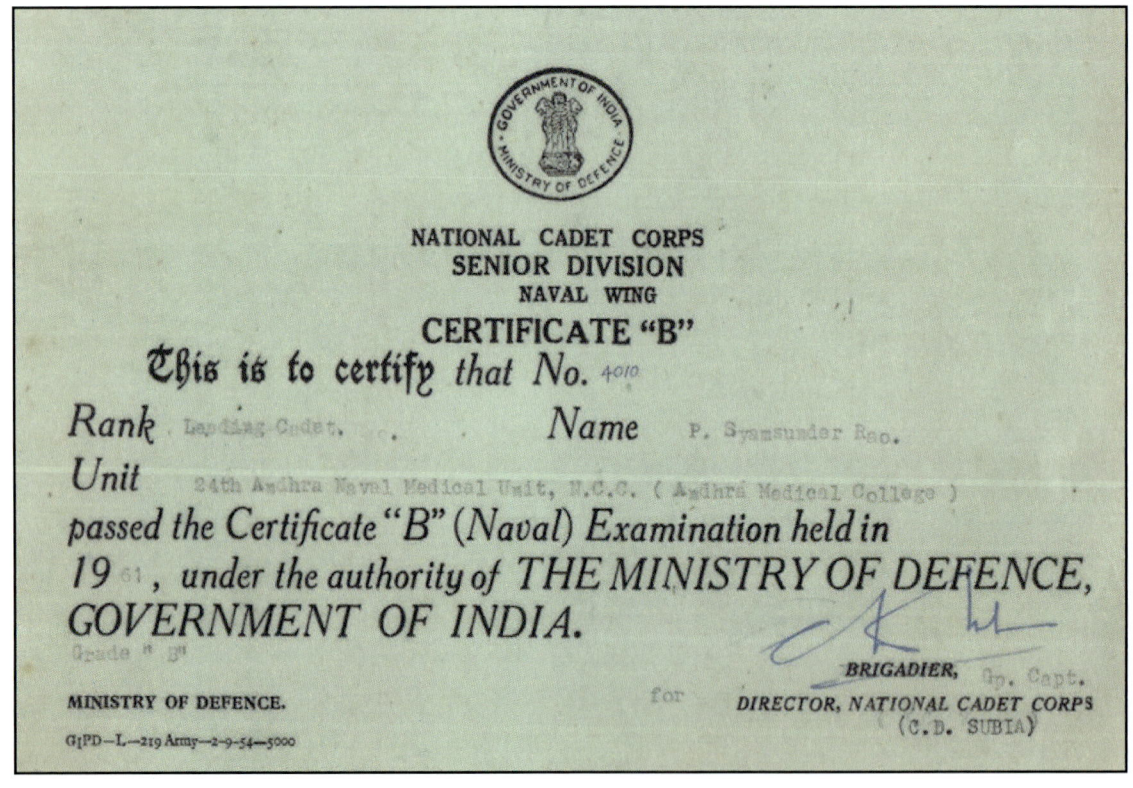

Figure 34. My Naval 'B' Certificate.

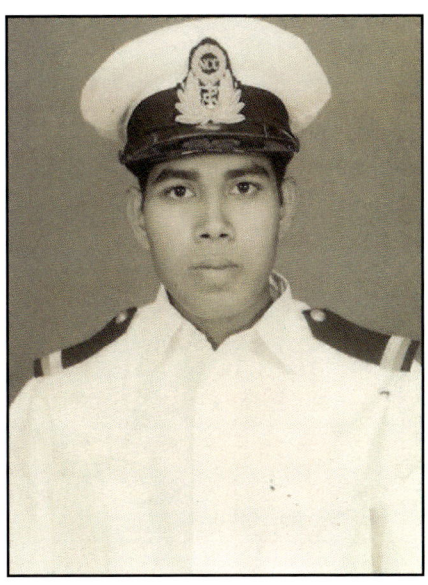

Figure 35. My photograph as a Cadet Captain.

During the following year, I also passed 'C' certificate (Figure 36), which resulted in my further promotion to Senior Cadet Captain (Figures 37, 38, and 39). I continued service as a Senior Cadet Captain until my discharge from the 24th Naval Medical Unit NCC in late August 1963 (Figure 40).

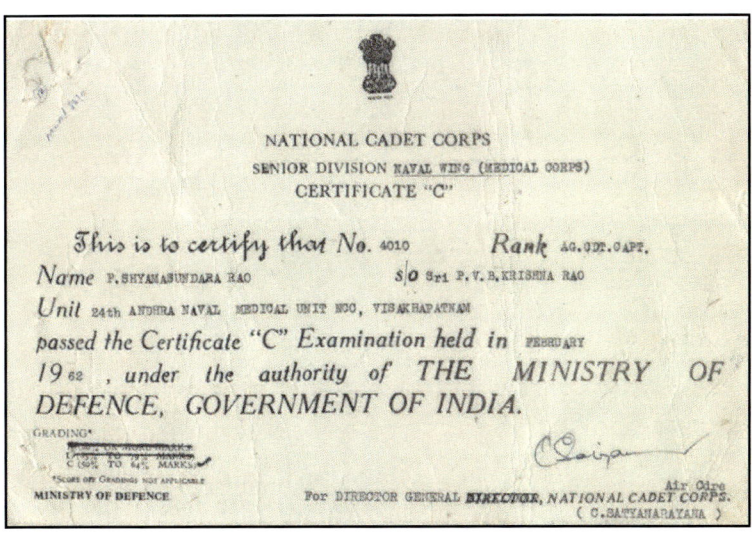

Figure 36. My Naval Medical 'C' Certificate.

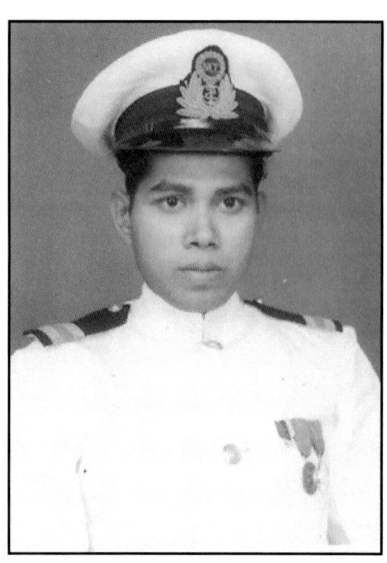

Figure 37. My photograph as a Senior Cadet Captain.

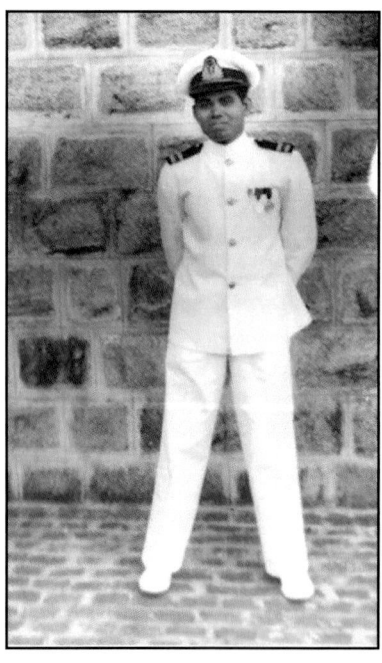

Figure 38. My photograph as a Senior Cadet Captain.

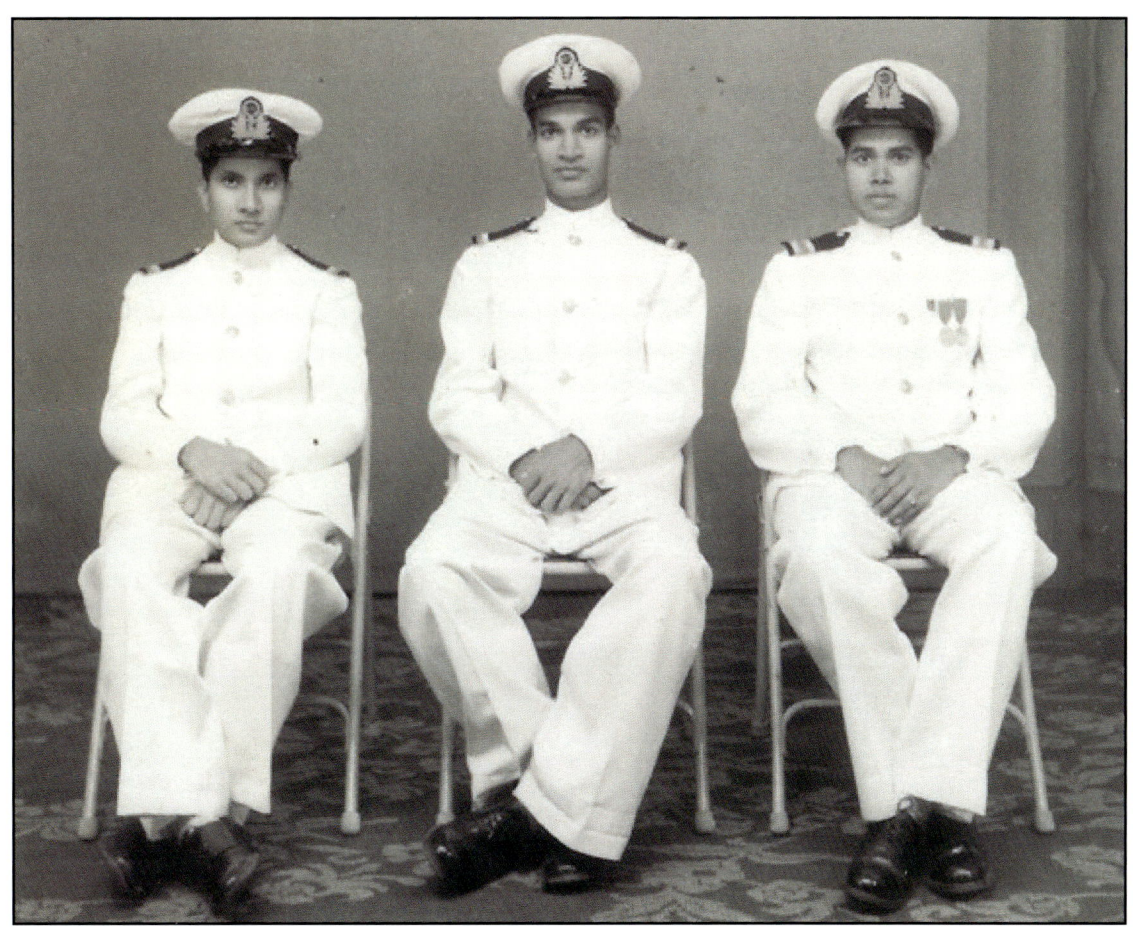

Figure 39. My (right) (Senior Cadet Captain) photograph with the Cadet Captains in the Navy Medical Unit.

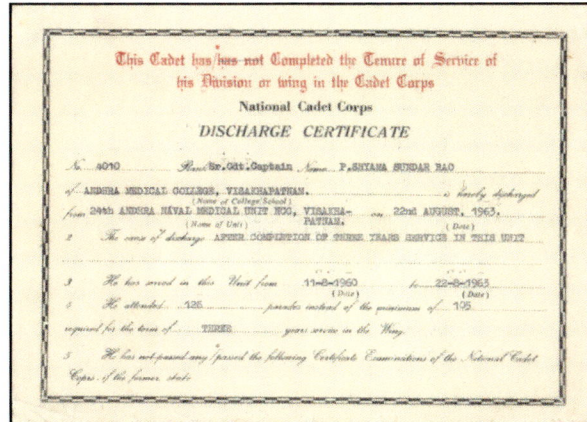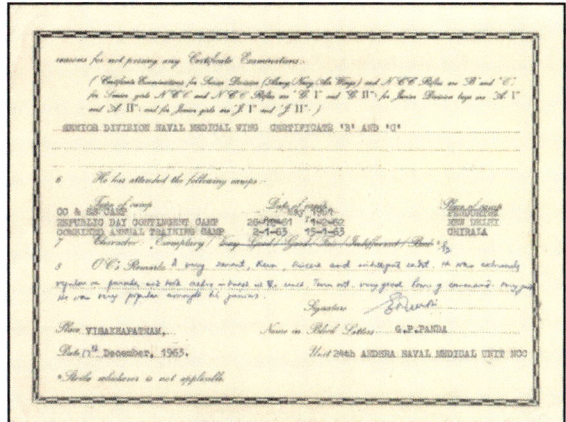

Figure 40. Discharge certificate from the 24th Naval Medical Unit NCC.

Republic Day Contingent

I was selected to participate in the Republic Day parade at New Delhi in January 1962. I was one of the three cadets (Figure 41) selected from Visakhapatnam region. Such selection was highly competitive and it is an honor for the selected candidate. Following a two-week intense training, the selected candidates participate in the march (Figures 42 and 43) on January 26, the Republic Day, along with the platoons of the regular Army, Navy and Air Force divisions. Following the parade and other celebrations, the participants had a chance to meet with the Camp Commandant (Figures 44 and 45), Defense Minister Krishna Menon (Figure 46), and Prime Minister Jawaharlal Nehru (Figure 47). Since the contingent from Andhra Pradesh won the first prize, we had the opportunity to have visits and photographs with dignitaries (Figures 46 and 47).

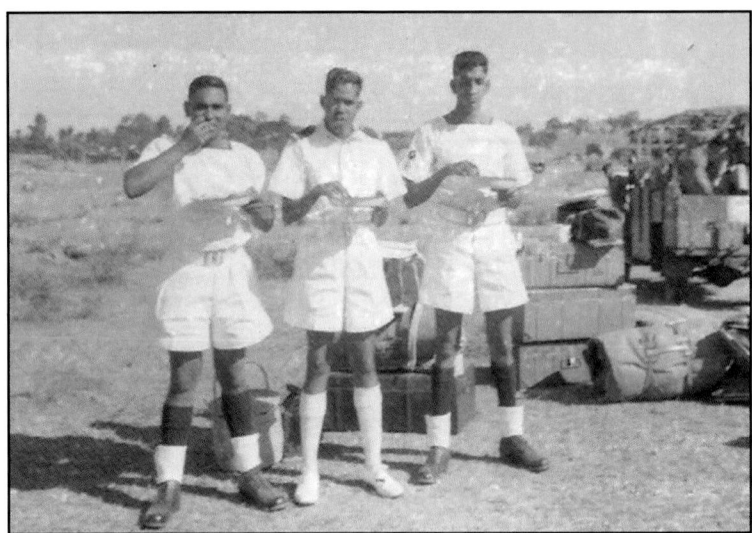

Figure 41. My photograph (center) with the other two cadets selected from Visakhapatnam region to participate in the Republic Day parade.

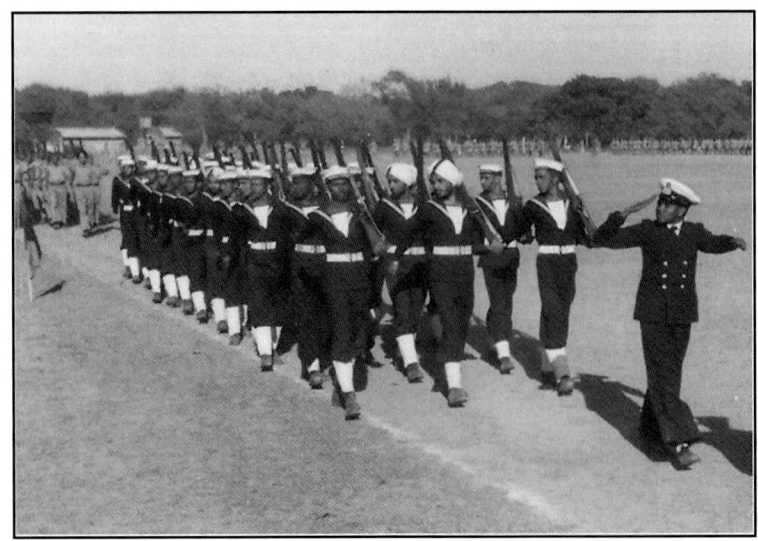

Figure 42. Photograph of my unit during a march.

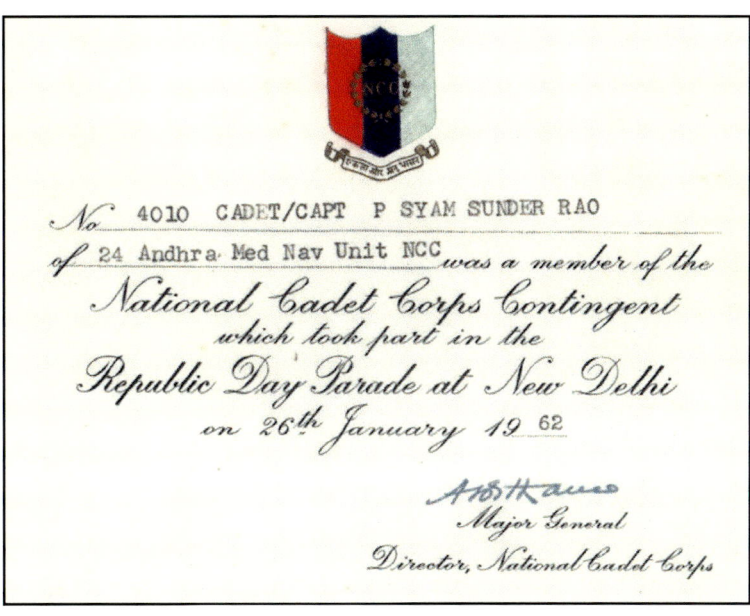

Figure 43. Certificate of participation in the Republic Day parade at New Delhi in January 1962.

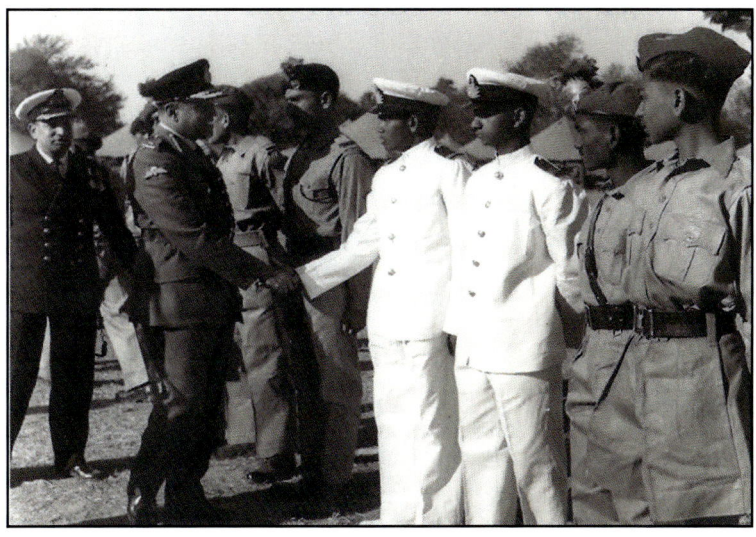

Figure 44. Shaking hands with the Camp Commandant.

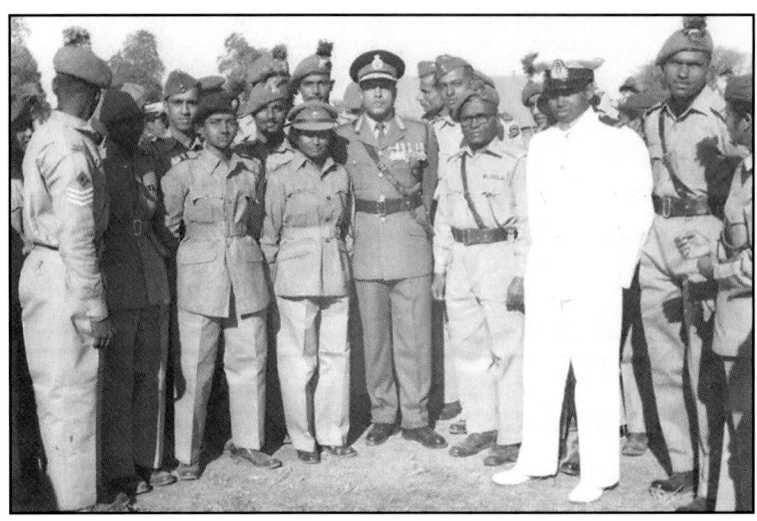

Figure 45. Photograph with the Camp Commandant and other cadets, officers, and staff.

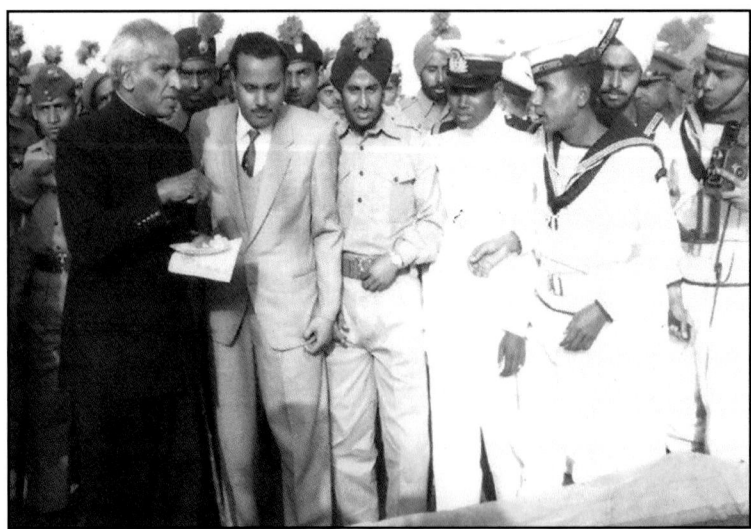

Figure 46. Photograph with the Defense Minister Krishna Menon.

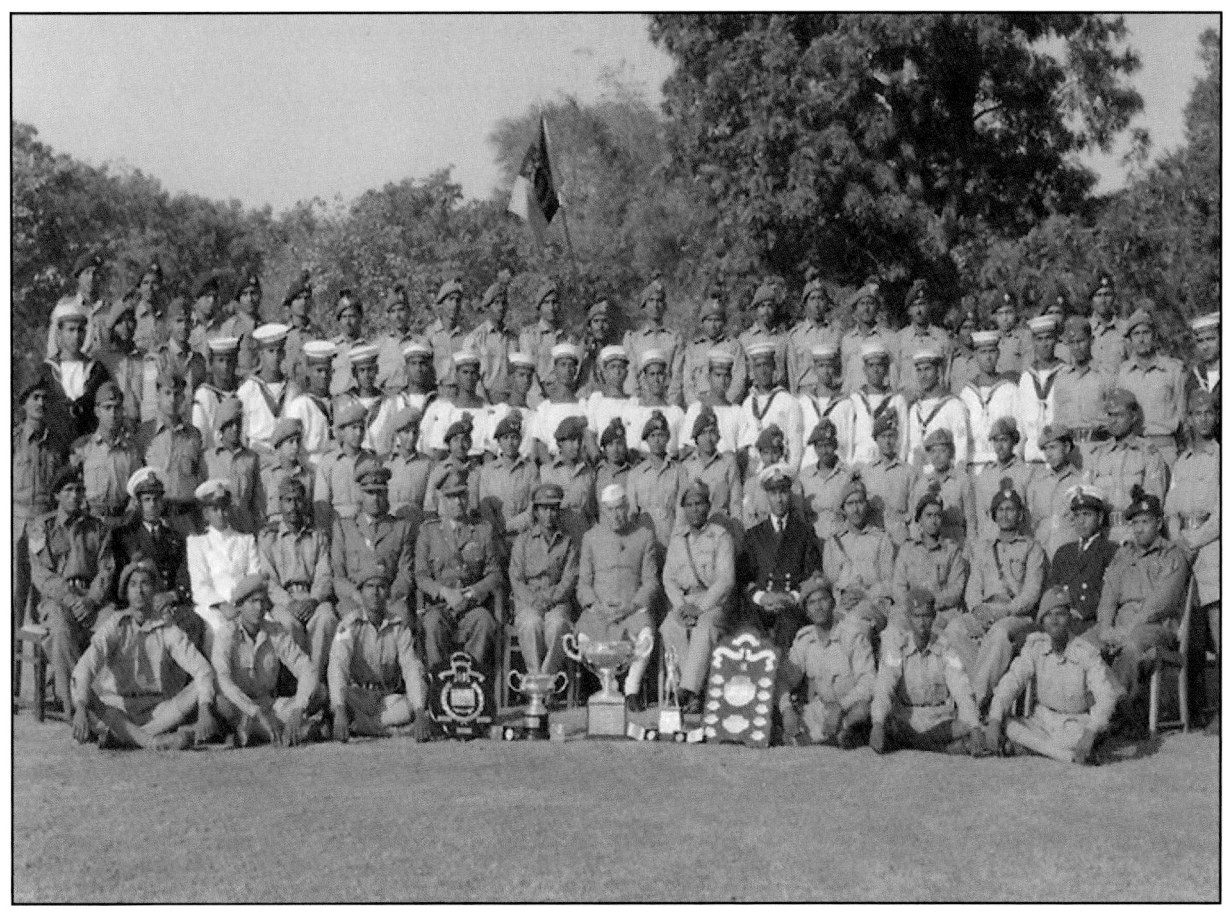

Figure. 47. Photograph of the entire Andhra Pradesh contingent with the
Prime Minister Jawaharlal Nehru.

After returning to Visakhapatnam, I was recognized by inspection of my unit by the Governor of Andhra Pradesh (Figure 48) and presentation of a medal by the Vice Chancellor of Andhra University (Figure 49).

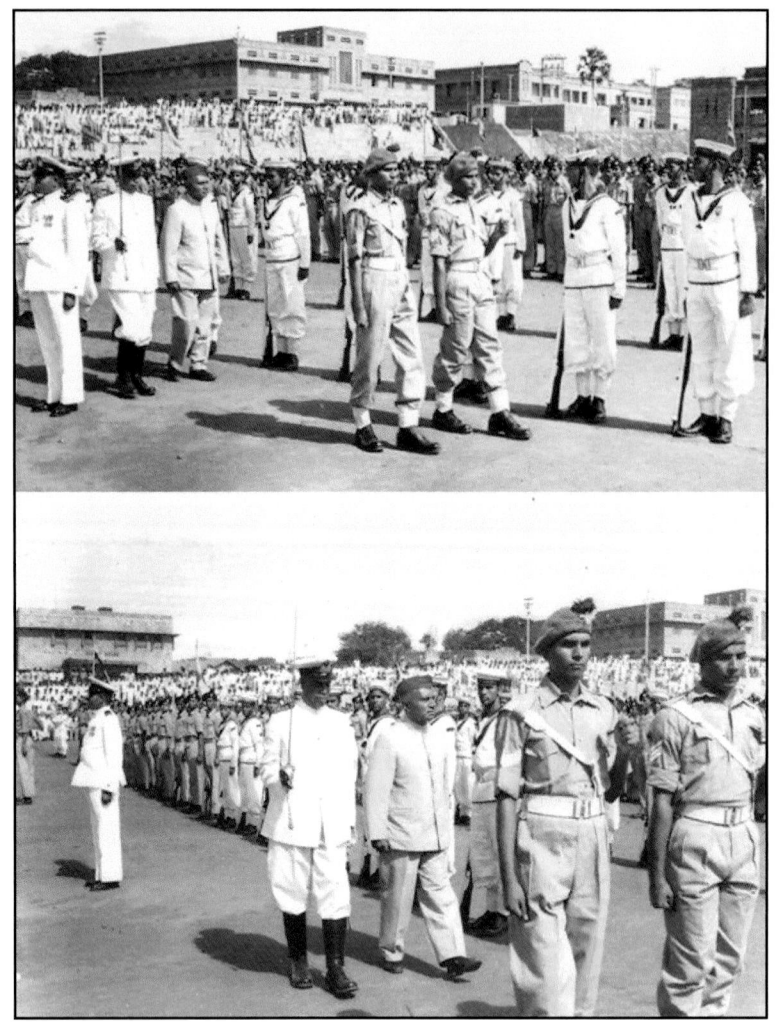

Figure 48. Inspection of my unit by the Governor of Andhra Pradesh.

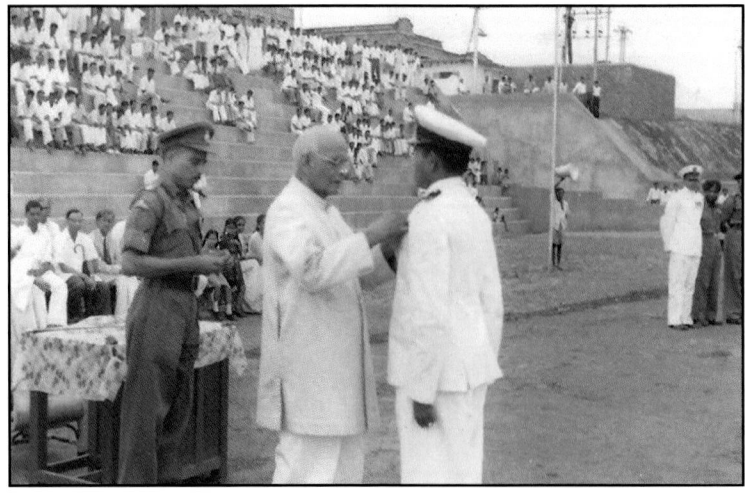

Figure 49. Presentation of medal of honor by the Vice Chancellor of Andhra University.

Postgraduate Studies

My election as the President of the House Surgeon's Association at the King George Hospital and as the President of the state-wide Andhra Pradesh House Surgeon's Association was already reviewed in the chapter on "The Journey Begins" and will not be repeated. As I began house surgeoncy, I was invited to become the NCC officer and was offered commission as the Navy Sub-Lieutenant without formal training (Figure 50) because of my prior NCC 'C' Certificate. I served as the NCC officer while a house surgeon and during DCH with a short break during my tenure as a medical officer in Kothapalli. After arriving in USA for additional postgraduate studies, I did not have the opportunity in participating in extracurricular activities, largely related getting adjusted to the new culture, demanding training requirements, including night-calls, and preparation for specialty and subspecialty board and state licensing examinations. However, I did serve as a team physician for the high school football teams while I was a pediatric resident at the Good Samaritan Hospital, Phoenix, AZ.

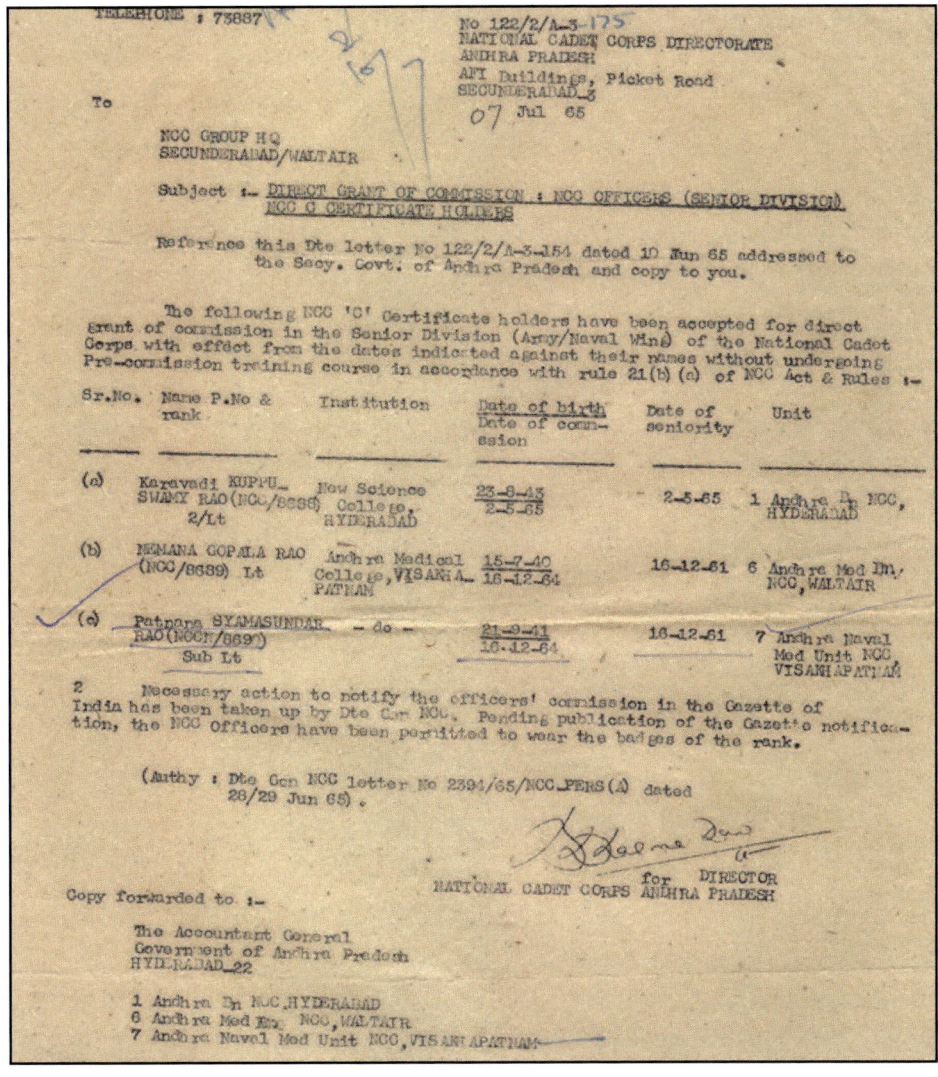

Figure 50. Letter of direct granting of commission as officer (Sub-Lieutenant).

Subsequent to Training

Subsequent to completion of my training, as mentioned in the preceding section on "Academic Career" of this chapter, I joined the Medical College of Georgia in Augusta, Georgia, as a faculty member. Shortly thereafter, in mid 1970s, I helped to form the Indian Association of Greater Augusta and was the founding Vice President and subsequently President of the Association. I also helped to organize and conduct cultural activities of the Association. Subsequently, in late 1970s, I also facilitated to form the Hindu Temple Society of Augusta and was also the founding Vice President and subsequently the President of the Association and was instrumental in acquiring site (with a small building) for the future temple (Figure 51). When I left Augusta to take a new position abroad in mid-1981, the reins were handed over to the incoming President and the Board of Directors. Subsequently, an orthodox multi-deity temple was constructed (Figures 52 and 53). While in Saudi Arabia, there was no additional time for extracurricular activities because of being busy establishing new services, administrative duties, and academic activities. However, I actively participated in tennis and indeed was the winner of the father-daughter tennis team competition. After returning to USA in 1987 to Madison, Wisconsin, I served as a member of the Executive Committee of the Indian Association of Madison for several years and helped organize cultural activities of the Association. I and my son, Vijay, were also winners of the father-son tennis tournament conducted by the Department of Pediatrics at the University of Wisconsin.

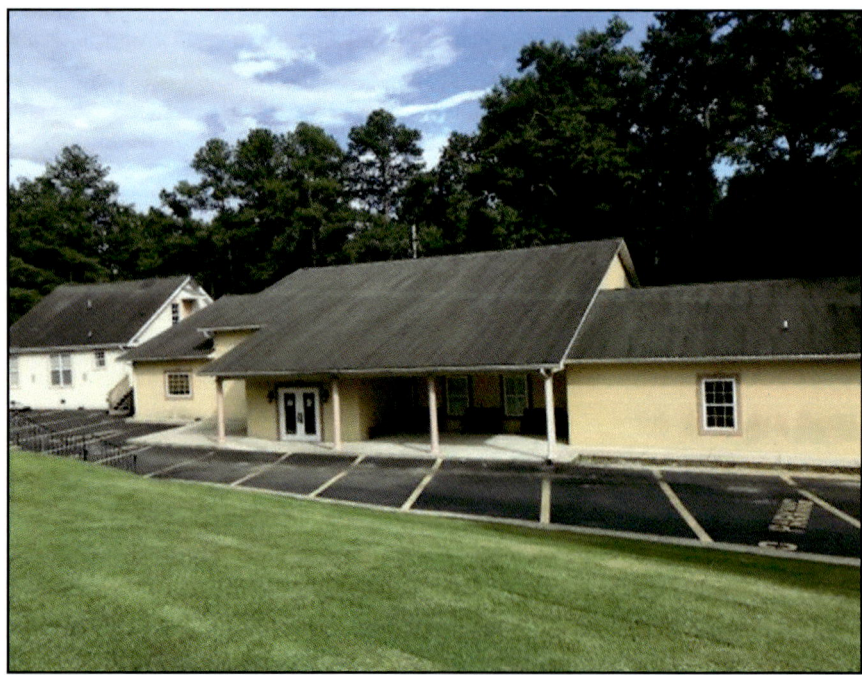

Figure 51. Site including a small building acquired/purchased by me (along with other members of the Board of Directors) when I was the President of the Hindu Temple Society of Augusta.

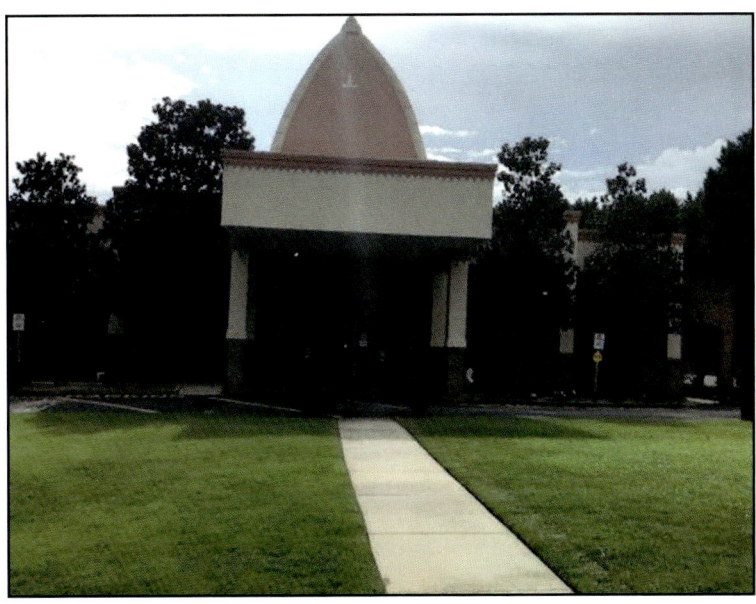

Figure 52. Photograph of the temple of the Hindu Temple Society of Augusta following the construction.

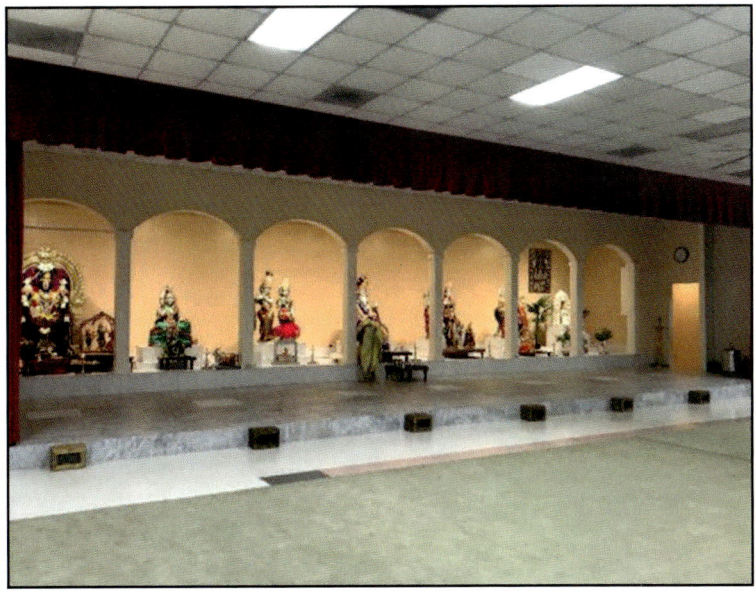

Figure 53. Photograph of a section of the interior of the multi-deity temple of the Hindu Temple Society of Augusta.

ATTEMPTS TO RETURN TO INDIA

I made multiple attempts to return to India and these will be reviewed in this section.

The First Attempt

As mentioned in the first chapter, "The Journey Begins," my intent was to get trained in pediatric cardiology in USA and return to India to serve people in India. In late 1960s and early 1970s, there were only few institutions in India that had facilities to perform cardiac catheterizations and other amenities to be able to care for children with congenital heart defects. As per my knowledge, All India Institute of Medical Sciences (AIMS) in New Delhi and Christian Medical College at Vellore, Madras State, were such institutions. There may have been other institutions in Bombay, Calcutta and other places, but I was unaware of such institutions at that time. At about the conclusion of my training, I contacted both these institutions, seeking for a position in pediatric cardiology. The Christian Medical College at Vellore responded and stated that they already have a pediatric cardiologist on their staff and that they are not looking to expand their program. However, the Head of Department of Cardiology at AIMS in New Delhi, Dr. Sujoy B. Roy, welcomed the idea and stated that they have only one pediatric cardiologist on their staff (Dr. Raj Tandon who was trained in Boston and returned to New Delhi) and encouraged me to pursue the possibility. I was optimistic and had letters of recommendation by Dr. Herman Lipow and Dr. Norman J. Sissman sent to Dr. Roy. Just prior to the completion of my training at the Case-Western Reserve University/University Hospitals of Cleveland (Figure 6), I went to New Delhi following the attendance of the World Congress of Cardiology in London to meet with Dr. Roy and his staff at AIMS in New Delhi to firm up of the offer of a position as Assistant Professor of Pediatric Cardiology. The trip included visit with my parents (Figure 54). Since the expectation for a position at the All India Institute of Medical Sciences was high, I purchased only one way tickets to India for my wife and son. Despite the prior arrangements made for the visit, Dr. Roy went away on a research trip to Kashmir. Therefore, I stopped in New Delhi on the way back to USA. After a long discussion, Dr. Roy told me that there was no vacant position of Assistant Professor of Pediatric Cardiology and if interested, I may come as a Scientific Pool Officer and take chances for future position at All India Institute of Medical Sciences. I respectfully declined the offer for Scientific Pool Officer and requested Dr. Roy to make his attempts to secure a more permanent position. A three-month period was requested so that I may make alternate career plans. No offer came during the set time resulting in me pursuing research fellowship at University of California at Los Angeles (UCLA), and a subsequent faculty position at the Medical College of Georgia, as detailed above in the sections on "Postgraduate Education" and "Academic Career" of this chapter, respectively.

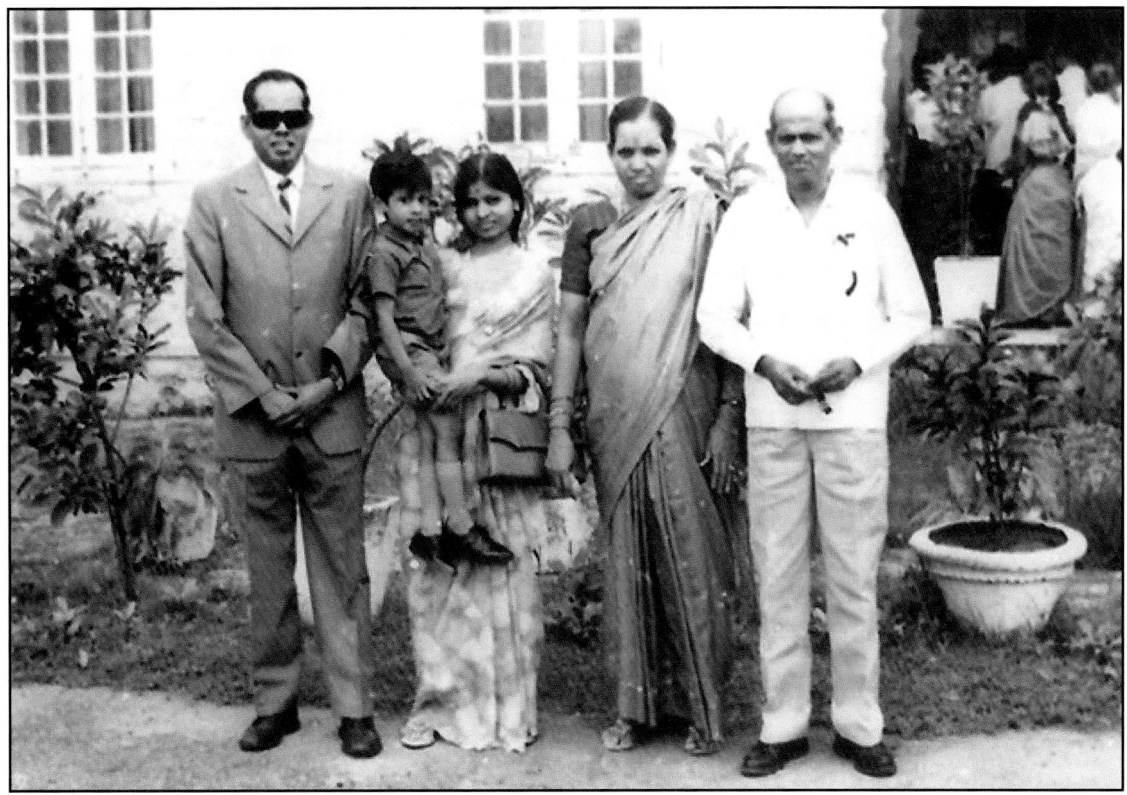

Figure 54. Photograph with my son (Vijay), wife (Hymavathi), mother (Savithramma) and father (PVB Krishna Rao) during a visit to India in 1970.

Second Attempt

The University System of Georgia including the Medical College of Georgia has had a sabbatical policy; following a continuous service of seven years, a faulty member may be granted one year leave with half salary (or six months leave with full salary) for pursuing academic interests. After seven years of service at the Medical College of Georgia as assistant/associate/full professor, I wanted to take advantage of this policy and corresponded with Dr. O. P. Ghai, Chairman of the Department of Pediatrics at the All Institute of Medical Sciences with request for sabbatical for one year with the provision that the institute does not have to pay me any financial remuneration. Dr. Ghai and the Dean appear to be interested (Figures 55 and 56) and further paperwork, as requested by the All Institute of Medical Sciences, was submitted. My intent was that if everything went well, I could permanently stay at All India Institute of Medical Sciences following the sabbatical. Despite the initial interest expressed by Dr. Ghai and Keswani (Figures 55 and 56) and the interest shown by the Professor and Head of the Department of Cardiothoracic and Vascular Surgery (Figure 57), and to my disappointment, after further consideration, the All India Institute of Medical Sciences declined to house me for the sabbatical.

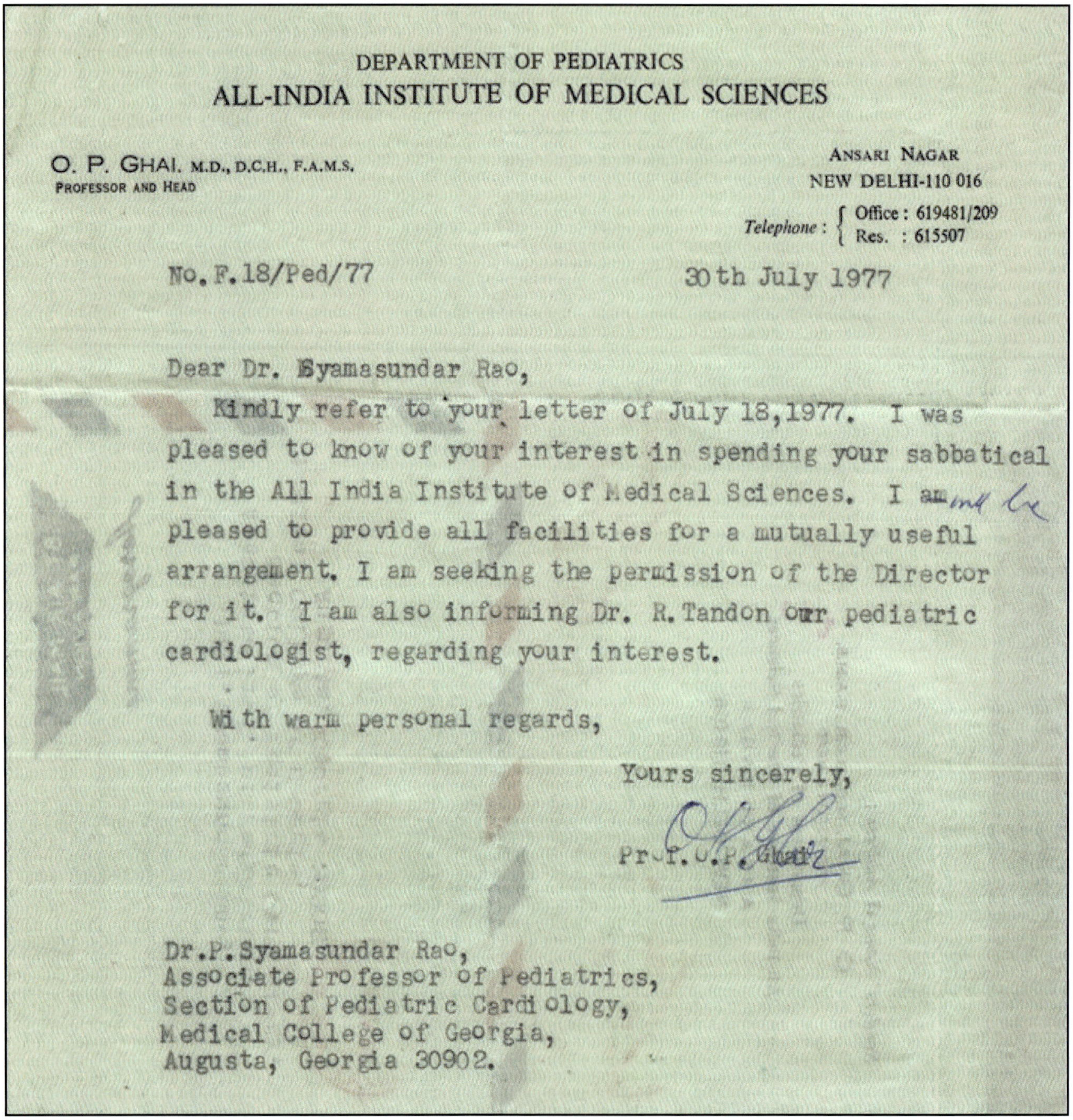

DEPARTMENT OF PEDIATRICS
ALL-INDIA INSTITUTE OF MEDICAL SCIENCES

O. P. GHAI, M.D., D.C.H., F.A.M.S.
PROFESSOR AND HEAD

ANSARI NAGAR
NEW DELHI-110 016

Telephone : { Office : 619481/209
              Res. : 615507

No. F.18/Ped/77   30th July 1977

Dear Dr. Syamasundar Rao,

Kindly refer to your letter of July 18, 1977. I was
pleased to know of your interest in spending your sabbatical
in the All India Institute of Medical Sciences. I am *and be*
pleased to provide all facilities for a mutually useful
arrangement. I am seeking the permission of the Director
for it. I am also informing Dr. R. Tandon our pediatric
cardiologist, regarding your interest.

With warm personal regards,

Yours sincerely,

Prof. O.P. Ghai

Dr. P. Syamasundar Rao,
Associate Professor of Pediatrics,
Section of Pediatric Cardiology,
Medical College of Georgia,
Augusta, Georgia 30902.

Figure 55. A copy of the letter from Dr. Ghai expressing interest in providing
facilities for my sabbatical at All India Institute of Medical Sciences.

ALL-INDIA INSTITUTE OF MEDICAL SCIENCES

No. 835/Acad.

Ansari Nagar, New Delhi-16.
Dated the 8th August, 1977.

PROF.N.H.KESWANI
DEAN

Dear Dr.Rao,

Kindly refer to your letter dated the 18th July, 1977 addressed to Dr.O.P.Ghai, Professor and Head of the Department of Paediatrics.

I am pleased to note that you would like to spend a part of your sabbatical leave with us at this Institute. We shall be glad to extend all possible facilities during your visit.

Please let us know the exact period you would like to spend at this Institute so that we may seek approval of the Government of India, which is mandatory for inviting a foreign national.

With kind regards,

Yours sincerely,

N.H. Keswani

(N.H. KESWANI)

Dr.P.Syamasundar Rao, M.B.
Associate Professor of Paediatrics
Section of Paediatric Cardiology,
Medical College of Georgia,
Augusta, Georgia 30902.

Figure 56. A copy of the letter from Dr. Keswani, Dean, expressing interest in providing facilities for my sabbatical at All India Institute of Medical Sciences.

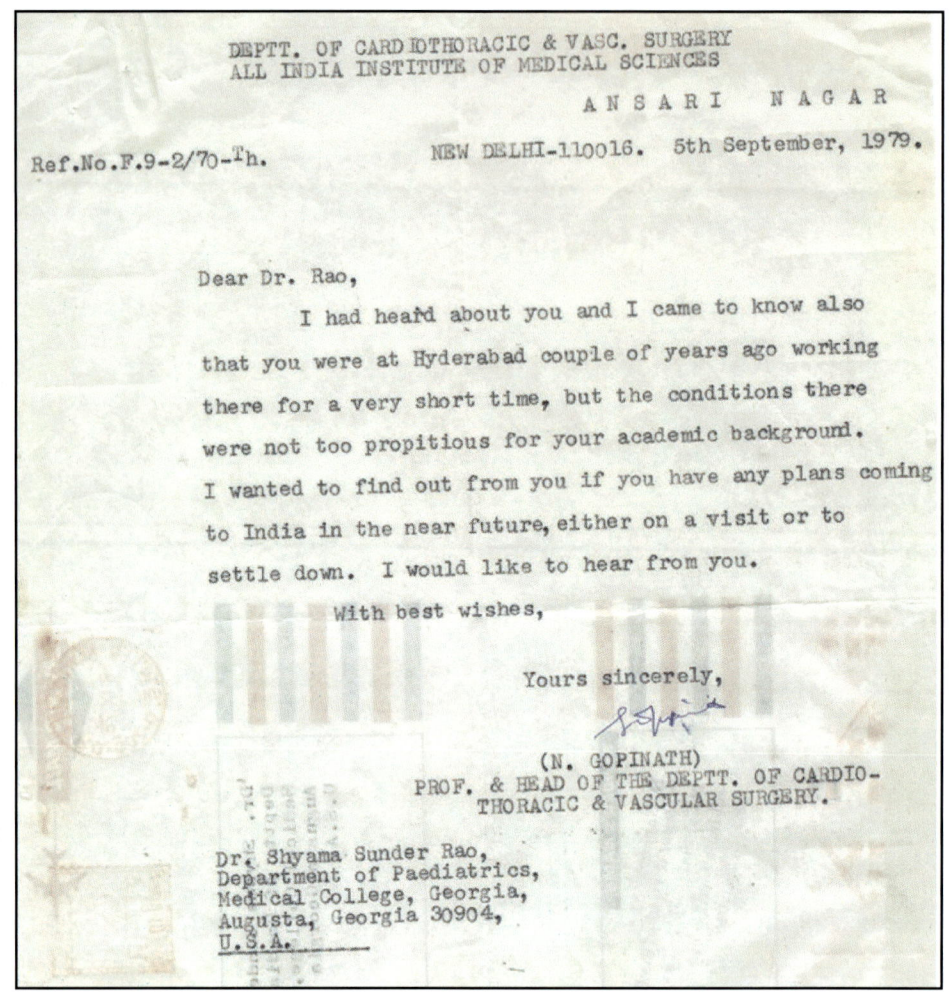

Figure 57. A copy of the letter from Dr. Gopinath, Professor and Head of the Department of Cardiothoracic and Vascular Surgery, showing interest in me in coming to All India Institute of Medical Sciences.

Subsequent Attempts

Following the above unsuccessful second attempt, I decided to pursue other academic ventures utilizing the sabbatical. The initial interest was to pursue research to investigate the cause(s) of congenital heart disease so that it may be prevented, it never materialized because of my inability to find a suitable mentor who was actively researching on embryology and causation of congenital heart defects. In retrospect, it was unfortunate that I failed to identify Dr. Margret Kirby[52-56] in the Department of Anatomy at the Medical College of Georgia itself who was actually investigating the subject of my interest. However, this pursuit resulted in the publication of multiple review papers,[57-60] including an excellent booklet (Figure 58).[61]

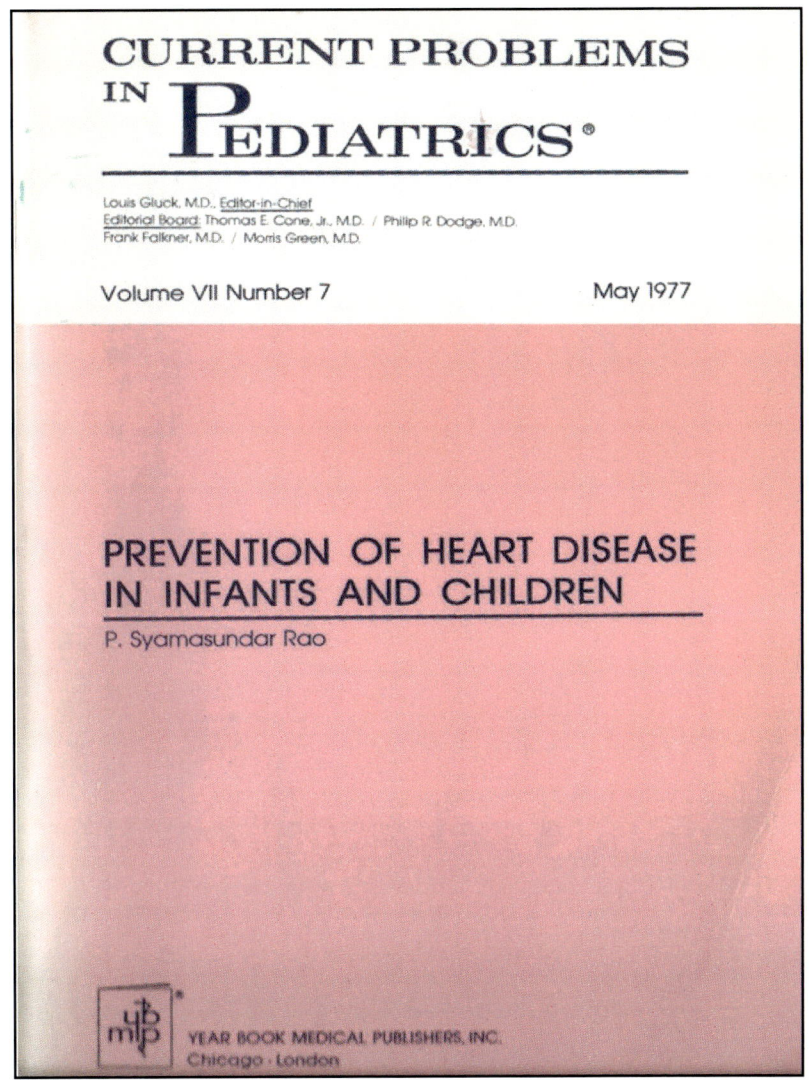

Figure 58. Photograph of monograph on "Prevention of Heart Disease in Infants and Children" published in Current Problems in Pediatrics.[61]

As the unsuccessful search for a mentor was concluded, an offer came from the Medical Director of the Hospital Corporation Association (HCA), International for the author to join the staff at the King Faisal Hospital & Research Center, Riyadh, Saudi Arabia as a pediatric cardiologist. A formal application for sabbatical with the objective of establishing pediatric cardiology service at the King Faisal Hospital & Research Center, and to write a book on Tricuspid Atresia was submitted. The sabbatical was approved by the Medical College of Georgia and the University System of Georgia administrations. I moved to Riyadh, Saudi Arabia in July 1981 to begin the sabbatical. I joined another pediatric cardiologist who was trained in USA and along with him, further strengthened the pediatric cardiology program at King Faisal Hospital & Research Center, initiated interventional pediatric cardiology program[32,62-69] and by the end of the year completed the book on Tricuspid Atresia (Figure 59).[70]

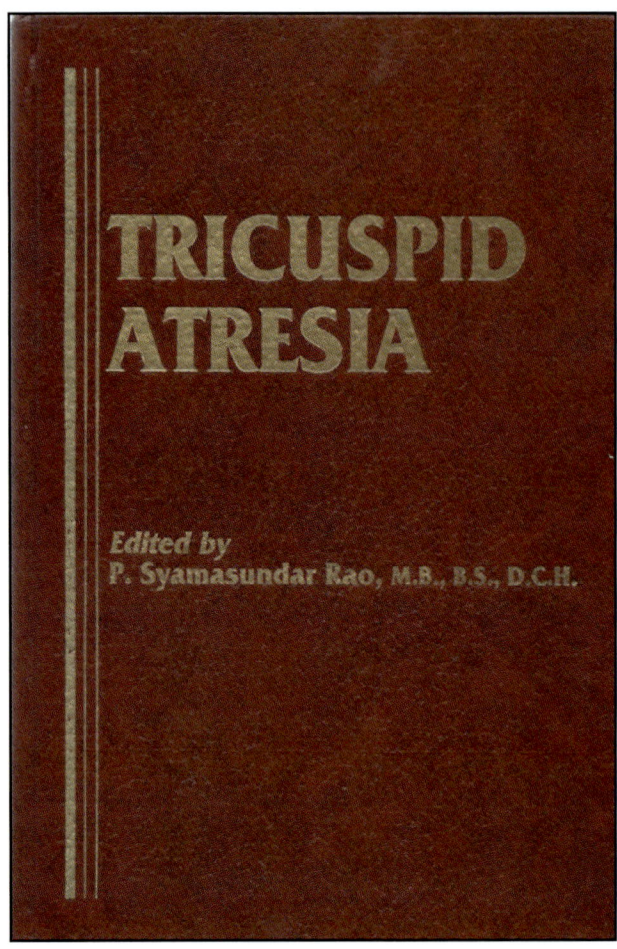

Figure 59. Photograph of the book on Tricuspid Atresia completed during the sabbatical.

While the objectives of the sabbatical program have been accomplished and plans to return to the Medical College of Georgia were being contemplated, my accountant in Georgia notified me of the tax liability. To claim any tax exemption for money earned both at the King Faisal Hospital & Research Center and sabbatical pay from the Medical College of Georgia, one must be out of the country (USA) for at least eighteen months. Given this huge financial burden, I requested the Department of Pediatrics' administration at the Medical College of Georgia to extend the sabbatical, this time without pay for another six months. They refused despite guaranty from me that I would return to the Medical College of Georgia after another six months. The decision was appealed to the Dean of the Medical School, the President of the Medical College of Georgia and finally to the Chancellor of the University System of Georgia without any favorable response from these higher authorities. I was then faced with the prospect of facing financial burden by returning to the Medical College of Georgia vs. resigning the professorial position at the Medical College of Georgia. After a long thought and consultation with members of my family, friends, and colleagues, I decided to resign the professorial position at the Medical College of Georgia. One of the major considerations was the initial desire to return to India; it was envisioned that I could stay in Riyadh for five years or so, and hopefully accumulate some wealth and return to India. This time, no attempt will be made to secure academic positions such as those made during my first and second attempts to return to India.

Work in interventional pediatric cardiology continued and I carried out administrative, clinical and academic responsibilities at the King Faisal Hospital & Research Center, as detailed in the section on "Academic Career." As the target date to return to India arrived, I made plans to build a Nursing Home/Small Hospital and was able have the Government of Andhra Pradesh allot a plot of land to construct a hospital in Muvvalivanipalem, a suburb of Visakhapatnam. The plan was to have my two brothers, who are physicians, and two brothers, who are accountants, to manage the hospital initially and then I would return a few years later. Unfortunately, two things happened. First, each of my brothers who were slated to run the hospital were unable to take the assigned task and more importantly, our children became young adults/teenagers and objected to return to India; they wanted to be in USA. Given these developments, plans to return to India were cancelled and job applications to return to USA began. I was fortunate in securing the position of Professor and Director of Pediatric Cardiology at the University of Wisconsin in Madison, Wisconsin, as detailed in the section on "Academic Career." No serious attempts to return to India were made following this; instead, yearly visits to India and making contributions to education of physicians in India (as reviewed in the next section) were planned.

CONTRIBUTIONS TO EDUCATION OF PHYSICIANS IN INDIA

Since my thought has always been about India, I have taken every available opportunity to make contributions to Indian physicians' education; this resulted in papers/publications in Indian journals (N=37),[6,64,71-105] book chapters in books edited by Indian authors (N=31) (Table I) and lectures/presentations at Indian institutions and scientific societies (N= 36) (Table II). I also organized and served as the Guest Editor for several symposia on behalf of the Indian Journal of Pediatrics (Table III).

Table I My Book Chapters in Books Edited by Indian Authors

---

1. Rao PS, *Doppler Echocardiography in Non-invasive Diagnosis of Congenital Heart Disease*, In: Current Trends in Pediatrics, Singh M. (ed.), Vanity Books, New Delhi, India, 1986, pp. 106-144.

2. Rao PS, *Non-Coronary Uses of Stents in Children and Adults*, In: Cardiology Update, 2002. Gambhir DS (ed.), Cardiological Society of India, New Delhi, 2002, pp. 268-282.

3. Rao PS, *Pediatric Cardiology – a Quarter Century of Progress*, In: Hridaya Sangamam – Souvenir – 2002. Manjuran RJ (ed.), CSI Kerala Chapter, Kochi, Kerala, 2002, pp. 43-48.

4. Gupta ML, Lantin-Hermosa MR, Rao PS, *What is New in Pediatric Cardiology?* In: Saxena A, Rao PS (ed.), Advances in Pediatrics – 1: Cardiology, Indian Journal of Pediatrics, New Delhi, India, 2005, pp. 10-26.

5. Rao PS, Gupta ML, Balaji S, *Recent Advances in Pediatric Cardiology – Electrophysiology, Transcatheter and Surgical Advances*, In: Saxena A, Rao PS (ed.). Advances in Pediatrics – 1: Cardiology, Indian Journal of Pediatrics, New Delhi, India, 2005, pp. 27-39.

6. Rao PS, *Diagnosis and Management of Acyanotic Heart Disease: Part I - Obstructive Lesions*, In: Rao PS, Saxena A (eds.), Recent Advances in Pediatric Cardiology, Indian Journal of Pediatrics, New Delhi, India, 2006, pp. 1-16.

7. Rao PS, *Diagnosis and Management of Acyanotic Heart Disease: Part II - Left-to-right Shunt Lesions*, In: Rao PS, Saxena A (eds.), Recent Advances in Pediatric Cardiology, Indian Journal of Pediatrics, New Delhi, India, 2006, pp. 17-36.

8. Gupta Malhotra, Rao PS, *Current Perspectives on Kawasaki Disease*, In: Rao PS, Saxena A (ed.), Recent Advances in Pediatric Cardiology, Indian Journal of Pediatrics, New Delhi, India, 2006, pp. 99-116.

9. Rao PS, Sharma SK, *Management of Patent Ductus Arteriosus with Particular Attention to Transcatheter Therapy*, In: Rao PS, Saxena A (eds.), Recent Advances in Pediatric Cardiology, Indian Journal of Pediatrics, New Delhi, India, 2006, pp. 125-139.

10. Gupta ML, Lantin-Hermoso R, Rao PS, *Recent Advances in Pediatric Cardiology: Part I – Medical Advances*, In: Rao PS, Saxena A (eds.), Recent Advances in Pediatric Cardiology, Indian Journal of Pediatrics, New Delhi, India, 2006, pp. 152-170.

11. Rao PS, Gupta ML, Balaji S., *Recent Advances in Pediatric Cardiology: Part II – Electrophysiology, Transcatheter and Surgical Advances*, In: Rao PS, Saxena A (eds.), Recent Advances in Pediatric Cardiology, Indian Journal of Pediatrics, New Delhi, India, 2006, pp. 171-190.

12. Rao PS., *Tricuspid Atresia*, In. Vijayalakshmi IB, Rao PS, Chugh R. (ed.), A Comprehensive Approach to Management of Congenital Heart Diseases, Jaypee Publications, New Delhi, India, 2013, pp. 397-413.

13. Balaguru D, Rao PS, *Diseases of the Tricuspid Valve (Ebstein's Anomaly, Tricuspid Stenosis and Regurgitation)*, In. Vijayalakshmi IB, Rao PS, Chugh R. (eds.), A Comprehensive Approach to Management of Congenital Heart Diseases, Jaypee Publications, New Delhi, India, 2013, pp. 414-433.

14. Balaguru D, Rao PS, *Mitral Atresia*, In. Vijayalakshmi IB, Rao PS, Chugh R. (eds.), A Comprehensive Approach to Management of Congenital Heart Diseases, Jaypee Publications, New Delhi, India, 2013, pp. 458-467.

15. Balaguru D, Rao PS, *Truncus Arteriosus*, In. Vijayalakshmi IB, Rao PS, Chugh R. (eds.), A Comprehensive Approach to Management of Congenital Heart Diseases, Jaypee Publications, New Delhi, India, 2013, pp. 600-613.

16. Rao PS, Alapati S., *Hypoplastic Left Heart Syndrome*, In. Vijayalakshmi IB, Rao PS, Chugh R. (eds.), A Comprehensive Approach to Management of Congenital Heart Diseases, Jaypee Publications, New Delhi, India, 2013, pp. 662-678.

17. Rao PS, *What the Adult Cardiologist Should Know About Cyanotic Congenital Heart Disease*, In: Chopra HK, et al. (eds.), State of Art CSI Cardiology Update 2014.

18. Rao PS, *History of Transcatheter Interventions in Pediatric Cardiology*, In. Vijayalakshmi IB, (ed.), Cardiac Catheterization and Imaging (From Pediatrics to Geriatrics), Jaypee Publications, New Delhi, India, 2015, pp. 3-20.

19. Rao PS, *Balloon Valvuloplasty for Pulmonary Stenosis*, In. Vijayalakshmi IB, (ed.), Cardiac Catheterization and Imaging (From Pediatrics to Geriatrics), Jaypee Publications, New Delhi, India, 2015, pp. 149-174.

20. Rao PS, *Neonatal Catheter Interventions*, In. Vijayalakshmi IB, (ed.), Cardiac Catheterization and Imaging (From Pediatrics to Geriatrics), Jaypee Publications, New Delhi, India, 2015, pp. 388-432.

21. Rao PS, *Percutaneous Management of Aortic Coarctation*, In. Vijayalakshmi IB, (ed.), *Cardiac Catheterization and Imaging (From Pediatrics to Geriatrics)*, Jaypee Publications, New Delhi, India, 2015, pp. 433-471.

22. Rao PS, *Stents in the Management of Vascular Obstructive Lesions Associated with Congenital Heart Disease*, In. Vijayalakshmi IB, (ed.), Cardiac Catheterization and Imaging (From Pediatrics to Geriatrics), Jaypee Publications, New Delhi, India, 2015, pp. 573-598.

23. Rao PS, *Cardiac Malposition*, In: Gupta P, Menon PSN, Ramji S, Lodha R (eds.), PG Textbook of Pediatrics, Jaypee Brothers Medical Publishers (P) Ltd., New Delhi, India, 2015, pp.1807-1816.

24. Rao PS, *Tricuspid Atresia*, In: Gupta P, Menon PSN, Ramji S, Lodha R (eds.), PG Textbook of Pediatrics, Jaypee Brothers Medical Publishers (P) Ltd., New Delhi, India, 2015, pp.1861-1870.

25. Rao PS, *Cardiac Malposition*, In: Gupta P, Menon PSN, Ramji S, Lodha R (eds.), PG Textbook of Pediatrics, 2nd edn., Jaypee Brothers Medical Publishers (P) Ltd., New Delhi, India, 2018, pp. 2134-2144.

26. Rao PS, *Tricuspid Atresia*, In: Gupta P, Menon PSN, Ramji S, Lodha R (eds.), PG Textbook of Pediatrics. 2nd edn., Jaypee Brothers Medical Publishers (P) Ltd., New Delhi, India, 2018, pp. 2189-2198.

27. Rao PS, *Tricuspid Atresia*, In. Vijayalakshmi IB, Rao PS, Chugh R. (eds.), A Comprehensive Approach to Management of Congenital Heart Diseases, 2nd edn., Jaypee Publications, New Delhi, India, 2019.

28. Balaguru D, Rao PS, *Diseases of the Tricuspid Valve (Ebstein's Anomaly, Tricuspid Stenosis and Regurgitation)*, In. Vijayalakshmi IB, Rao PS, Chugh R. (eds.), A Comprehensive Approach to Management of Congenital Heart Diseases, 2nd edn., Jaypee Publications, New Delhi, India, 2019.

29. Balaguru D, Rao PS, *Mitral Atresia*, In. Vijayalakshmi IB, Rao PS, Chugh R. (eds.), A Comprehensive Approach to Management of Congenital Heart Diseases, 2nd edn., Jaypee Publications, New Delhi, India, 2019.

30. Balaguru D, Rao PS, *Truncus Arteriosus*, In. Vijayalakshmi IB, Rao PS, Chugh R. (eds.), A Comprehensive Approach to Management of Congenital Heart Diseases, 2nd edn., Jaypee Publications, New Delhi, India, 2019.

31. Rao PS, Alapati S., *Hypoplastic Left Heart Syndrome*, In. Vijayalakshmi IB, Rao PS, Chugh R. (eds.), A Comprehensive Approach to Management of Congenital Heart Diseases, 2nd edn., Jaypee Publications, New Delhi, India, 2019.

Table II. Lectures/Presentations in India

---

1. Visiting Professor, Department of Pediatrics, Andhra Medical College, Visakhapatnam, India, September 1973. Presented "Natural History of Ventricular Septal Defects" and "Treatment of Ventricular Septal Defect."

2. Visiting Professor, Department of Pediatrics, Andhra Medical College, Visakhapatnam, India, September 1977. Presented "Cyanotic Newborn: Diagnosis and Treatment," "Differential Diagnosis of Congenital Heart Defects," and others.

3. Visiting Professor, Department of Cardiology, All India Institute of Medical Sciences (AIMS), New Delhi, India, October 1977. Presented "Natural History of Ventricular Septal Defect in Tricuspid Atresia and Its Surgical Implications."

4. Visiting Professor, Nilufur Hospital for Women and Children, Osmania University Medical School, Hyderabad, India, September 27 and 28, 1978. Presented "Diagnosis and Management of Neonates with Cyanosis" and participated in several conferences.

5. Visiting Lecturer, Indian Medical Association, Visakhapatnam Industrial Branch, Visakhapatnam, Andhra Pradesh, India, March 1983. Presented "Recent Advances in Therapy for Congenital Heart Disease."

6. Visiting Professor, Department of Pediatrics, Andhra Medical College, Visakhapatnam, Andra Pradesh, India, March 1983. Case presentations and discussion.

7. Visiting Professor, Department of Pediatrics, Osmania University Medical School and Nilufur Hospital for Women and Children, Hyderabad, India. January 24, 1984. Presented "Recent Advances in Therapy for Congenital Heart Disease."

8. Visiting Professor, Apollo Hospital, Madras, India, July 1984. Presented "Recent Advances in Therapy for Congenital Heart Disease," "Neonate with Heart Disease - Diagnosis and Management," "Systematic Approach to the Differential Diagnosis of Dextrocardia" and "Present Status of Surgery in Congenital Heart Disease."

9. Visiting Professor, Department of Pediatrics and Department of Cardiology, Kusturba Medical College, Manipal, Karnataka State, India. August 7, 1984. Presented "Recent Advances in the Therapy for Heart Disease in Infants and Children."

10. Visiting Professor, Department of Pediatrics, M.R. Medical College, Gulbarga, Karnataka State, India, June 24, 1985. Presented "Neonate with Heart Disease: Diagnosis and Management" and participated in case discussions.

11. Guest Speaker, 23rd National Conference of Pediatrics, Indian Academy of Pediatrics, New Delhi, India, November 14-16, 1986. Presented "Doppler in Noninvasive Diagnosis of Congenital Heart Disease."

12. Visiting Professor, Department of Pediatrics, M.R. Medical College, Gulbarga, Karnataka State, India, November 1986. Presented "Transcatheter Management of Heart Disease in Infancy and Childhood," and participated in case discussions.

13. Faculty Lecturer, Continuing Medical Education Program, Andhra Medical College, Visakhapatnam, Andhra Pradesh, India, December 17, 1988. Presented "Transcatheter Management of Heart Disease in Children."

14. Faculty Lecturer, International Pediatric Update, Mudurai, Madras, India, February 10-12, 1990. Presented "Doppler Echocardiography in Children with Congenital Heart Disease" and "Transcatheter Management of Heart Disease in Infants and Children."

15. Visiting Professor, Department of Pediatrics, All India Institute of Medical Science (AIMS), New Delhi, India, February 10, 1993. Presented "Diagnosis and Management of Congenital Heart Disease in the Neonate."

16. Visiting Professor, Department of Cardiology, Batra Hospital and Medical Research Center, New Delhi, India, February 11-15, 1993. Presented "Transcatheter Occlusion of Cardiac Septal Defects" and several other conferences. Also, conducted a workshop on transcatheter closure of atrial septal defects and patent ductus arteriosus.

17. Visiting Professor, Department of Cardiology, Apollo Hospital and Medical Center, Hyderabad, India, April 10-12, 1993. Presented "Role of Balloon Angioplasty/Valvuloplasty in the Treatment of Congenital Heart Defects" and "Catheter Closure of Cardiac Septal Defects" and conducted a workshop on transcatheter closure of patent ductus arteriosus and atrial septal defect.

18. Visiting Professor, Osmania General Hospital and Osmania Medical College, Hyderabad, India, April 13, 1993. Presented "Transcatheter Therapy of Congenital Heart Defects."

19. Visiting Professor, Nilufar Hospital for Women and Children, Hyderabad, India, April 13, 1993. Presented "The Role of Transcatheter Techniques in the Management of Heart Defects in Children."

20. Visiting Professor, Department of Cardiology, Nizam's Institute of Medical Sciences, Hyderabad, India, April 14, 1993. Presented "Catheter Methods in the Treatment of Heart Defects-State of the Art."

21. Faculty Lecturer, IX Annual Conference of Cardiological Society of India, New Delhi, India, August 21-22, 1993. Presented "Role of Occlusive Devices in Cardiology."

22. Visiting Professor, Department of Cardiology, All India Institute of Medical Sciences (AIMS), New Delhi, India, August 23-26, 1993. Presented several lectures, group discussions and conducted a workshop on Transcatheter Occlusion of Patent Ductus Arteriosus and Atrial Septal Defect.

23. Visiting Professor, Department of Pediatrics, All India Institute of Medical Sciences (AIMS), New Delhi, India, August 25, 1993. Presented "Transcatheter Therapy in Pediatric Heart Disease-State of the Art."

24. Visiting Professor, Department of Cardiology, G.B. Pant Hospital, New Delhi, India, August 26, 1993. Presented and lead group discussions on "Interventional Pediatric Cardiology Techniques."

25. Visiting Professor, Department of Cardiology, Sri Ramachandra Medical College, Chennai, India, November 15, 1999. Presented a lecture titled "Non-Coronary Interventional Cardiology." Also, participated in case discussions.

26. Visiting Professor, Sri Satya Sai Institute of Higher Medical Sciences, Prasanthigram, Andhra Pradesh, India, February 8-12, 2002. Presented "Transcatheter approaches in the management of interatrial septal communications," "Percutaneous occlusion of patent ductus arteriosus," "Balloon valvuloplasty/ angioplasty (Long-term results) and performed case demonstrations of transcatheter occlusion of patent ductus arteriosus and coronary arteriovenous fistula."

27. Visiting Professor and Guest Lecturer, Jayadev Institute of Cardiology, Bangalore, India, February 13-14, 2002. Presented "Stents in the management of vascular obstructive lesions associated with congenital heart defects" and "Transcatheter Management of Cardiac Defects in Children and Adults." Also, demonstrated a number of interventional pediatric cardiology techniques.

28. International Faculty, 54th Annual Conference of Cardiological Society of India, Kochi, Kerala, India, December 1-4, 2002. Chaired a session on "Technical Session: How to Do it? – Interventions in Congenital Heart Disease" and delivered a guest lecture titled "Non-Coronary Applications of Stents in Children and Adults."

29. Visiting Professor, Sri Satya Sai Institute of Higher Medical Sciences, Prasanthigram, Andhra Pradesh, India, December 5-9, 2002. Presented "Non-Coronary Applications of Stents in Children and Adults," "Catheter-Based Treatment of Heart Defects in Children and Adults," and performed case demonstrations of transcatheter occlusion of patent ductus arteriosus and atrial septal defects and stent implantation for treatment of branch pulmonary artery stenosis and aortic coarctation.

30. Visiting Professor, Andhra Medical College/King George Hospital/Indian Academy of Pediatrics, Visakhapatnam, A.P., India, December 13, 2002 and presented a lecture titled "Interventional Pediatric Cardiology – State of the Art."

31. Visiting Professor, Sri Satya Sai Institute of Higher Medical Sciences, Prasanthigram, Andhra Pradesh, India, October 17-20, 2004. Presented "Transcatheter Closure of Atrial Septal Defects and Patent Ductus Arteriosus with Amplatzer Devices," "Applications of Pediatric Interventional Technology to Adult heart Disease", and performed case demonstrations of transcatheter occlusion of patent ductus arteriosus and atrial septal defects, stent implantation for treatment of branch pulmonary artery stenosis and balloon angioplasty/valvuloplasty of aortic coarctation, aortic stenosis and tetralogy of Fallot.

32. Visiting Professor, Sri Satya Sai Institute of Higher Medical Sciences, Prasanthigram, Andhra Pradesh, India, January 26-31, 2006. Presented "Cyanotic Neonate: Diagnosis and Management," "Pediatric Cardiac Interventions, Past, Present and Future," "Acyanotic Heart Defects: Diagnosis and Treatment Approach," and performed case demonstrations of transcatheter occlusion of patent ductus arteriosus and balloon angioplasty/valvuloplasty.

33. Member of the Organizing Committee, OMICS Group 2nd International Conference on Pediatrics and Gynecology, Keynote Speaker and Session Chair, Track 3-4: Pediatric Cardiology and presented two talks titled "Noninvasive evaluation of neonates with suspected heart disease" and "Interventional pediatric cardiology – State of the art," Marriott Hotel and Convention Center, Hyderabad, India, September 24-26, 2012.

34. Guest Speaker at the 66th Annual Scientific Conference of the Cardiac Society of India, Hyderabad, December 4-7, 2014 and served as Chairman for the session on "The ubiquitous VSD" and delivered a State of the Art lecture titled "What the Adult Cardiologist Should Know About Cyanotic Congenital Heart Disease"

35. Visiting Professor, Sri Satya Sai Institute of Higher Medical Sciences, Prasanthigram, Andhra Pradesh, India, December 22-27, 2014. Presented "Acyanotic Heart Defects," "Cyanotic Heart Defects," "Pulmonary Hypertension," "Dextrocardia," "Cyanotic Neonate: Diagnosis and Management" and "Principles of Surgical Management of Congenital Heart Disease," and performed case demonstrations of transcatheter interventions of several types of congenital heart defects.

36. Orator, Dr. K. C. Chaudhuri Lifetime Achievement Award Oration at All India Institute of Medical Sciences, New Delhi, India, September 10, 2017. Title of the talk: The Journey of an Indian Pediatric Cardiologist.

Table III. Service as Editor for Seminars Organized by the Indian Journal of Pediatrics.

1. Rao PS (Guest Editor), Pediatric Cardiology Seminar, Indian Journal of Pediatrics, Vol. 55, No. 1, January-February 1988.

2. Rao PS (Guest Editor), Pediatric Cardiology Seminar, Indian Journal of Pediatrics, Vol. 58, Nos. 4 and 5, 1991.

3. Rao PS, Saxena A (Guest Editors), Pediatric Cardiology Symposium – Part I, Indian Journal of Pediatrics, Vol. 65, No. 1, January-February 1998.

4. Rao PS, Saxena A (Guest Editors), Pediatric Cardiology Symposium – Part II, Indian Journal of Pediatrics, Vol. 65, No. 2, March-April 1998.

5. Saxena A, Rao PS (Guest Editors), Symposium on Pediatric Cardiology – Part I, Indian Journal of Pediatrics, Vol. 69, No. 4, April 2002.

6. Saxena A, Rao PS (Guest Editors), Symposium on Pediatric Cardiology – Part II, Indian Journal of Pediatrics, Vol. 69, No. 5, May 2002.

7. Rao PS, Saxena A (Guest Editors), Symposium on Pediatric Cardiology - Part I, Indian Journal of Pediatrics, Vol. 72, No. 6, June 2005.

8. Rao PS, Saxena A (Guest Editors): Symposium on Pediatric Cardiology - Part II, Indian Journal of Pediatrics, Vol. 72, No. 7, July 2005.

9. Saxena A, Rao PS, Kohli V. (Guest Editors), Symposium on Advances in Cardiology - Part I, Indian Journal of Pediatrics, Vol. 76, Nos. 1, 2 and 3, January, February and March 2009.

10. Rao PS, Saxena A (Guest Editors), Symposium on Pediatric Cardiology, Indian Journal of Pediatrics, Vol. 22, Nos. 11 and 12, November and December 2015.

TEACHING

As reviewed in the "Academic Career" section above, I have actively participated in teaching trainees and practicing physicians and these activities will be reviewed in this section.

Medical Students

Beginning as a faculty member at the Medical College of Georgia, Augusta, Georgia, I presented lectures to the second and third year medical students, involved in one-to-one bed-side in-patient and out-patient clinic teaching of Junior (third year) and Senior (fourth year) medical students and served as a mentor in their research projects.

Similar active medical student teaching activities continued at the University of Wisconsin Medical School in Madison, Wisconsin, the St. Louis University School of Medicine, St. Louis, Missouri and the University of Texas at Houston Medical School, Houston, Texas. When I arrived at the University of Texas at Houston Medical School in 2002, there were no established senior medical student electives. I took active role in formally establishing a new senior medical student pediatric cardiology elective in 2003. A few years later, I also established a new junior medical student pediatric cardiology elective.

Residents

I have actively participated in teaching of pediatric and medicine-pediatric residents at the Medical College of Georgia, Augusta, Georgia; the King Faisal Specialist Hospital & Research Center, Riyadh, Saudi Arabia; the University of Wisconsin Medical School in Madison, Wisconsin; the St. Louis University School of Medicine, St. Louis, Missouri; the University of Texas at Houston Medical School, Houston, Texas. At institutions where the Pediatric Residency Program Directors were not in favor of having the pediatric residents rotating in the pediatric cardiology service during their tenure as residents, I advocated and fought for required rotation in pediatric cardiology and was successful in doing so. Though limited number of residents were interested in participating in research activities (presumably related very busy clinical service), I served as a mentor to few such residents.

Fellows

At all the four institutions mentioned above, I have actively participated in teaching the fellows; these are the physicians who are fully trained pediatricians who are interested in becoming pediatric cardiologists. At the Medical College of Georgia, Augusta, Georgia, I actively taught and guided the fellows, served as the Associate Program Director and provided mentorship for their research projects. At the King Faisal Specialist Hospital & Research Center, Riyadh, Saudi Arabia, there was no pediatric cardiology fellowship program when I arrived there. Shortly thereafter, I established an Arab Board-approved pediatric cardiology fellowship program. Recruitment of fellows and their training ensued. When I assumed Directorship of Pediatric Cardiology programs at the University of Wisconsin Medical School in Madison, Wisconsin, the St. Louis University School of Medicine, St. Louis, Missouri, and the University of Texas at Houston Medical School, Houston, Texas, there were no ACGME-accredited pediatric cardiology fellowship programs. At all these three institutions, I established interventional pediatric cardiology fellowship programs; several fellows joined the program both from abroad and from other University Medical Centers in USA. I also established ACGME-accredited pediatric cardiology fellowship program at the University of Texas at Houston Medical School, Houston, Texas with three fellows at each of first, second and third year levels. The program was very competitive with more than hundred candidates applying for three positions each year. I also established a Texas State Medical Board-approved interventional pediatric cardiology fellowship program. I provided clinical and research mentorship to all the fellows at these above four institutions; the later activity resulted in numerous publications which will be reviewed in detail in the forthcoming chapters and in the book titled, "Pediatric Cardiology: How It Has Evolved Over the last 50 Years." The fellows trained under my guidance are listed in table IV.

Table IV. Fellows trained.

1. Ow Bong Kwon, MD – 1972-1974

2. Judy J. Rigby, MD – 1974-1976

3. Mansur Salehbhai, MD – 1975-1977

4. James H. Rogers, Jr., MD – 1976-1978

5. Allen H. Rees, MD – 1977-1979

6. Tadashi Hayashidera, MD – 1978-1980

7. Mohinder K. Thapar, MD – 1977-1980

8. Carlos N. Monarrez, MD – 1979-1981

9. Timothy A. Truman, MD – 1979-1980

10. Raju J. Kulangara, MD – 1980-1982

11. Robert J. Voller, MD – 1980-1981

12. Ian C. Balfour, MD – 1980-1982

13. Saadeh B. Jureidini, MD – 1980-1982

14. Haitham N. Najjar, MD – 1983-1985

15. Subash C. Reddy, MD – 1992-1993

16. H. Y. Lee, MD – 1993-1994

17. Ghasan Siblini, MD – 1997-1998

18. Kevin Wyle, DO – 1999-2000

19. Ashraf M. Nagm, MD – 2003-2004

20. Rabbi Hamza, MD – 2004-2005

21. William Wang, MD – 2005-2006

22. Jennifer Blake, MD – 2006-2008

23. Sumeet K. Sharma – 2007-2008

24. Georgios A. Hartas, MD – 2007-2010

25. Emmanouil Tsounias, MD – 2007-2010

26. Srilatha Alapati, MD – 2008-2012

27. Henry Burkholder, MD – 2009-2012

28. Tharak R. Yarrabolu, MD – 2009-2013

29. Raj Sahu, DO – 2010-2013

30. N. C. Agu, MD – 2010-2013

31. Arpan R. Doshi, MD – 2011-2014

32. Unnati R. Doshi, MD – 2012 -2015

33. Claudeen Whitfield, MD – 2013-2014

34. Ashish Banker, DO – 2012-2015

35. Maria C. Yates, MD – 2012-2015

36. Yuliya Turiy, MD – 2012-2015

37. Elizabeth W. Wang, DO – 2013-2016

38. Durga P. Naidu, MD – 2013-2016

39. Ankur B. Shah, MD – 2013-2016

40. Christina T. Dang, MD – 2014-2017

41. Jyoti Bhatia-Barnes, MD – 2014-2017

42. Andrea Harris, MD – 2014-2017

43. Geetha Radhakrishnan, MD – 2015-2018

44. Jenna L. Aldinger, MD – 2015-2018

45. Siddharth Dubey, MD – 2015- 2018

CONTINUING MEDICAL EDUCATION

I have organized and conducted a number of continuing medical educational events throughout my career that are listed in Table V.

Table V. Continuing Medical Education

1. Organized and Chaired Round Table Session on "Tricuspid Atresia" at the Section of Cardiology, American Academy of Pediatrics, 46th Annual Scientific Session, November 4-10, 1977, New York City, New York.

2. Course Director and Co-Chairman, King Faisal Specialist Hospital and Research Center's Pediatric Symposium: Recent Advances, Riyadh, Saudi Arabia, November 30 to December 1, 1983.

3. Course Director, King Faisal Specialist Hospital and Research Center's Second Annual Pediatric Symposium: Recent Advances, Riyadh, Saudi Arabia, April 24-25, 1985.

4. Course Director, Pediatric Cardiology Symposium: Recent Advances, King Faisal Specialist Hospital and Research Centre, Riyadh, Saudi Arabia, April 21-22, 1987.

5. Course Director, Pediatric Cardiology Mini-Symposium, University of Wisconsin, School of Medicine, Madison, WI, November 12, 1988.

6. Course Director, Progress in Pediatrics: Pediatric Cardiology, University of Wisconsin Children's Hospital, Madison, WI, May 19, 1994.

7. Course Director, Pediatric Cardiology Update - 1996, Saint Louis University School of Medicine/Cardinal Glennon Children's Hospital, Ritz-Carlton, St. Louis, MO, November 1, 1996.

8. Course Director, Pediatric Cardiology for the Primary Care Physician, October 21, 2005, Hermann Pavilion Conference Center, Memorial Hermann Hospital, Houston, TX.

9. Course Director, Second Annual Pediatric Cardiology Symposium for the Primary Care Physician, October 20, 2006, Hermann Pavilion Conference Center, Memorial Hermann Hospital - TMC, Houston, TX.

10. Course Director, Third Annual Pediatric Cardiology Symposium for the Primary Care Physician, October 26, 2007, Hermann Pavilion Conference Center, Memorial Hermann Hospital - TMC, Houston, TX.

11. Course Director, Fourth Annual Pediatric Cardiology Symposium for the Primary Care Physician, October 31, 2008, Hermann Pavilion Conference Center, Memorial Hermann Hospital - TMC, Houston, TX.

12. Course Director, Fifth Annual Pediatric Cardiology Symposium for the Primary Care Physician, October 30, 2009, Hermann Pavilion Conference Center, Memorial Hermann Hospital - TMC, Houston, TX.

13. Course Director, Sixth Annual Pediatric Cardiology Symposium for the Primary Care Physician, October 29, 2010, Children's Memorial Hermann Hospital Conference Center, Memorial Hermann Hospital - TMC, Houston, TX.

14. Course Director, Seventh Annual Pediatric Cardiology Symposium for the Primary Care Physician, October 14, 2011, Children's Memorial Hermann Hospital Conference Center, Memorial Hermann Hospital - TMC, Houston, TX.

15. Course Director, Eighth Annual Pediatric Cardiology Symposium for the Primary Care Physician, November 17, 2012, Memorial Hermann Hospital Conference Center, Memorial Hermann Hospital - TMC, Houston, TX.

16. Course Director, Ninth Annual Pediatric Cardiology Symposium for the Primary Care Physician, November 2, 2013, Memorial Hermann Hospital Conference Center, Memorial Hermann Hospital - TMC, Houston, TX.

17. Course Director, Tenth Annual Pediatric Cardiology Symposium for the Primary Care Physician, October 18, 2014, Memorial Hermann Hospital Conference Center, Memorial Hermann Hospital - TMC, Houston, TX.

Teaching Physicians in India

This subject was reviewed in the preceding section on "Contributions to Education of Physicians in India."

Visiting Professorships/Lectureships

I also served as visiting professor, invited lecturer/faculty at many institutions, local, regional, national and international scientific societies in USA and aboard with the express intent of teaching/training these physicians and these are listed in Table VI.

Table VI. Visiting Professorships/Lectureships

---

1. Visiting Professorships/Lectureships at Indian institutions listed in Table II.

2. Faculty Lecturer, Georgia Heart Association, Annual Scientific Session, Atlanta, GA, September 1975. Presented "Recognition and Management of the Infants with Congenital Heart Disease."

3. Faculty Lecturer, Critical Care Seminar, University Hospital, Augusta, GA, March 1977. Presented "Introduction to Pediatric Cardiology," "Recognition and Management of Congestive Heart Failure," and "Cardiac Sounds: Theory and Practice."

4. Faculty Lecturer, Neonatal Nurse Clinician Program, Medical College of Georgia, Augusta, GA, March 1978. Presented "Congestive Heart Failure," "Patent Ductus Arteriosus," and "Neonatal Arrhythmias."

5. Visiting Professor, National Cardiovascular Center, Osaka, Japan, September 21-22, 1978. Presented "Surgical Implications of Spontaneous Closure of Ventricular Septal Defects in Tricuspid Atresia" and participated in several conferences.

6. Visiting Professor, Queen Pahlavi Cardiovascular Medical Center, Tehran, Iran, October 18-19, 1978. Presented "Fate of the Ventricular Septal Defect in Tricuspid Atresia and Its Surgical Implications."

7. Chairman, Session II, Pediatric Update - 1979. Presented by School of Medicine, Medical College of Georgia, Augusta, GA, at Kiawah Island, South Carolina, August 6-8, 1979.

8. Faculty Lecturer, Pediatric Update - 1979. Presented by School of Medicine, Medical College of Georgia, Augusta, GA, at Kiawah Island, South Carolina, August 6-8, 1979. Presented "New Therapies in Cardiology."

9. Consultant Pediatric Cardiologist and Visiting Professor, King Faisal Specialist Hospital and Research Centre, Riyadh, Saudi Arabia, July to August 1980. Presented "Treatment of Congestive Heart Failure in Infants and Children," "Recent Therapeutic Advances in Pediatric Cardiology," "Natural History of Ventricular Septal Defect," and "Interpretation of Electrocardiograms in Infants and Children" and participated in several conferences.

10. Visiting Professor, Vanderbilt University School of Medicine, Nashville, Tennessee, April 1981. Presented "Tricuspid Atresia: Classification and Natural History of the Ventricular Septal Defect."

11. Faculty Lecturer, Critical Care Medicine, Presented by School of Medicine, Medical College of Georgia, Augusta, GA, May 18-22, 1981. Presented "Acute Heart Failure in Childhood."

12. Faculty Lecturer, Critical Care Medicine, Presented by School of Medicine, Medical College of Georgia, Augusta, GA, May 18-22, 1981. Presented "The Differential Diagnosis of Cardiopulmonary Disease in Infancy and Childhood."

13. Faculty Lecturer, Pediatric Update - 1981. Presented by School of Medicine, Medical College of Georgia, Augusta, GA, Kiawah Island, South Carolina, July 27-29, 1981. Presented "The Ductus to Be or Not to Be."

14. Visiting Professor, Department of Pediatrics, Kurashiki Central Hospital, Kurashiki, Japan, August 17, 1983. Presented "Neonate with Heart Disease - Diagnosis and Management."

15. Visiting Professor, Department of Pediatrics, National Cardiovascular Center, Osaka, Japan, August 19, 1983. Presented "Tricuspid Atresia - Selected Aspects."

16. Co-Chairman, Session III, King Faisal Specialist Hospital and Research Center's Pediatric Symposium: Recent Advances, Riyadh, Saudi Arabia, November 30-December 1, 1983.

17. Moderator, Panel Discussion, King Faisal Specialist Hospital and Research Center's Pediatric Symposium: Recent Advances, Riyadh, Saudi Arabia, November 30-December 1, 1983.

18. Faculty Lecturer and Moderator, Simultaneous Group Session titled "Cardiac Emergencies in Pediatric Practice'" at the King Faisal Specialist Hospital and Research Center's Pediatric Symposium: Recent Advances, Riyadh, Saudi Arabia.

19. Faculty Lecturer, International Symposium: Heart Disease in Neonates and Children, Presented by Riyadh Armed Forces Hospital, Riyadh, Saudi Arabia, November 27-28, 1984. Presented "Pulmonary Stenosis and Atresia with Intact Septum: Current Management."

20. Faculty Lecturer, King Faisal Specialist Hospital and Research Center's Second Annual Pediatric Symposium: Recent Advances, Riyadh, Saudi Arabia, April 24-25, 1985. Presented "Transcatheter Management of Heart Disease in Children."

21. Moderator, Panel Discussion, King Faisal Specialist Hospital and Research Center's Second Annual Pediatric Symposium: Recent Advances, Riyadh, Saudi Arabia, April 24-25, 1985.

22. Faculty Lecturer, King Fahd Hospital at Al Baha and Ministry of Health Symposium "Cardiology in the Kingdom," Al Baha, Saudi Arabia, May 11-14, 1985. Presented "Diagnostic Approach to a Pediatric Cardiac Patient" and "Cardiac Disease in the Neonate."

23. Faculty Lecturer, Riyadh Cardiology Technologists Association's Educational Seminar, Riyadh, Saudi Arabia, July 12, 1985. Presented "Introduction to Pediatric Cardiology."

24. Visiting Professor, Department of Pediatrics & Likoff Cardiovascular Institute, Hanneman Medical College, Philadelphia, PA, October 1985. Presented "Diagnosis and Management of the Neonate with Heart Disease."

25. Visiting Professor, Department of Pediatrics, Medical College of Georgia, Augusta, Georgia, October 1985. Presented Pediatric Grant Rounds, "Transcatheter Management of Heart Disease in Infancy and Childhood."

26. Faculty Lecturer, MRCP, Part II (Pediatrics) Course, College of Medicine, King Saud University, Riyadh, Saudi Arabia, February 28 to March 11, 1987.

27. Guest Speaker, Symposium on New Modalities in the Management of Myocardiopathy, Sponsored by Joint Board of Postgraduate Medical Education and King Faisal Specialist Hospital and Research Centre, Riyadh, Saudi Arabia, April 19-20, 1987. Presented "Cardiomyopathy in the Pediatric Age Group" and "Vasodilators in Cardiomyopathy in the Pediatric Age Group."

28. Member, Panel Discussion, Session VI, Dilated Cardiomyopathy, Symposium on New Modalities in the Management of Myocardiopathy, Joint Board of Postgraduate Medical Education, Riyadh, Saudi Arabia, April 19-20, 1987.

29. Faculty Lecturer, Pediatric Cardiology Symposium: Recent Advances, King Faisal Specialist Hospital and Research Centre, Riyadh Saudi Arabia, April 21-22, 1987. Presented "Transcatheter Management of Heart Disease in Children," "Selected Aspects of Tricuspid Atresia," "Pulmonary Atresia with Intact Ventricular Septum" and "Doppler Echocardiography in Congenital Heart Disease."

30. Moderator, Session on Pulmonary Atresia, Pediatric Cardiology Symposium: Recent Advances, King Faisal Specialist Hospital and Research Centre, Riyadh, Saudi Arabia, April 21-22, 1987.

31. Chairman and Discussant, Round Table Session on Evaluation of Cardiac Murmurs, Pediatric Cardiology Symposium: Recent Advances, King Faisal Specialist Hospital and Research Center, Riyadh, Saudi Arabia, April 21-22, 1987.

32. Faculty Lecturer, Riyadh Cardiology Technologists Association's Seminar on Pediatric Cardiology, Riyadh, Saudi Arabia, June 19, 1987. Presented "Interventional Techniques for Congenital Heart Disease."

33. Faculty Lecturer, Update in Medicine, Oakland University, Rochester, Michigan, July 2, 1988. Presented "Transcatheter Management of Heart Disease in Children."

34. Faculty Lecturer, University of Wisconsin-Madison, Continuing Medical Education's 1988-1989 Teleconferences for MD's in Wisconsin. Presented "Congestive Heart Failure in Infants and Children - Causes and Management," September 13, 1988.

35. Visiting Professor, Department of Pediatrics, The University of Texas Medical School at Houston, Houston, Texas, September 29, 1988. Presented Pediatric Grand Rounds titled "Pediatric Catheter Interventions."

36. Moderator, Session on Pediatric Intervention on September 30, 1988 at Texas Heart Institute's Symposium on Cardiology and Cardiovascular Surgery: Interventions, 1988 at Houston, Texas, September 28 to October 1, 1988.

37. Faculty Lecturer, University of Wisconsin-Madison, Continuing Medical Education's 1988-1989 Teleconferences for MD's in Wisconsin. Presented "Congestive Heart Failure in Infants and Children - Causes and Management," September 13, 1988.

38. Speaker, Health Matters Series, October to December 1988, University of Wisconsin Hospital and Clinics, Madison, Wisconsin. Presented "Pediatric Cardiology: Early Diagnosis and Treatment of Heart Defects in Children" on October 11, 1988.

39. Moderator, Cardiovascular Session II, MSPR/AFCR/CSCR Annual Meeting in Chicago, IL, November 8-10, 1989.

40. Visiting Professor, Division of Pediatric Cardiology, Department of Pediatrics, University of Iowa Hospitals, Iowa City, IA, January 18, 1990. Presented "Balloon Valvuloplasty/Angioplasty in Infants, Children and Adolescents."

41. Faculty Lecturer, 3rd Annual Scientific Session of the Saudi Heart Association, Jeddah, Saudi Arabia, February 20-22, 1990. Presented "Balloon Valvuloplasty and Angioplasty for Congenital and Acquired Heart Defects in Children."

42. Faculty Lecturer, 39th Annual Scientific Session of the American College of Cardiology, Presented "Should Balloon Angioplasty be Used Instead of Surgery for Native Coarctation" at a Symposium on Controversies in Pediatric Cardiology, New Orleans, LA, March 18-22, 1990.

43. Chairman, Session on Interventional Cardiology, Midwest Pediatric Cardiology Society Meeting, St. Louis, Missouri, September 13-14, 1990.

44. Faculty Lecturer, Seminars in Pediatrics, Madison, Wisconsin, October 26-27, 1990. Presented "Non-Surgical Correction of Congenital Heart Defects."

45. Visiting Professor, Department of Pediatrics and Department of Medicine, Facultad de Ciencias Medicas, Universidad Nacional Autonomia de Nicaragua, Leon, Nicaragua, December 1-8, 1990.

Presented "Neonate with Cyanosis: Diagnosis and Management," "Transcatheter Management of Heart Defects," "Evaluation of Cardiac Murmurs," and "Cardiac Emergencies in Pediatric Practice."

46. Faculty Lecturer, Specialty Review in Neonatology/Perinatology, Cook County Graduate School of Medicine, Chicago, Illinois, August 12-17, 1991. Presented "Diagnosis of Congenital Heart Disease," "Neonatal Echocardiography" and "Operative and Transcatheter Treatment of Congenital Heart Disease."

47. Visiting Professor, Department of Pediatrics, Valley Children's Hospital, Fresno, California, November 15, 1991. Presented "Transcatheter Management of Congenital Heart Disease."

48. Visiting Professor, Division of Pediatric Cardiology, Department of Pediatrics. Indiana University Medical Center, Riley Children's Hospital, Indianapolis, Indiana, January 16-17, 1992. Presented "Balloon Angioplasty of Aortic Coarctation" and participated in several conferences.

49. Visiting Professor, Institute "Dante Pazzanese" de Cardiologia, Sao Paulo, Brazil, June 17, 1992. Presented "Balloon Angioplasty and Valvuloplasty in the Treatment of Congenital Heart Defects in Children," and participated in several case discussions.

50. Faculty Lecturer, XIV Brazilian Angiography Congress, Sao Paulo, Brazil, June 18-20, 1992. Presented "Interventional Cardiology in Congenital Heart Disease" and "Practical Aspects of Interventional Procedures in Congenital Heart Disease" and participated in Panel Discussions.

51. Visiting Professor, Department of Pediatrics, Gothenburg University and East Hospital, Gothenburg, Sweden, October 15-16, 1992. Presented "Emergencies in Pediatric Cardiology" at their post-graduate training course and participated in several case discussions.

52. Faculty Lecturer, Swedish Pediatric Association's Scientific Session, Gothenburg, Sweden, October 17, 1992. Presented John Lind's lecture on "Interventional Pediatric Cardiology-State of the Art."

53. Visiting Lecturer, Department of Pediatrics, UCLA/Harbor Medical Center, Torrance, CA, July 27, 1993. Presented Pediatric Critical Care Conference on "Transcatheter Management of Congenital Heart Defects."

54. Visiting Lecturer, Division of Pediatric Cardiology, UCLA School of Medicine, Los Angeles, CA, July 27, 1993. Presented a lecture titled "Balloon Angioplasty of Native Coarctation."

55. Visiting Lecturer, Department of Pediatrics, St. Louis University School of Medicine/Cardinal Glennon Children's Hospital, St. Louis, MO, February 18, 1994. Presented "Transcatheter Management of Heart Defects in Infants and Children."

56. Faculty Lecturer, Clinical Cardiology Symposium, Oshkosh Hilton and Convention Center, Oshkosh, WI, April 14, 1994. Presented "Transcatheter Treatment of Heart Defects in Children."

57. Faculty Lecturer and Course Director, Progress in Pediatrics: Pediatric Cardiology, University of Wisconsin Children's Hospital, Madison, WI, May 19, 1994. Presented "Decade of Advances in the

Transcatheter Management of Cardiac Defects in Children," "Evaluation of Cardiac Murmurs in Children," and "Arrhythmias."

58. Faculty Lecturer, Neonatal, Perinatal Pediatric Progress – 1994, St. Luke's Hospital, Racine, WI, May 21, 1994. Presented "Transcatheter Management of Congenital Heart Disease."

59. Faculty Lecturer at a Symposium on Interventional Techniques in Pediatric Cardiology at Joint XIIth World Congress of Cardiology and XVIth Congress of the European Society of Cardiology, Berlin, Germany, September 10-16, 1994 and delivered a lecture titled "Balloon Dilatation of Native Coarctations: Long-term Follow-up."

60. Visiting Professor, Department of Pediatrics/Division of Pediatric Cardiology, University of Alberta Hospitals/Walter C. Mackenzie Health Sciences Center, Edmonton, Alberta, Canada, October 26, 1994, and delivered a Special Guest Lecture titled "Transcatheter Therapy in Pediatric Cardiology."

61. Faculty Lecturer/Panelist at Workshop titled "Interventional Cardiology for Congenital Heart Disease" at the 47th Annual Meeting of the Canadian Cardiovascular Society, October 25-29, 1994, and presented "Treatment of Coarctation of the Aorta" and participated in panel discussion.

62. Faculty Lecturer, Cardinal Glennon Children's Hospital's Continuing Medical Education Series, Frontenac Hilton, St. Louis, MO, January 16, 1995. Presented "Evaluation of Cardiac Murmurs in Children: The Role of Current Technology in Diagnosis and Management."

63. Co-Chairman, Meet-The-Expert session titled "Percutaneous Closure of Interatrial Septal Communications" at the American College of Cardiology, 44th Annual Scientific Session, New Orleans, LA, March 19-22, 1995.

64. Visiting Professor, Department of Pediatrics/Division of Pediatric Cardiology, University of Miami/ Jackson Memorial Medical Center/Children's Hospital Center, Miami, FL, April 24-26, 1995, and presented: (1) Pediatric Grand Rounds titled "Recent Advances in Transcatheter Therapy in Pediatric Cardiology," (2) "Practical Issues Related to Atrial Septal Defect Closure," and (3) "Device Closure of Cardiac Septal Defects."

65. Visiting Professor, Department of Pediatrics/Division of Pediatric Cardiology, Children's Hospital, University of Helsinki, Helsinki, Finland, June 12-14, 1995. Delivered a lecture titled "Transcatheter Management of Heart Defects in Children" and conducted a workshop on transcatheter closure of atrial septal defects and implantation of stents.

66. Visiting Professor, Department of Cardiology, Green Lane Hospital, Auckland, New Zealand, July 31 to August 3, 1995, and presented a lecture titled "Transcatheter Closure of Cardiac Septal Defects with Buttoned Devices" and conducted workshop on Transcatheter Occlusion of Atrial Septal Defect and Patent Ductus Arteriosus.

67. Guest Speaker at Royal Children's Hospital's 1995 Cardiac Symposium, Melbourne, Australia, August 10, 1995, and gave a lecture titled "Device Closure of Cardiac Septal Defects."

68. Visiting Professor, Royal Children's Hospital, Melbourne, Australia, August 11, 1995, and participated in case discussions and conducted practical demonstration of implantation of stents.

69. Faculty Lecturer, Cardinal Glennon Children's Hospital: Continuing Medical Education Series, Frontenac Hilton, St. Louis, MO, January 11, 1996. Presented "Early Intervention in Heart Disease in Children."

70. Faculty Lecturer, St. John's Regional Health Center Continuing Medical Education Series, Springfield, MO, January 1996. Presented "Transcatheter Therapy in Neonates, Infants and Children."

71. Principal Guest Speaker, 7th Annual Meeting of the Japan Pediatric Interventional Cardiology Society, Tokyo, Japan, January 19-20, 1996. The major lectures given include "Should Balloon Angioplasty Be Used as a Treatment of Choice of Native Aortic Coarctation" and "Transcatheter Occlusion of Atrial Septal Defects." Also, presented, "Transcatheter Closure of Patent Ductus Arteriosus - The Buttoned Device Experience" and "Balloon Dilatation of Right and Left Ventricular Outflow Tract Obstructions - Where do we Need Surgeons?" during the symposia.

72. Faculty Lecturer, Good Samaritan Hospital Continuing Medical Education Series, Ramada Inn, Mount Vernon, IL, April 1996. Presented "Evaluation of Cardiac Murmurs in Children."

73. Faculty Lecturer, Cardinal Glennon Children's Hospital's Continuing Medical Education Series, Bogey Hills Country Club, St. Charles, MO, April 18, 1996. Presented "Recent Advances in the Treatment of Heart Disease in Children."

74. Moderator, Morning Session, Pediatric Cardiology Update - 1996, Ritz-Carlton, St. Louis, MO, November 1, 1996.

75. Faculty Lecturer, Pediatric Cardiology Update - 1996, Ritz-Carlton, St. Louis, MO, November 1, 1996. Presented "Evaluation of Cardiac Murmur in Children" and "Non-Surgical (Transcatheter) Management of Heart Defects in Children: State of the Art."

76. Visiting Professor, National Cardiovascular Center, Osaka, Japan, January 22, 1996. Presented a lecture titled "Transcatheter Occlusion of Cardiac Septal Defects in Children."

77. Faculty Lecturer, Good Samaritan Hospital Continuing Medical Education Series, Ramada Inn, Mount Vernon, IL, April 1996. Presented "Evaluation of Cardiac Murmurs in Children."

78. Chairman, Abstract Session on Catheter Intervention on May 14, 1997 at the 2nd World Congress of Pediatric Cardiology and Cardiac Surgery, May 11-15, 1997, Honolulu, Hawaii.

79. Guest Speaker and Course Director, Transcatheter Devices for Congenital Heart Disease 1997, Minneapolis, MN, August 6-8, 1997. Served as a Co-Chairman for the following sessions:

    a. Intracardiac Occlusion Devices: Session I - ASD Occlusion Devices,

    b. Intracardiac Occlusion Devices: Session II - VSD Occlusion Devices,

    c. Balloon Technology in Congenital Heart Disease, and

d. Interactive Dynamic Case Illustrations.

80. Presented "The Buttoned ASD Device," "The Buttoned Devices for VSDs," "The Buttoned PDA Occluder: Technique and Results" and "Balloon Angioplasty of Native Aortic Coarctation Should Replace Surgical Correction."

   a. Course faculty, The Inaugural New England Pediatric Interventional Cardiac Symposium, Boston, MA.

   b. Live case demonstrations.

   c. Guest Lecturer: Balloon Valvuloplasty.

   d. Guest Lecturer: Buttoned Device ASD Closure.

81. Guest Lecturer, SSM Cardinal Glennon Children's Hospital's Physician Recognition Program, October 9-10, 1997. Presented "Transcatheter Closure of the Congenital Heart Defects."

82. Guest Speaker, The 25th Annual Scientific Meeting of the Egyptian Society of Cardiology, Cairo, Egypt, February 22-27, 1998. Delivered the following lectures: "State of the Art Lecture on Interventional Pediatric Cardiology: Long Term Results of Balloon Dilatation of Coarctation of the Aorta," "Aortic Stenosis" and "Pulmonary Stenosis and Transcatheter Occlusion of Atrial Septal Defects."

83. Continuing Medical Education Program of St. Mary's Hospital, Jefferson City, Missouri, March 24, 1998. Presented "Evaluation of Cardiac Murmurs in Children: The Role of Current Technology in the Diagnosis and Management."

84. Course faculty, Pediatric Interventional Cardiac Symposium II, Boston, MA, August 30-September 2, 1998 and participated as follows:

   Guest lecture 1: "Coarctation of the Aorta in Older Children: Balloon Angioplasty is the Preferred Method."

   Guest lecture 2: "Buttoned Device for Septal Repair. Transcatheter Closure of Ostium Secundum Atrial Septal Defects with 4th Generation Buttoned Device."

   Guest lecture 3: "Transcatheter Buttoned Device Occlusion of Patent Ductus Arteriosus and Panelist for live case demonstrations."

85. Visiting Professor, Department of Physiology, St. George's University Medical School, Grenada, West Indies, October 1998 and participated in Laboratory demonstration of blood pressure regulation. Also, delivered the following lectures:

   "Transcatheter Management Cardiac Defects in Children," and

   "Perinatal Circulatory Physiology: It's Role in Clinical Manifestations of Heart Disease in the Neonate."

86. Guest Speaker, Cardiology at the Bix, Davenport, Iowa, July 30, 1999. Presented "Applications of Pediatric Interventional Technology to Adult Disease."

87. Visiting Lecturer, Department of Anesthesiology, Washington University School of Medicine/Barnes-Jewish Hospital, St. Louis, MO, September 1, 1999. Presented Anesthesiology Grand rounds titled "Catheter-based Therapy of Heart Defects in Children."

88. Guest Faculty, The Third Pediatric Interventional Cardiac Symposium (PICS-III), Chicago, IL, September 7-10, 1999, Sponsored by the University of Chicago Children's Hospital and the Pritzker School of Medicine, Chicago. Participated as follows:

    Panelist: Live Case Demonstration

    Lecture: "ASD Devices – The Buttoned Device: Late Follow-up."

    Lecture: "PDA Devices – PDA Buttoned Device: Late Results."

89. Guest Speaker, The Fifth International Conference of the Jordanian Cardiac Society, Amman, Jordan, April 19-22, 2000. Presented the following lectures:

    "Role of Stents in the Management of Heart Defects in Children,"

    "Application of Pediatric Interventional Technology to Adult Disease," and

    "Transcatheter Management of Aortic Coarctation."

90. Visiting Professor, Louisiana State University Medical School/Children's Hospital, New Orleans, LA. June 1 and June 2, 2000. Participated in case discussions and demonstration of transcatheter closure of atrial septal defects.

91. Guest Faculty, The Fourth Pediatric Interventional Cardiac Symposium (PICS-IV), Chicago, IL, September 24-27, 2000. Sponsored by the University of Chicago Hospital and New York Columbia Presbyterian Hospital. Participated as follows:

    Nightmare Case Presentation

    Lecture: "COD Buttoned Device for ASD Closure."

    Panelist: Live Case Demonstrations (9/27/00)

    Lecture: "PDA Devices," and "Sideris' Buttoned Device."

92. Faculty, The Fifth Pediatric Interventional Cardiac Symposium (PICS-V), Toronto, Canada, May 22-25, 2001. Sponsored by the University of Chicago Children's Hospital, Chicago, IL, Columbia Presbyterian Hospital, New York, NY and The Hospital for Sick Children, Toronto, Canada. Participation is as follows:

    Poster Session With Masters: Catheter Closure of Secundum Atrial Septal Defects with Centering-on-Demand Device.

    Panelist: Live Case Demonstration (5/23/01)

Lecture: "Balloon Valvuloplasty: What is New and Long-term Results?"

93. Chairman, Moderated Poster Session, 3rd World Congress of Pediatric Cardiology & Cardiac Surgery, May 27-31, 2001, Toronto, Canada.

94. Faculty Lecturer, 15th Annual Scientific Session of the Association of Black Cardiologists, Sheraton Atlanta Hotel, Atlanta, GA, March 16, 2002. Presented "Transcatheter Management of Congenital Heart Lesions in Children and Adults."

95. Faculty Lecturer, 51st Annual Scientific Session of the American College of Cardiology, Atlanta, GA, March 16-20, 2002. Presented "Buttoned Device Closure of Atrial Septal Defects" in a Symposium on New Methods of ASD Closure.

96. Faculty, The Sixth Pediatric Interventional Cardiac Symposium (PICS-VI), The Chicago Marriott Downtown Hotel, Chicago, IL, September 22-25, 2002. Chaired Moderated Poster Session on September 22, 2002 and Platform Abstract Session on September 25, 2002.

97. Invited Faculty, Concepts in Contemporary Cardiology, Inter-Continental Hotel, Houston, Texas, October 23-26, 2002. Presented live case demonstration of transcatheter occlusion of patent ductus arteriosus.

98. Invited Faculty, 26th Annual Scientific Sessions of the Society of Cardiac Angiography and Interventions, Westin Copley Place, Boston, MA, May 7-10, 2003. Presented "Advanced Interventional Procedures in Congenital Heart Disease - Valvuloplasty Techniques".

99. Visiting Professor, St. Luke's Hospital/Baylor College of Medicine/Texas Heart Institute, Houston, Texas, July 11, 2003. Presented "The Art and Science of Balloon Angioplasty/Valvuloplasty in Congenital Heart Disease" and "Applications of Pediatric Interventional Technology to Adult Heart Disease" and participated in case discussions.

100. Faculty, The Seventh Pediatric Interventional Cardiac Symposium (PICS-VII), Orlando, Florida, September 21-24, 2003. Sponsored by the University of Chicago Children's Hospital, Chicago, IL. Participation is as follows:

    Chairman, Abstract Session, September 21, 2003

    Panelist: Live Case Demonstration, September 22, 2003

101. Invited Faculty, 27th Annual Scientific Sessions of the Society of Cardiac Angiography and Interventions. San Diego, CA, April 2-May 1, 2004. Moderator, Scientific Abstract Session, April 30, 2004.

102. Visiting Professor, Department of Pediatrics, University of Texas Medical Branch, Galveston, Texas, presented Pediatric Grand Rounds titled "Interventional Pediatric Cardiology – State of the Art," May 14, 2004.

103. Visiting Professor, Department of Pediatrics, University of Texas Medical Branch, Galveston, Texas, presented Pediatric Grand Rounds titled "Cyanotic Neonate: Diagnosis and Management," September 10, 2004.

104. Faculty, The Eighth Pediatric Interventional Cardiac Symposium (PICS-VIII), The Chicago Marriott Downtown Hotel, Chicago, IL, September 19-22, 2004. Chaired Abstract Session on September 19, 2004 and Luncheon Session titled "Everything You Need to Know About Stents" on September 20, 2004.

105. Invited Faculty, Concepts in Contemporary Cardiology, George R. Brown Convention Center, Houston, Texas, April 14-16, 2005. Served as Panelist for the session titled "Management of the Failing Heart" and Live case demonstrations and Moderator of interesting case presentation session of "The Agony of Defeat vs. The Ecstasy of Unsuspected Success," both on April 15, 2005.

106. Visiting Professor, Tufts University, New England Medical Center, Boston, MA, delivered Kreidberg's Lecture titled "Pediatric Cardiac Interventions: Past, Present and Future," May 18, 2005. Also, participated in case presentations and discussions.

107. Faculty, The Ninth Pediatric Interventional Cardiac Symposium (PICS-IX) and Emerging New Technologies in Congenital Heart Surgery (ENTICHS) - 2005, The Hilton Buenos Aires, Buenos Aires, Argentina, September 15-18, 2005. Chaired Meet the Experts session on September 15, 2005.

108. Program Faculty and Course Director, Pediatric Cardiology for the Primary Care Physician, October 21, 2005, Hermann Pavilion Conference Center, Memorial Hermann Hospital, Houston, TX. Served as a Moderator for the Morning Session and presented "Evaluation of Cardiac Murmur in Children" and "Non-Surgical (Transcatheter) Management of Heart Defects in Children: State of the Art."

109. Invited Faculty, Concepts in Contemporary Cardiology, Omni Houston Hotel, Houston, Texas, April 20-22, 2006. Served as Panelist for the session titled "Congenital Heart Disease in the Adult" and presented "When and how should atrial septal defects be closed in adults" and "ASD Closure and coarctation of the aorta" on April 20 and April 21, 2006, respectively.

110. Faculty, The Tenth Pediatric Interventional Cardiac Symposium (PICS-X) and Emerging New Technologies in Congenital Heart Surgery (ENTICHS) - 2006, The Bellagio, Las Vegas, NV, September 10-13, 2006. Chaired the Abstract session on September 10, 2006 and served as Panelist: Live Case Demonstration, September 13, 2006.

111. Program Faculty and Course Director, Second Annual Pediatric Cardiology Symposium for the Primary Care Physician, October 20, 2006, Hermann Pavilion Conference Center, Memorial Hermann Hospital, Houston, TX. Served as a Moderator for the Morning Session and presented "Prevention of Sudden Death in Athletes," "The Cyanotic Neonate: Diagnosis and Management" and "Principles of Surgical Management of Congenital Heart Defects."

112. Invited Faculty, Concepts in Contemporary Cardiology, George R. Brown Convention Center, Houston, Texas, April 18-21, 2007 and presented "Percutaneous Closure of PDA and Coronary AV Fistulae" on Friday April 20, 2007.

113. Faculty, Eleventh Pediatric Interventional Cardiac Symposium (PICS-X) and Emerging New Technologies in Congenital Heart Surgery (ENTICHS) - 2007, The Bellagio, Las Vegas, NV, July 22-25, 2007. Chaired the Abstract session on July 22, 2007.

114. Program Faculty and Course Director, Third Annual Pediatric Cardiology Symposium for the Primary Care Physician, October 26, 2007, Hermann Pavilion Conference Center, Memorial Hermann Hospital, Houston, TX. Served as a Moderator for the Morning Session and presented "Evaluation of Cardiac Murmur in Children," "Prevention of Sudden Death in Athletes."

115. Invited Faculty, Concepts in Contemporary Cardiology, Hilton of America Hotel, Houston, Texas, April 06-09, 2008. Presented a lecture entitled "What interventionalist should know about congenital heart disease" on April 08, 2008.

116. Program Faculty and Course Director, Fourth Annual Pediatric Cardiology Symposium for the Primary Care Physician, October 31, 2008, Hermann Pavilion Conference Center, Memorial Hermann Hospital, Houston, TX. Served as a Moderator for the Morning Session and presented "Evaluation of Cardiac Murmur in Children," "The Cyanotic Neonate: Diagnosis and Management" and "Echocardiography for the Primary Care Physician."

117. Invited Faculty, Concepts in Contemporary Cardiology, Hilton of America Hotel, Houston, Texas, April 14-17, 2009. Presented a lecture titled "What interventionalist should know about congenital heart disease" on April 16, 2009.

118. Program Faculty and Course Director, Fifth Annual Pediatric Cardiology Symposium for the Primary Care Physician, October 30, 2009, Hermann Pavilion Conference Center, Memorial Hermann Hospital, Houston, TX. Served as a Moderator for the Morning Session and presented "Evaluation of Cardiac Murmur in Children."

119. Invited Faculty, Concepts in Contemporary Cardiology, Hilton of America Hotel, Houston, Texas, April 2010.

120. Program Faculty and Course Director, Sixth Annual Pediatric Cardiology Symposium for the Primary Care Physician, October 29, 2010, Hermann Pavilion Conference Center, Memorial Hermann Hospital, Houston, TX. Served as a Moderator for the Morning Session and presented "Prevention of Sudden Death in Athletes."

121. Program Faculty and Course Director, Seventh Annual Pediatric Cardiology Symposium for the Primary Care Physician, October 14, 2011, Hermann Pavilion Conference Center, Memorial Hermann Hospital, Houston, TX. Served as a Moderator for the Afternoon Session and presented "Evaluation of Cardiac Murmur in Children."

122. Invited Faculty, CME Program, 12th American Telugu Association Conference and Youth Convention, Georgia World Congress Center, Atlanta, Georgia, July 6-8, 2012 and presented a talk titled "What the Practicing Physician Should Know About Congenital Heart Disease."

123. Program Faculty and Course Director, Eighth Annual Pediatric Cardiology Symposium for the Primary Care Physician, November 17, 2012, Hermann Pavilion Conference Center, Memorial Hermann Hospital, Houston, TX. Served as a Moderator for the Afternoon Session and presented "Evaluation of Cardiac Murmur in Children" and "Prevention of Sudden Death in Athletes."

124. Program Faculty and Course Director, Ninth Annual Pediatric Cardiology Symposium for the Primary Care Physician, November 2, 2013, Hermann Pavilion Conference Center, Memorial Hermann Hospital, Houston, TX. Served as a Moderator for the Afternoon Session and presented "Evaluation of Cardiac Murmur in Children" and "Cyanotic Neonate."

125. Program Faculty and Course Director, Tenth Annual Pediatric Cardiology Symposium for the Primary Care Physician, October 18, 2014, Hermann Pavilion Conference Center, Memorial Hermann Hospital, Houston, TX. Served as a Moderator for the Afternoon Session and presented "Evaluation of Cardiac Murmur in Children" and "Prevention of Sudden Death in Athletes."

LEADERSHIP ROLES

The author is the eldest of nine children of his parents and eldest grandson of more than fifty grandchildren of his grandparents. Consequently, he had a leadership role in addressing family issues and indeed was helpful financially or otherwise to those in need. As mentioned in the "College, Medical School, and DCH" section of Chapter 1, the author failed to get elected as class representative while in medical school, but achieved leadership role as President of the House Surgeon's Association and formed state-wide House Surgeon's Association and became its President. Also, while in the medical school, as detailed in "Extracurricular Activities" section of this chapter, I served leadership role for the entire Navy Medical NCC wing by being its Cadet Captain and Senior Cadet Captain. The leadership role continued as an NCC Officer during House-Surgeoncy and DCH. In early 1970s, I was founding Vice-President and subsequently President of the Indian Association of Greater Augusta and Hindu Temple Society of Augusta. I also served as Associate Director of Pediatric Cardiology and Director of Pediatric Cardiac Catheterization Laboratory during late 1970s. Service as Associate Chief of Staff for Inpatient Affairs, Chairman of the Department of Pediatrics and Chairman of several important Committees at the King Faisal Hospital and Research Center, Riyadh, Saudi Arabia attests to my leadership roles. After returning to USA, I served as Director, Division of Pediatric Cardiology at University of Wisconsin Medical School, Madison, Wisconsin, St. Louis University School of Medicine, St. Louis, Missouri, and University of Texas McGovern Medical School, Houston, Texas. Additional leadership roles include serving as the Director of Pediatric Cardiology and Interventional Pediatric Cardiology fellowship programs at several of the above Universities.

REFERENCES

1. Rao PS, "Congenital pulmonary cyst," *Amer J Dis Child* 1970; 119:341-2.

2. Rao PS, "Late respiratory distress in a premature infant," *Chest 1970*; 57:495-6. Available at https://doi.org/10.1378/chest.57.5.495

3. Rao PS, Patel JK, "Fever, vomiting and dome shaped density in right thorax," *Chest 1970*; 58:89-90. Available at https://doi.org/10.1378/chest.58.1.89

4. Rao PS, Alva J, Lipow HW, "Foreign body (peanut) in the left main stem bronchus," *Amer J Dis Child 1970*; 120:51-2.

5. Rao PS, Molthan ME, Lipow HW, "Cor pulmonale as a complication of ventriculoatrial shunts," *J Neurosurg 1970*; 33:221-5.

6. Rao PS, "Physiological basis of diuretic drugs," *J Indian Med Ass*, 56:100-107, 1971.

7. Rao PS, Lipow HW, "Growth retardation in steroid dependent asthma - Management by corticotrophin (ACTH)," *Clin Pediat 1972*; 11:93-7.

8. Rao PS, Molthan ME, "Systemic venous anomalies and partial heterotaxia with normal heart," *Amer J Dis Child* 1973; 125:749-52.

9. Rao PS, Sissman NJ, "Spontaneous closure of physiologically advantageous ventricular septal defects," *Circulation 1971*; 43:83-90.

10. Rao PS, Sissman NJ, "The relationship of pulmonary venous wedge to pulmonary arterial pressures," *Circulation 1971*; 44:565-74.

11. Rao PS, Sissman NJ, "Congenital heart disease in the de Lange syndrome," *J Pediatr 1971*; 79:674-7.

12. Rao PS, "Left ventricular obstruction in double outlet right ventricle (Letter)," *Amer Heart J 1972*; 83:389-90.

13. Rao PS, "The femoral route for cardiac catheterization in infants and children," *Chest 1973*; 63:239-41.

14. Rao PS, Sissman NJ, "The significance of pulmonary venous wedge pressure, Proceedings of the XIII International Congress of Pediatrics," Wien, Osterreich, August 29-September 4, 1971, Vol. IX, *Cardiology and Pneumology*, pp. 55-60.

15. Rao PS, "Physiologically advantageous ventricular septal defects and their spontaneous closure," *Abstracts of the VI World Congress of Cardiology*, September 1974, Buenos Aires, Argentina, p. 396.

16. Liebman J, Lee MH, Rao PS and Mackay W, "Quantitation of the normal Frank and McFee Parungao orthogonal electrocardiogram in the adolescent," *Circulation 1973*; 48:735-52.

17. Rao PS, Linde LM, Liebman J, and Perrin E, "Functional closure of physiologically advantageous ventricular septal defects: Observations in three cases with tricuspid atresia," *Amer J Dis Child 1974*; 127:36-40.

18. Rao PS, Silbert DR, "Superior vena caval obstruction in total anomalous pulmonary venous return," *Brit Heart J 1974*; 36:228-32.

19. Rao PS, Liebman J, Borkat G., "Right ventricular growth in a case of pulmonic stenosis with intact ventricular septum and hypoplastic right ventricle," *Circulation 1976*; 53:389-94.

20. Rao PS, Awa S, Linde LM, "Role of kinetic energy in pulmonary valvar pressure gradients," *Circulation 1973*; 48:65-73.

21. Linde LM, Rao PS, "A modern view of infective endocarditis," *Cardiovasc Clinics 1973*; Vol. 5, No. 2:15-34.

22. Rao PS, Jue KL, Isabel-Jones J, Ruttenberg HD, "Ebstein's malformation of the tricuspid valve with atresia," *Amer J Cardiol 1973*; 32:1004-9.

23. Vincent WR, Rao PS, "Early identification of the neonate with suspected serious heart disease," *Paediatrician 1973*; 2:239-50.

24. Rao PS, Linde LM, "Pressure and energy in cardiovascular chambers," *Chest 1974*; 66:176-8.

25. Rao PS, "Imperforate Ebstein's anomaly of the tricuspid valve (Letter)," *Brit Heart J 1976*; 38:1108.

26. Rao PS, "Valve gradients and kinetic energy, Presented at the Southeastern Pediatric Cardiology Society," Fifth Annual Meeting, Williamsburg, Virginia, September 15-16, 1972.

27. Rao PS, "Ebstein's Anomaly of the Tricuspid Valve with Atresia - A Surgically Correctable Form of Physiologic Tricuspid Atresia," Presented at the Southeastern Pediatric Cardiology Society, Sixth Annual Meeting, New Orleans, Louisiana, September 21-22, 1973.

28. Rao PS, Awa S, Linde LM, "Valve gradients and kinetic energy." Presented at the 41st Annual Meeting of the American Academy of Pediatrics, Section on Cardiology, October 1972, New York City, New York.

29. Rao PS, Linde LM, "Isoproterenol and right ventricular obstruction, Proceedings of the XIV International Congress of Pediatrics," October 1974, Buenos Aires, Argentina, Vol. VIII, Cardiology-Nephrology, pp. 47-49.

30. Rao PS, "Effect of acute increase in stroke volume on pulmonary vascular impedance," *Pediatr Res 1980*; 14:449.

31. Rao PS, "Transcatheter Management of Heart Disease in Infants and Children," *Pediat Rev Comm 1987*; 1:1-18.

32. Rao PS, "Balloons, blades, plugs and umbrellas in the treatment of heart disease in infants and children (Editorial)," *Ann Saudi Med 1987*; 7:85-87.

33. Rao PS, "Balloon Angioplasty and Valvuloplasty in Infants, Children and Adolescents, Current Problems in Cardiology," *YearBook Medical Publishers, Inc.*, Chicago, 1989; 14(8): 419-497.

34. Rao PS, "Transcatheter treatment of heart disease in infancy and childhood," *Wisconsin Med J 1988*, 87:28-30.

35. Rao PS, "Medical progress: Balloon valvuloplasty and angioplasty in infants and children," *J Pediat 1989*; 114:907-914.

36. Rao PS, "Balloon dilatation in infants and children with cardiac defects," *Cath Cardiovasc Diagn 1989*; 18:136-149.

37. Rao PS, "Balloon valvuloplasty and angioplasty for congenital and acquired heart defects in children," Bull Saudi Heart Assoc 1990; 2:10-22.

38. Rao PS, "Balloon angioplasty/valvuloplasty in congenital heart disease (Editorial)," *J Invasive Cardiol*, 1990; 2:129-136.

39. Rao PS, "Balloon valvuloplasty and angioplasty of stenotic lesions of the heart and great vessels in children," *In. Advances in Pediatrics*, Barness LA; DeVivo DC, Morrow G, III, Oski F, Rudolph AM; (eds.), Year Book Medical Publishers, Inc., Chicago, IL, Vol. 37, 1990; pp. 33-76.

40. Rao PS, "Percutaneous balloon valvuloplasty/angioplasty in congenital heart disease," *In. Percutaneous Valvuloplasty and Related Techniques*, Bashore TM and Davidson CT (eds.), Williams & Wilkins, Baltimore, MD, 1990, pp. 251-277.

41. Rao PS (Editor), "Transcatheter Therapy in Pediatric Cardiology," *Wiley-Liss, Inc.*, New York, 1993.

42. Rao PS, Sideris EB, Chopra PS, "Catheter closure of atrial septal defect: Successful use in a 3.6 kg infant," *Am Heart J 1991*; 121:1826-1829.

43. Rao PS, Wilson AD, Levy JM, Chopra PS, "Role of 'buttoned' double-disk device in the management of atrial septal defects," *Am Heart J 1992*; 123:191-200.

44. Rao PS, Wilson AD, Chopra PS, "Transcatheter closure of atrial septal defect by 'buttoned' devices," *Am J Cardiol* 1992; 69:1056-1061.

45. Rao PS, Sideris EB, Hausdorf G, et al, "International experience with secundum atrial septal defect occlusion by the buttoned device," *Am Heart J 1994*; 128:1022-35.

46. Ende DJ, Chopra PS, Rao PS, "Transcatheter closure of atrial septal defect or patent foramen ovale with the buttoned device for prevention of recurrence of paradoxic embolism," *Am J Cardiol 1996*; 78:233-6.

47. Rao PS, Wilson AD, Sideris EB, Chopra PS, "Transcatheter closure of patent ductus arteriosus with buttoned device: First successful clinical application in a child," *Am Heart J* 1991; 121:1799-1802.

48. Rao PS, Sideris EB, Haddad J, et al, "Transcatheter occlusion of patent ductus arteriosus with adjustable buttoned device: Initial clinical experience," *Circulation 1993*; 88:1119-1126.

49. Lochan R, Rao PS, Samal AK, et al, "Transcatheter closure of patent ductus arteriosus with an adjustable buttoned device in an adult patient," *Am Heart J 1994*; 127:941-943.

50. Rao PS, "Interventional pediatric cardiology: State of the art and future directions," *Pediat Cardiol 1998*; 19:107-124.

51. Rao PS, Kern MJ (eds.), "Catheter Based Devices for Treatment of Noncoronary Cardiovascular Disease in Adults and Children," *Lippincott, Williams & Wilkins*, Philadelphia, PA, 2003.

52. Kirby ML, Weidman TA, McKenzie JW, "An ultrastructural study of the cardiac ganglia in the bulbar plexus of the developing chick heart," *Dev Neurosci 1980*; 3:174-84.

53. Kirby ML, McKenzie JW, Weidman TA, "Developing innervation of the chick heart: a histofluorescence and light microscopic study of sympathetic innervation," Anat Rec 1980; 196:333-40.

54. Kirby ML, "Alteration of cardiogenesis after neural crest ablation," *Ann N Y Acad Sci 1990*; 588:289-95, PMID: 2192647.

55. Kirby ML, Gale TF, Stewart DE, "Neural crest cells contribute to normal aorticopulmonary septation," *Science, 1983*; 220:1059-61, PMID: 6844926

56. Kirby ML, Waldo KL, "Role of neural crest in congenital heart disease," *Circulation 1990*; 82:332-40, PMID: 2197017.

57. Rao PS, "Preventive aspects of congenital heart disease," *Paediatrician 1973*; 2:224-38.

58. Strong WB, Rao PS, Steinbauch M, "Primary prevention of atherosclerosis: A challenge to the physician caring for children," *Southern Med J 1975*; 68:319-27.

59. Rao PS, "Prevention of pediatric heart disease," *Paediatrician 1975*; 4:320-42.

60. Rao PS, "Preventive aspects of heart disease in infants and children," *South Med J 1977*; 70:728-40.

61. Rao PS, "Prevention of Heart Disease in Infants and Children, Current Problems in Pediatrics," Vol. 7, May 1977, pp. 1-48, *Yearbook Medical Publisher, Inc.*, Chicago, U.S.A.

62. Rao PS, Mardini MK, "Atrial septostomy without thoracotomy: The experience with transcatheter knife atrial septostomy," *King Faisal Specialist Hospital Medical Journal 1983*; 3:165-171.

63. Rao PS, "Transcatheter blade atrial septostomy," *Cath Cardiovasc Dgn 1984*; 10:335-342.

64. Rao PS, "Surgery without thoracotomy: transcatheter management of pediatric heart disease," *Indian J Pediatr 1984*; 51:703-714.

65. Rao PS, Mardini MK, "Pulmonary valvotomy without thoracotomy: The experience with percutaneous balloon pulmonary valvuloplasty," *Ann Saudi Med 1985*; 5:149-155.

66. Rao PS, Mardini MK, Najjar HN, "Relief of coarctation of the aorta without thoracotomy: The experience with percutaneous balloon angioplasty," *Ann Saudi Med 1986*; 6:193-203.

67. Rao PS, "Transcatheter treatment of pulmonic stenosis and coarctation of the aorta: The experience with percutaneous balloon dilatation," *Brit Heart J 1986*; 56:250-258.

68. Rao PS, "Balloon angioplasty for coarctation of the aorta in infancy," *J Pediat 1987*; 110:713-718.

69. Rao PS, "Influence of balloon size on the short-term and long-term results of balloon pulmonary valvuloplasty," *Texas Heart Institute J 1987*; 14:57-61.

70. Rao PS, "Tricuspid Atresia," *Futura Publishing Co.*, Mount Kisco, New York, 1982.

71. Rao PS, "Present status of surgery in congenital heart disease," *Indian J Pediatr 1981*; 49:349-363.

72. Rao PS, Kulangara RJ, "Echocardiographic evaluation of global left ventricular performance in infants and children," *Indian Pediat 1982*; 19:21-32.

73. Rao PS, "Vasodilator therapy for cardiac failure in pediatric practice," *Indian J Pediat 1982*; 49:843-848.

74. Rao PS, "Pathophysiologic consequences of cyanotic heart disease," *Indian J Pediat 1983*; 50:479-487.

75. Rao PS, "Mitral valve prolapse síndrome," *Indian J Pediat 1987*; 54:140-144.

76. Rao PS, "Preface to the pediatric cardiology issue," *Indian J. Pediatr 1988*; 55:7-9.

77. Rao PS, "Transcatheter therapy of cardiac defects in infants and children," *Indian J Pediatr 1988*; 44:137-140.

78. Rao PS, "Doppler echocardiography in non-invasive diagnosis of heart disease in infants and children," *Indian J. Pediatr 1988*; 55:80-95.

79. Rao PS, "Pediatric cardiology symposium (Editorial)," *Indian J Pediat 1991*; 58:439-440.

80. Rao PS, "Perinatal circulatory physiology," *Indian J Pediat 1991*; 58:441-451.

81. Rao PS, "Evaluation of cardiac murmurs in children," *Indian J Pediat 1991*; 58:471-489.

82. Rao PS, "Transcatheter occlusion of cardiac septal defects," *Indian J Pediat 1991*; 58:605-621.

83. Chopra PS, Rao PS, "Surgical management of congenital heart disease: Current trends," *Indian J Pediat 1991*; 58:623-640.

84. Rao PS, "Transcatheter Occlusion of atrial septal defects and patent ductus arteriosus: Now a reality in India," *Indian J Pediat 1993*; 60:615-623.

85. Rao PS, "Symposium on pediatric cardiology (Editorial)," *Indian J Pediat 1998*; 65:11-12.

86. Balfour IC, Rao PS, "Chest Pain in Children," *Indian J Pediat 1998*; 65:21-26.

87. Jureidini SB, Marino CJ, Rao PS, "Congenital coronary artery anomalies," Indian J Pediat 1998; 65:217-229.

88. Rao PS, "Closure devices for atrial septal defect: Which one to choose? (Editorial)," *Indian Heart J 1998*; 50:379-383.

89. Rao PS, "Stents in the management of congenital heart disease in the pediatric and adult patients," *Indian Heart J 2001*; 53:714-730.

90. Saxena A, Rao PS, "The practice of pediatric cardiology – Symposium on pediatric cardiology (Editorial)," *Indian J Pediat 2002*; 69:313-314.

91. Gupta ML, Lantin-Hermosa MR, Rao PS, "What is new in pediatric cardiology?" *Indian J Pediat 2003*; 70:41-49.

92. Rao PS, Gupta ML, Balaji S, "Recent Advances in Pediatric Cardiology - Electrophysiology, Transcatheter and Surgical Advances," *Indian J Pediat 2003*; 70:557-564.

93. Rao PS, "Current status of cardiac interventions for pediatric congenital heart disease – Part I: Balloon valvuloplasty/angioplasty," *Pediatric Cardiology Newsletter 6* (No.1 January-June):1-4, 2004.

94. Rao PS, "Current status of cardiac interventions for pediatric congenital heart disease – Part II: Percutaneous closure of cardiac septal defects," *Pediatric Cardiology Newsletter 6* (No. 2, July-December):1-5, 2004.

95. Rao PS, "Introduction of pediatric cardiology symposium – I: Pediatric Cardiology," *Indian J Pediatr 2005*; 72:493.

96. Rao PS, "Diagnosis and management of acyanotic heart disease: Part I - obstructive lesions," *Indian J Pediatr 2005*; 72:496-502.

97. Rao PS, "Diagnosis and management of acyanotic heart disease: Part II - left-to-right shunt lesions," *Indian J Pediatr 2005*; 72:503-512.

98. Gupta-Malhotra M, Rao PS, "Current perspectives on Kawasaki disease," *Indian J Pediatr 2005*; 72:621-629.

99. Rao PS, "Transcatheter interventions in critically ill neonates and infants with aortic coarctation (Editorial)," *Annals of Pediat Cardiol 2009*; 2:116-119.

100. Rao PS, "Consensus on timing of intervention for common congenital heart diseases: Part I - Acyanotic heart defects," *Indian J Pediatr 2013*; 80:72-78.

101. Rao PS, "Consensus on timing of intervention for common congenital heart diseases: Part II - Cyanotic heart defects," *Indian J Pediatr*, Volume 2013; 80: 663-674.

102. Rao PS, "Editorial: What does the pediatrician needs to know about heart defects in children?" *Indian J Pediatr 2015*; 82:1019-20.

103. Rao PS, "Fontan operation: Indications, short and long term outcomes," *Indian J Pediatr 2015*; 82:1147-1156.

104. Rao PS, Balloon aortic valvuloplasty (Editorial), Indian Heart Journal. 2016; 68: 592–595.

105. Rao PS, The Journey of an Indian Pediatric Cardiologist Dr. K. C. Chaudhuri Lifetime Achievement Award/Oration at AIIMS, New Delhi, September 2017. Indian J Pediat 2017; DOI 10.1007/s12098-017-2452-8.

CHAPTER 4

OTHER EVENTS DURING THE JOURNEY

INTRODUCTION

In this chapter, I will review other events that occurred during the journey and will include Awards and Honors as well as disappointments. This is followed by presentation of my activities that made significant contributions, resulting in creation of news, the newsworthy events.

AWARDS AND HONORS

I was bestowed with a number of awards and honors during my career, which will be reviewed in this section. The first was a distinction by standing first in the Andhra University at Diploma in Child Health (DCH) examinations (Chapter 1, Figure 18) in 1966. The next is a selection for fellowship at Stanford University by Evelyn L. Nizer Foundation (1969-1970), which made it possible to undertake the fellowship at Stanford University. This was particularly important in that the National Institutes of Health (NIH) required citizenship or US immigrant visa to qualify for funding. By the time I joined University of California in Los Angeles (UCLA), I secured immigrant visa and consequently, my fellowship at UCLA could be supported by NIH (1971-1972). I was selected as Finalist for the Best Teacher Award in the Department of Pediatrics, Medical College of Georgia, Augusta, GA (1979-1980). In the same year, I was chosen as one of the investigators to test the Rashkind Occluder device to non-surgically close atrial septal defects and patent ductus arteriosus; this is particularly noteworthy in that only seven centers were designated in the entire USA for clinical testing of the device. I was a participant in a course titled, "Introduction to Clinical Medicine," which was chosen by the M.D. class of 1983 at the School of Medicine, Medical College of Georgia, Augusta, as the most outstanding course in the first two years of medical school (Figure 1). I was a subject of biographic record in Who's Who in the World, Seventh (1984-1985) Edition (Figure 2) and in several subsequent editions (Figure 3). I was conferred with an Award for Outstanding Contribution to Pediatric Cardiology by the Telugu Association of North America (TANA) in July 1989, at their annual meeting in Houston, TX (Figure 4).

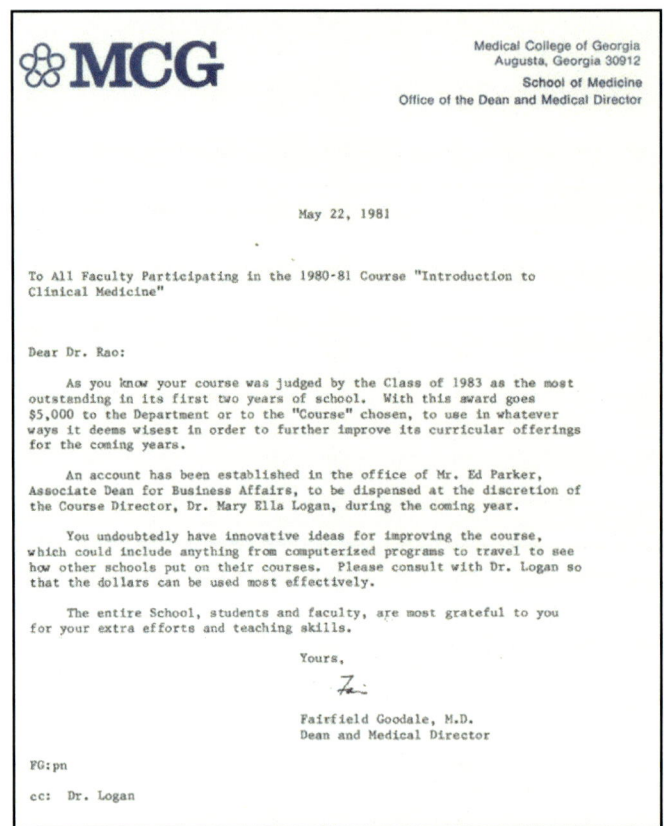

Figure 1. A copy of the letter from the Dean of the Medical School stating that my course was judged as the most outstanding course in the first two years of medical school.

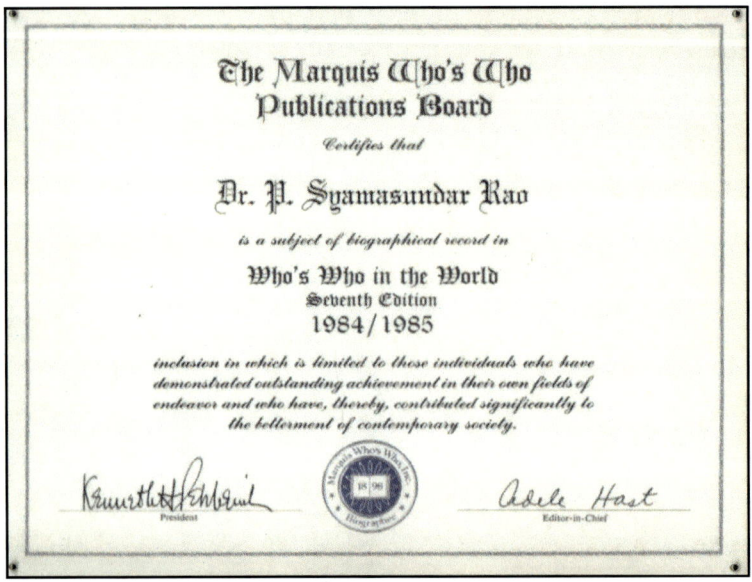

Figure 2. Certificate stating that I was a subject of biographic record in Who's Who in the World, Seventh (1984-1985) Edition.

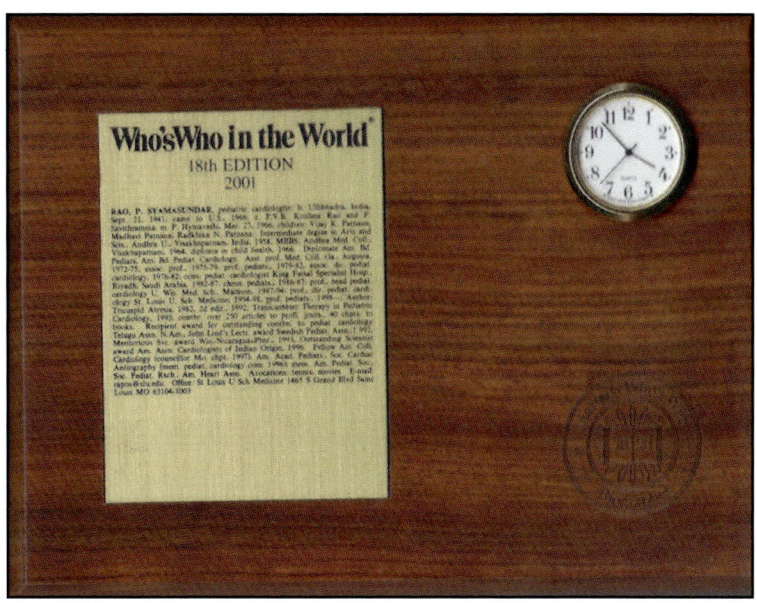

Figure 3. Wall plaque from Who's Who in the World certifying that I was a subject of biographic record in Who's Who in the World, 18th (2001) Edition.

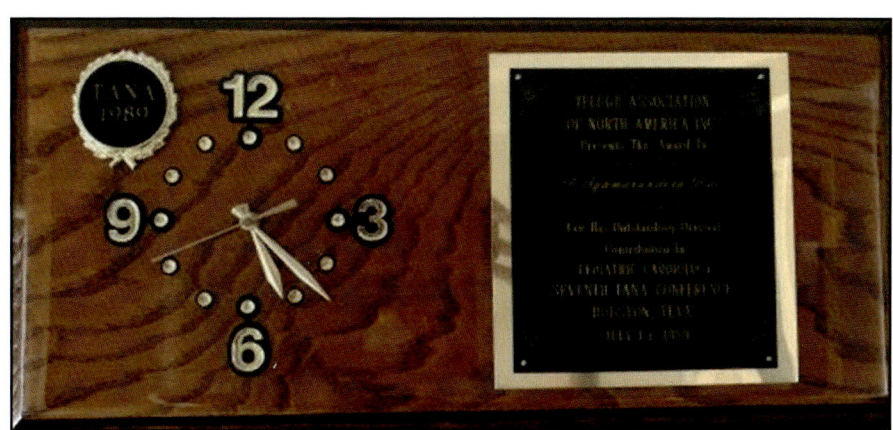

Figure 4. Wall plaque indicating that I was bestowed with an Award for Outstanding Contribution to Pediatric Cardiology by the Telugu Association of North America (TANA) in July 1989.

In 1991, I was chosen as the monitor for US trial for trans-catheter button device occlusion of cardiac septal defects. In 1992, I was invited to present John Lind's Lecture at the Swedish Pediatric Association, Gothenburg, Sweden. In 1993, Meritorious Service Award from Wisconsin Nicaragua Partners of the Americas was presented to me (Figure 5). Also, in the same year, Outstanding Service Award from Healing the Children of Wisconsin was conferred to me (Figure 6). In 1994, my book titled, "Transcatheter Therapy in Pediatric Cardiology," Rao PS (ed.), was selected as one of the best health sciences books published in 1993 (Figure 7). The Outstanding Scientist Award was presented to me by the American Association of Cardiologists of Indian Origin at the American College of Cardiology meeting in Orlando, Florida on March 24, 1996 (Figure 8).

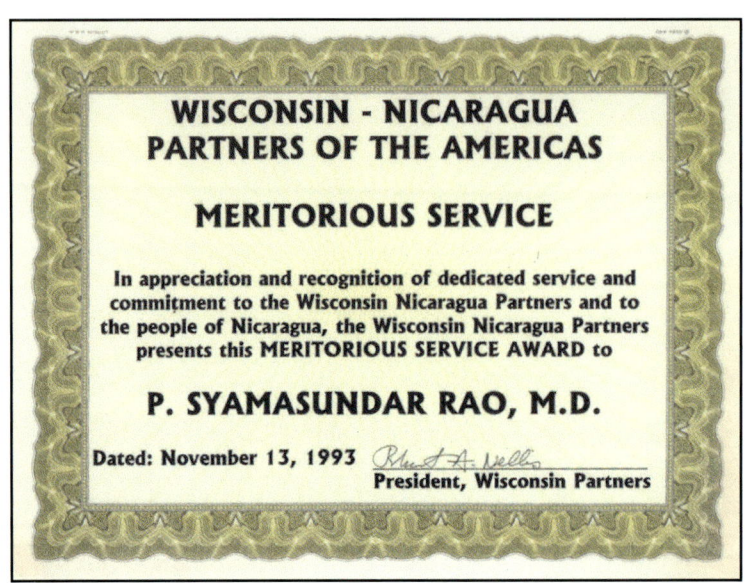

Figure 5. Meritorious Service Award from Wisconsin Nicaragua
Partners of the Americas.

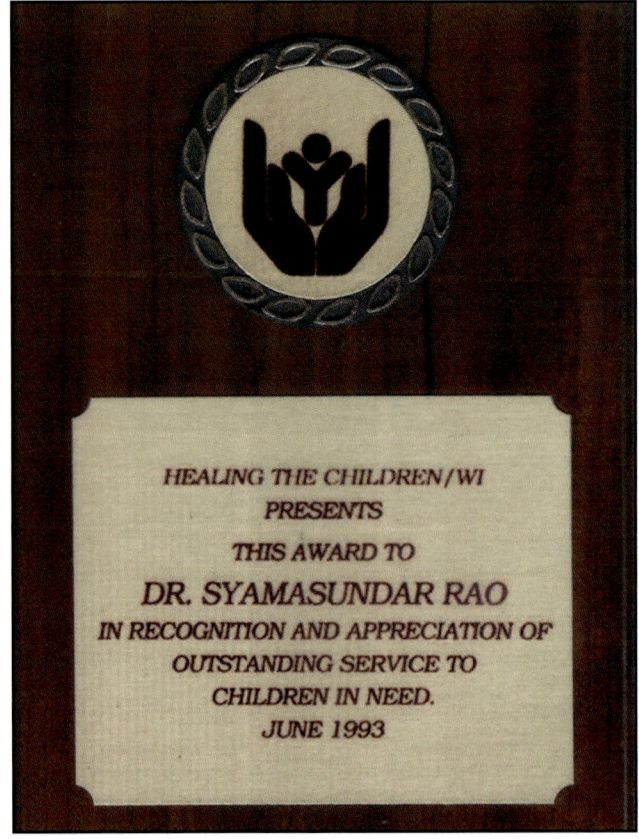

Figure 6. Outstanding Service Award from Healing the
Children of Wisconsin presented to me in 1993.

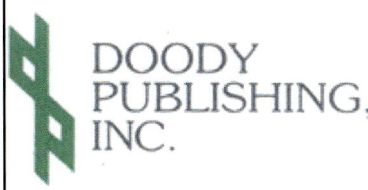

DOODY
PUBLISHING,
INC.

May 31, 1994

P. Syamasundar Rao, MD
University of Wisconsin Medical School
1300 University Avenue
Madison, Wisconsin 53706

Dear Dr. Rao:

Congratulations! *Transcatheter Therapy in Pediatric Cardiology* has been selected as one of the 250 best health sciences books published in 1993.

It appears in a new reference book we have just published, **Doody's Rating Service: A Buyer's Guide to the 250 Best Health Sciences Books, 1993.** The winning titles were selected from a field of 1,620 books we received during 1993 from more than 70 publishers across 87 specialties.

Award-winning titles represent the consensus opinion of health sciences publishers, Doody Publishing's reviewer network of more than 600 academic health sciences professionals, and members of the Medical Library Association. "Best" means most important to the individual book's target audience or most innovative.

Your book has been selected to appear in the inaugural volume of **Doody's Rating Service**, which will be published every spring to identify and celebrate the best books of the previous copyright year.

You are to be commended for the commitment it took to put together a book of this importance. We hope this honor rewards that commitment, in some small degree. Congratulations, once again, for this singular honor.

Cordially,

Daniel J. Doody
President & Publisher

P.S. The list price of **Doody's Rating Service, 1993** is $49.50. But we are extending a limited-time 20% discount to all authors of award winning books. To place your order, simply phone us at 1-800-219-9500. To take advantage of this special author's discount, we must receive your order by July 31, 1994.

cc: Larry Olson

Westgate Professional Building • 1145 Westgate, Suite 200 • Oak Park, Illinois 60301 • 708-386-9500 • 708-386-0860 Fax

Figure 7. Letter from Doody Publishing Inc. indicating that my book titled, "Transcatheter Therapy in Pediatric Cardiology," Rao PS (ed.), was selected as one of the best health sciences books published in 1993.

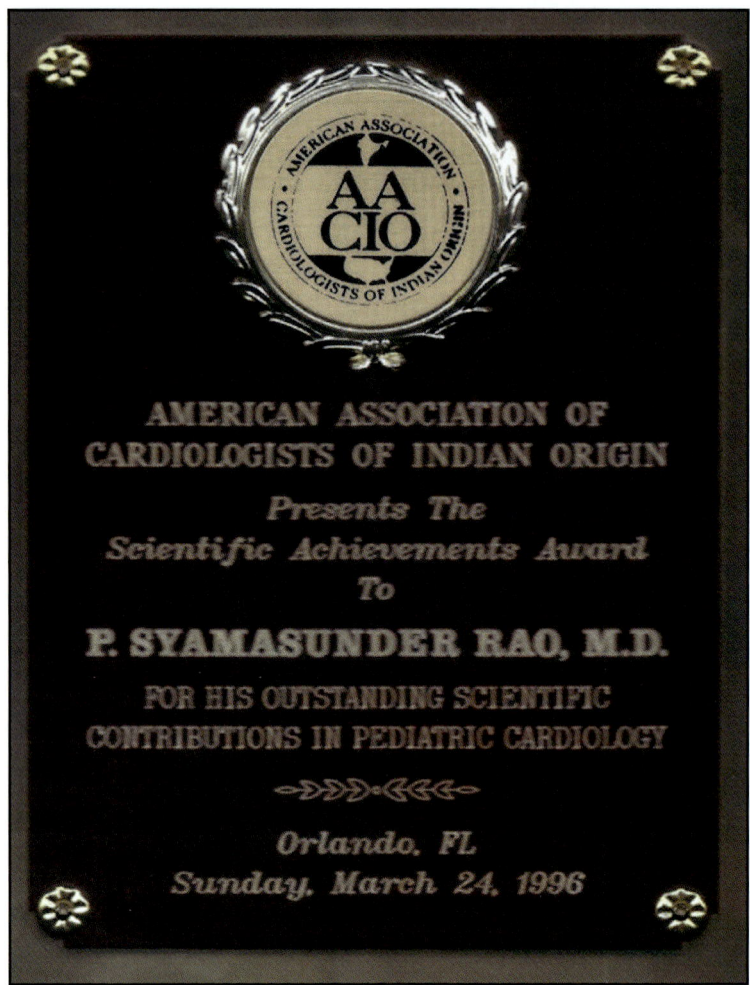

Figure 8. Outstanding Scientist Award presented by the American Association
of Cardiologists of Indian Origin at the American College of Cardiology
meeting in Orlando, Florida in 1996.

I was invited to present Kreidberg's Lecture, titled "Pediatric Cardiac Interventions: Past, Present and Future," at Tufts University, New England Medical Center, Boston, MA, on May 18, 2005. In 2012, the Outstanding Scientist Award (Figure 9) was presented to me by the North American Telugu Association (NATA) at George R. Brown Convention Center, Houston, Texas, on July 2-4, 2012. Shortly thereafter, the ATA Distinguished Award in Medicine (Figure 10) was conferred by the American Telugu Association (ATA) at Georgia World Congress Center, Atlanta, Georgia on July 6, 2012. In 2014, I was selected for the Dean's Teaching Excellence Award, 2013-2014 (Figure 11) at the UT Health, University of Texas at Houston McGovern Medical School, Houston, TX. In 2017, I was conferred with the Dr. K. C. Chaudhuri Lifetime Achievement Award (Figures 12, 13 and 14), which was presented at All India Institute of Medical Sciences, New Delhi, India on September 10, 2017. The final award was another Lifetime Achievement Award (Figure 15) by the Telugu Cultural Association of Houston in early 2018.

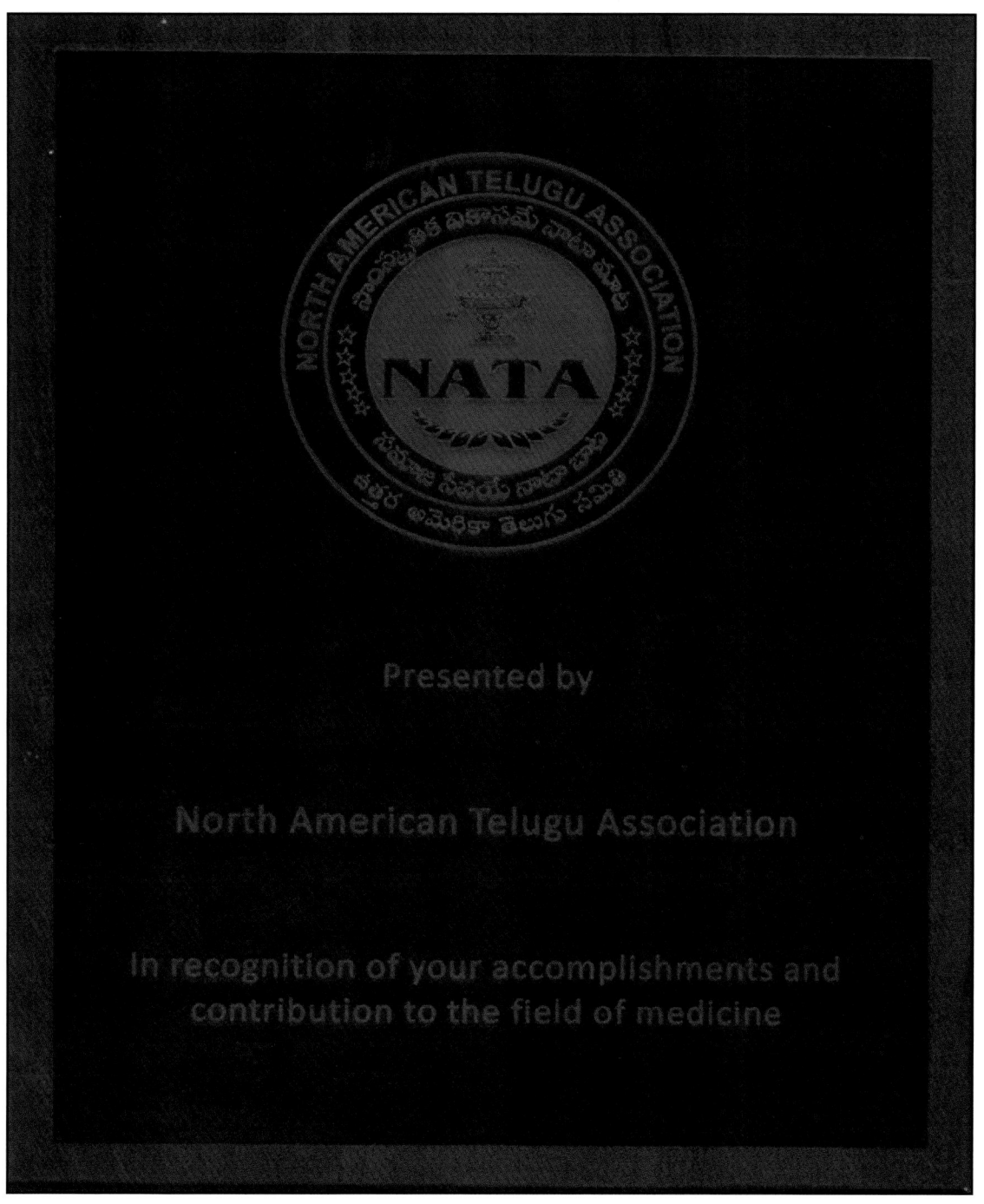

Figure 9. Outstanding Scientist Award presented by the North American Telugu
Association (NATA) at George R. Brown Convention Center, Houston, Texas,
in 2012.

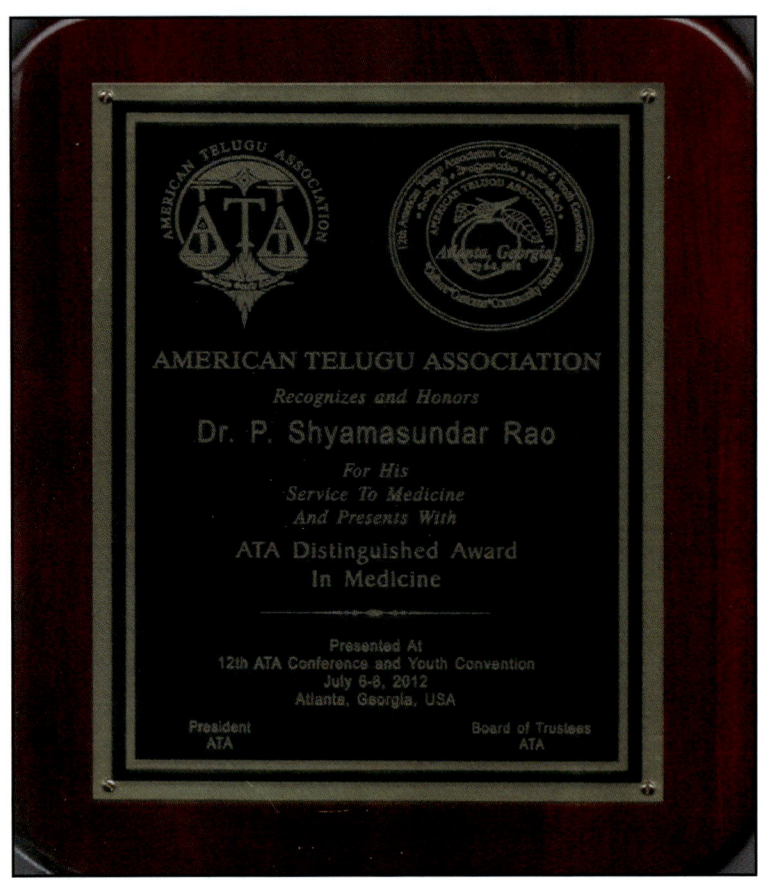

Figure 10. ATA Distinguished Award by the American Telugu Association (ATA) at Georgia World Congress Center, Atlanta, Georgia in 2012.

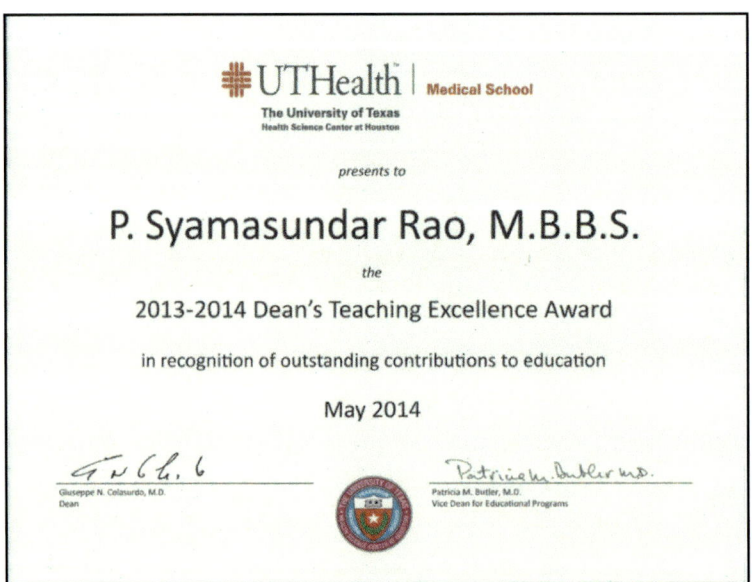

Figure 11. Dean's Teaching Excellence Award, 2013-2014, presented by the UT Health, University of Texas at Houston Medical School, Houston, Texas in 2014.

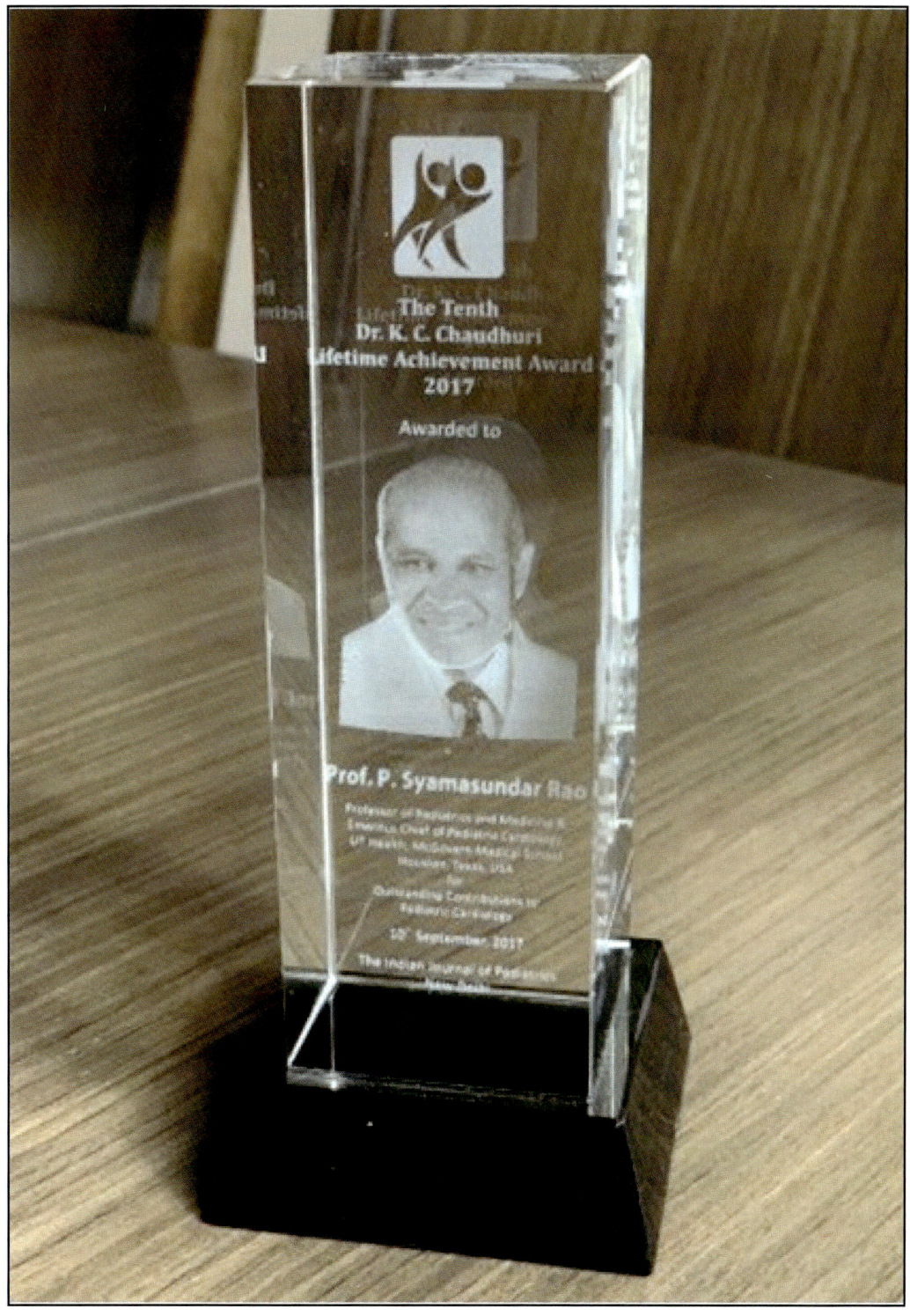

Figure 12. Dr. K. C. Chaudhuri Lifetime Achievement Award by the Indian
Journal of Pediatrics/All India Institute of Medical Sciences in New Delhi
in 2017.

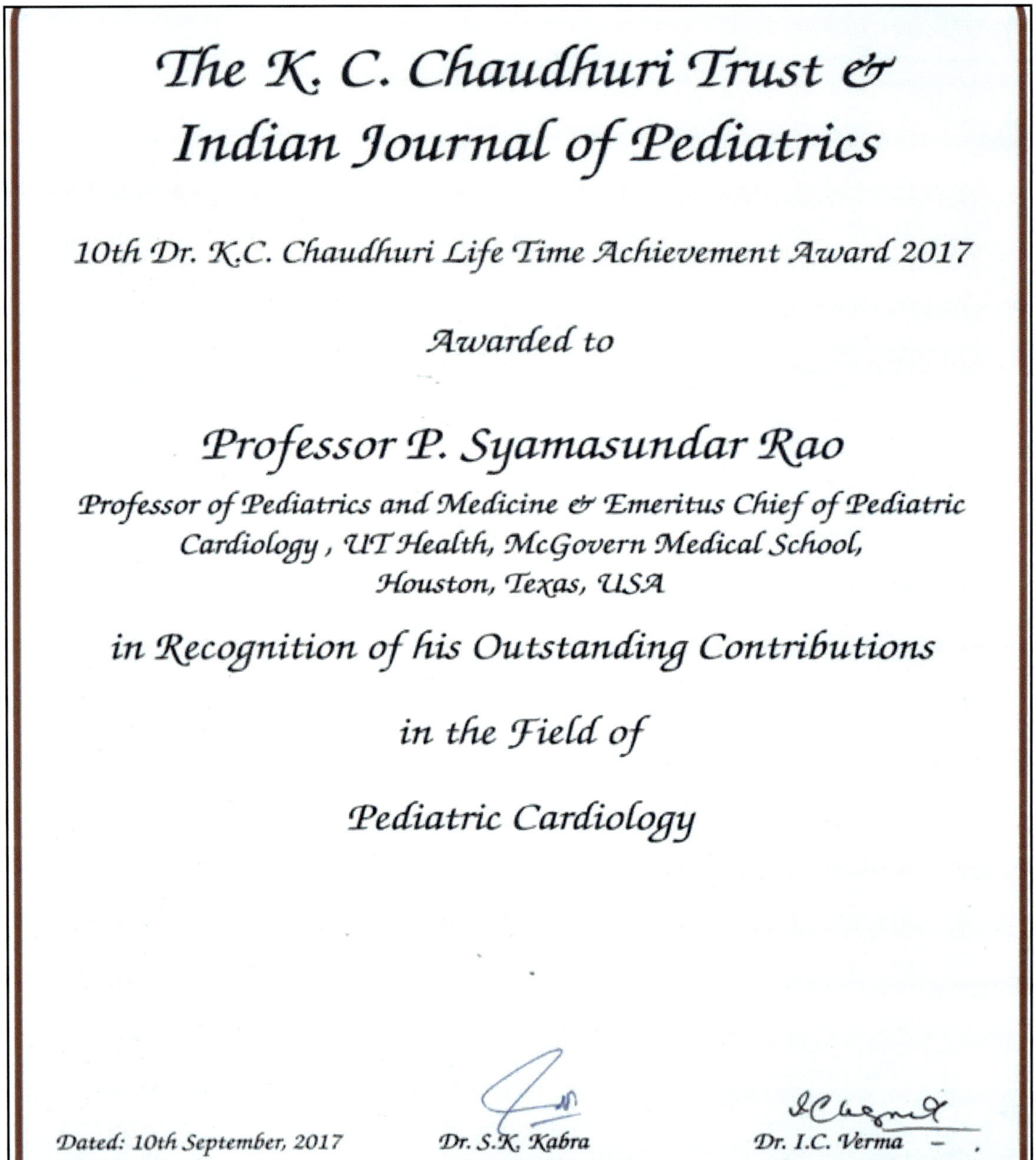

The K. C. Chaudhuri Trust &
Indian Journal of Pediatrics

10th Dr. K.C. Chaudhuri Life Time Achievement Award 2017

Awarded to

Professor P. Syamasundar Rao

Professor of Pediatrics and Medicine & Emeritus Chief of Pediatric
Cardiology , UT Health, McGovern Medical School,
Houston, Texas, USA

in Recognition of his Outstanding Contributions

in the Field of

Pediatric Cardiology

Dated: 10th September, 2017   Dr. S.K. Kabra   Dr. I.C. Verma
New Delhi   Editor-in-Chief, IJP   Editor Emeritus, IJP

Figure 13. Dr. K. C. Chaudhuri Lifetime Achievement Award by the Indian
Journal of Pediatrics/All India Institute of Medical Sciences in New Delhi
in 2017.

IJP Annual Scientific Day

10th September 2017

10th Dr. K. C. Chaudhuri Oration:
Prof. P. Syamasundar Rao
The Journey of An Indian Pediatric Cardiologist

5th Dr. I. C. Verma Excellence Oration:
Prof. Joseph L. Mathew
Etiology of Childhood Pneumonia: What We Know and What We Need to Know!

Competitive Grand Rounds & Best Thesis Awards

Venue:
Dr. Ramalingaswami Board Room,
All India Institute of Medical Sciences, New Delhi

Organized by
The Indian Journal of Pediatrics
&
Dept. of Pediatrics, AIIMS, New Delhi

Professor P. Syamasundar Rao

Dr. P. Syamasundar Rao is the Professor of Pediatrics and Medicine & Emeritus Chief of Pediatric Cardiology, UT Health, McGovern Medical School, Houston, Texas, USA. He obtained MBBS from Andhra Medical College, Visakhapatnam. He went to USA and worked in prestigious universities such as Stanford, Case-Western Reserve and UCLA. Dr. Rao served as Professor of Pediatrics and Director of Pediatric Cardiology at several major Universities including Medical College of Georgia, Augusta, University of Wisconsin, Madison, St. Louis University School of Medicine, and UT Health, McGovern Medical School, Houston, TX. He trained more than 45 post-doctoral fellows in Pediatric Cardiology.

He is an acknowledged pioneer in interventional pediatric cardiology. He made major contributions to catheterization and angiography in 1970s, balloon angioplasty /valvuloplasty in 1980s and transcatheter closure of cardiac defects in 1990s. He developed new pediatric cardiology/cardiovascular surgery programs in 2000s and educational and teaching material for physicians in 2010s.

For his remarkable achievements in Pediatric Cardiology he received multiple awards: by Telugu Association of North America; Wisconsin Nicaragua Partners of the Americas; Swedish Pediatric Association, Healing the Children of Wisconsin; American Association of Cardiologists of Indian Origin; Tufts University/New England Medical Center, and ATA Distinguished Award in Medicine by American Telugu Association, Atlanta, GA.

He has published more than 380 papers in Journals, 230 Abstracts, 150 Invited Presentations & Lectureships, and 17 Monographs and Books. He has served as Editorial Board Member for >10 Journals, Reviewer >20 Journals, and Section Editor for Pediatric Interventional Cardiology, Current Intervention Cardiology Reports and Journal of Invasive Cardiology.

He has been greatly involved in the education of pediatricians in India through innumerable lectures and workshops at Indian Institutions and Scientific Societies. In recognition of his lifetime contributions to developing Pediatric Cardiology, the Indian Journal of Pediatrics is proud to present its most prestigious Dr. K.C. Chaudhuri Life Time Achievement award 2017 to Professor Syamasundar Rao.

Program

10th September 2017

9:00 AM – 9:15 AM	Registration
9:15 AM –11:00 AM	Clinical Grand Rounds (Four Best Submissions) Presentations by Senior Residents of Holy Family Hospital, New Delhi; Jaslok Hospital & Research Centre, Mumbai; PGIMER, Chandigarh; PGIMER & Assoc. Dr. RML Hospital, New Delhi
11:00 AM –11:30 AM	Tea
11:30 AM –12:30 PM	10th Dr. K. C. Chaudhuri Life Time Achievement Award 2017 Oration by Prof. P.Syamasundar Rao Chairpersons : Dr. I.C. Verma & Dr. Anita Saxena
12:30 PM – 1:15 PM	5th Dr. I.C. Verma Excellence Award 2017 Oration by Prof. Joseph L. Mathew Chairpersons : Dr. Madhulika Kabra & Dr. S.K. Mittal
1:15 PM – 2:15 PM	Lunch
2:15 PM – 3:30 PM	Thesis Presentations (Six Top Submissions)
	Dr. Ramakrishnan A.P, ESIC Medical College & PGIMSR, Chennai; Dr. Bindu Deopa, Dr. S.N. Medical College, Jodhpur; Dr. Bikrant Bihari Lal, Institute of Liver & Biliary Sciences, New Delhi; Dr. Kaustuv Mitra, CNBC, Delhi; Dr. A. Murugesan, MAMC, New Delhi; Dr. Sricharantheja Nalisetty, Dr. Mehta's Children's Hospital, Chennai
3:30 PM onwards	Award Presentations
	Chief Guest : Dr. Santosh T. Soans, President-Elect IAP

Figure 14. Program of Dr. K. C. Chaudhuri Lifetime Achievement Award presentation by the Indian Journal of Pediatrics/All India Institute of Medical Sciences in New Delhi in 2017.

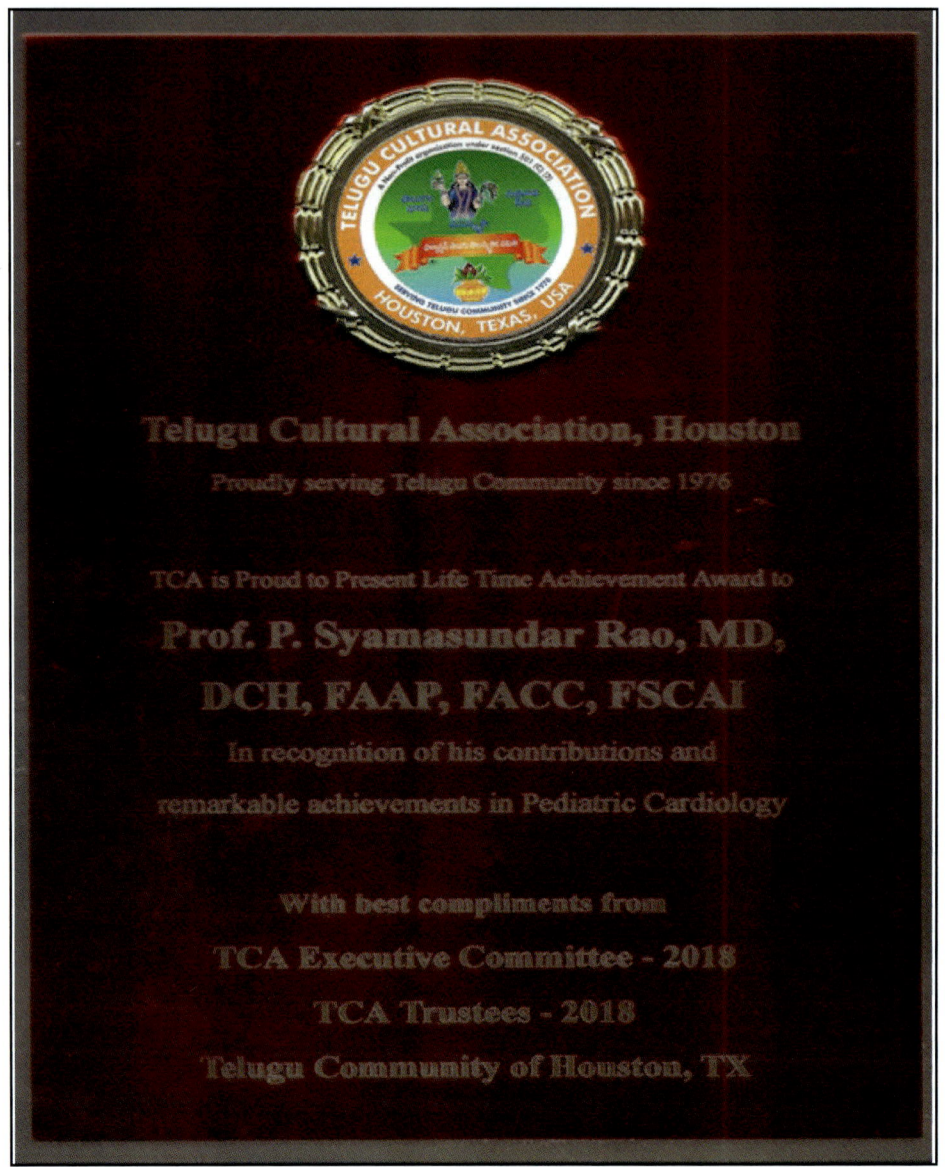

Figure 15. Lifetime Achievement Award by the Telugu Cultural Association of Houston in 2018.

DISAPPOINTMENTS

While majority of my journey is remarkable with successful events, there are some disappointments too and will be reviewed in this section. While in medical school, I contested for Class President for second and fourth year classes and lost both elections, but fortunately, two years later I was successful in winning the contest for President of the House Surgeon's Association. The next disappointments were my inability to return to India and refusal by the Medical College of Georgia administration to extend the sabbatical, as reviewed in the "Attempts to Return to India" section of Chapter 3 on "The Journey Continues."

The most painful disappointment was when the Chairman of Pediatrics at the St. Louis University asked me to resign from my position as Director of Pediatric Cardiology. When I refused to resign, I was forcefully removed by the Chairman. The disagreement arose initially when I tried to recruit a pediatric electro-physiologist to the staff of the Division of Pediatric Cardiology; the Chairman's major argument against such recruitment was that it is not financially feasible, despite providing evidence to the contrary. Indeed, the pediatric electro-physiology physicians brought in more revenues than the other pediatric cardiology sub-specialists. I appealed to the Dean of the School of Medicine and President and Provost of the St. Louis University providing evidence of my accomplishments in terms increasing the volume of patients seen in the outpatient clinics (Figure 16), number of general pediatric cardiology clinics (Figure 17), number of pediatric cardiology outreach clinics (Figure 18), number of echocardiograms (Figure 19), cardiac catheterizations (Figure 20), trans-catheter interventional procedures performed (Figure 21), and the number of publications (Figure 22), abstract presentations (Figure 23), invited scientific presentations (Figure 24) by the pediatric cardiology faculty although the number of faculty remained relatively constant (Figure 25). In addition, I attracted patient referrals from several states in the US and abroad (Figure 26), outside the conventional drawing area of the Cardinal Glennon Children's Hospital/St. Louis University because of my expertise in transcatheter interventional procedures in children. The financial position (Figure 27) of the Division of Pediatric Cardiology also improved remarkably. Despite presentation of my achievements, my appeal to the Dean of the School of Medicine and President and Provost of the St. Louis University did not reverse my dismissal as Division Director; the Chairman's wish prevailed.

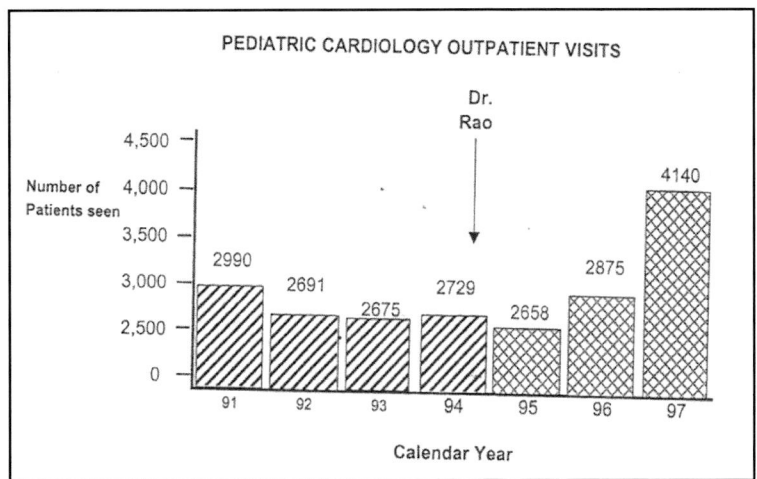

Figure 16. Bar graph of volume of patients seen in the outpatient clinics demonstrating increase in the number of outpatient pediatric cardiology visits after my arrival (arrow).

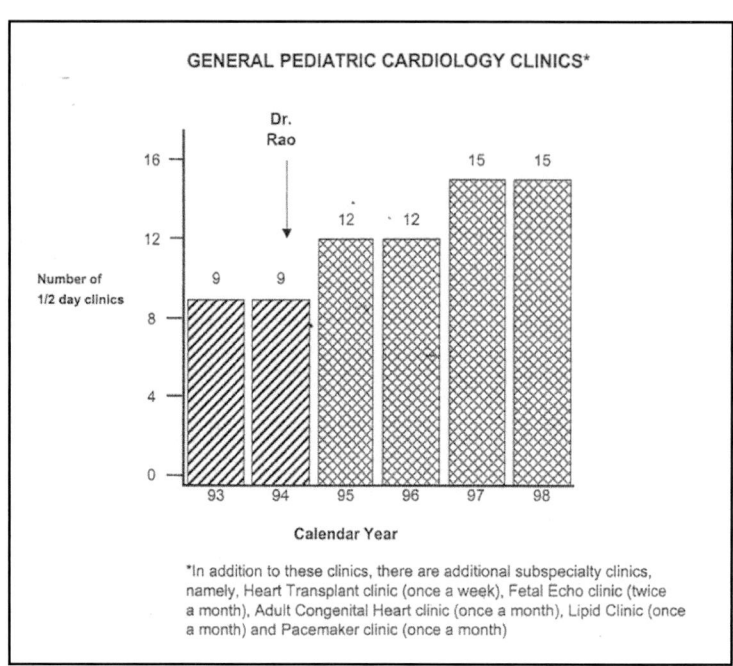

Figure 17. Bar graph of number of half-day outpatient clinics demonstrating increase in the number of outpatient pediatric cardiology clinics after my arrival (arrow).

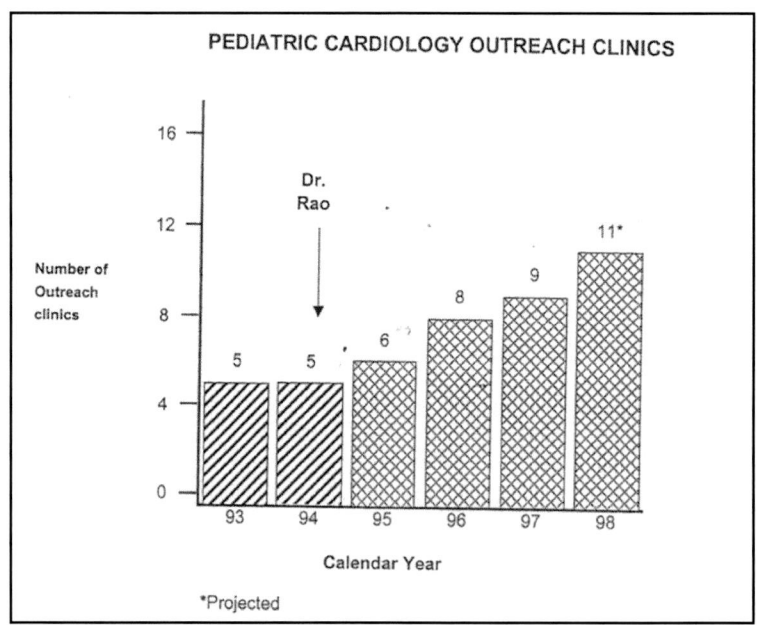

Figure 18. Bar graph of number of pediatric cardiology outreach clinics demonstrating increase in the number of outreach pediatric cardiology clinics after my arrival (arrow).

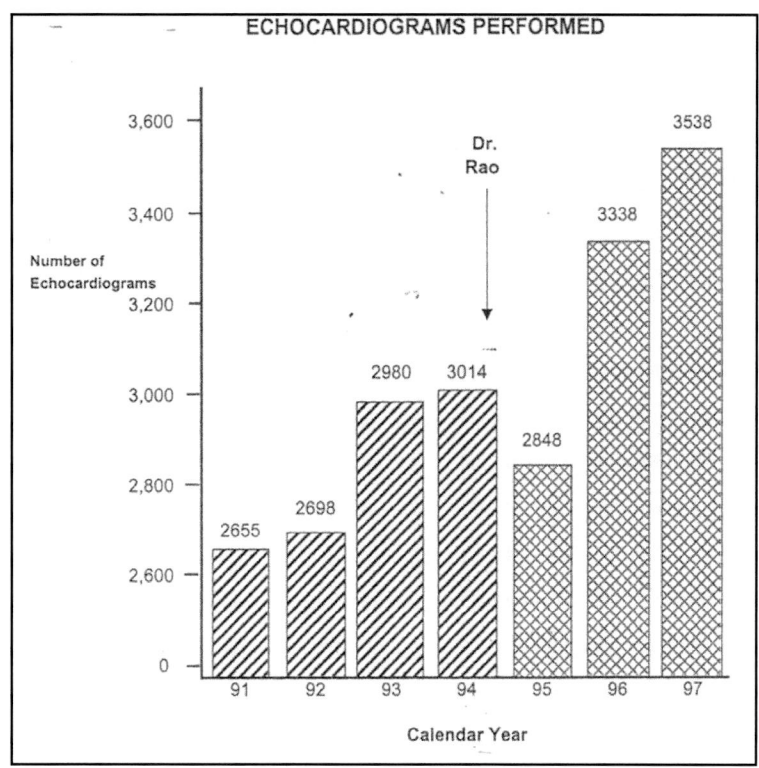

Figure 19. Bar graph of number of echocardiograms performed demonstrating increase in the number of echocardiograms performed since my arrival (arrow).

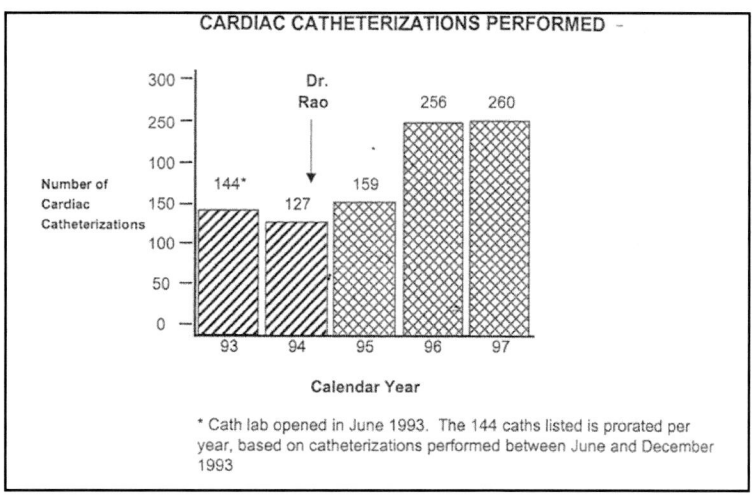

Figure 20. Bar graph of number of cardiac catheterizations performed demonstrating increase in the number of cardiac catheterizations performed since my arrival (arrow).

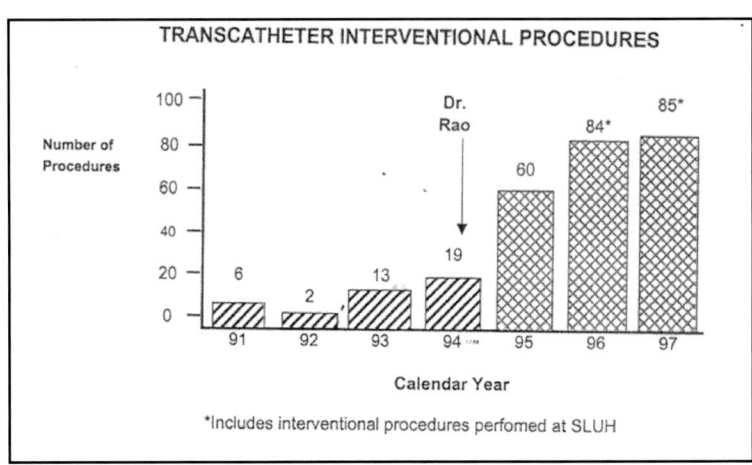

Figure 21. Bar graph of number of trans-catheter interventional procedures performed demonstrating increase in the number of these procedures performed since my arrival (arrow).

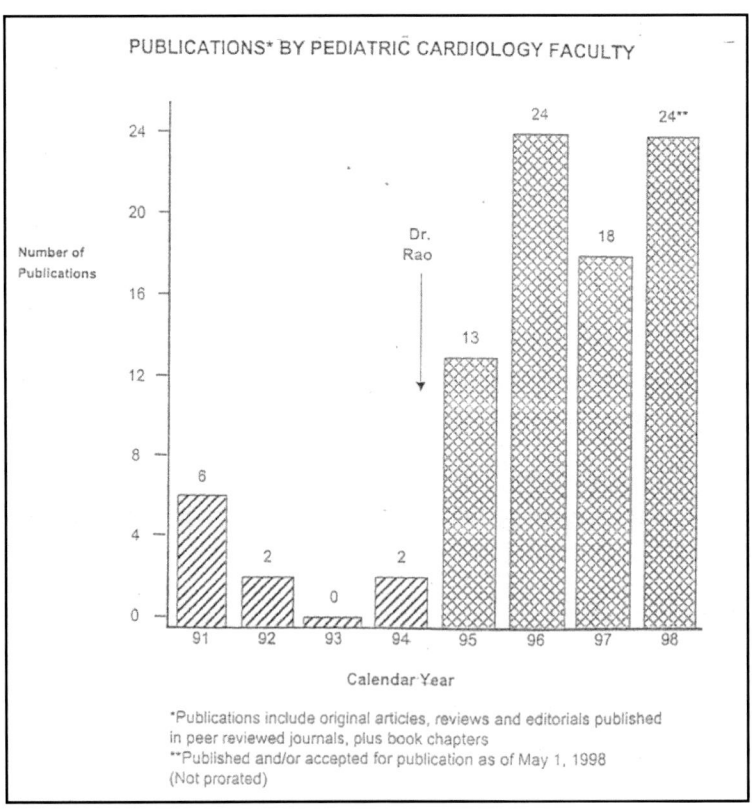

Figure 22. Bar graph of number of publications published by the members of the pediatric cardiology division demonstrating substantial increase in the number of the publications since my arrival (arrow).

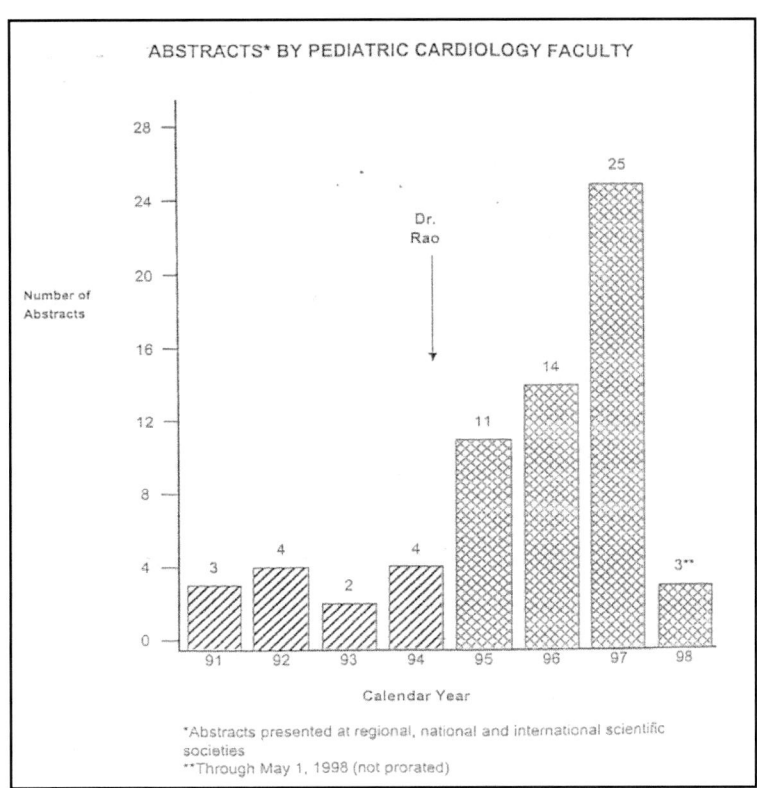

Figure 23. Bar graph of number of abstracts presented at regional, national and international scientific societies by the members of the pediatric cardiology division demonstrating substantial increase in the number of abstract presentations since my arrival (arrow).

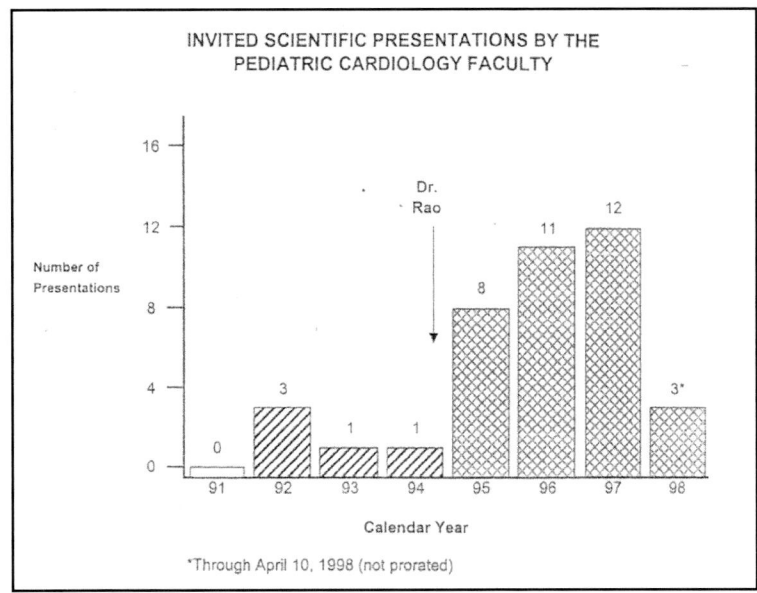

Figure 24. Bar graph of number of invited scientific presentations at regional, national and international scientific societies by the members of the pediatric cardiology division demonstrating substantial increase in the number of such presentations since my arrival (arrow).

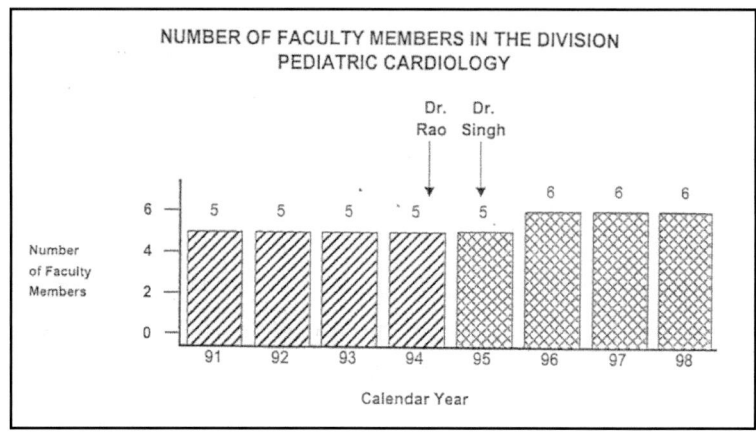

Figure 25. Bar graph of number of faculty members in pediatric cardiology division showing no substantial change despite increase in clinical and academic productivity of the Division under my direction.

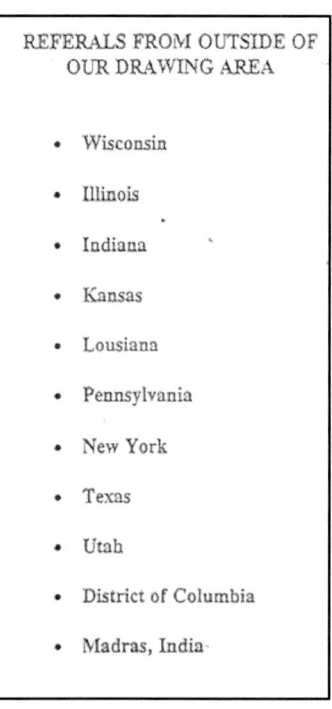

Figure 26. This figure lists referrals to me from outside the drawing area of the Cardinal Glennon Children's Hospital/St. Louis University.

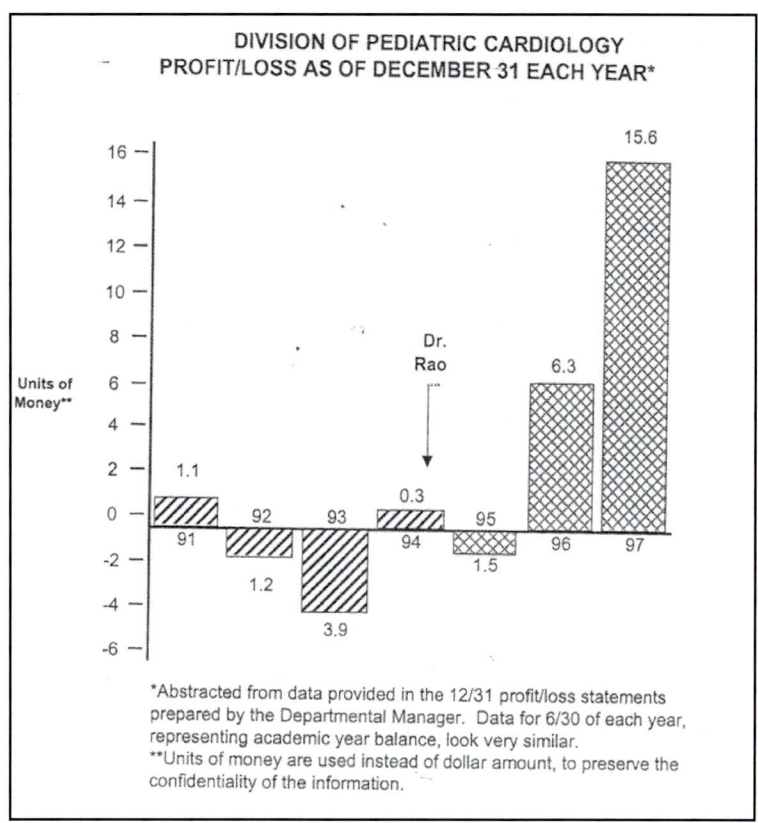

Figure 27. Bar graph of the financial position of the Division of Pediatric Cardiology demonstrating remarkable improvement since my arrival.

Consequently, I decided to leave the St. Louis University and applied to several institutions; positions as Professor and Director of Division of Pediatric Cardiology were offered almost simultaneously from the Medical College of Georgia, Augusta, GA, the Tufts University/New England Medical Center, Boston, MA and the University of Texas at Houston Medical School. I accepted the position at the University of Texas in Houston as reviewed in the section on "Academic Career" of the chapter on "The Journey Continues."

LOCAL, REGIONAL, NATIONAL, AND INTERNATIONAL CONFERENCES

I was a speaker at several local, regional, national and international conferences. Most of these are listed in Tables II and VI of the chapter on "The Journey Continues" and will not be repeated. However, copies of conference brochures or proceedings, or certificates of attendance at these conferences are presented in figures 28 through 34; unfortunately, not all brochures were available.

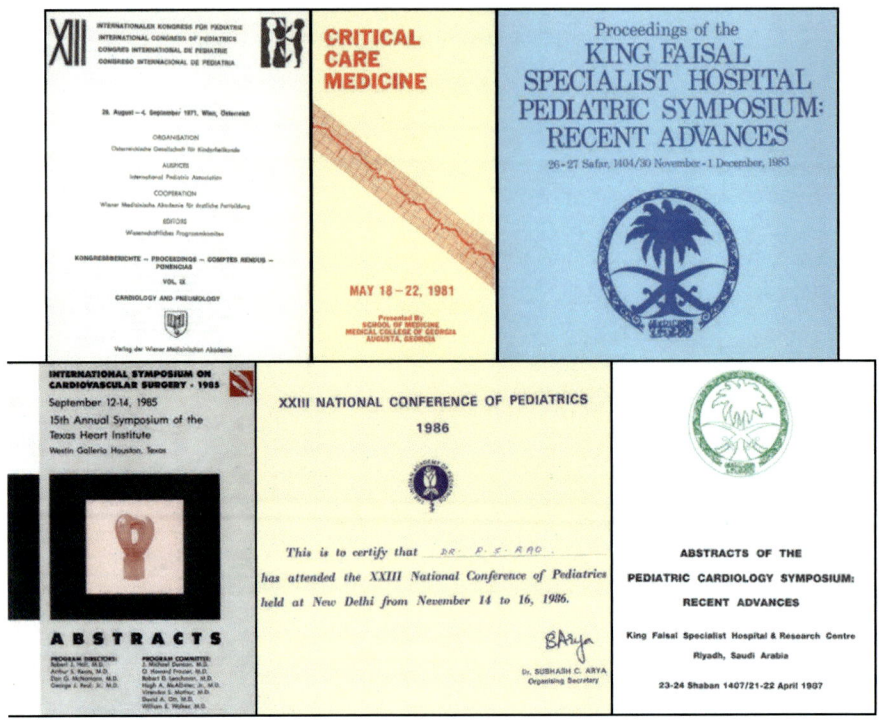

Figure 28. Copies of conference brochures or proceedings, or certificates of attendance (1971-1987).

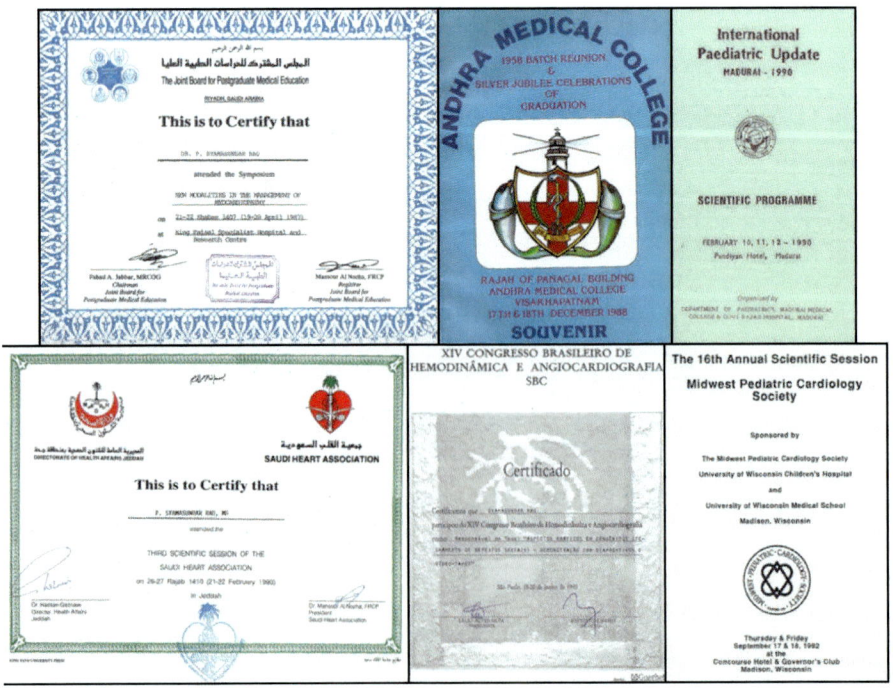

Figure 29. Copies of conference brochures or proceedings, or certificates of attendance (1987-1992).

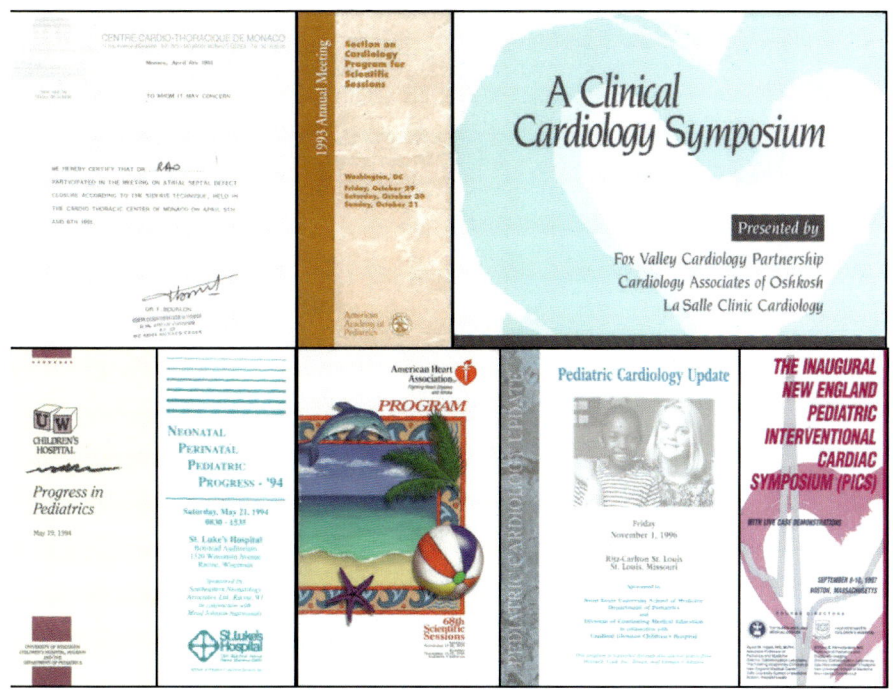

Figure 30. Copies of conference brochures or proceedings, or certificates of attendance (1993-1997).

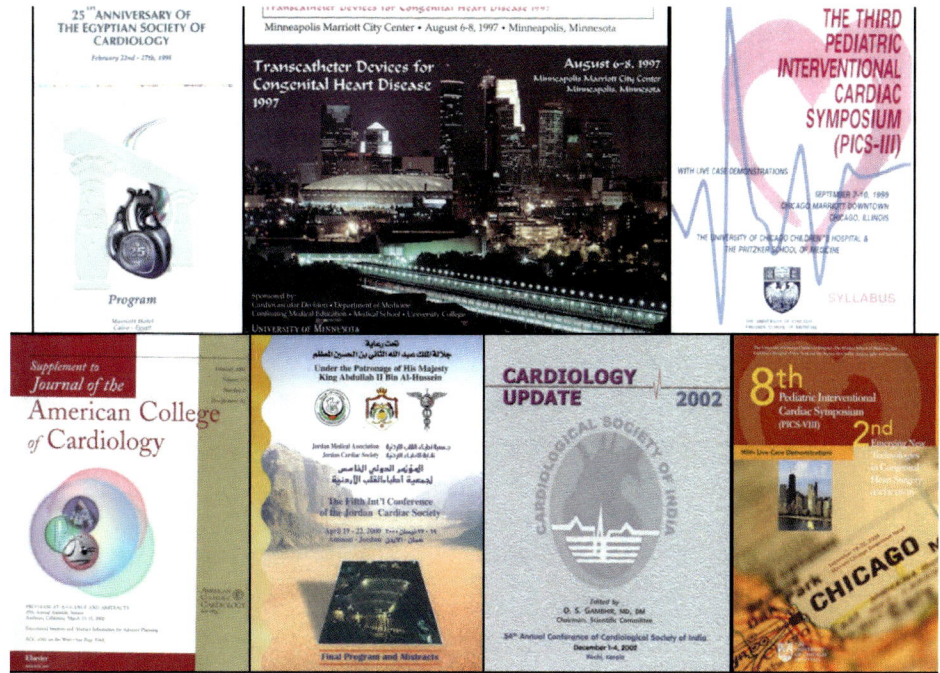

Figure 31. Copies of conference brochures or proceedings (1998-2004).

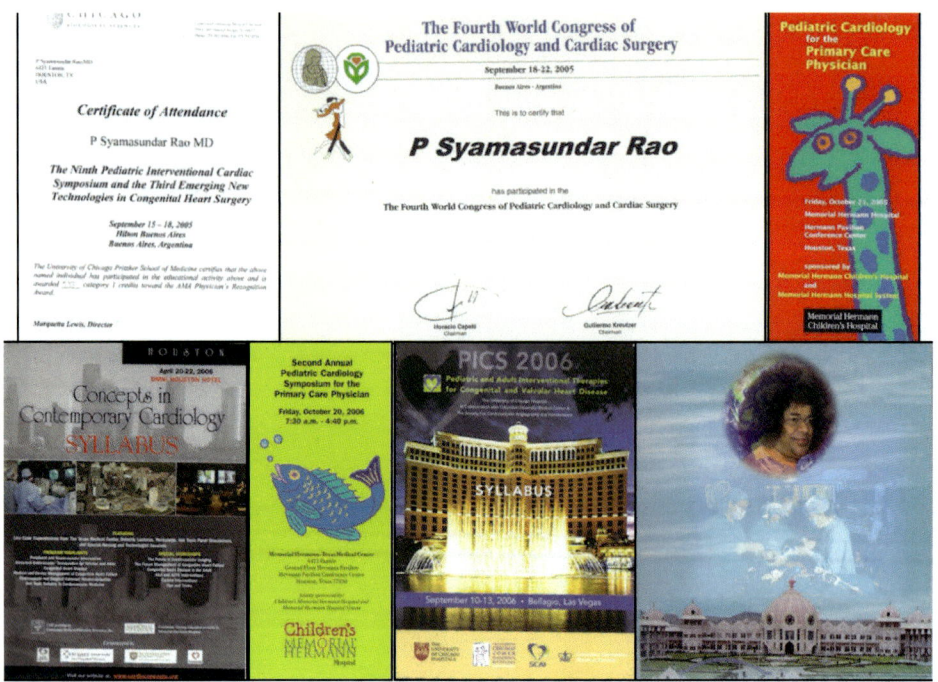

Figure 32. Copies of conference brochures or proceedings, or certificates of attendance (2005-2007).

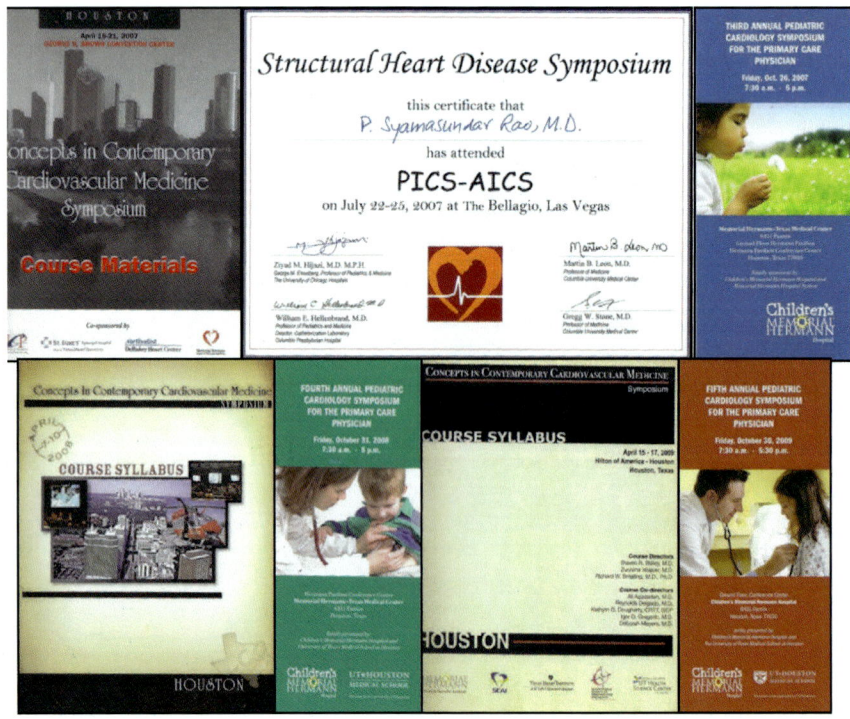

Figure 33. Copies of conference brochures or proceedings, or certificates of attendance (2007-2009).

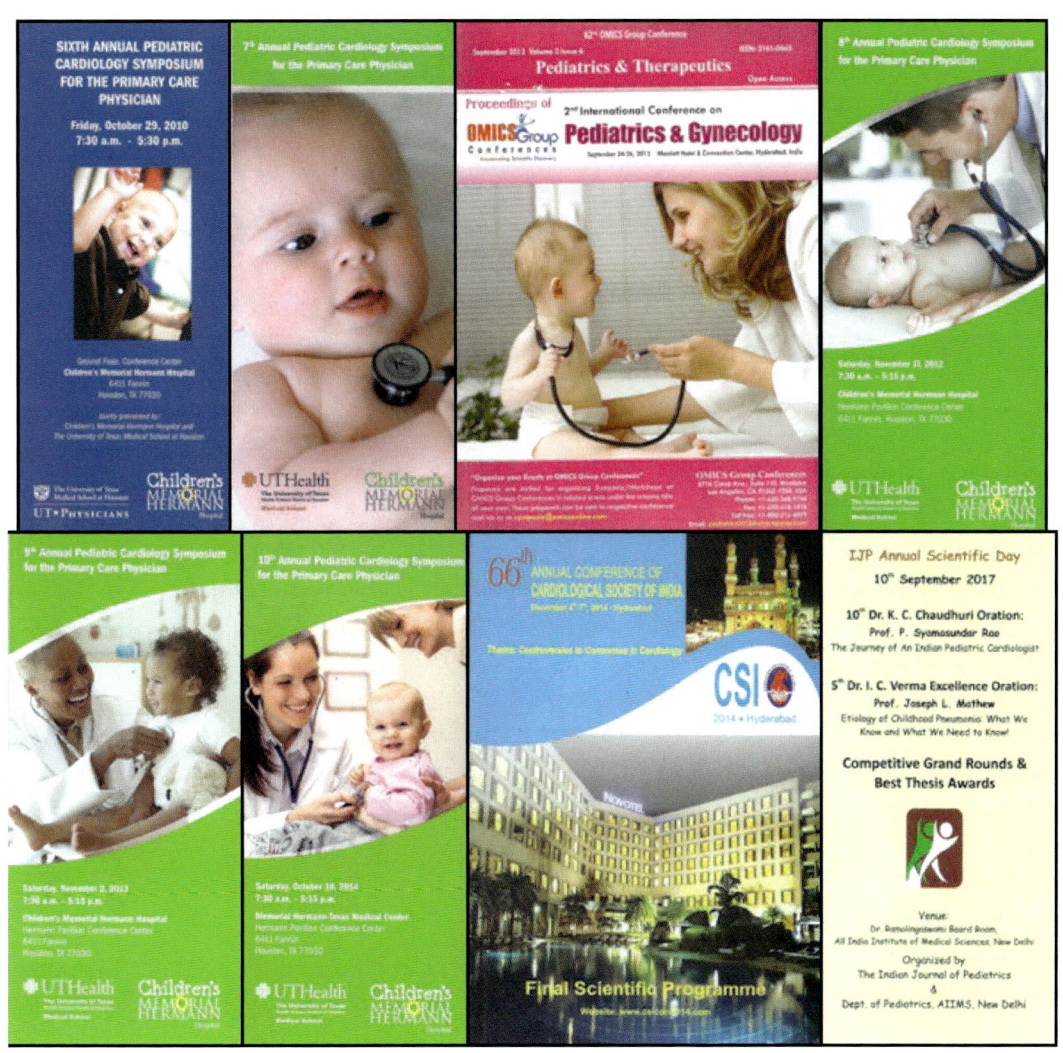

Figure 34. Copies of conference brochures or proceedings (2010-2017).

NEWSWORTHY EVENTS

Some of the activities of the author made significant contributions, resulting in creation of news. Some of these were reported in print form and others in television format. The television events could not be preserved in a form that could be reproduced in print format and therefore, will not be included. However, some of the news paper clippings were preserved and an attempt will be made to present these events.

As mentioned in the "Extracurricular Activities" section of the chapter on "The Journey Continues", I was selected to participate in the Republic Day parade in New Delhi in January 1962 and the contingent from Andhra Pradesh won first prize. The photographs of the participants with the Defense Minister, Krishna Menon; Prime Minister, Jawaharlal Nehru; other dignitaries, were published in Indian Express, as shown in figures 37 through 40 of the chapter on "The Journey Continues."

Following a mini-sabbatical with Dr. William B. Rashkind at the Children's Hospital of Philadelphia, PA, in June 1976, as described in the "Academic Career" section of the chapter on "The Journey Continues," I was selected as an investigator to test the Rashkind Occluder device to non-surgically close the atrial septal defects and patent ductus arteriosus; this became newsworthy and the story was published in The Augusta Chronicle in January 1981 (Figures 35 and 36).

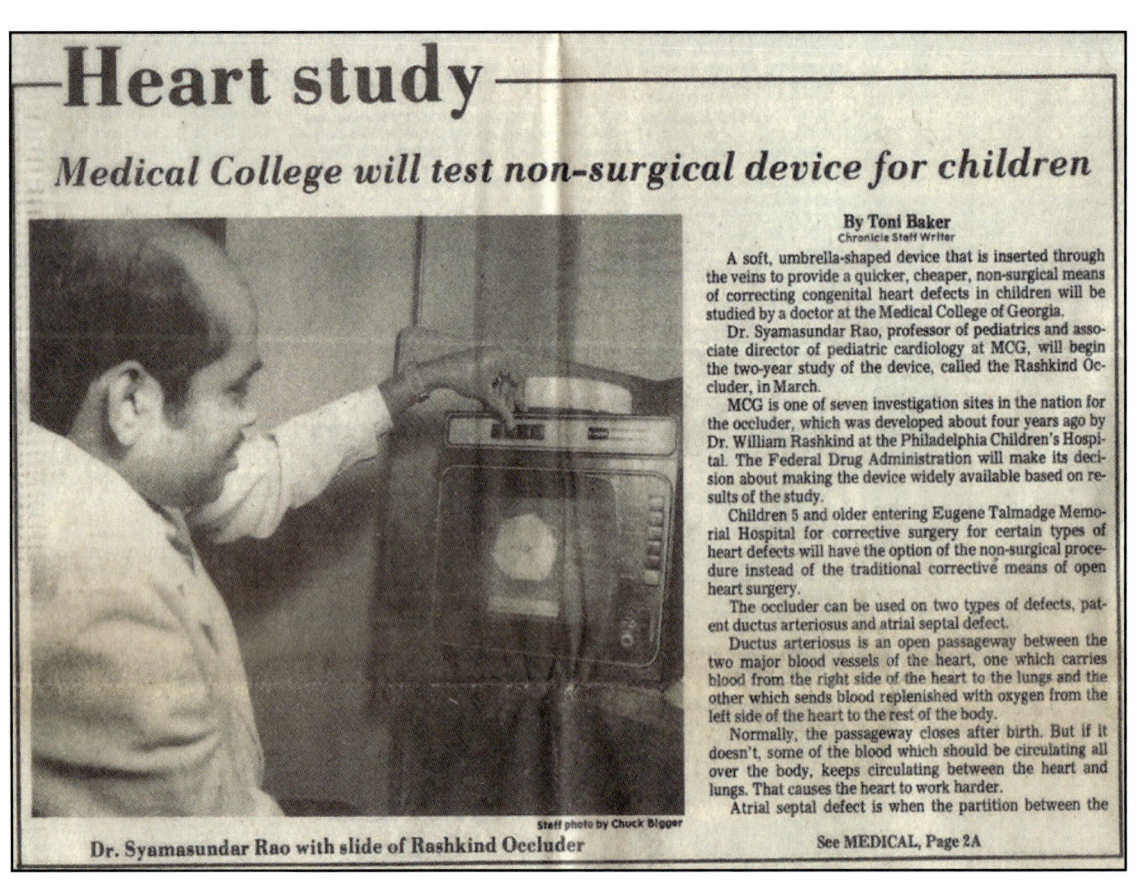

Heart study

Medical College will test non-surgical device for children

By Toni Baker
Chronicle Staff Writer

A soft, umbrella-shaped device that is inserted through the veins to provide a quicker, cheaper, non-surgical means of correcting congenital heart defects in children will be studied by a doctor at the Medical College of Georgia.

Dr. Syamasundar Rao, professor of pediatrics and associate director of pediatric cardiology at MCG, will begin the two-year study of the device, called the Rashkind Occluder, in March.

MCG is one of seven investigation sites in the nation for the occluder, which was developed about four years ago by Dr. William Rashkind at the Philadelphia Children's Hospital. The Federal Drug Administration will make its decision about making the device widely available based on results of the study.

Children 5 and older entering Eugene Talmadge Memorial Hospital for corrective surgery for certain types of heart defects will have the option of the non-surgical procedure instead of the traditional corrective means of open heart surgery.

The occluder can be used on two types of defects, patent ductus arteriosus and atrial septal defect.

Ductus arteriosus is an open passageway between the two major blood vessels of the heart, one which carries blood from the right side of the heart to the lungs and the other which sends blood replenished with oxygen from the left side of the heart to the rest of the body.

Normally, the passageway closes after birth. But if it doesn't, some of the blood which should be circulating all over the body, keeps circulating between the heart and lungs. That causes the heart to work harder.

Atrial septal defect is when the partition between the

Staff photo by Chuck Bigger

Dr. Syamasundar Rao with slide of Rashkind Occluder

See MEDICAL, Page 2A

Medical College will study heart device

Continued from Page 1A

two upper chambers of the heart doesn't develop. That defect also causes circulation problems.

The congenital defects can result in heart failure, heart infection and damage to the lungs — all of which are potentially fatal.

With open-heart surgery, the open passageway is sutured or the ill-developed partition is sewn together or patched with a piece of Dacron.

Open-heart surgery is a safe procedure for any age person, Rao said. But, it involves putting the patient to sleep and opening up the chest and heart. That chest incision leaves a large scar, something which can be traumatic, especially for a young person. Plus, the procedure costs the patient between $4,000 and $5,000 and keeps him in the hospital from seven to 10 days.

But the occluder is folded up and placed in a catheter — a long, thin tube which can be inserted in the vein. The catheter is pushed to the heart and through the area which is causing the problem. Then, the occluder is opened by a device in the physicians hand outside the body.

The soft device, made of polyurethane foam with three small stainless steel hooks, is pulled back against the opening. The hooks hold the occluder in place and within a month, a thin layer of tissue grows over it.

The virutally painless procedure costs about $2,000, requires from three to five days of hospitalization and the patient remains awake. Improved techniques might reduce hospitalization to only a day, Rao said.

Risks are slight, Rao said. Doctors will be observing the insertion of the device with a fluoroscope. But there is a chance that the device could be put in the wrong place. In that case, the open-heart surgery would have to be performed. During the surgery, the occluder could be removed.

Also, there is a small chance — about one in 100 — that the occluder could get dislodged. The loose occluder wouldn't pose any danger to the patient and could be retreived with another catheter, Rao said.

The Augusta Chronicle
(USPS 037-380)
AN INDEPENDENT PAPER
Printed daily (except Sunday and holidays) by Southeastern Newspapers Corporation, News Building, Augusta, Georgia 30913. POSTMASTER: Send address changes to The Augusta Chronicle, P.O. Box 1928(13), Augusta, Ga. 30913.
MEMBER OF THE ASSOCIATED PRESS
The Associated Press is entitled exclusively to the use of publication of all the local news printed in this newspaper as well as AP news dispatches.

Figures 35 and 36. Copy of story published in The Augusta Chronicle in January 1981 following my selection as an investigator to test the Rashkind Occluder device to non-surgically close the atrial septal defects and patent ductus arteriosus.

My colleague, Dr. Mardini, and I at the King Faisal Hospital and Research Center in Riyadh, Saudi Arabia, performed balloon dilatation of the pulmonary valve; this was the first time the procedure was performed in the Kingdom of Saudi Arabia prompting publication of this event in Arab News in May 1984 (Figure 37). The results in a larger number of patients was later published in medical Journals.[1,2]

Dilatation of pulmonary valve without surgery performed

By Wafa Al Wasif

RIYADH, May 5 — A rare medical feat — balloon dilatation of the pulmonary valve without surgery — was performed "for the first time in the Kingdom," at King Faisal Specialist Hospital here recently.

The surgery known in medical terminology as "transluminal percutaneous valvulopasty" was performed by two pediatric cardiologists — Dr. Mardini and Dr. Rao. They were able to split and dilate a severely destructive valve of the pulmonary artery (lung vessel) in two children, of one year and four years—during cardiac catheterization, under mild sedation not requiring anesthesia, surgery or even a cut down on any vessel.

The procedure was successful in both took only a few minutes after completing the diagnostic cardiac catheterization. Both children were transferred to their rooms without the need for staying in the recovery room or intensive care unit and both were discharged home the following day.

Explaining the procedure, Dr. Mardini said that it consists of percutaneous introduction through the skin without a cut down of a synthetic catheter containing a deflated balloon attached to its tip via the femoral vein into the right ventricle and then into the pulmonary artery through the obstructive pulmonary valve. Once the position of the balloon catheter is identified by the fluoroscopy, the balloon is inflated with special paque material under a high pressure using a pretested special equipment connected with the other end of the catheter. The inflation of the balloon should not last more than seven to 10 seconds while monitoring the heart rhythm and systemic pressure.

The same technique is repeated two to three times as required to assure adequate split and dilatation of the stenosed pulmonary valve by measuring a significant drop in the right ventricular pressure. This new method of treatment eliminates the need for open heart surgery using the cardio pulmonary bypass for surgical division of the stenosed pulmonary valve (pulmonary valvatomy) with its risk and complication. Furthermore, this modern technique shortens the period of hospitalization to about two days instead of 10 to 15 days allowing better utilization of beds.

Figure 37. A copy of story published in The Arab News in May 1984 following performance of balloon dilatation of the pulmonary valve by my colleague, Dr. Mardini, and I at the King Faisal Hospital and Research Center, Riyadh, Saudi Arabia; this was the first time the procedure was performed in the Kingdom of Saudi Arabia.

When I assumed the position of Professor of Pediatrics and Director, Division of Pediatric Cardiology at the University of Wisconsin, School of Medicine/University of Wisconsin Hospital and Clinics, it became instant news with publication in Wisconsin State Journal (Figure 38). Subsequent write-ups appeared in CenterLifelines (Figure 39) in December 1987, and Medical Directions (Figure 40) in Winter of 1988.

Pediatric heart doctor brings pioneering skill

By William R. Wineke

Medical reporter

Out of every 100 babies born in the United States, one will have some kind of congenital heart defect, and half of these babies — one of every 200 born — will need some major kind of medical intervention to save its life.

What that means is there will be between 25,000 and 30,000 babies born in the United States this year who may be good candidates for open-heart surgery.

A pediatric cardiologist who just joined the staff of the UW-Madison Medical School, however, hopes he can spare hundreds of Madison-area babies the danger and discomfort of such major surgery.

Dr. P. Syam Rao is a pioneer in a technique of sending a tiny catheter into the sick baby's heart and inflating a balloon that will repair the damaged heart.

It is a technique very similar to the popular balloon angioplasty procedure used by many Madison cardiologists to unclog arteries as an alternative to coronary bypass surgery.

But rather than opening arteries supplying the heart with blood, Rao's procedure is used to separate leaflets

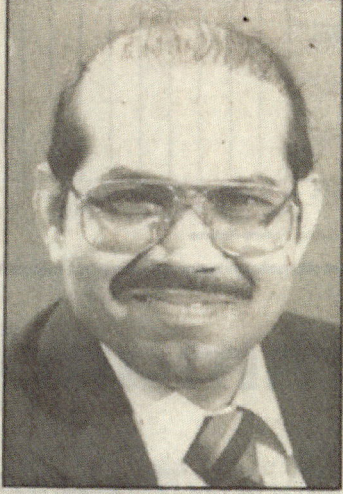

P. Syam Rao

that narrow a valve in the heart.

He says he can also plug holes in a baby's heart by using the catheter to deliver an "umbrella" to the hole.

The advantage is simple: The baby doesn't undergo surgery and, consequently, is far less likely to suffer complications, Rao says.

The baby is hospitalized for two days, rather than two to three weeks, according to Dr. Philip Farrell, chairman of the pediatrics department at UW.

The idea sounds simple, but it isn't. There are only about a half-dozen medical centers in the country that use a balloon catheter approach to pediatric heart cases, Farrell continued.

Farrell said he expects Rao will be able to perform about 75 procedures a year, and he said the recruitment of Rao "is a major development for the whole upper midwest in the field of congenital heart disease."

What makes use of the balloon catheter so rare is, of course, the fact that babies are so tiny.

The catheters and the balloons must be very small and must be very strong, Rao said. The cardiologist's skill must be very high.

A native of India who later served as associate director of pediatric cardiology at the Medical College of Georgia and as chairman of pediatrics at King Faisal Specialist Hospital in Saudi Arabia, Rao said he became a physician because of his grandfather's influence.

Farrell, who is obviously pleased at being able to recruit Rao — he advertised internationally for a pediatric cardiologist — and calls Rao "one of the best pediatric cardiologists in the world" — says Rao's work is a "key event in the field of pediatrics. It brings us to a national, even an international standard of pediatric cardiology."

Figure 38. A copy of the story published in the Wisconsin State Journal after I assumed the position of Professor of Pediatrics and Director, Division of Pediatric Cardiology at the University of Wisconsin, School of Medicine/ University of Wisconsin Hospital and Clinics, Madison, Wisconsin.

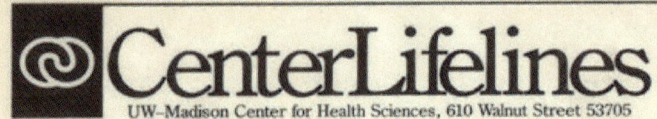

CenterLifelines

UW–Madison Center for Health Sciences, 610 Walnut Street 53705

December 1987

Treatments for patients young at heart

by Mark L. Hendrickson

At the time, his patients don't understand the profound effect he has on their lives. They're children—from a day to just a few years old—and they have congenital heart defects.

Dr. Syam Rao corrects many heart flaws that once required open heart surgery. Today he corrects them without raising a scalpel. Rao, professor of pediatrics at the UW Medical School and director of pediatric cardiology at UW Hospital and Clinics, uses tiny balloon catheters and careful maneuvering to repair common pediatric heart defects. It's a unique procedure, performed at fewer than a dozen medical centers in the United States. And it offers his young patients a life full of normal activity, work and play.

The benefits for patients are significant. Instead of open heart surgery, defects are corrected via catheterization, a diagnostic procedure all patients would have undergone anyway. Instead of a huge scar on the chest, the catheter incision leaves a two to three millimeter mark, and the children are hospitalized for just three days, rather than 10 days following surgery.

Types of defects

Three of the most common and most threatening congenital heart defects are treatable via catheter. They include:

- Pulmonic stenosis—narrowing of the pulmonic valve that regulates blood flow from heart to lungs.
- Aortic stenosis—narrowing of the aortic valve that regulates blood flow from the heart to the rest of the body.
- Coarctation of the aorta—narrowing of the aorta, the main blood vessel that

carries blood from the heart to the rest of the body.

If not corrected, narrow valves and blood vessels cause the heart to pump harder to maintain normal blood pressure beyond the obstruction. Many years of this exertion would lead to heart problems such as hypertrophy—or overgrowth—of the heart, restricting the child's activity.

Treating valvular defects

Pulmonic and aortic valves consist of three leaflets that open and close, regulating blood flow. In a defect, two leaflets may be fused together, reducing the volume of blood allowed to pass through the valve. To correct it, Rao carefully guides a balloon catheter through the valve and inflates the balloon for a few seconds, tearing the fused leaflets. In most cases, the tear helps restore near normal blood flow.

Treating coarctation of the aorta

In treating this defect, Rao positions the balloon catheter precisely at the narrow portion of the aorta. The balloon is inflated, stretching the tissue to make a wider blood vessel.

The balloon technique for coarctation of the aorta is a bit more difficult than those used for other problems, says Rao. If the balloon isn't inflated enough, it will not tear the tissue to relieve coarctation. If the balloon is inflated too much, it may tear excessively and cause swelling or a dangerous aneurysm of the blood vessel. "We match the size of the balloon to the size of the aorta, and monitor the procedure closely with special X-ray cameras and monitors in the catheterization laboratory," Rao explains.

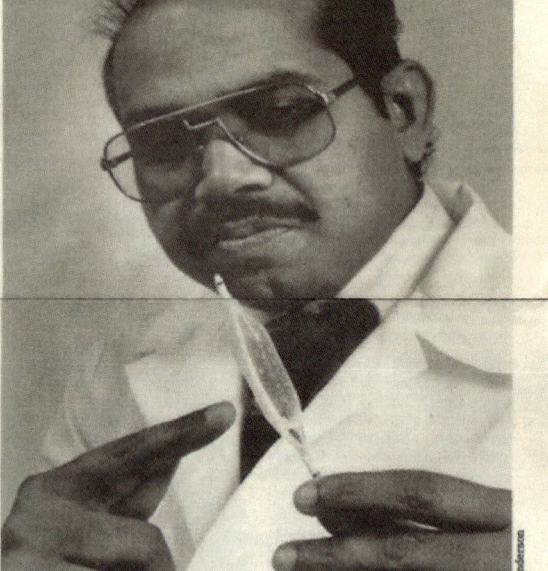

Dr. Syam Rao examines the type of inflated balloon he uses during catheterization to correct pediatric heart defects.

After the procedures, children soon regain their health and become more energetic. Even if defects are only partially corrected, patients can usually be much more active. While Rao's patients may not understand the effect of catheter treatment at the time, the results are readily apparent as they grow.

Figure 39. A copy of write-up published in the CenterLifelines in December 1987, following my arrival at the University of Wisconsin, School of Medicine, Madison, Wisconsin.

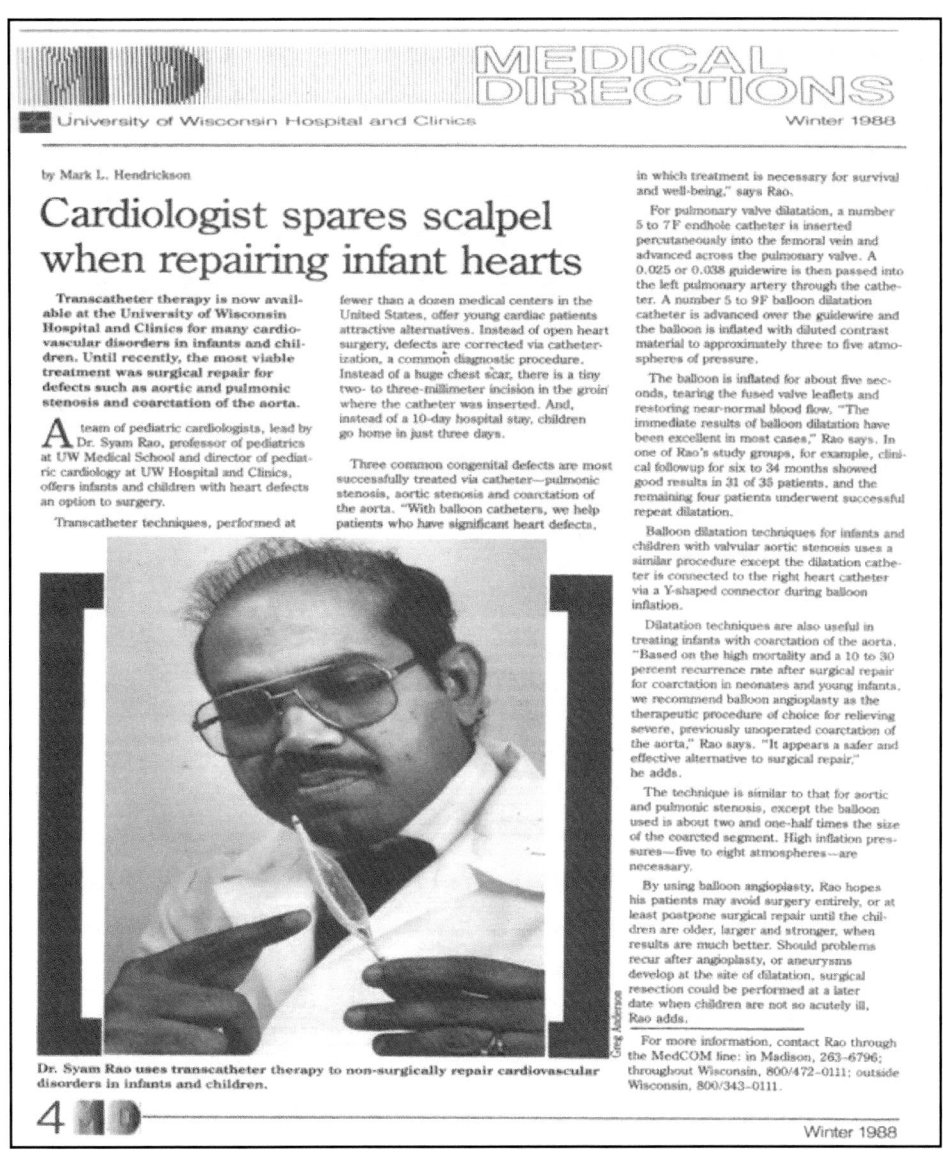

Figure 40. A copy of write-up published in the Medical Directions in Winter of 1988, following my arrival at the University of Wisconsin, School of Medicine, Madison, Wisconsin.

In August 1989, I was invited to serve as a protagonist for the topic, "Balloon Angioplasty Should be Used Instead of Surgery for Native Coarctation," in the session titled "Controversies in Pediatric Cardiology" at the Thirty Ninth Annual Scientific Session of the American College of Cardiology (ACC) to be held in New Orleans in March 1990 (Figure 41). I accepted the invitation and made a presentation supporting that balloon angioplasty should be used instead of surgery for native coarctation. A few months later, in November 1990, I presented an original paper on "Balloon Angioplasty of Native Aortic Coarctations in Neonates and Infants < 1 year: Follow-up Results" at the Sixty-Third Scientific Sessions of the American Heart Association (AHA), Dallas, Texas.[3] The Pediatric News published a summary of this presentation in their March 1991 issue (Figure 42). Although the presented AHA paper is largely unrelated to "Controversies in Pediatric Cardiology" discussion at ACC in March 1990, Dr. Gessner, the antagonist at the "Controversies in Pediatric Cardiology," chose to critique my presentation and Pediatric News' portrayal of my presentation (Figures 43 and 44). In the reply (Figures 43 and 44), I fully supported the Pediatric News' portrayal of the presentation and that it did not mislead. In addition, both side of the issue were adequately discussed. In addition, Dr. Gessner's support for surgical Dacron patch angioplasty is not warranted because of definitive development of aneurysms at follow-up. However, I did not object to waiting until all the data is in prior to making a final decision, especially when experienced clinicians and researchers like Dr. Gessner make such recommendations.

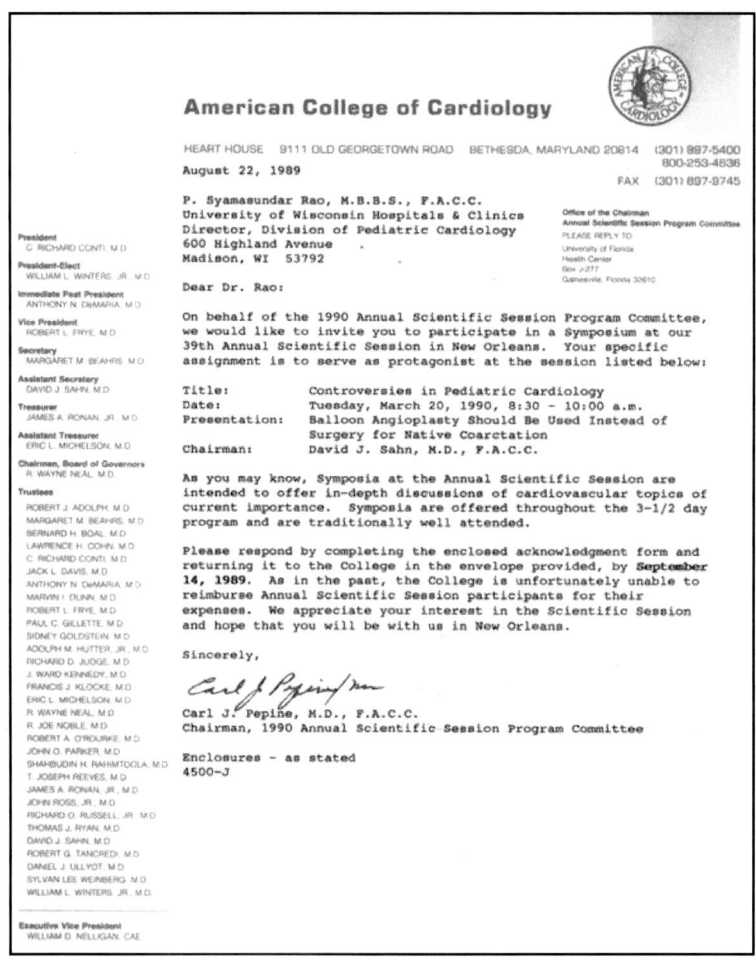

Figure 41. Letter of invitation asking me to serve as a protagonist for the topic, "Balloon Angioplasty Should be Used Instead of Surgery for Native Coarctation" in the session titled "Controversies in Pediatric Cardiology" at the Thirty-Ninth Annual Scientific Session of the American College of Cardiology in New Orleans in March 1990.

Balloon Angioplasty Is Advised for Native Coarctation in Infant

DALLAS — The low risk and excellent results of balloon angioplasty make this the procedure of choice for relief of symptomatic native coarctation in neonates and infants under age 1 year, Dr. P. Syamasundar Rao said at the annual scientific sessions of the American Heart Association.

Balloon angioplasty is just as successful as surgical repair, yet poses much less risk of morbidity and mortality in neonates and young children, said Dr. Rao, director of the division of pediatric cardiology at the University of Wisconsin Children's Hospital, Madison.

The residual coarctation gradient and coarcted segment size remain improved in 16 infants who underwent balloon angioplasty at the hospital during a 60-month period ending January 1990. None of the children developed aneurysms, and the five who had evidence of recoarctation were successfully managed with surgery or repeat balloon angioplasty.

When data from the literature were compared for 25 reports on balloon angioplasty from 1982 to 1989 and 5 reports on surgical repair from 1979 to 1986, balloon angioplasty had significantly lower rates of initial and late mortality (4 of 57, or 7%, and 1 of 55, or 2%, respectively) than did surgery (30 of 204, or 15%, and 26 of 174, or 15%), Dr. Rao said.

Although earlier reports on surgical repair indicated a recoarctation rate of 18%, more recent reports show a lower rate. In the pooled studies Dr. Rao cited, recoarctation occurred in 6 of 55 (11%) cases managed with balloon angioplasty and 14 of 174 (8%) managed surgically.

Dr. Rao's associates in this study were Drs. Mohinder K. Thapar, Omar Galal, and Allen D. Wilson.

Figure 42. Summary of original paper presented on "Balloon Angioplasty of Native Aortic Coarctations in Neonates and Infants < 1 year: Follow-up Results" at the Sixty-Third Scientific Sessions of the American Heart Association , Dallas, Texas, as published by The Pediatric News in their March 1991 issue.

Pediatric Forum

...plasty, Cholesterol Testing

...March 1991 issue of PEDIATRIC ...contains two items that I believe ...sleading in that they present only ...de of a controversial issue. One ...se items, particularly, has poten-...erious ramifications for the pedi-...ommunity.

...first, and less substantial, issue ...to your report on p. 8, "Balloon ...plasty Is Advised for Native ...ation in Infant." The article, re-...g a presentation by Dr. P. Sya-...dar Rao, presents limited data ...elatively short follow-up times ...early, as indicated in the next-to-...aragraph, uncertain conclusions ...ing efficacy.

...y pediatric cardiologists do not ...with Dr. Rao's recommendation. ...t, this issue was debated at the ...g of the American College of ...logy in March 1990 and the ma-...felt that surgery was the prefer-...eatment for native coarctation.

...appropriate, it seems to me, for ...workers to be investigating this ...ethod of therapy to determine its ...place in management of this ...ion. I think that it is unfortunate

the Muscatine study are among the leading authorities who say that manda-tory screening should not be done.

Creating an imperative that all chil-dren over the age of two should have their cholesterol measured is, I believe, a significant disservice. At the least, be-fore presenting this issue in your news-paper, I believe that you should seek to present both sides.

It seems to me these two examples cast substantial doubt on the validity of the word "accurate" on your front page.

Ira H. Gessner, M.D.
Gainesville, Fla.

Dr. Rao replies:

I do not agree with Dr. Gessner's as-sessment that your coverage is mislead-ing and presents only one side of the is-sue. Your article is a reasonably accurate account of what I presented in Dallas. I do not believe that every item abstracted in PEDIATRIC NEWS should be independently researched, editorialized, and polled for consensus.

I agree with Dr. Gessner that there is not complete agreement among pedi-atric cardiologists with regard to whether balloon angioplasty is the treatment of choice for native aortic

markedly lesser incidence of a... have been documented.

I receive numerous inquiri... cardiologists around the countr... ing clarification of the concept... technical aspects of balloon coa... angioplasty; these cardiologists... ther started to perform or hav... performing the procedure.

There seems to be a trend t... using balloon angioplasty in a... number of patients. However, I... object to someone, like Dr. G... who wants to wait until all the ... in before making a final decis... his or her patients.

Dr. Kashani replies:

I thank Dr. Gessner for hi... ments. No one doubts that the ... cholesterol screening in childre... resolved and that many unsettle... tions remain. The National Inst... Health pediatric guidelines rele... April 8, 1991 only recommend... ing children with a family histor...

The focus of my talk was on ... cents and I have not implied "m... ry screening"; perhaps the hea... misleading. Dr. Gessner prese... opposing view, one that is not ... by many experts in the field. I... aware of a consensus in any di... Therefore, calling cholesterol sc... "a significant disservice" repres... Gessner's personal point of vi... time may prove the contrary.

Despite the debate, there is ...

...ning.

...is issue was presented in debate ...at the ACC meeting in Atlanta in ...h and the majority of the pediatric ...logists and other workers present ...audience agreed with the position ...andatory screening is inappropri-...he major objection to mandatory ...ning—creating a population of ...nts" when no disease is present-...ot discussed in your article.

...e implications of mandatory ...ing of all children over 2 years of ...re enormous and the pressure on ...ricians to accomplish this task is ...sed by the type of article that you ...ated. Your article, while it does at-...to present some balance, clearly ...ressure on the general pediatri-...o accept the value of mandatory ...ing when the information in the ...is relatively meager.

...article, in fact, uses the Musca-...ata to support its conclusion, but ...th of the matter is the directors of

aneurysms develop in a significant

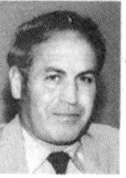

Dr. Kashani

number of patients following Dacron patch angioplasty, albeit several years later. It is not yet known whether or not a significant number of patients develop aneurysms following balloon angioplasty of native coarctation. These considerations suggest that Dacron patch angioplasty, as advocat-ed by Dr. Gessner, should not be used.

It also should be noted that my pre-sentation at the American Heart Asso-ciation meeting dealt with balloon an-gioplasty in neonates and infants (not children) and that, to my knowledge, no aneurysms were documented following balloon angioplasty in the neonatal and infant groups.

The controversy stems from two sources: a negative recommendation by one investigator based on balloon an-gioplasty of native coarctation in three infants; and two reports of a high inci-dence of aneurysms following balloon angioplasty in children.

Now that a large number of balloon dilatations have been performed worldwide.

...healthy eating habits in childr...

If one was to use the arg... "creating a population of patie... no disease is present," then ... cholesterol should be measur... hardly any child has corona... disease; this stands true for m... types of screening in pediatric...

It is the prudent hea... provider's job to make sure t... ease state is not created and, ... cated by the just-released NIH ... guidelines, promoting a ... lifestyle in children is the goal.

There is no potential harm ... dren from expert guidance on ... diet, exercise, and no smo... cholesterol value may provi... centive. The debate is a health...

Editor's note:

Although Dr. Rao answers ... tion of what "accurate" should... we'd like to restate our editori... ophy: When we started P... NEWS, we were determined to ... the truth. We soon ran into the ... of "whose truth?" so we set the ... alistic goal of printing the facts...

We tell you what reputabl... are saying at legitimate forum... every meeting presentation is ... view paper, neither are our ... Over the course of a year we ... sent many different viewpoints... ous issues. We count on ou... edgeable and medically soph... pediatrician readers to evalua...

...s is your page, a place where ...can voice your opinions. You ...welcome, but not limited, to ...ment on articles that we pub-...t. You're also invited to ex-...ss your views on anything of ...rest and concern to pediatri-...ns. Send your letters, subject ...editing, to us at Pediatric ...vs, 12230 Wilkins Ave., Rock-...Md. 20852

Figures 43 and 44. Dr. Gessner's critique of my presentation at the American Heart Association meeting and of the Pediatric News' portrayal of my presentation as well as my reply fully supporting the Pediatric News' portrayal of the presentation and of course, of my presentation. The Pediatric News' article also includes Dr. Gessner's critique of Dr. Kashani and his response.

Subsequent papers/editorials detail all the issues comparing the two techniques to address aortic coarctation.[4,5] More recent evaluation suggests the effective palliative role of balloon angioplasty in the neonate and small infant.[6,7] As more data were accumulated, our views evolved and the type of intervention now depends upon age at presentation, type of coarctation (discrete vs. long segment), nature of the coarctation (native, post-surgical or post-balloon re-coarctation) or a combination thereof (Figure 45).[8]

Age	Anatomy of the Coarctation	Mode of Intervention
Neonates and infants < six months	Irrespective of anatomy	Surgery
Infants and young children	Post-surgical recoarctation	Balloon angioplasty
Children older than 6 months and adults	Discrete native coarctation	Balloon angioplasty
Older children, adolescents and adults	Long-segment coarctation or significant isthmic hypoplasia	Stent placement
Older children, adolescents and adults	Post-surgical recoarctation, post-balloon recoarctation and aneurysms after surgical or balloon therapy	Stent placement

Figure 45. The type of intervention for aortic coarctations at the present time depends upon age at presentation, type of coarctation (discrete vs. long segment), nature of the coarctation (native, post-surgical or post-balloon re-coarctation) or a combination thereof.8

The AHA presentation was also reviewed by Cardiology World News in their May 1991 issue (Figures 46 and 47).

Relieving aortic obstruction
in neonates

Sleep apnea: Raising
the mortality risk of CVD

Advancing ultrasonic
angioplasty

Exercise echocardiography:
Improving CAD outcomes

MAY 1991

Cardiology World News™

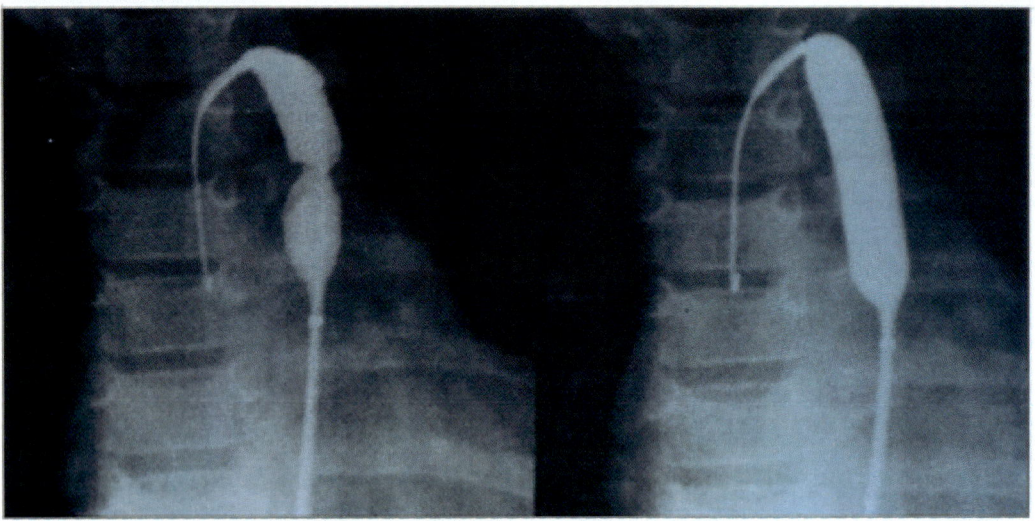

On the left, the radiograph shows the position of the balloon across the coarctation, in the initial phase of inflation. The right image shows complete balloon inflation (in a 3-month-old infant).

Relieving aortic obstruction in neonates

By Stephen A. Rothman

Balloon angioplasty is effective in relieving aortic obstruction in neonates and young infants, with an acceptable complication rate. Although the recoarctation rate is high, it can be relieved by repeat angioplasty or surgery when the infant is stable and less acutely ill.

Based on these findings and the high mortality and morbidity after surgical repair in neonates and young infants, "we recommend balloon angioplasty as the procedure of choice for relief of symptomatic native coarctation in neonates and infants," says Dr. P. Syamasundar Rao, head of pediatric cardiology at University of Wisconsin Medical School, Madison. Rao's study included 19 neonates and infants aged three days to one year who underwent balloon angioplasty of unoperated aortic coarctation over 60 months ending January 1990.

Indications for balloon angioplasty were congestive heart failure and/or hypertension not controlled by conventional medical management. Of those studied, three had no cardiac defect, three had a small patent ductus arteriosus, and the remaining 13 had significant associated defects.

THE AUTHOR is a health care writer based in the South and a frequent contributor to CARDIOLOGY WORLD NEWS.

Rao says the team used the balloon procedure with the following modifications:

▪ Addition of 100 units per kilogram of heparin administered immediately after the introduction of the arterial catheter; the heparin effect was neither reversed nor continued after balloon angioplasty.

▪ The size of the balloon chosen was two or more times the size of the coarcted segment but no larger than the size of the descending aorta at the level of the diaphragm, as measured from a frozen frame of the video recording.

▪ At no time was a catheter or guidewire manipulated over the area of freshly dilated aortic coarctation.

Several complications were encountered during and following the procedure. One balloon ruptured during angioplasty when the inflation pressure reached nine atmospheres. However, no adverse effects were noted.

Six infants sustained significant blood loss during catheter/guidewire exchanges and required transfusions. One infant lost the femoral pulse but had good perfusion. In another infant, low-molecular-weight dextran was administered because of poor perfusion in the catheterized limb. Perfusion improved by the morning following catheterization.

Despite these problems, all patients had good collateral circulation based on long-term follow-up, Rao says. Most of the patients were discharged home within 24 to 48 hours following the procedure. One 11-day-old infant died two days

Part II

Rao presented his conclusions at an American Heart Association scientific meeting. He cited eight previous papers reporting on studies of a total of 39 neonates and infants under one year. In 25 of these 39, the peak-to-peak systolic pressure gradient across the aortic coarctation was reduced from 64 ± 34 to 23 ± 26 mm Hg immediately after angioplasty, he says. Of the 39, he notes that surgical intervention was required in only two (5 percent).

after angioplasty while awaiting surgical palliation for double inlet left ventricle. The death resulted in a mortality rate of 5 percent.

None of the patients required immediate surgical intervention for aortic coarctation. With the exception of one infant who was lost to follow-up and one it was too soon to restudy, the remaining 16 had repeat cardiac angiography six to 15 months following angioplasty.

Despite improvements as a group, five of the 16 infants developed recoarctation, defined as peak-to-peak gradient of greater than 20 mm Hg. The residual gradients in these five were 39 ± 7 mm Hg. Four of the five were neonates at the time of angioplasty. Two underwent surgical repair early on. The other three had repeat angioplasty, with reduction of gradients from 30, 39, and 48 mm Hg respectively to 0, 10, and 8 mm Hg.

None of the 16 infants with follow-up angiographic study developed an aneurysm.

In clinical follow-up, three patients underwent surgical closure of ventricular septal defects after the follow-up catheterization. Two increased the severity of aortic valve obstruction and underwent successful balloon aortic valvuloplasty. Two had residual small patent ductus arteriosus, and no treatment was recommended.

One infant with cardiomyopathy improved left ventricular size and function. The remaining children were clinically well.

Equally impressive reductions of pressure gradient across the coarctation following angioplasty were achieved in 27 of 39 infants under 1 year who were reported on in the Valvuloplasty and Angioplasty of Congenital Anomalies (VACA) Registry. "Thus, immediate results of balloon angioplasty in infants are excellent," he says. "Balloon angioplasty appears to be an effective method of treatment for relief of symptomatic aortic coarctation."

In a previous study, Rao says he identified four factors for recurrence following angioplasty: Age under 12 months; aortic isthmus less than $^2/_3$ size of the ascending aorta; coarctation segment less than 3.5 mm before angioplasty; and coarcted aortic segment less than 6 mm after dilatation.

"We also observed that the higher the number of risk factors, the higher the chance for recurrence," Rao adds, noting that many of the infants in the series had several risk factors. "Despite this high recurrence rate, we believe balloon angioplasty is a worthwhile procedure," he says, "because repeat intervention to relieve residual or recurrent obstruction can be safely undertaken when the infant is older and is not acutely ill."

While recommendation for use of the procedure with native aortic coarctations has been clouded by reports of aneurysms developing at the site of dilatation, Rao says he knows of none reported after balloon angioplasty in infants under one year. The VACA Registry also does not list any children under age four who developed aneurysms, he says.

Although the data are encouraging, Rao cautions, longer-term follow-up results should be scrutinized prior to declaring freedom from aneurysm development in this age group. ♥

Figures 46 and 47. My AHA presentation was also reviewed by the Cardiology World News in their May 1991 issue.

In early May 1990, I performed button device closure of an atrial septal defect in a four-year-old girl by the name of Tammy Bitterman; this was the first time such a procedure was performed in the state of Wisconsin. The Public Affairs Department of the University of Wisconsin called for a news conference and a room-full of television and newspaper reporters attended and asked appropriate questions. The story was published in Wisconsin State Journal (Figure 48), the Capital Times (Figure 49), Adams County Times (Figures 50 and 51) and multiple other Wisconsin Newspaper Association affiliated papers (Figure 52).

METRO
■ Players plead innocent/2D
■ DEATH NOTICES/4D
■ CLASSIFIED ADS/4D

1D

●● Wisconsin State Journal
Wednesday, May 2, 1990

Birthday girl, 4, has reason to celebrate

By William R. Wineke
Medical reporter

Tammy Bitterman celebrated her fourth birthday on Tuesday and made medical history, too.

The daughter of James and Linda Bitterman, of Friendship, was born with a hole between the upper chambers of her heart.

The defect is usually closed in open-heart surgery but on Tuesday, University Hospital pediatric cardiologist Dr. P.S. Rao used a catheter and a device resembling an umbrella to close the hole with-

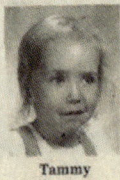

Tammy

out surgery.

Tammy, who entered the hospital Monday, is scheduled to leave today and should never again be bothered by the heart condition.

Had she received open heart surgery — the standard treatment for her condition — she would

have likely been hospitalized for seven to 10 days.

Her only scar will be from a small incision in her groin, where Rao inserted the catheter.

Rao said the procedure, called "transcatheter closure" has never before been done in Wisconsin. Eventually, however, he said he expects UW cardiologists to perform it on children about once a week on average.

The procedure involves threading a tiny catheter that carries with it tiny foam umbrellas

through a vein to the heart. When the catheter reaches the hole in the heart, the umbrellas open and plug the hole.

Within a few weeks, heart tissue grows across the umbrellas and, in effect, heals the heart defect permanently, Rao said.

He said Tammy was diagnosed at birth with the hole in her heart, an "atrial septal defect." Without treatment, about a third of persons with the defect develop a fatal disease of the blood vessels of the lungs during childhood. They also have problems with nor-

mal exercise and with childbirth.

Tammy, on the other hand, should be able to resume normal 4-year-old activity today.

Her parents said she celebrated her fourth birthday with a party Sunday.

The Bittermans have 11 other children between them, four of whom live at home. Tammy is their youngest. Linda Bitterman works for the Adams-Friendship Emergency Medical Service. James Bitterman is disabled and cares for the children.

Figure 48. A copy of the story published in the Wisconsin State Journal in May 1990 describing button device closure of an atrial septal defect in a four-year-old girl performed by me; this was first time such a procedure was performed in the state of Wisconsin.

UW fixes tot's heart without surgery

From staff, news service reports

A Friendship girl who celebrated her fourth birthday Tuesday by undergoing a new procedure that closed a hole in her heart will be back home with her family by tonight.

Tammy Bitterman, the daughter of James and Linda Bitterman, was born with a hole between the upper chambers of her heart. On Tuesday, she had it repaired without surgery at University of Wisconsin Hospital in a procedure never before used in Wisconsin, said Dr. P.S. Rao.

Rao, who is director of pediatric cardiology at UW Children's Hospital, used a catheter and a device resembling an umbrella to close the hole without the open heart surgery that is the standard treatment for the problem.

Tammy was scheduled to

leave the hospital today with the hope she never again will be bothered by the heart condition.

Rao said the new procedure, called transcatheter closure, has never before been done in Wisconsin but eventually could be performed on children about once a week by UW Hospital cardiologists.

The procedure involved making a 2-millimeter incision in the right groin and using a catheter to follow the vein up to the heart. The catheter carried with it small foam umbrella devices that opened up when the catheter reached the hole in the heart. Those umbrella devices were used to plug the hole.

Within a few weeks, heart tissue will grow across the umbrellas and, in effect, heal the heart defect permanently, Rao said. Tammy was sedated during the

procedure, which took about two hours.

Rao said Tammy was diagnosed shortly after birth with the hole in her heart, also called atrial septal defect. Without treatment, he said, about a third of the people with that particular defect develop a fatal disease of the blood vessels of the lungs during adulthood. They also have problems with normal exercise and with childbirth.

Tammy, however, should be able to resume normal 4-year-old activity immediately.

Her parents said she celebrated her fourth birthday with a party Sunday.

The Bittermans have 10 other children. James Bitterman cares for the four children who live at home. Linda Bitterman works for the Adams-Friendship Emergency Medical Service.

Figure 49. A copy of the story published in the Capital Times on May 2, 1990 describing button device closure of an atrial septal defect in a four-year-old girl performed by me.

Friendship girl scores a first

by David Steinkraus

On her fourth birthday, Tammy Bitterman received the most precious gift anyone could get.

Lying on a table at the University of Wisconsin Children's Hospital last Monday, April 30, she received a healthier life through "transcatheter closure," a new medical procedure that closed a hole in her heart yet had her out of the hospital just two days later. She is the first person in the state to be cured with the new technique.

The hole was a half-inch opening between the left and right atriums, the upper two of the human heart's four chambers. Though the problem had been diagnosed shortly after Tammy's birth, said her mother Linda, doctors waited until this year to see if the problem would correct itself. Originally, Tammy had another hole in her heart between the ventricles, the two lower chambers. But that hole sealed itself, Linda said.

Through the hole connecting the atriums, two and a half times more blood than normal flowed to Tammy's lungs, said Dr. P.S. Rao, professor of pediatrics and director of pediatric cardiology at the hospital and the physician who performed the transcatheter closure. Left uncorrected, the defect could cause pulmonary vascular obstructive disease, Rao said, in which the lung's blood vessels, swollen with too much blood, contract and thereby reduce the amount of oxygen supplied to the body.

But while transcatheter closure promised much, it is still an experimental procedure, approved only for limited use on humans. The only alternative for Tammy was the common one of open heart surgery which would have involved splitting open her chest and which would have required a seven- to 10-day hospital stay after the operation. For Jim Bitterman, transcatheter closure sounded worthwhile. His wife took a different view.

"It sounded too good to be true at first," said Linda, who works at Adams County Memorial Hospital as an emergency room technician and is studying to become a registered nurse.

So instead of giving immediate consent, the Bittermans returned to Friendship and consulted their pediatrician. He talked with Rao and

See Heart on page 11A

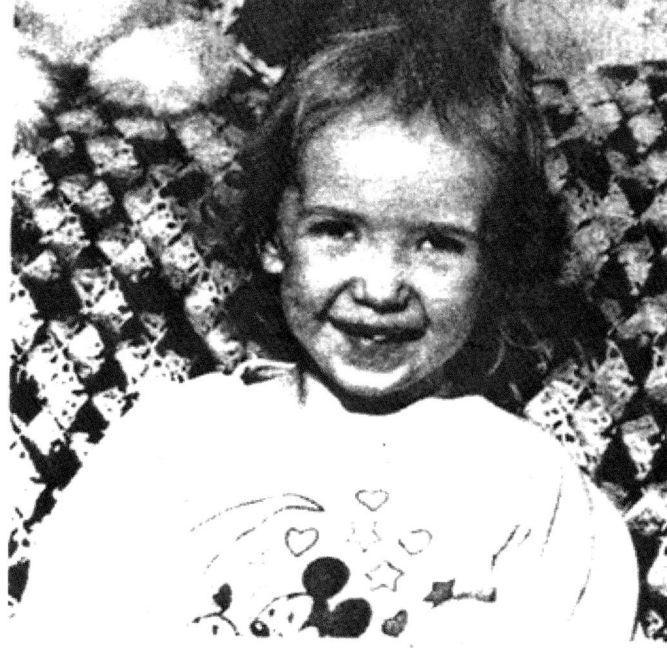

Adam County Times

Figure 50. A copy of the story published in the Adams County Times in May 1990 describing button device closure of an atrial septal defect in a four-year-old girl performed by me (Part I).

Heart

Continued from page 1A

then with the Bittermans. Given the extra advice, they decided to have Rao try the transcatheter closure.

Last Monday, Tammy was placed under simple sedation (not the full anesthesia needed for surgery) and Rao inserted a catheter into her abdomen through an opening about one-tenth of an inch in diameter. Using a fluoroscope, he maneuvered the catheter through Tammy's veins and into the left atrium of her heart.

Through the catheter, he inserted a small umbrella-like device made of polyurethane plastic with Teflon-coated wire spokes. He pushed the device through the hole and into the left atrium, expanded it, and pulled it back against the wall of the heart. A second umbrella was placed in the right atrium and connected to the first umbrella. With the plastic as a base, the tissue inside Tammy's heart will grow over the plastic like moss over a stone, providing an unbroken natural lining inside the atriums.

Outside the operating room, the Bittermans waited.

"It's a very traumatic experience," Jim said.

Adding to the tension was the presence of an open heart surgical team, which the Bittermans knew was standing by in case something went wrong with the transcatheter closure. Finally word came; the procedure had been a success.

In the future there may be other cases like Tammy's.

Once doctors gain more experience with transcatheter closure, they can ask the U.S. Food and Drug Administration to approve the technique for common use. Such approval may take about five years, Rao said.

But he doesn't see this procedure as the beginning of a trend that will make open heart surgery a rare event.

Of all the children born, about 1 percent have heart defects, Rao said. Half of those defects will cure themselves. Of the other half, the transcatheter technique will cure about one-third. The rest are too complex and will still require open heart surgery, he said.

But in cases like Tammy's, the new procedure means an end to the need for expensive open heart surgery, an end to the prominent scars typical of heart surgery, and an end to long hospital stays. The only facet of the whole procedure that bothered Tammy, Linda said, was the need to keep her one leg immobile for a day so the catheter wound could begin healing.

Last Friday, four days after the repair of her heart, Tammy was in the panelled den of the Bitterman's Lake Street home. Through the door into the Bitterman's kitchen came the cry of "momeee!" as Tammy tried to gain possession of one of the family cats from her 5-year-old brother Ricky.

"It's hard to keep her down," Linda said. "It's hard because she feels so good."

Figure 51. A copy of the story published in the Adams County Times in May 1990 describing button device closure of an atrial septal defect in a four-year-old girl performed by me (Part II).

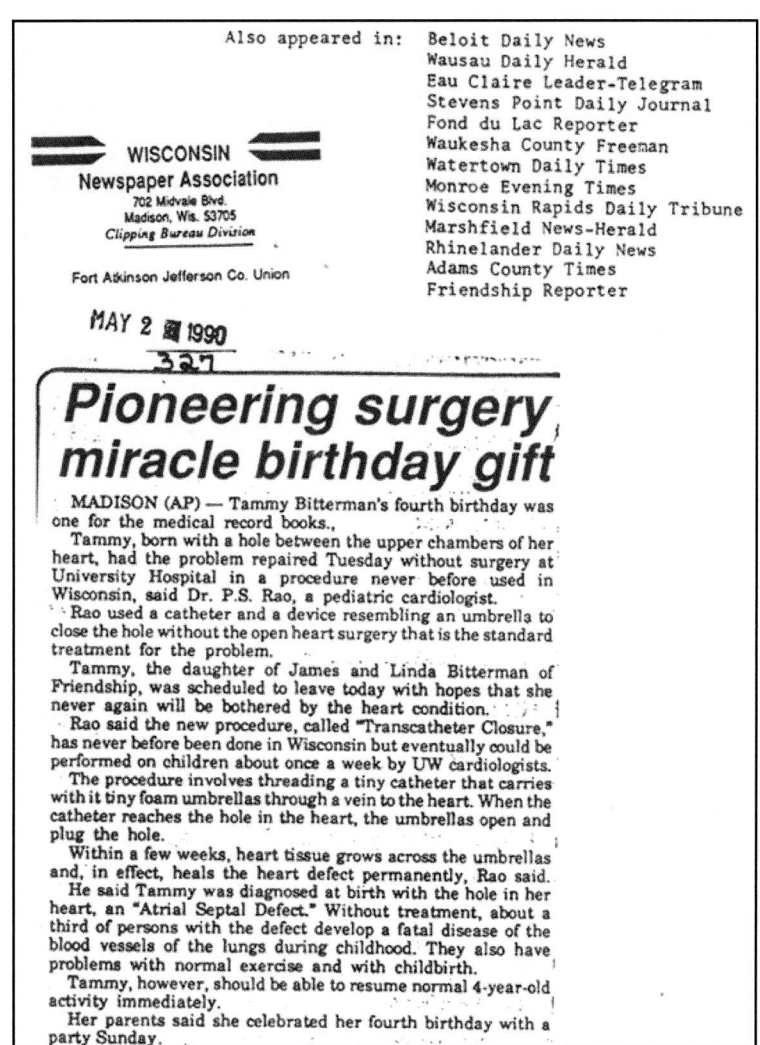

Figure 52. A copy of the story published in multiple other Wisconsin Newspaper Association affiliated papers in May 1990 describing button device closure of an atrial septal defect in a four-year-old girl performed by me.

Shortly after the publication of the above newspaper articles, I received a phone call from Mr. Le Roy Tietz who stated that his wife, Christine, had a stroke and her cardiologists and neurologists determined that Christine has a hole in her heart and needs open-heart surgery to repair the hole in the heart and asked if I could do the same procedure as I performed on Tammy and save his wife from open-heart surgery. I said, we could do it and Christine's data was evaluated and her hole in the heart (patent foramen ovale [PFO]) was closed with a buttoned device; the story was picked up by the Capital Times (Figure 53) on July 3, 1990.

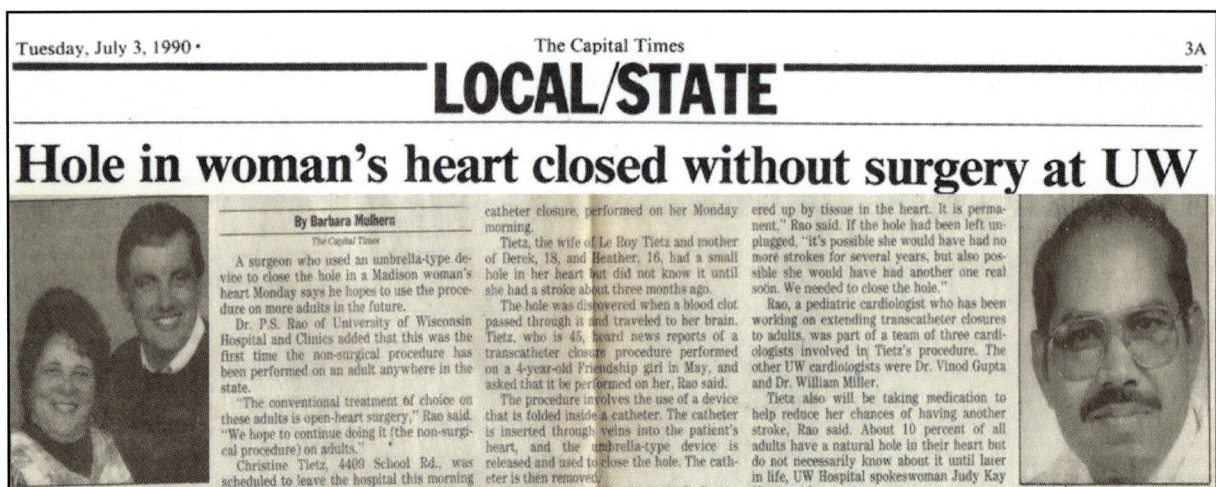

Figure 53. A copy of story published in the Capital Times on July 3, 1990 describing button device closure of a patent foramen ovale in a forty-four-year old lady performed by me for prevention of recurrence of stroke.

More than hundred children who had catheter-based interventional procedures and their families were invited to a picnic in August 1990, where an opportunity was provided for the families to exchange their stories with each other and a chance to interact with their doctors and nurses at a social level. This event was covered by multiple news organizations and one such story is shown in figure 54.

Reuniting in gratitude

By W.P. Norton

Correspondent for The Capital Times

More than 100 children and their families were part of the state's first-ever reunion of recipients of a unique treatment that eliminates the need for open-heart surgery in about 40 percent of coronary patients.

The event at Garner Park on Saturday, sponsored by the University of Wisconsin-Madison Children's Hospital, brought together the kids and their families so they could share stories, talk and just have a good time.

An 8-year-old technique known as transcatheterization allows doctors to bypass the open-heart procedure by use of a tube inserted in the groin.

The tube carries a device somewhat like an umbrella or balloon to the heart, where it corrects defects such as narrowed valves or holes between one of the heart's four chambers, said Dr. P. Syamasundar Rao, professor of pediatrics at the UW-Madison Medical School.

"The idea is to repair these defects by less-invasive means," Rao said.

Not only is the treatment less "invasive," it's also a lot easier on the pocketbook. Open heart surgery can cost between $40,000 to $50,000, while the catheterization costs only $5,000 to $8,000.

Not every patient with a heart defect can be helped by this technique, Rao said. But of the 1 percent of live births that have a congenital heart defect — about 25,000 to 31,000 each year — about half can be helped.

Ken Fenton is one father of a child that has been helped. A Waupaca salesman, his first child, Jaymes, had to have open chest surgery about a day after he was born in 1985. The first operation corrected the immediate problem, but was not a long-term cure.

Two years ago they went back to correct the problem with the balloon repair.

"It made us feel great," Fenton said. "This spring we went back and they did another (treatment) just to check. It looked the best it's ever been."

Figure 54. A copy of the story published in the Capital Times in August 1990 covering a picnic organized by me and the University of Wisconsin Children's Hospital to encourage social interaction of more than hundred children (and their parents) that had catheter-based interventional procedures.

I continued to use the techniques of balloon angioplasty/valvuloplasty and transcatheter closure of cardiac septal defects to address cardiac defects resulting in review of these procedures in the CenterLifelines (Figure 55) and the UW Building Blocks (Figures 56 and 57) in the Spring of 1991.

⊚ CenterLifelines
UW–Madison Center for Health Sciences, 610 Walnut Street 53705

7

March/April 1991

Balloons and umbrellas mend tiny hearts

by Kris Whitman

A miniature catheter may eventually replace the scalpel for thousands of infants and children with heart defects, says Dr. P. Syamasundar Rao, professor of pediatrics at the University of Wisconsin Medical School and director of pediatric cardiology at UW Children's Hospital.

Of the 35,000 infants with congenital heart defects born each year in the United States, about half heal spontaneously or with conventional management with heart medications. According to Rao, another quarter are likely candidates for non-surgical techniques to mend their defects.

Recognized as a pioneer in pediatric cardiology, Rao has fashioned procedures akin to those using catheters to remove plaque from the arteries of adults. He says two such techniques show particular promise with infants and children. The first, balloon angioplasty, uses a tiny balloon apparatus mounted on a catheter to separate small tissue flaps, called leaflets, that can narrow a heart valve. The second, transcatheter closure, uses an umbrella-like device to seal a hole in the wall between chambers of the heart.

"Compared to the surgical procedures they replace, both techniques offer many advantages for patients and their parents," says Rao. These benefits include:

* a two-day hospital stay rather than the seven to 10 days required for surgery;
* no general anesthesia or intubation;
* no intensive care unit stay;
* no surgical scar;
* less psychological trauma to the child and parents; and
* considerably less expense.

Rao says balloon angioplasty offers immediate results for patients with narrowing of the heart valve, narrowing of an artery near the heart and other lesions. In the last eight years, he has performed 300 such procedures. "Of these patients, only 10 to 15 required repeat catheterization procedures, and less than five went on to need surgery," he says.

During balloon angioplasty, Rao guides a catheter through the major vein or artery leading from the child's thigh to the heart. He then repeatedly inflates a balloon mounted on the tip of the catheter. "Our goal is to tear the valve leaflets precisely to allow the valve to open

fully and increase blood flow," explains Rao. If the defect is in an artery, the inflated balloon breaks through constrictions on the inner two layers of the vessel wall, again increasing blood flow. The technique requires precision to avoid damaging the outermost layer of the vessel wall, which would result in internal bleeding.

According to Rao, several medical centers in the United States use balloon angioplasty to treat pediatric patients with

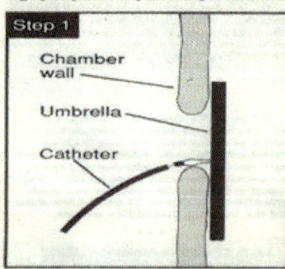
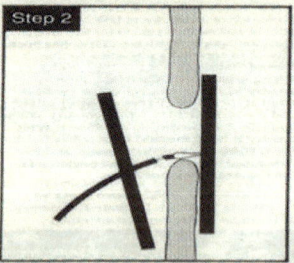

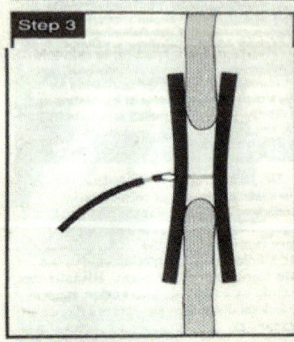
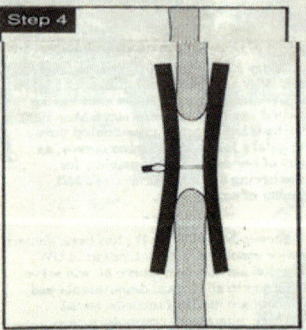

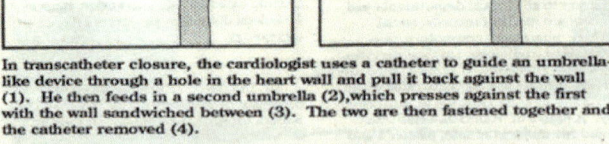

In transcatheter closure, the cardiologist uses a catheter to guide an umbrella-like device through a hole in the heart wall and pull it back against the wall (1). He then feeds in a second umbrella (2), which presses against the first with the wall sandwiched between (3). The two are then fastened together and the catheter removed (4).

defects in the pulmonary artery, the vessel that carries blood from the heart to the lungs. He is, however, one of few practitioners in Wisconsin to treat lesions in the aorta and aortic valve in this way. In addition, Rao is the only pediatric cardiologist in the state skilled in transcatheter closure, a procedure still in clinical trials.

Transcatheter closure benefits certain patients with abnormal openings between the left and right heart chambers, or between the aorta and pulmonary artery,

says Rao. "The size and location of the defect determines whether this technique or traditional surgical methods are most suitable," he adds.

During this type of defect closure, Rao "patches" the hole in a chamber or artery wall. After threading a catheter through the femoral vein from the thigh into the heart, he feeds an umbrella-shaped polyurethane device from the catheter through the hole and pulls it back against the wall (see diagram). Next, he feeds in a second umbrella, which presses against the first, with the wall sandwiched between the two. The two umbrellas are then "riveted" together, and the catheter removed. Within a few weeks, normal tissue grows over the umbrellas, which remain in place indefinitely.

Rao has performed six transcatheter closures, with the first in Wisconsin about a year ago. Most patients are six months to 10 years old, but Rao has used the procedure successfully on a 3.6-kg baby and a 45-year-old woman—the first adult to undergo the procedure in Wisconsin. "The conventional treatment for adults is open-heart surgery, but in this case catheterization closure was applicable and the patient preferred it," says Rao.

"Using balloon angioplasty and transcatheter closure, we'll be able to correct more and more types of heart defects and to reduce the number of patients who need surgery or repeated non-surgical treatments," says Rao. Nevertheless, he points out, surgery remains the appropri-

Like any medical procedure, catheterization techniques carry risks and disadvantages as well as advantages. Possible complications include temporarily irregular heartbeats, rupture or bulging of the vessel wall or re-narrowing of a vessel or valve after the procedure. Also, because the techniques are new, physicians have little information about patients' long-term medical needs. "We know, however, that total complications for these procedures affect only about 5 to 10 percent of patients, and follow-up results for the first five years are encouraging," says Rao.

The future success of these procedures depends on the availability and miniaturization of equipment. "The catheters must be minuscule for use on tiny infants, but the devices are getting better all the time. I anticipate continued advances and improvements in results," Rao concludes.

Figure 55. A copy of the write-up published in CenterLifelines in 1991 describing the use of techniques of balloon angioplasty/valvuloplasty and transcatheter closure of cardiac septal defects to treat cardiac defects at University of Wisconsin.

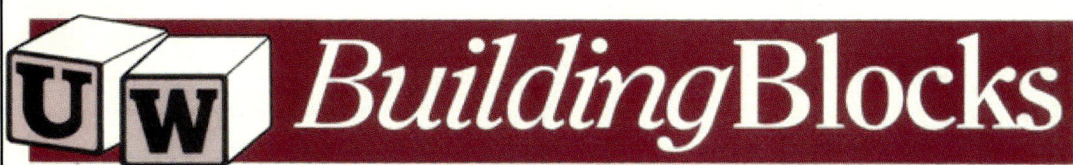

UNIVERSITY OF WISCONSIN CHILDREN'S HOSPITAL MADISON

Presenting issues and advances in the care of children

Spring 1991

Young patients benefit from non-surgical heart defect repair

by Kris Whitman

A miniature catheter may eventually replace the scalpel for thousands of pediatric heart surgery candidates, says P. Syamasundar Rao, M.D., professor of pediatrics at the University of Wisconsin Medical School and director of the division of pediatric cardiology at UW Children's Hospital.

Of the 35,000 infants with congenital heart defects born each year in the United States, about half heal spontaneously or with medical management. Another quarter are likely candidates for non-surgical techniques rather than traditional open or closed heart surgery to mend defects.

Rao has adapted catheterization procedures similar to those used in adults to combat arterial plaque. He says two such techniques for pediatric patients deserve particular note: balloon angioplasty to separate leaflets that narrow a heart valve; and transcatheter closure of a hole in the wall between chambers in the heart. "Compared to the surgical procedures they replace, both techniques offer many advantages," says Rao. These benefits include:

- a two-day hospital stay rather than the seven to 10 days required for surgery;
- no general anesthesia or intubation;
- no intensive care unit stay;
- no scar of cardiac surgery;
- less psychological trauma to the child and parents; and
- considerably less expense.

He explains that balloon angioplasty offers immediate results for patients with pulmonic or aortic stenosis, aortic coarctation and other lesions. In the last eight years, Rao has performed 300 such procedures with great success. "Of these patients, only 10 to 15 required repeat catheterization procedures, and less than five went on to need surgery," he explains.

Continued on page 4

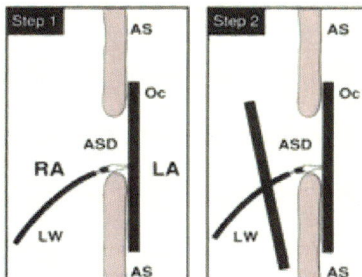

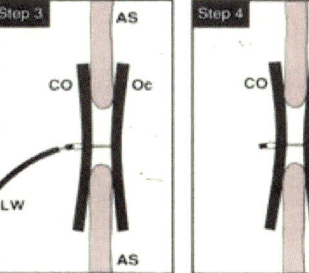

AS, atrial septum;
ASD, atrial septal defect;
CO, counter-occluder (second umbrella);
LA, left atrium;
LW, loading wire;
Oc, occluder (first umbrella);
RA, right atrium.

Transcatheter closure—a non-invasive procedure that repairs atrial and ventricular septal defects, patent ductus arteriosus and other heart defects in infants and children—offers many benefits over the open heart surgery it replaces. During this yet-experimental procedure, a polyurethane umbrella is fed from a catheter through the hole in the septum and pulled back toward the chamber wall. The chamber wall is then sandwiched between this and a second umbrella. Both become encompassed by normal tissue and remain in place indefinitely. P. Syamasundar Rao, M.D., a UW Children's Hospital pediatric cardiologist, is the only practitioner in Wisconsin skilled in transcatheter closure.

*Spring
1991*

Non-surgical heart repair

from page 1

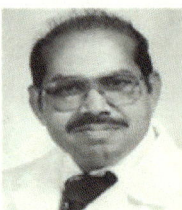

P. Symasundar Rao, M.D., graduated from the Andhra Medical College in India, and obtained pediatric cardiology training at Stanford University, University of California at Los Angeles and Case Western Reserve University. Board certified in pediatrics and pediatric cardiology, Rao joined UW Children's Hospital in 1987.

Once a heart defect has been diagnosed by conventional studies, the indications for using balloon angioplasty are the same as for surgery, explains Rao. The blood pressure gradient across the obstruction is the key to determining whether the condition is severe enough to justify intervention.

During balloon angioplasty, Rao guides a catheter through the infant or child's femoral vein or artery to the lesion. Then, the balloon is inflated with contrast agent three to four times for five seconds each, with five minutes between inflations.

"Our goal is to precisely tear the commissures of the valve leaflets to allow the valve to open fully, decreasing the pressure difference and increasing blood flow to a normal level," explains Rao. If the lesion is in an artery, the inflated balloon breaks strictures on the inner two layers of the vessel wall; the technique requires precision to avoid damage to the outermost layer of the vessel.

According to Rao, several medical centers in the United States use balloon dilatation to treat pulmonic stenosis in children; he is, however, one of few practitioners in Wisconsin to treat aortic stenosis and other conditions in this way. In addition, Rao is the only pediatric cardiologist in the state skilled in transcatheter closure, a procedure still under experimental protocol.

Transcatheter closure benefits certain patients with atrial or ventricular septal defects or patent ductus arteriosus, says Rao. "The size and location of the defect determines whether this technique or traditional surgery is most suitable."

During this type of defect closure, Rao threads a catheter through the femoral vein into the heart. An umbrella-shaped polyurethane device is fed from the catheter through the hole in the septum and pulled back toward the chamber wall. A second umbrella is pressed against the first, with the chamber wall sandwiched between the umbrellas. The two umbrellas are connected, and the catheter removed. Within a few weeks, normal tissue grows over the umbrellas, which remain in place. (See diagram on page 1.)

Rao has performed six transcatheter closures, with the first in Wisconsin about a year ago. Most patients are between ages six months and 10 years, but have included a 3.6-kilogram baby and a 45-year-old woman—the first adult to undergo this procedure in Wisconsin.

"Balloon angioplasty and transcatheter closure offer great potential to improve more and more types of heart defects," says Rao. However, surgery remains the appropriate choice for certain conditions, including transposition of the great arteries, tetralogy of Fallot and other complex defects.

As with any medical procedure, non-surgical techniques carry risks and disadvantages. Possible complications include temporary arrhythmias, rupture of the vessel wall, aneurysm formation or re-narrowing of a vessel or valve. Also, because the techniques are new, statistics for long-term follow-up are not available. "However, total complications for these procedures affect only about 5 to 10 percent of patients, and follow-up results for the first five years are encouraging," says Rao.

The future success of these procedures depends on the availability and miniaturization of the equipment.

"These procedures and the devices are getting better all the time," Rao concludes. "I'd say the techniques will only improve."

For more information, contact Rao via MedCOM: in Madison, 263-6796; throughout Wisconsin, (800) 472-0111; outside Wisconsin, (800) 343-0111.

Rao PS: Balloon valvuloplasty and angioplasty in infants and children. *Journal of Pediatrics* 1989;114(6):907-914.

Rao PS: Transcatheter management of heart disease in infants and children. *Pediatric Res. Commun.* 1987;1:1-18.

Figures 56 and 57. A copy of the write-up published in the UW Building Blocks in the spring of 1991 describing the use of techniques of balloon angioplasty/valvuloplasty and transcatheter closure of cardiac septal defects to treat cardiac defects at University of Wisconsin.

Establishment of satellite Pediatric Cardiology clinic at Wausau Hospital (Figures 58 and 59) and formation of Adult Congenital Heart Disease Clinic at the Center for Health Sciences in Madison (Figures 60 and 61) were publicized.

Pediatric cardiology services to be offered here

Pediatric cardiologists from the University of Wisconsin-Madison will hold office hours one day a month at Wausau Hospital Center beginning August 12.

Bringing this subspecialty service to Wausau is an outgrowth of the affiliation agreement between Wausau Hospital Center and the University of Wisconsin Hospital and Clinics.

One of the objectives of the affiliation is to bring to Wausau specialized medical services not currently available locally in order to enhance the accessibility, quality and depth of health care to residents of Central and Northern Wisconsin.

"We developed this new service after receiving encouragement from local pediatricians, family practice physicians, cardiologists and cardiovascular surgeons," said Lee Olkowski, Vice President of Corporate Services.

Two Pediatric Cardiologists will be sharing visits to Wausau.

Dr. P. Syamasundar Rao is internationally recognized in the field having done extensive research in congential heart disease, electrophysiology and echocardiography. He is a leading authority on Tricuspid Atresia, a type of heart birth defect. He has also done research in the development of catheters and other devices to provide nonsurgical correction of congenital heart disease.

Dr. Rao received his Medical Degree from Andhra Medical College in India. He served his residency in Pediatrics at Good Samaritan Hospital, Phoenix, Arizona, and served fellowships in Pediatric Cardiology at Stanford University School of Medicine, Stanford, California and the University Hospitals of Cleveland and Case-Western Reserve University School of Medicine, Cleveland, Ohio.

In addition, he served a research fellowship in Pediatric Cardiology and Cardiovascular Physiology at U.C.L.A. School of Medicine in Los Angeles, California. Dr. Rao was also a Professor of Pediatrics in the Pediatric Cardiology Section of the Medical College of Georgia, Augusta, Georgia.

Last August, Dr. Rao spoke at a Wausau Hospital Center Medical Surgical Conference on the identification of newborns with heart defects, cardiac diagnosis and new methods of treating heart defects.

Dr. Allen Wilson is an Associate Professor of Pediatrics at the University of Wisconsin Hospital and Clinics and serves as Director of Pediatric and Fetal Echocardiography.

He received his Medical Degree from Abraham Lincoln School of Medicine, University of Illinois. He is board certified in Pediatrics and Pediatric Cardiology and has published several papers in the field of Pediatric Cardiology.

Appointments with the physicians can be arranged by calling 847-2349.

insights

Published by the Wausau Hospital Center for its employees, medical staff, volunteers and friends.

Donald C. Sibery
President

Kenneth L. Day, Ph.D.
Vice President for Marketing

Paul Jaeger
Director of Public Relations

Don Oakland
Writer/Editor

Leon Tietyen
Photographer

Wausau Hospital Center,
333 Pine Ridge Blvd.
Wausau, WI 54401. 847-2255

Figures 58. A copy of the write-up published in the Insights of Wausau Hospital announcing the establishment of satellite Pediatric Cardiology clinic at the Wausau Hospital.

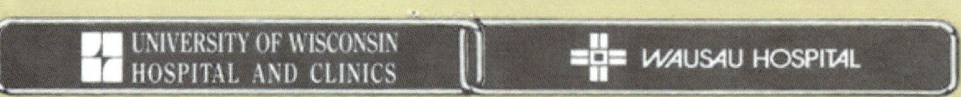

Working together on specialty care.

For the parents of a three-year-old child with a congenital heart condition or for a grandmother suffering from emphysema, the need for convenient specialty care is vital – no matter where they live. As a result of the five-year affiliation between UW Hospital and Clinics and Wausau Hospital, many residents in north and central Wisconsin now have greater access to a wider range of specialties. By working together on specialty care, UW Hospital and Clinics and Wausau Hospital have achieved these major accomplishments:

A pediatric cardiology clinic has been established at Wausau Hospital.

Dr. P. Syamasundar Rao, a professor of pediatrics and division head of pediatric cardiology at UW Children's Hospital, has conducted a pediatric cardiology clinic in Wausau for the past four years. During visits to Wausau, Dr. Rao consults with several area physicians and sees eight to 12 patients each month. In the past two years, he has conducted approximately 200 evaluations on more than 100 patients.

An endocrinology clinic has been developed.

Two endocrinology physicians who are professors at the UW Medical School, Dr. Wolfram Nolten and Dr. Don Schalch, share monthly visits to the clinic. They consult with area physicians and see patients with disorders including diabetes mellitus and its complications,

and specific endocrine disorders including the pituitary, hypothalamus, thyroid and adrenal glands, and the gonads. The clinic also is staffed by a Wausau Hospital registered nurse and a registered dietitian who received training in working with endocrinology patients at UW Hospital and Clinics. In addition, the clinic serves as a

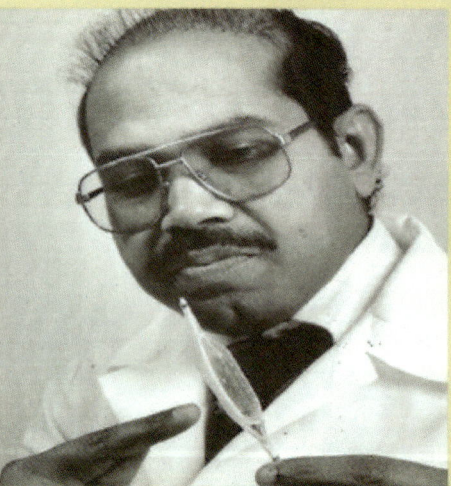

When Dr. P. Syamasundar Rao sees patients at Wausau Hospital's Pediatric Cardiology Clinic, he brings with him extensive knowledge of congenital heart defects in infants and children. Rao is skilled in non-surgical techniques such as balloon angioplasty and transcatheter closure to repair certain defects.

training site for residents in the Wausau-based UW Family Practice Residency Program.

The organ donation and transplant program has been expanded.

UW Hospital and Clinics offers one of the largest and most

successful organ transplant centers in the United States, according to a recent report released by the Health Resources and Services Administration, the federal agency responsible for the nation's organ donation and transplant programs. As a result of the affiliation, residents in north and central Wisconsin are benefiting from and supporting this program more than ever. UW Hospital and Clinics has trained several individuals in the area to serve as organ procurement coordinators, and organ procurement teams from UW Hospital fly to Wausau Hospital when donor organs become available.

Patients with chronic pulmonary disease in north and central Wisconsin receive better care.

In 1978, UW Hospital and Clinics started RESTOR, which stands for Respiratory Education and Services Through Organized Resources. In April 1992, UW Hospital named Wausau Hospital a regional center for the program. Members of the RESTOR staff teach people with respiratory problems (such as bronchitis, asthma and emphysema) how to better manage their diseases and live fuller, more active lives.

Figures 59. A copy of the write-up published in University of Wisconsin Hospital and Clinic and Wausau Hospital publication announcing the establishment of satellite Pediatric Cardiology clinic at Wausau Hospital.

Public Affairs Department
758 WARF Building
610 Walnut Street
Madison, WI 53705
Ph. (608) 262–6343
FAX (608) 263–6394

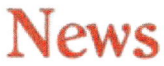

Center for Health Sciences
University of Wisconsin–Madison

FOR RELEASE UPON RECEIPT   CONTACT: Judy Kay Moore or
                                            Amy Hiesberg

Date mailed: August 23, 1993   Phone: (608) 262-6343

UW OPENS ADULT CONGENITAL HEART DISEASE CLINIC

MADISON, Wis. — To better serve adults with congenital heart defects, cardiologists at UW Children's Hospital and UW Hospital and Clinics have teamed up to open the Adult Congenital Heart Disease Clinic.

The clinic offers expertise in congenital heart defects and coronary artery disease, according to Dr. P.S. Rao, cardiologist at UW Children's Hospital and professor of pediatrics at UW Medical School. Rao co-directs the clinic with Dr. Ford Ballantyne, cardiologist at UW Hospital and Clinics and associate professor of medicine at UW Medical School.

About one in 100 children is born with a congenital heart defect. The clinic assists those who need additional care for their condition as they become adults and also treats those born with heart conditions that were not diagnosed until adulthood.

Some simpler defects, such an abnormal connection between the pulmonary artery and the aorta, may be cured in childhood, according to Rao and Ballantyne. But many other congenital heart defects need continual follow-up, either because there are residual problems, or the natural history of those defects indicates that they may get worse with time.

For more information on the clinic, call the Adult Cardiology Clinic at (608) 263-1530 and ask for the Adult Congenital Heart Disease Clinic appointment desk.

Figure 60. Center for Health Sciences of University of Wisconsin announcing the formation of the Adult Congenital Heart Disease Clinic at the Center for Health Sciences in Madison, which will be co-directed by me and Dr. Ford Ballantyne.

**Wisconsin Week
9-2-93**

■ UW opens heart clinic — To better serve adults with congenital heart defects, cardiologists at UW Children's Hospital and

UW Hospital and Clinics have teamed up to open the Adult Congenital Heart Disease Clinic.

The clinic offers expertise in congenital heart defects and coronary artery disease, according to P.S. Rao, cardiologist at UW Children's Hospital and professor of pediatrics at UW Medical School. Rao co-directs the clinic with Ford Ballantyne, cardiologist at UW Hospital and Clinics and associate professor of medicine at UW Medical School.

About one in 100 children is born with a congenital heart defect. The clinic assists those who need additional care for their condition as they become adults and also treats those born with heart conditions that were not diagnosed until adulthood.

Some simpler defects, such as an abnormal connection between the pulmonary artery and the aorta, may be cured in childhood, according to Rao and Ballantyne. But many other congenital heart defects need continual follow-up, either because there are residual problems, or the natural history of those defects indicates that they may get worse with time.

For more information on the clinic, call 263-1530 and ask for the Adult Congenital Heart Disease Clinic appointment desk.

Figure 61. Wisconsin Week announcing the formation of the Adult Congenital Heart Disease Clinic at the Center for Health Sciences in Madison, which will be co-directed by me and Dr. Ford Ballantyne.

I was invited to conduct a workshop to non-surgically close atrial septal defects and patent ductus arteriosus. Drs. Allan Cribier and Brice Letac from France were also invited to concurrently demonstrate modern techniques in the treatment of coronary artery disease. These activities started with lecture series followed by case demonstrations from April 7 through April 13, 1993. The announcements (Figures 62 and 63), photograph of faculty and staff (Figure 64), the coverage in the Indian Express (Figure 65), and the Deccan Chronicle (Figure 66) are shown.

Figure 62. Announcing the conduct of a workshop to non-surgically close atrial septal defects and patent ductus arteriosus in the Indian Express.

HYDERABAD – APOLLO HOSPITAL
INSTITUTE OF CARDIOLOGY & CARDIOVASCULAR SURGERY
Jubilee Hills, Hyderabad-500 034 Phone: 238857/59/61 Telex: 0425-6097 DHC IN FAX-0842 - 238050

Dear Doctor,

CARDIOLOGY
Dr. P.S. Rao, MD, DM
Dr. P.C. Rath, MD, DM
Dr.(Mrs.) T. Deb MD, DNB

CARDIOVASCULAR SURGERY
Dr.Vijay Dikshit Mch.
Dr. Sitaram Reddy FRCS.
Dr.Rajendra Prasad Mch.

CARDIAC ANAESTHESIA
Dr.A. Sathpathy MD
Dr. G.N. Reddy DA

We are pleased to inform you that a team of Internationally renowned Interventional cardiologists from France and USA are coming to Apollo Hospital, Hyderabad from 8th April to 12th April '93. The distinguished Cardiologists are **Prof. Allan Cribier, Prof. Brice Letac** from the University of Rouen, France and **Prof. P.Syamasundar Rao,** from the University of Wisconsin, USA.

Dr. Allan Cribier needs no introduction. He is the Professor of Cardiology and Director, Cardiac Catheterization Laboratory of the prestigious University of Rouen, France. He is a pioneer in the field of Interventional Cardiology and has got many innovative original work in Coronary angioplasty(PTCA), Atherectomy, Rotablator, Angioscopy, stent and Valvuloplasty to his credit.

He came to India for the first time to Apollo Hospital, Hyderabad in 1990 and conducted a workshop on Interventional Cardiology. Subsequently he conducted workshops in Bombay and Delhi. He is a visiting interventional cardiologist to many institutes in USA, Europe and regularly conducts workshops and live demostration courses in different parts of the world. This time he will be demonstrating the use of Coronary angioscopy for the first time in India. By Coronary angioscopy, one can directly visualise the lumen of the coronary arteries & the lesion. Subsequently he will be using the appropriate methods of treating the lesion like Balloon angioplasty, Artherectomy or Rotablation. Coronary stents will also be used when indicated.

Dr. Brice Letac is the Prof & Chairman of the Dept of Cardiology of the University of Rouen, France. He along with Dr. Cribier did the first Aortic Valvuloplasty in adults. He has designed Catheters for Aortic Valvuloplasty called "Cribier Letac" Balloon Aortic Valvuloplasty catheter. He is now concentrating on developing coronary Artery stents and Auto perfusion device to be used for PTCA. Besides doing many original work in the field of interventional cardiology and basic Cardiology, he is a highly respected teacher and clinical cardiologist in Europe.

Dr.P. Syamasunder Rao is the Professor and Head of the Department of Paediatric Cardiology of the University of Wisconsin, USA. He along with **Dr. Sideris** has done the largest number of ASD and PDA closures in children and adults by using buttoned umbrella device designed by them with 98% success rate. Besides umbrella closure he will also demonstrate the dilatation of Coarctation of Aorta and Congenital valvular stenosis in Children.

If you feel any of your patients are going to be benefited by the expertise of these eminent cardiologists then please send them as soon as possible to any of us in the department of Cardiology for preliminary investigations which may include Catheterisation and Angiography. As they are staying for a short period the number of patients taken by them will be very limited. Priority will be given to the patients on first come first basis. We are also organising a workshop and seminar during their stay here. (Details including the Brochure will be sent to you soon.)

If you need any further information, please don't hesitate to write to us or call us over phone to the Department or at our Residence.

With personal regards,

Dr. P. SESHAGIRI RAO, MD. DM
Head of the Dept., Cardiology
Phone : Res: 228822

Dr. P.C.RATH, MD. DM
Director Cardiac Cath Lab
Phone : Res: 247596.

Figure 63. Announcing the conduct of a workshop to non-surgically close atrial septal defects and patent ductus arteriosus.

224

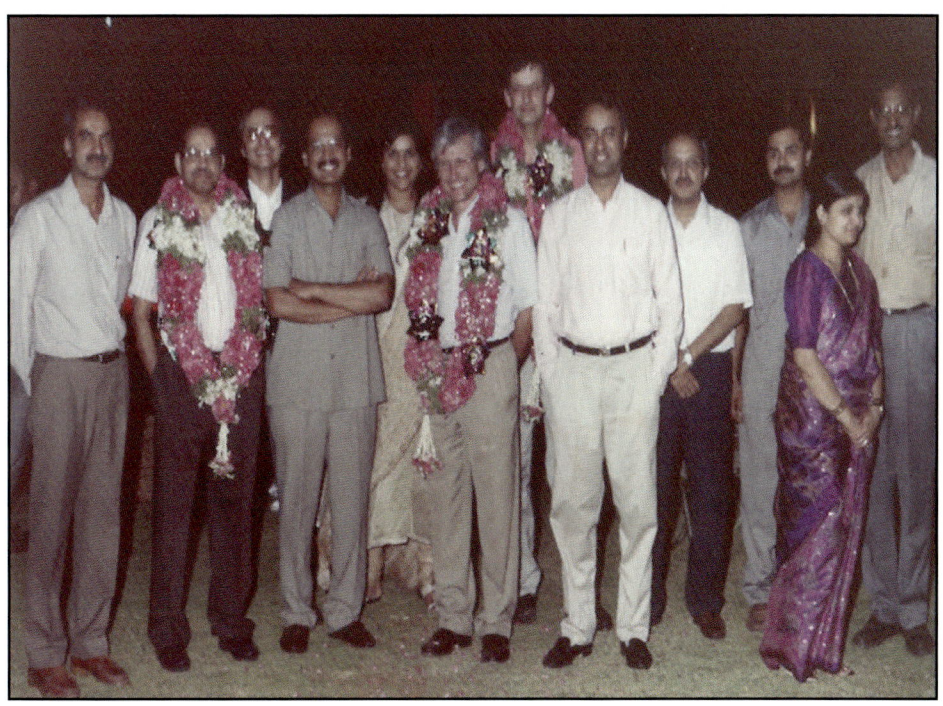

Figure 64. Photograph of the faculty and staff participating in the conference and workshop conducted at the Apollo Hospital, Hyderabad, India in April 1993.

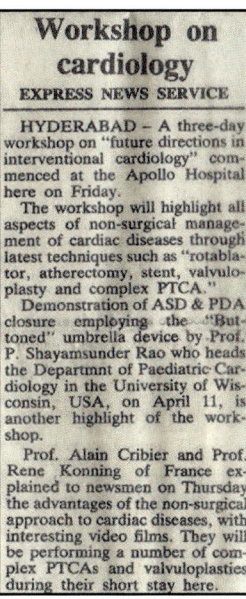

Workshop on cardiology

EXPRESS NEWS SERVICE

HYDERABAD – A three-day workshop on "future directions in interventional cardiology" commenced at the Apollo Hospital here on Friday.

The workshop will highlight all aspects of non-surgical management of cardiac diseases through latest techniques such as "rotablator, atherectomy, stent, valvuloplasty and complex PTCA."

Demonstration of ASD & PDA closure employing the "Buttoned" umbrella device by Prof. P. Shayamsunder Rao who heads the Department of Paediatric Cardiology in the University of Wisconsin, USA, on April 11, is another highlight of the workshop.

Prof. Alain Cribier and Prof. Rene Konning of France explained to newsmen on Thursday the advantages of the non-surgical approach to cardiac diseases, with interesting video films. They will be performing a number of complex PTCAs and valvuloplasties during their short stay here.

Figure 65. A copy of the write-up in the Indian Express (Saturday, April 10, 1993) about the workshop on non-surgical management of cardiac disease.

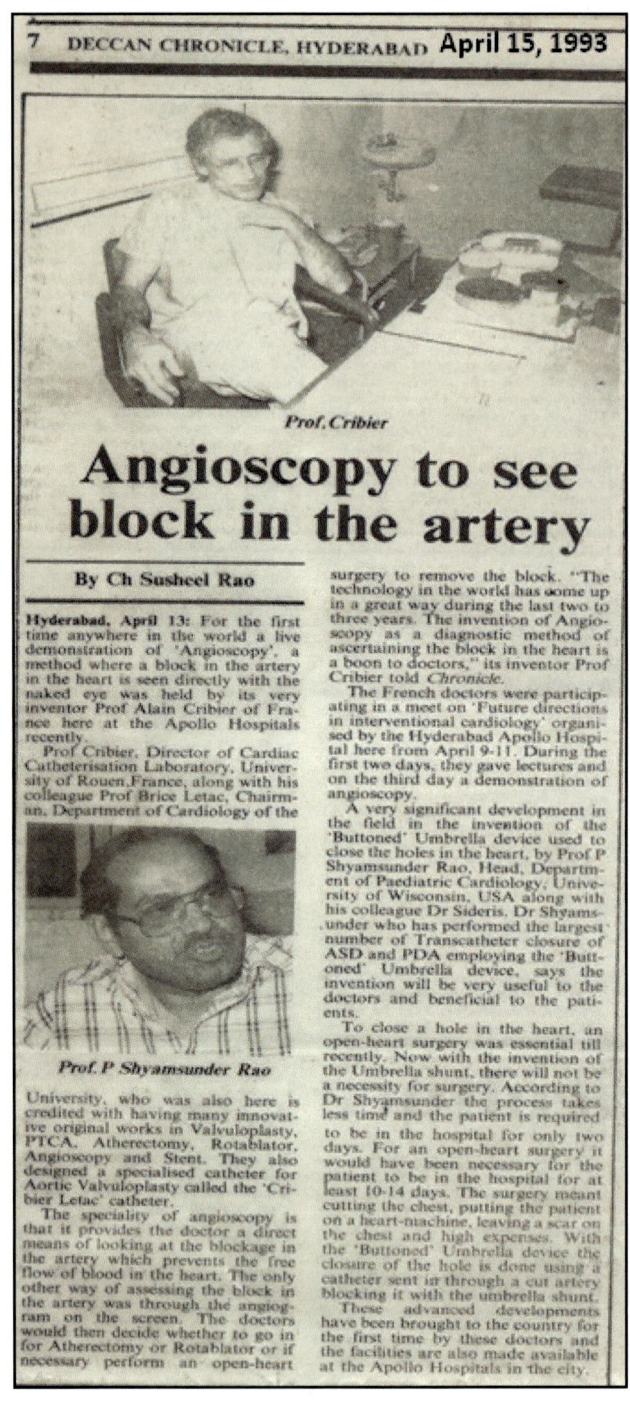

Figure 66. A copy of the write-up in the Deccan Chronicle (April 15, 1993) about the workshop on non-surgical management of cardiac disease.

As reviewed in the "Academic Carreer" section of the chapter on "The Journey Continues," I moved to the St. Louis University, School of Medicine/Cardinal Glennon Children's Hospital in October 1994, prompting the publication of my profile (Figure 67) in the Cardinal Glennon Children's Hospital's publication, "FOCU ON PEDIATRICS."

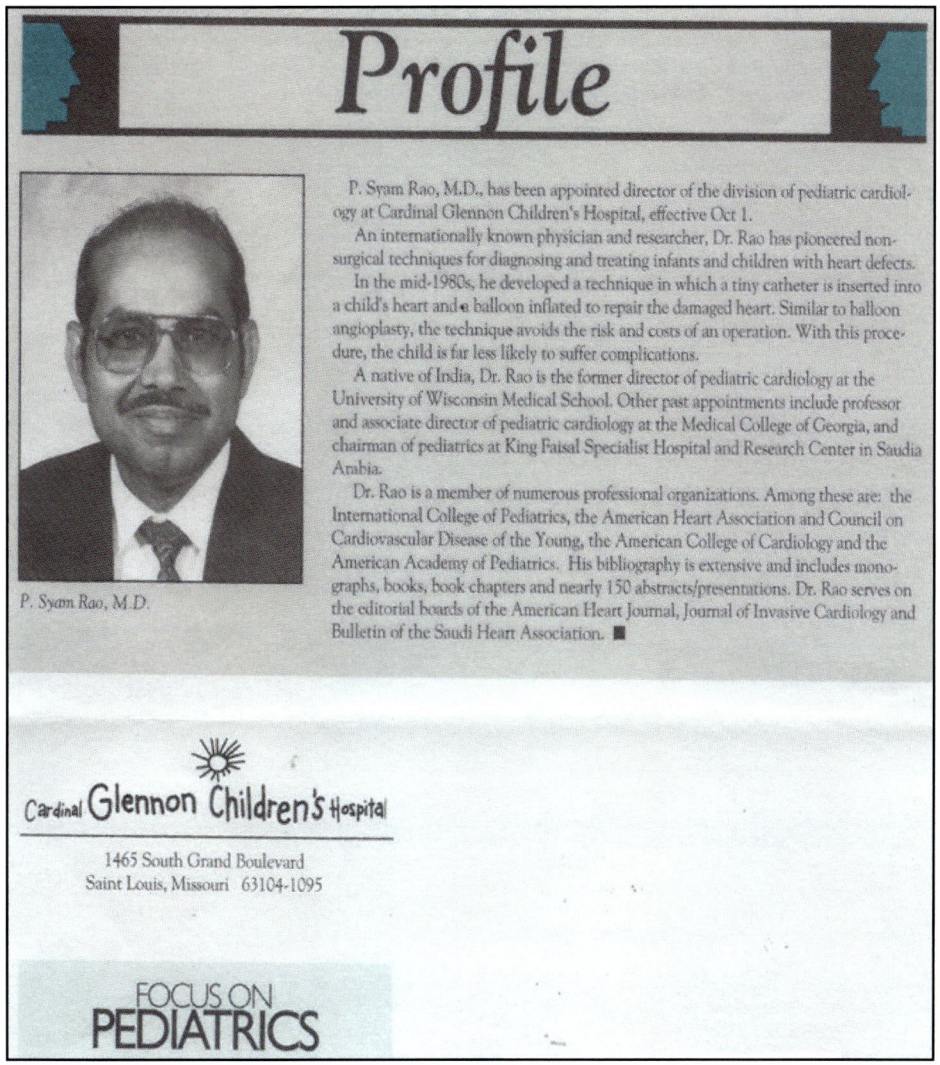

Profile

P. Syam Rao, M.D., has been appointed director of the division of pediatric cardiology at Cardinal Glennon Children's Hospital, effective Oct 1.

An internationally known physician and researcher, Dr. Rao has pioneered non-surgical techniques for diagnosing and treating infants and children with heart defects.

In the mid-1980s, he developed a technique in which a tiny catheter is inserted into a child's heart and a balloon inflated to repair the damaged heart. Similar to balloon angioplasty, the technique avoids the risk and costs of an operation. With this procedure, the child is far less likely to suffer complications.

A native of India, Dr. Rao is the former director of pediatric cardiology at the University of Wisconsin Medical School. Other past appointments include professor and associate director of pediatric cardiology at the Medical College of Georgia, and chairman of pediatrics at King Faisal Specialist Hospital and Research Center in Saudia Arabia.

Dr. Rao is a member of numerous professional organizations. Among these are: the International College of Pediatrics, the American Heart Association and Council on Cardiovascular Disease of the Young, the American College of Cardiology and the American Academy of Pediatrics. His bibliography is extensive and includes monographs, books, book chapters and nearly 150 abstracts/presentations. Dr. Rao serves on the editorial boards of the American Heart Journal, Journal of Invasive Cardiology and Bulletin of the Saudi Heart Association. ∎

P. Syam Rao, M.D.

Cardinal Glennon Children's Hospital

1465 South Grand Boulevard
Saint Louis, Missouri 63104-1095

FOCUS ON
PEDIATRICS

Figure 67. A copy of the story published in the Cardinal Glennon Children's Hospital's publication, "FOCU ON PEDIATRICS" after I assumed the position of Professor of Pediatrics and Director, Division of Pediatric Cardiology at the St. Louis University/Cardinal Glennon Children's Hospital, St Louis, Missouri.

In early April 1995, I transcatheter occluded a patent ductus arteriosus with the buttoned device in a one-year baby by the name of Veneka Harris; this was the first time such a procedure was performed in the state of Missouri and became newsworthy (Figures 68 and 69), although such procedures were successfully performed by me in Wisconsin.[9,10] The story was again reviewed in the May issue of "Expanded Update," which is another publication of the Cardinal Glennon Children's Hospital (Figure 70); the story was picked up by several newspapers across the country, including Chicago Tribune (Figure 71).

ST. LOUIS POST-DISPATCH

Copyright 1995 • MONDAY, APRIL 17, 1995 (5) 5-STAR ● ●

New Heart-Patch Method Offers Hope For Children

Cardinal Glennon Hospital Helps Break New Ground

By Roger Signor
Post-Dispatch Science-Medicine Editor

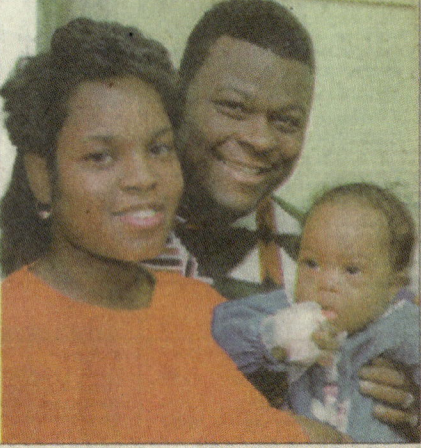

Renyold Ferguson/Post-Dispatch
Davangela Jones and Reginald Harris with their daughter, Veneka Harris, 1.

Veneka Harris, 1, seemed just a bump in a blanket while she slept beneath a huge camera that was sending pictures of the inside of her heart to a nearby array of video screens.

Veneka was making local history in the midst of all the high technology last week at Cardinal Glennon Children's Hospital. She was the first child to have a hole in her heart — a congenital defect — repaired by a technique called "transcatheter closure." The experimental technique to close such holes is used in place of major open heart surgery.

Dr. Syam Rao patched up Veneka's heart by manipulating minute tools inside a catheter. Two hours earlier, he'd threaded the lightweight catheter into the large femoral vein of Veneka's thigh, then slowly edged it up to the site of the defect in her heart.

Radio-opaque coating in the probes permitted the camera to map out the anatomy of Veneka's heart and the precise location of the defect. Then, Rao used a thin wire inside the catheter to deliver two tiny pieces of plastic to "button up" the hole in her heart.

Veneka, the daughter of Davangela Jones and Reginald Harris of Spanish Lake, tolerated the 2 ½-hour procedure so well that she was discharged from the hospital the next morning.

A nationwide trial of the technique is being overseen by Rao and Dr. Terry Sideris of Amarillo, Texas, who invented the button device. If it proves effective in treating 300

See SURGERY, Page 5

Surgery

From page one

to 400 children nationwide, thousands of children will benefit from the technique each year. Aside from bypassing the trauma of major surgery, the procedure could save about $200 million annually.

It costs about $5,000, compared to $30,000 for surgery, Rao said in an interview Friday.

Eventually, the technique may be applied to premature infants with heart defects, if smaller catheters can be made to fit inside their small veins, he said. If that happens, the technique will have even broader application.

Foremost, others see the technique as a breakthrough in patient care. "One goal of medicine is to fix problems without having to cut patients open — and Dr. Rao is one of many helping to do just that," said Dr. Gregory Launius, staff radiologist at Cardinal Glennon Hospital.

The morning after Veneka's heart was repaired, she ate a breakfast of oatmeal, eggs, toast and juice. At noon, her parents took her home.

Davangela Jones, 21, was amazed at her daughter's speedy recovery. "It was unbelievable to watch her eating well and playing patty-cake the night after her heart was repaired," Jones said.

On Friday, Veneka awoke at 6 a.m., ate breakfast and played with her brother, Reginald, 2, until 11 a.m. "She has more energy than before," Jones said. Before the defect was corrected, Veneka woke up at 6 a.m., but she had to sleep another hour or two after breakfast.

"We were blessed to have this option available to us," Jones said.

The technique is being used to repair two kinds of congenital heart defects, Rao said. Veneka's defect is called "patent ductus artery." Ductus refers to a normal vein that forms in all fetuses. Unborn babies do not breathe until birth because their lungs are collapsed. A duct or vein connects the two great arteries of the baby's heart to help carry oxygen from the placenta to the fetus.

After birth, the baby breathes and the duct isn't needed; it closes up naturally within a day or two after birth. But that does not happen in 3,000 babies born each year in this country, Rao said.

Because of a congenital defect, the duct fails to close. That connection spells trouble. It enables blood to leak back into the child's heart and lung. Over time, this can lead to heart failure or lung problems.

A similar number of babies are born with a hole in the partition between the upper chambers of the heart — the atrium and the ventricle — that also causes a potentially dangerous leaking of blood. This is called "atrial septal defect." Fortunately, it also is repairable by the simple catheter technique.

Rao has had a lot of experience using the technique. Sideris recruited him several years ago to begin the current clinical trial. To train other cardiologists for the trial, he has performed the catheter technique on about 100 children in this country. He also has done the procedure on about 400 babies and young children in Europe and Asia.

As yet, no manufacturer of medical equipment has shown interest in making the button devices, so Sideris has manufactured them in his office, Rao said.

Rao has no financial stake in the devices or the equipment to put them in place.

"I want this made available to everyone because it can avoid the trauma of major surgery and long hospital stays for children," he said.

Figures 68 and 69. A copy of the story published in the St. Louis Post-Dispatch in April 1995 describing button device closure of a patent ductus arteriosus in a one-year-old girl performed by me; this was the first time such a procedure was performed in the state of Missouri.

May 1995
volume 2
no. 5

employee newsletter

New Procedure Offers Hope for Children
Glennon Breaks Ground With Heart-Patch Method

In April 1995, P. Syam Rao, M.D., director of pediatric cardiology, Cardinal Glennon, made local medical history when he repaired a hole in the heart of a 1-year-old child using a new technique called transcatheter closure.

The child tolerated the 2-1/2 hour procedure so well that she was discharged from the hospital the morning following the procedure.

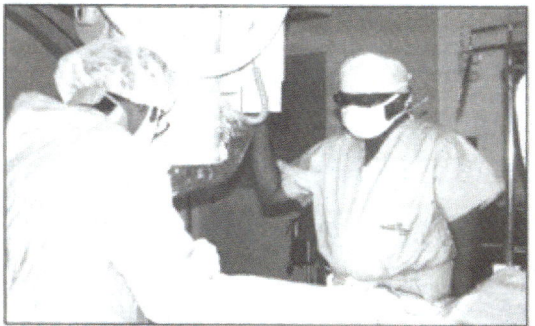

P. Syam Rao, M.D., (right) observes a procedure being performed by cardiologist Saadeh Jureidini, M.D., in the hospital's cardiac catheterization lab.

Transcatheter closure involves manipulating a minute device inside a catheter. The lightweight catheter is threaded into the femoral vein in the groin region, then slowly edged up to the site of the defect in the heart.

Injection of radio-opaque material into the heart permits the camera to map out the anatomy of the heart and the precise location of the defect. A thin wire inside the catheter is used to deliver two tiny pieces of plastic to "button up" the hole in the heart.

A nationwide trial of the technique is being overseen by Dr. Rao and Terry Sideris, M.D., of Amarillo, Texas, who invented the button device. If transcatheter closure proves effective in treating 300 to 400 children nationwide in the trial, thousands of children will benefit from the technique each year. Aside from bypassing the trauma of major surgery, the procedure could save about $200 million annually.

Dr. Rao said the procedure costs about $5,000 compared to $30,000 for surgery. "Eventually, the technology may be applied to premature infants with heart defects, if smaller devices can be made to fit inside their small veins," Dr. Rao said. If that happens, he predicts the technique will have even broader application.

Currently, transcatheter closure is being used to repair two kinds of congenital heart defects — patent ductus arteriosus and atrial septal defect. "Ductus refers to a normal blood vessel that forms in all fetuses. In most instances, after birth, when the baby breathes, the duct isn't needed; it closes up naturally in a few days," Dr. Rao said. But, in 3,000 babies born each year in this country, that doesn't happen, he added.

"Because of a congenital defect, the duct fails to close, enabling blood to leak back into the child's heart and lungs. This can lead to heart failure or lung problems," Dr. Rao said.

A similar number of babies are born with a hole in the partition between the upper chambers of the heart. That also causes a potentially dangerous shunting of blood. This is known as atrial septal defect. Fortunately, it also is repairable by the simple catheter technique.

Although this is the first time Dr. Rao has used this technique on a patient since joining Cardinal Glennon late last year, he was recruited several years ago by Dr. Sideris to begin the current transcatheter closure clinical trial. The catheter technique has been used in approximately 100 children in this country and approximately 400 children and adults in Europe and Asia.

"I want this technology made available to everyone because it can avoid the trauma of major surgery and long hospital stays for children," Dr. Rao said.

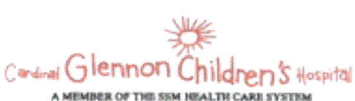

Cardinal Glennon Children's Hospital
A MEMBER OF THE SSM HEALTH CARE SYSTEM
AND THE ST. LOUIS HEALTH CARE NETWORK

Figures 70. A copy of the story reviewed in May 1995 issue of "Expanded Update," a publication of the Cardinal Glennon Children's Hospital.

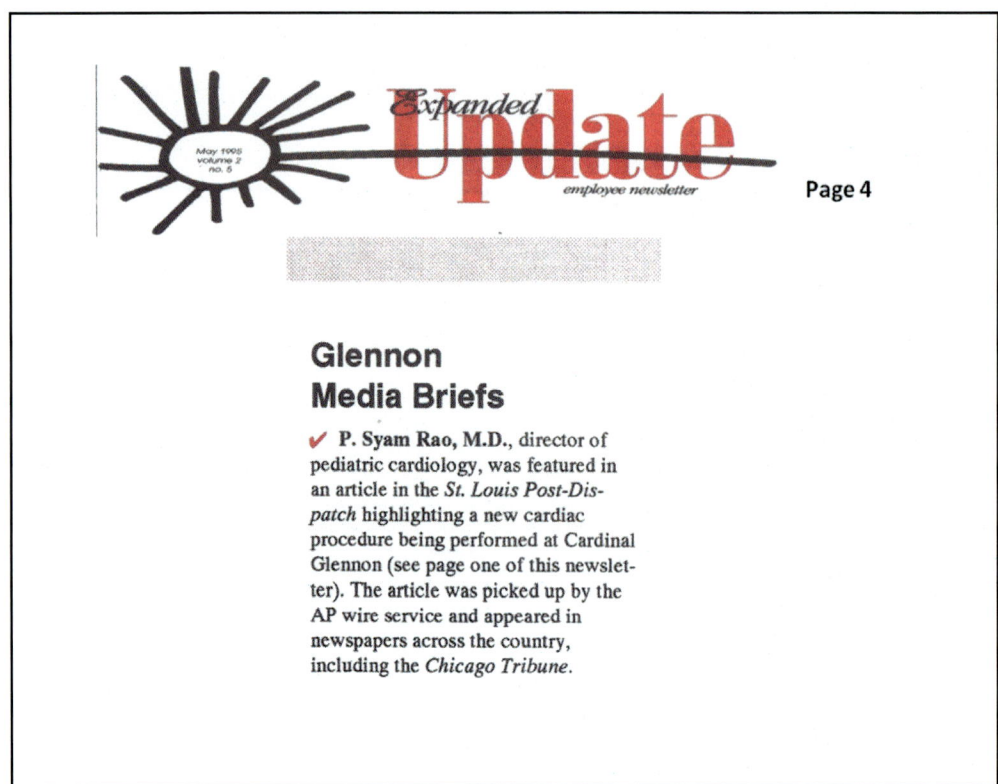

Figures 71. The story was picked up by several newspapers across the country, including the Chicago Tribune.

A few months later, I performed button device closure of an atrial septal defect in a three-year-old girl by the name of Emily Bauer; this was again the first time such a procedure was performed in the state of Missouri and was the subject of extensive review in the fall 1995 issue of the Magazine of the Cardinal Glennon Children's Hospital (Figures 72 through 77). However, it should be noted that such procedures were successfully performed in Wisconsin as reviewed above and published in medical journals.[11-13]

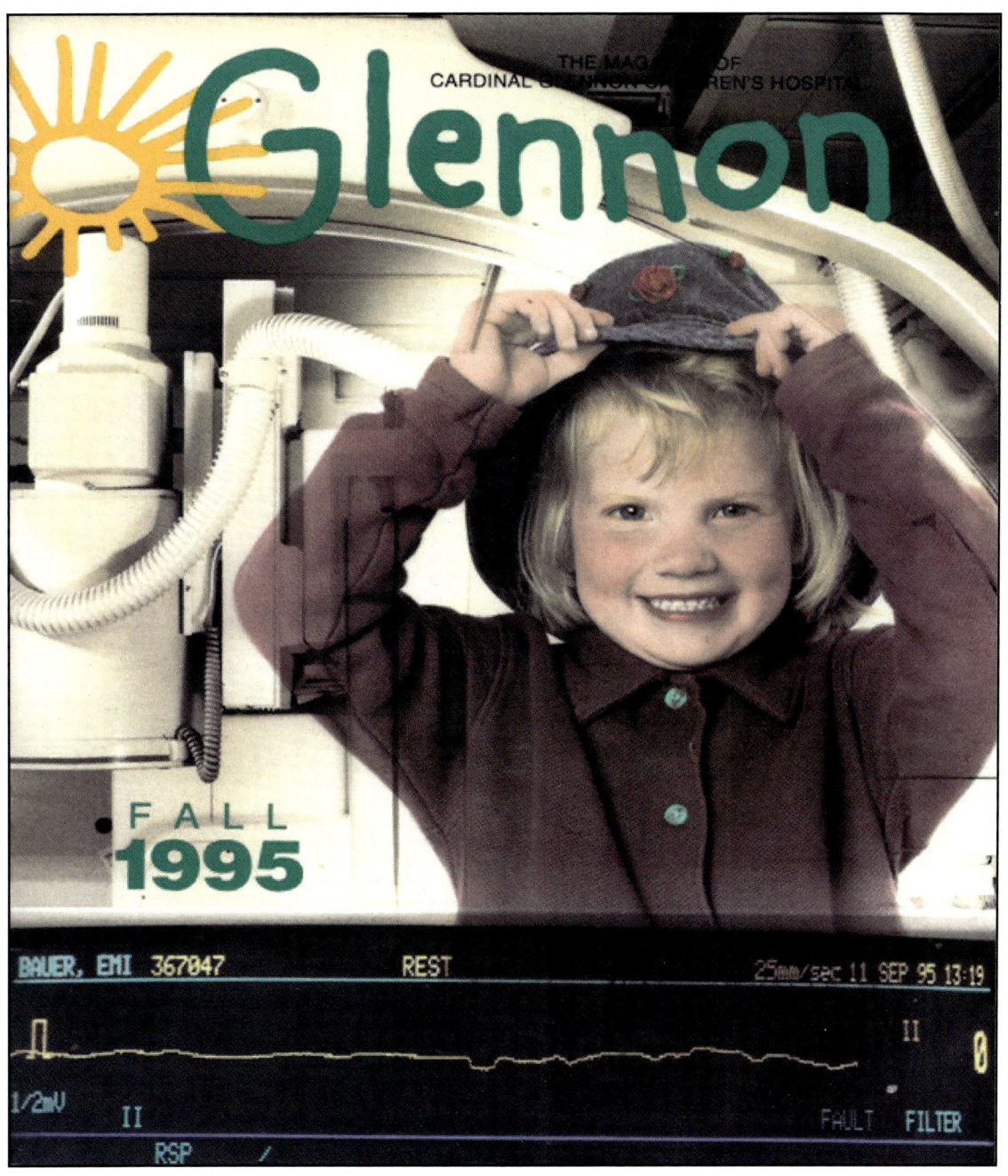

Glennon

THE MAGAZINE OF
CARDINAL GLENNON CHILDREN'S HOSPITAL

FALL
1995

BAUER, EMI   367047   REST   25mm/sec 11 SEP 95 13:19

1/2mV   II   FAULT   FILTER

II   0

RSP   /

HEARTening DEVELOPMENT

Watching 3-year-old Emily Bauer chase her sister around the backyard of her home in New Haven, Missouri, it's hard to imagine that just one month ago, the child was treated to correct a serious heart defect.

That's exactly what her parents and the doctors at Cardinal Glennon Children's Hospital had hoped for this spirited little girl when they scheduled her to undergo a new procedure to correct a heart defect she had been living with since birth.

In July, Emily became one of fewer than 700 children worldwide to undergo transcatheter closure, an experimental, non-surgical procedure to correct congenital heart defects in children. Cardinal Glennon is one of only five pediatric centers in the country that is able to offer transcatheter closure as a non-invasive alternative to open heart surgery.

Emily was referred to the cardiology department at Cardinal Glennon three years ago when her pediatrician detected a heart murmur resulting from an atrial septal defect, a malformation consisting of abnormal holes in the walls that separate the chambers of the heart. These holes impede the normal flow of oxygenated blood through the body and can cause a variety of complications.

Glennon Pioneers Non-Surgical Procedure To Correct Children's Heart Defect

Doctors at Glennon monitored Emily since birth, hoping that the holes would close on their own.

"We were waiting to see if the holes would close by themselves," said Kelly Bauer, Emily's mother. "If not, they told us Emily would need surgery. The idea of having Emily undergo major surgery was scary for us."

4

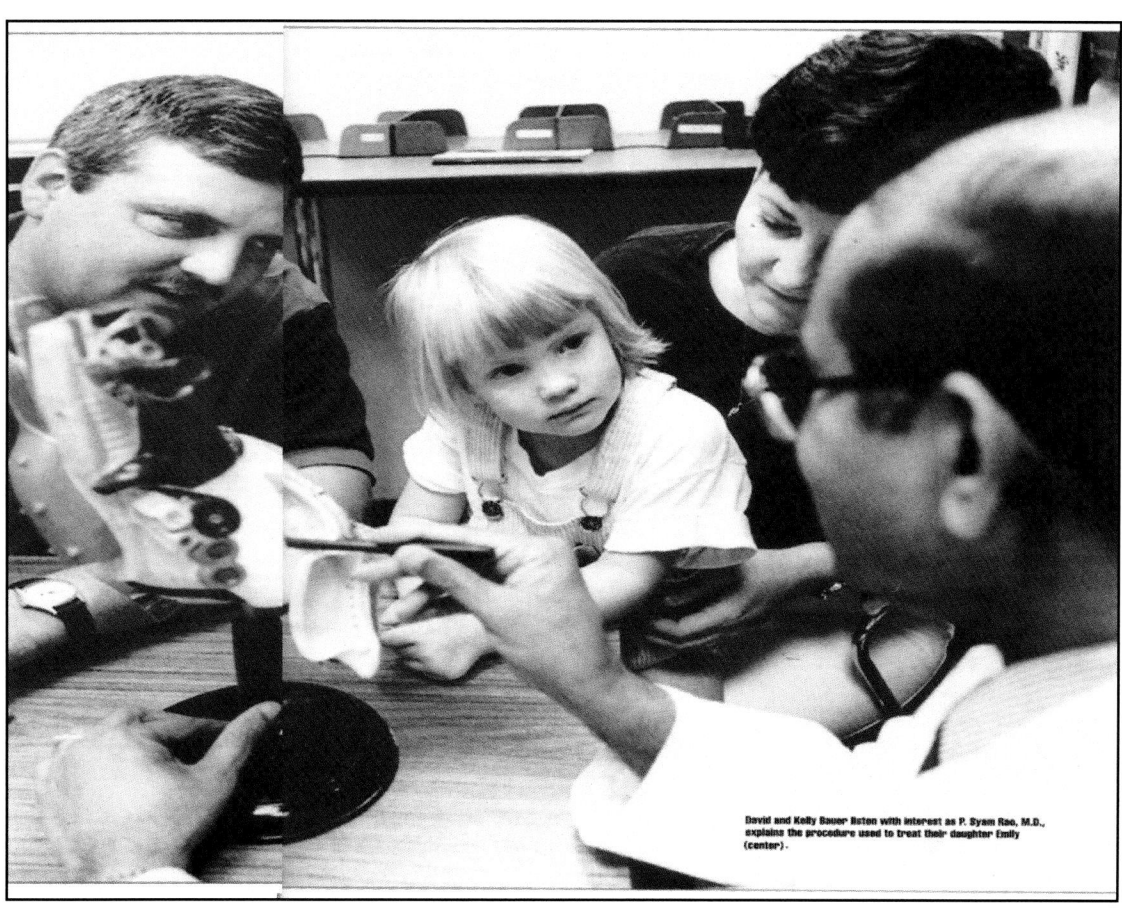

David and Kelly Bauer listen with interest as P. Syam Rao, M.D., explains the procedure used to treat their daughter Emily (center).

However, when P. Syam Rao, M.D., arrived at Cardinal Glennon last spring as director of pediatric cardiology, Kelly Bauer and her husband, David , were made aware of an option that would repair the defects, but would not require surgery, the transcatheter closure.

The procedure promises to spare many children from open-heart surgery and save thousands of dollars in medical expenses.

Dr. Rao is one of the procedure's pioneers. He is an internationally known physician and researcher who has developed several non-surgical techniques for the diagnosis and treatment of pediatric heart defects.

Since 1988, Dr. Rao has been collaborating with Terry Sideris, M.D., of Amarillo, Texas, on transcatheter closure, which uses a device invented by Dr. Sideris.

Dr. Rao views transcatheter closure as an evolutionary step in the treatment of two common congenital heart defects, atrial septal defect and patent ductus arteriosus, that account for about one in five congenital heart problems.

"Fifty years ago there were no operations available for these defects," Dr. Rao said. "Then there was considerable development of surgical procedures to take care of them. Once the defects were conquered surgically, we began to think of ways to do them with fewer risks to the patients."

Dr. Rao believes that 99 out of 100 patients he sees with holes in the heart can be treated successfully using just the transcatheter closure procedure.

Before the technique was available, all 100 would require surgery. Some types of heart defects, he cautions, cannot be treated using the procedure because of the size and location of the holes within the heart.

The transcatheter closure technique uses two tiny, umbrella-like devices that are inserted through a catheter placed in the patient's thigh. The devices are made of an extremely fine wire skeleton covered with polyurethane foam.

The devices remain flat as they pass through the catheter and are guided at the end of a slender wire through blood vessels into the patient's heart. After reaching the heart, the skeleton is pulled open to an x-shape that forms a button.The buttons are about twice the size of the hole in the heart. They range in size from one-half inch to two inches. Two of the buttons are precisely positioned on opposite sides of the hole. They then are pulled into

Dr. Rao and associates conferring on a patient's x-rays.

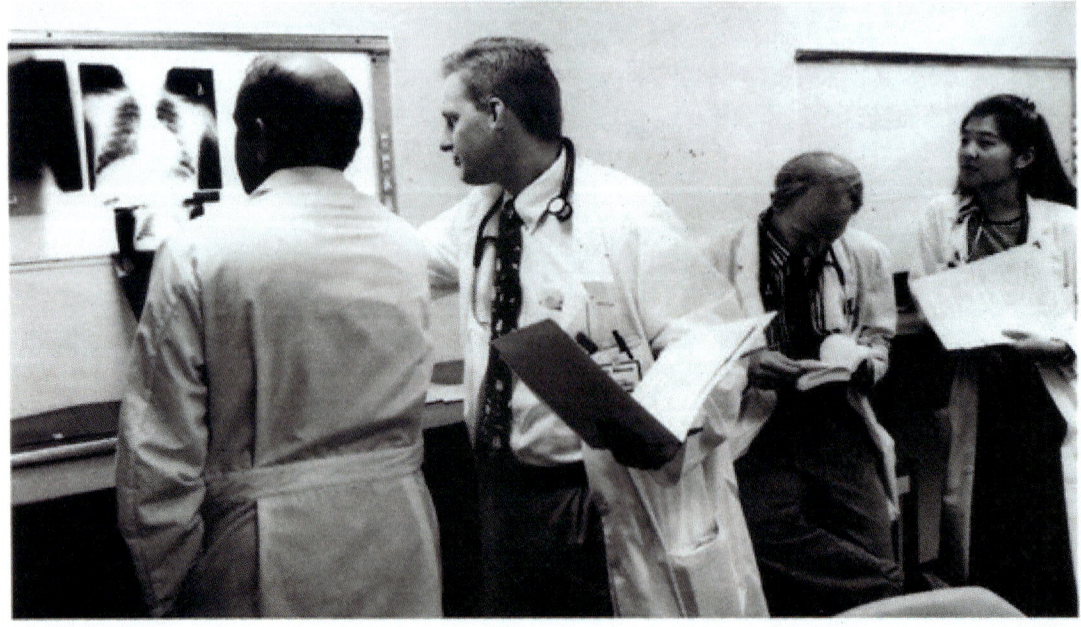

6

place against each other and secured with a knot to press against tissue surrounding the hole.

Placement of the device takes about two hours. The patient is sedated but remains awake while the cardiologist guides the tiny device into the heart. After the two halves are in place, the patient remains under observation for a few hours or overnight.

"Most patients feel like new the next morning," Dr. Rao said.

Within a few weeks, normal heart lining tissue grows over the buttons to close the defect permanently, sparing the patient the complications of a major surgical procedure.

In addition to fewer medical risks, the transcatheter closure is also less expensive. "Open-chest heart surgery might cost between $25,000 to $30,000. The patient undergoes anesthesia, receives an endotracheal tube and goes on a heart/lung machine during the operation. The chest is opened and there is a stay in the intensive care unit afterwards. The whole hospitalization might take five to six days," Dr. Rao said.

"The transcatheter procedure costs around $5,000 to $8,000. It is performed through a two-millimeter incision. The patient is hospitalized less than a day."

About one in every 125 children are born with heart defects. Many of these will heal naturally or with the aid of medication, but about half of the children born with them require further treatment.

Because the U.S. Food and Drug Administration still classifies the device as experimental, it may be used only on a select group of patients

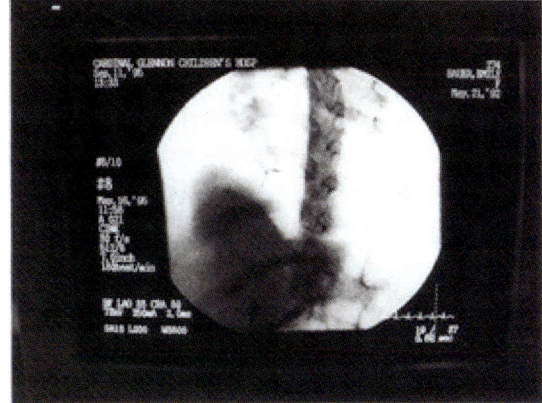

A close-up of the video monitor which allows physicians to observe and direct the catheter during the procedure.

The catheter laboratory where Transcatheter Closure is performed.

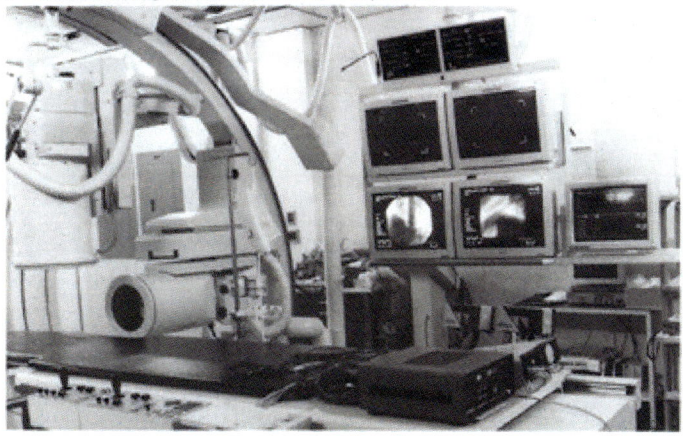

meeting narrow criteria. The device is now undergoing materials and engineering testing required by the FDA. Drs. Rao and Sideris are awaiting government permission to use the procedure on a broader patient population as the next step toward its adoption for widespread use.

As for Emily, life is back to normal. Hours after undergoing the procedure she was eating anything the nurses put on her tray. She went home the next day, wearing only three band-aids as indications that she had just

undergone correction of a serious heart problem.

"You'd never know she had anything done," Mrs. Bauer said. "She didn't have very many symptoms before, and she doesn't have any of those now. She's a real go-getter. She loves to climb, ride her tricycle, play on the swing set and bug her big sister.

"She had a lot of energy before, and this procedure certainly didn't slow her down. The doctors say there is no need to consider doing anything else for her. We couldn't be happier." ■

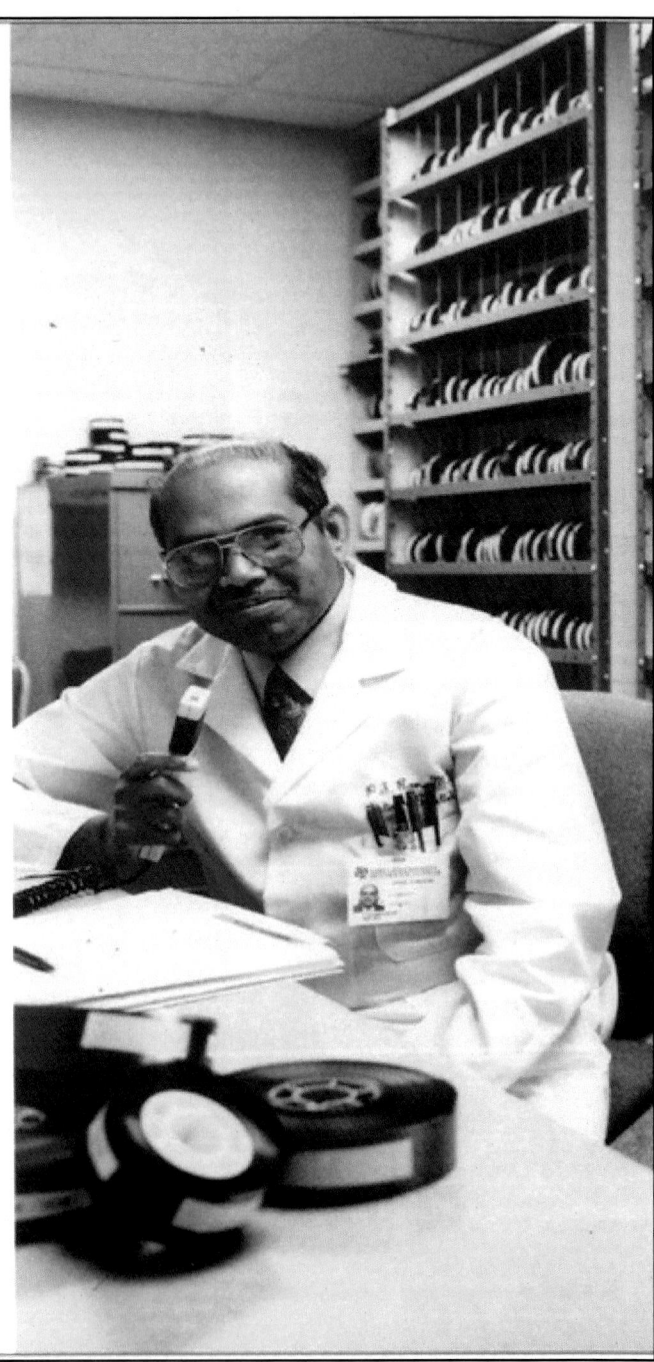

PIONEER IN PEDIATRIC CARDIOLOGY

P. Syam Rao, M.D., joined Cardinal Glennon Children's Hospital last October as director of the division of pediatric cardiology. An internationally known physician and researcher, Rao has pioneered non-surgical techniques for diagnosing and treating infants and children with heart defects.

In the mid-1980s, he developed a technique, transcatheter closure (see accompanying article), in which a tiny catheter is inserted into a child's heart and a balloon is inflated to repair the damaged heart. Similar to balloon angio-plasty, the technique avoids the risk, cost and complications of an operation.

A native of India, Rao is the former director of pediatric cardiology at the University of Wisconsin Medical School. He is a member of numerous professional organizations. Among these are: the International College of Pediatrics, the American Heart Association's Council on Cardiovascular Disease of the Young, the American College of Cardiology and the American Academy of Pediatrics. His bibliography is extensive and includes several books, book chapters and nearly 150 abstracts and presentations. Dr. Rao serves on the editorial boards of the American Heart Journal, the Journal of Invasive Cardiology and Bulletin of the Saudi Heart Association.

Figures 72 through 77. A copy of the extensive review of the story of Emily, the procedure of closure of atrial septal defect and of me, published in the fall 1995 issue of the Magazine of the Cardinal Glennon Children's Hospital.

The Outstanding Scientist Award by the American Association of Cardiologists of Indian Origin at the American College of Cardiology meeting in Orlando, Florida, in March 1996 was featured in the March 1996 Newsletter of the American Association of Cardiologists of Indian Origin (Figure 78).

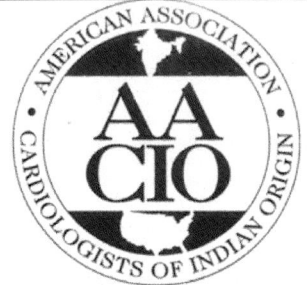

AMERICAN ASSOCIATION OF CARDIOLOGISTS OF INDIAN ORIGIN

MARCH 1996 NEWSLETTER

SPRING 1996 A.A.C.I.O. AWARDS

A.A.C.I.O. is proud to present the following awards during the semi-annual Spring Meeting on March 24th, 1996, at Orlando, Florida.

Our Young Investigators Award program appears to be catching up and we received four abstracts out of which two were chosen. The other two are of such good merit that we have decided to reconsider them with other entries for the Fall semi-annual Meeting in November 1996 in New Orleans. The following are the Young Investigators Awardees:

1) Prasad Chalasani, M.D., Emory University, Atlanta, Ga. "Five year Hemodynamic Follow Up After Heterotopic Heart Transplantation, Emory Experience."

2) Anil Nanda and Anita Nanda. "Transesophageal Three Dimensional Assessment of Normal and Stenosed Coronary Arteries."

Anita Nanda is a Freshman at Medical College of University of South Alabama, and Anil Nanda is a Freshman at Meharry Medical College, Nashville, Tennessee.

Each of the above presentations will last for 10 minutes and will receive remuneration of $500 and a plaque.

Two outstanding Scientists will be honored for their scientific achievements:

1) Pitambar Somani, M.D., Ph.D., is author of more than 100 articles in professional journals, holds 4 US patents, and serves on several editorial boards. He has served on numerous N.I.H. Study Sections and most recently served as U.N. Technical Advisor to the Government of Thailand. He taught at several medical schools in the US. including University of Miami and Marquette University. He joined Voinovich Administration in the State of Ohio in February 1991 and was nominated Director of Health for the State of Ohio. He has major interest in the health care of Asian Americans.

2) P. Syamasunder Rao, M.D. is an outstanding Pediatric Cardiologist. He has published more than 200 scientific papers, 160 abstracts, and contributed chapters in many books and monograms and has written a book on Tricuspid Atresia. He has held chairmanships of Pediatric Cardiology at three U.S. Universities. A.A.C.I.O. feels privileged to honor these two outstanding scientists.

Figure 78. A copy of the March 1996 Newsletter of the American Association of Cardiologists of Indian Origin featuring my Outstanding Scientist Award by the American Association of Cardiologists of Indian Origin at the American College of Cardiology meeting in Orlando, Florida, in March 1996.

The Pediatric Grand Rounds in March 1997 on "Perinatal circulatory physiology: Its role in clinical manifestation of heart disease" given by me on Doctor's Day was attended by more than 200 physicians (Figures 79 and 80) and was reviewed in "FOCU ON PEDIATRICS," a publication of the Cardinal Glennon Children's Hospital.

April 1997
Vol 4, No. 4

FOCUS ON
PEDIATRICS

Medical News From Cardinal Glennon Children's Hospital

"Thanks" to Doctors on Their Day

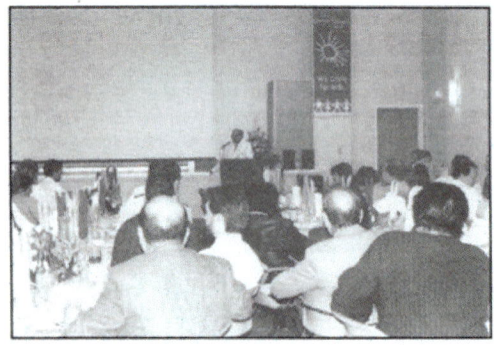

More than 200 physicians attended Grand Rounds on Wednesday, March 19, in Cardinal Glennon's Danis Auditorium. In addition to an enlightening presentation, "Perinatal Circulatory Physiology: It's Role in Clinical Manifestations of Heart Disease" (a synopsis may be found on page 6) by P. Syamasundar Rao, M.D., director of the Division of Cardiology, attendees were treated to breakfast in honor of Doctors Day. As a remembrance of the day, participants also received a red golf umbrella bearing the hospital's logo.

Grand Rounds
Synopsis

Grand Rounds presentations are offered from 8-9 a.m. each Wednesday, late August through June, in Danis Auditorium. AMA Category I CME credits are offered to those registered.

"Perinatal Circulatory Physiology: Its Role in Clinical Manifestations of Heart Disease in the Neonate"
Presented by
P. Syamasundar Rao, M.D.
Director, Pediatric Cardiology
Cardinal Glennon Children's Hospital
Professor, Department of Pediatrics
Saint Louis University
School of Medicine

The objectives of this presentation were: a) outline the fetal circulation, b) describe the changes at birth, and c) discuss circulatory adaptation to important congenital heart defects.

The fetal circulation is designed to utilize the placenta for gas exchange, whereas the postnatal circulation uses lungs for gas exchange. Fetal circulatory pathways, namely umbilical vessels, foramen ovale and ductus venosus along with high pulmonary vascular resistance and low placental vascular resistance facilitates placental gas exchange and promote distribution of oxygenated blood to the vital organs of the fetus. Mechanical factors appear to keep the umbilical vessels, ductus venosus and foramen ovale open.

The ductus arteriosus seems to be actively kept open by locally produced and circulating prostaglandins. While it is not entirely clear, the low PO_2 to which the pulmonary arterioles are exposed may be responsible for maintaining high pulmonary resistance. The role of a variety of other substances has been investigated and none could explain the phenomenon completely; however, recent evidence suggests an important role of leukotrions. Placenta, because of the arteriovenous nature of the connections, has low resistance.

Postnatal circulatory changes include elimination of the placenta, development of pulmonary circulation and closure of fetal circulatory pathways. Rapid reduction of pulmonary vascular resistance is related to spontaneous breathing and lung expansion at birth. Mechanical expansion of lung per se has a vasodilatory effect independent of oxygen; this appears to be related to release of PGD_2 and histamine from mast cells. The increase in pulmonary flow may also release PGI2 from vascular endothelium which, in turn, further relaxes pulmonary arterioles.

The role of EDRF (endothelium-derived relaxing factor) or EDNO (endothelium-derived nitric oxide), ATP — dependent K+ channel activation and endothelin-1 (Et-1) have not been clearly elucidated. In summary, there seems to be a decrease in pulmonary vascular resistance secondary to ventilation, which may be mediated through prostacyclins, and the decrease secondary to O_2 may be related to EDRF. With the increase of pulmonary flow secondary to reduction of pulmonary resistance, the left atrial volume increases and concomitantly the right atrial volume decreases, causing apposition of septum primum and septum secundum and resulting in functional closure of foramen ovale.

The ductus venosus closes because of the abrupt fall in flow after disconnection of placenta. Mechanisms similar to ductus arteriosus closure also may be involved in ductus venosus closure. The ductus arteriosus closes primarily due to the direct effect of oxygen. The oxygen effect may be accentuated by the decreasing sensitivity of ductal musculature to prostaglandins with increasing gestational age.

In hypoplastic left heart syndrome, presence of patent foramen ovale to allow egress of left atrial blood and of the patent ductus arteriosus to facilitate systemic perfusion is important. In addition, maintenance of high pulmonary resistance to promote systemic perfusion also is important. In hypoplastic right heart

syndrome (pulmonary atresia, tricuspid atresia) atrial right-to-left shunt and ductal left-to-right shunt are important to reroute the circulation. In total anomalous pulmonary venous connection, systemic and pulmonary venous returns empty into the right atrium and the presence of an unrestricted atrial defect is essential. In the infradiaphragmatic type, constriction of ductus venosus, in addition, may cause pulmonary venous obstruction. In transposition of the great arteries, because parallel circulation instead of normal in-series circulation, patency of the foramen ovale and/or ductus arteriosus is essential for patient survival. Finally, in aortic arch obstructions, such as severe coarctation and interrupted aortic arch, patency of ductus arteriosus facilitates systemic perfusion.

Despite the fact that persistence of some of the fetal circulatory pathways may be beneficial in most congenital heart defects, just reviewed, these pathways go ahead and close spontaneously, thus causing significant hemodynamic burden. Based on this information, development of therapeutic modalities has been undertaken by several groups of workers and include PGE_1 administration to keep open the ductus arteriosus, placement of intravascular stents to produce longer-lasting ductal patency and balloon or blade septostomy or static balloon dilatation to augment shunting of blood across the atrial septum.

Postnatal circulatory changes markedly influence the clinical presentation of congenital heart defects in the neonate. Knowledge of these changes results in better understanding of the disease itself and in the undertaking medical transcatheter and surgical therapy. ■

6

Figures 79 and 80. A copy of the write-up of the Pediatric Grand Rounds in March 1997 on "Perinatal circulatory physiology: Its role in clinical manifestation of heart disease" given on Doctor's Day was reviewed in "FOCU ON PEDIATRICS," a publication of the Cardinal Glennon Children's Hospital.

At the time of publication of our paper on transcatheter occlusion of patent ductus arteriosus (PDA) in 1999,[14] the Editor-in-Chief of the Journal of American College of Cardiology recognized our publication by placing the figure demonstrating occlusion of the PDA on the cover page of the journal (Figure 81).

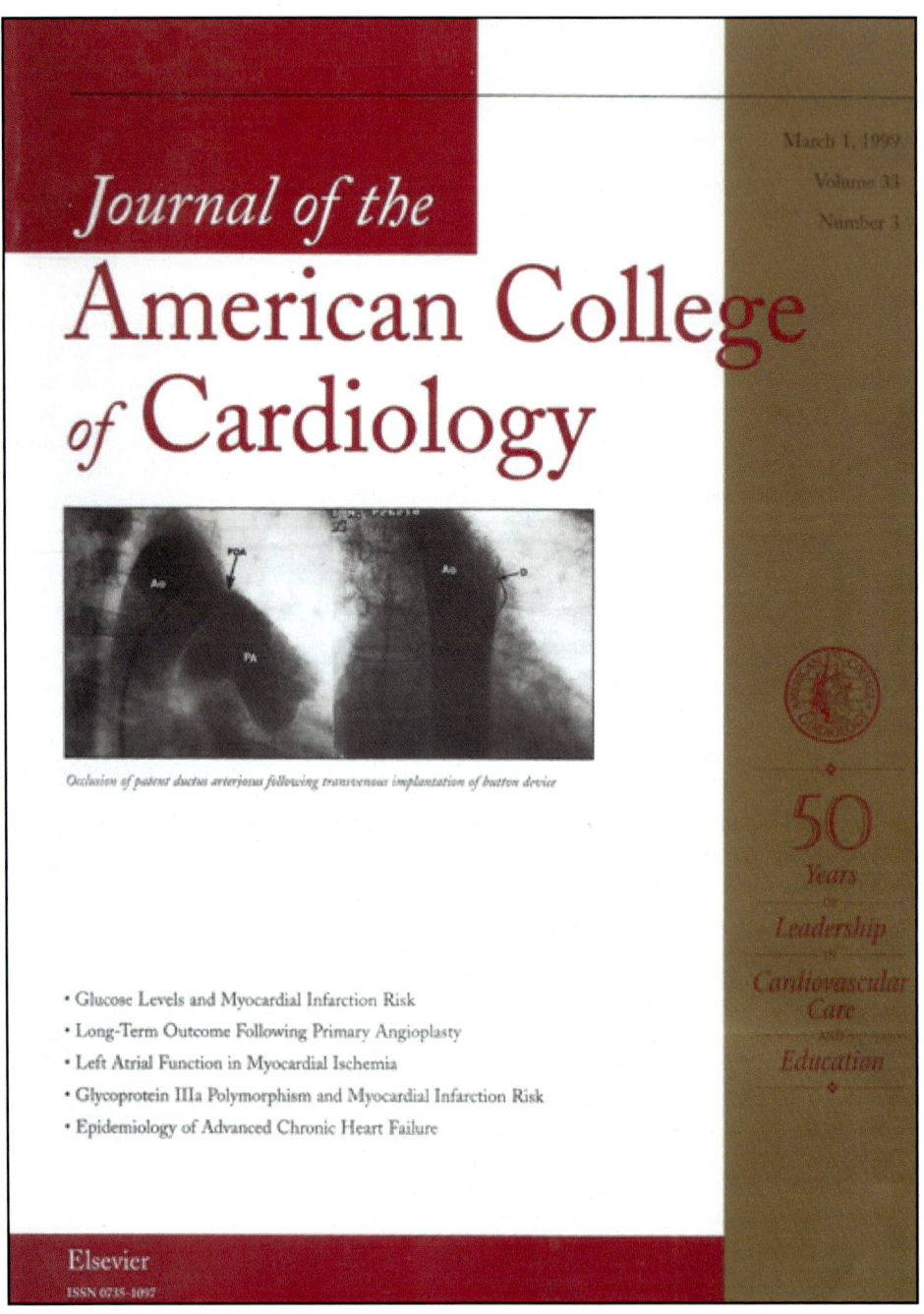

Figure 81. Cover page of the Journal of American College of Cardiology demonstrating occlusion of the PDA with buttoned device.

Again, as reviewed in the "Academic Career" section of the chapter on "The Journey Continues," my final move was to the University of Texas Medical School/Children's Memorial Hermann Hospital, Houston, Texas, in 2002 resulting in write-ups in the Scoop, a publication of the University of Texas Medical School at Houston in June 2002 (Figure 82); the Distinctions, a publication of the University of Texas Health Science Center at Houston in October 2002 (Figure 83); also in the Physicians Practice of UT Physicians in 2004 (Figure 84, 85 and 86).

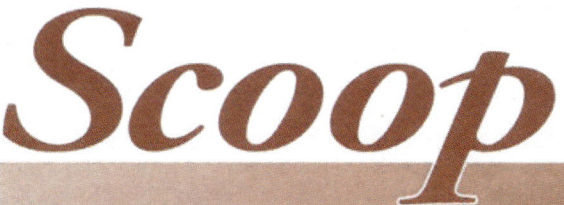

Scoop

June 28, 2002

THE UNIVERSITY OF TEXAS MEDICAL SCHOOL AT HOUSTON

RAO CHARTS COURSE AS PEDIATRIC CARDIOLOGY DIRECTOR

Dr. P. Syamasundar Rao, director, Division of Pediatric Cardiology, recently came on board with the UT-Houston Medical School. He is charged with developing a pediatric cardiology program here by **Dr. John Sparks**, chairman, Department of Pediatrics, and **Dean Max Buja**. Rao came from the Division of Pediatric Cardiology at St. Louis University School of Medicine. He is a pioneer in using catheter-directed interventional procedures to treat heart problems in children. He received his medical degree in India and became interested in the field of pediatric cardiology as he witnessed first-hand, surgeons at a loss to save the lives of babies with sick hearts back in the 1960s.

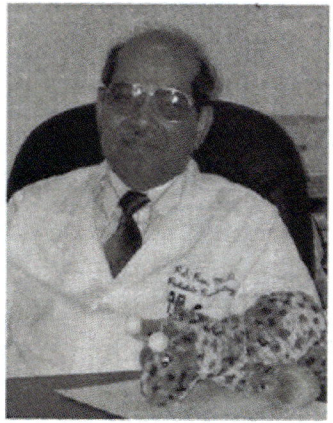

Dr. P. S. Rao and his buddy Topper, a Memorial Hermann Children's mascot.

Early in his career, he experienced a three-day workshop with Dr. Helen Taussig, the "mother of pediatric cardiology." He became convinced that he should seek further training in the field and came to the U.S., completing his pediatric cardiology training at Stanford, Case-Western Reserve, and UCLA in the early 1970s. Dr. Andreas Gruntzig, a Swiss cardiologist, began working with a balloon angioplasty technique in the mid to late 1970s, and Rao wondered if the technique could be applied to children. In the late 1970s, Rao undertook a mini-sabbatical with Dr. William Rashkind, learning and researching transcatheter closure of heart defects. By 1982, Rao was working with balloon angioplasty techniques on pediatric patients.

One baby out of 100 is born with congenital heart problems. That translates into 30-35,000 babies each year in the U.S. alone. With catheter-based interventional pediatric cardiology procedures, up to 50 percent of babies who would normally need open or closed heart surgery, have been able to receive the catheter interventional procedures instead. Less time in the hospital, less money spent on procedures, no surgical scar on the chest, and most importantly Rao said, a better psychological outcome for both his small patient and his patient's parents, are the fruits of these less invasive procedures.

Figure 82. A copy of the story published in the Scoop, a publication of the University of Texas Medical School at Houston after I assumed the position of Professor of Pediatrics and Director, Division of Pediatric Cardiology at the University of Texas Medical School at Houston/Children's Memorial Hermann Hospital, Houston, TX.

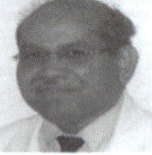

Figure 83. A copy of the story published in the Distinctions, a publication of the University of Texas Health Sciences Center at Houston after I assumed the position of Professor of Pediatrics and Director, Division of Pediatric Cardiology at the University of Texas Medical School at Houston/Children's Memorial Hermann Hospital, Houston, Texas.

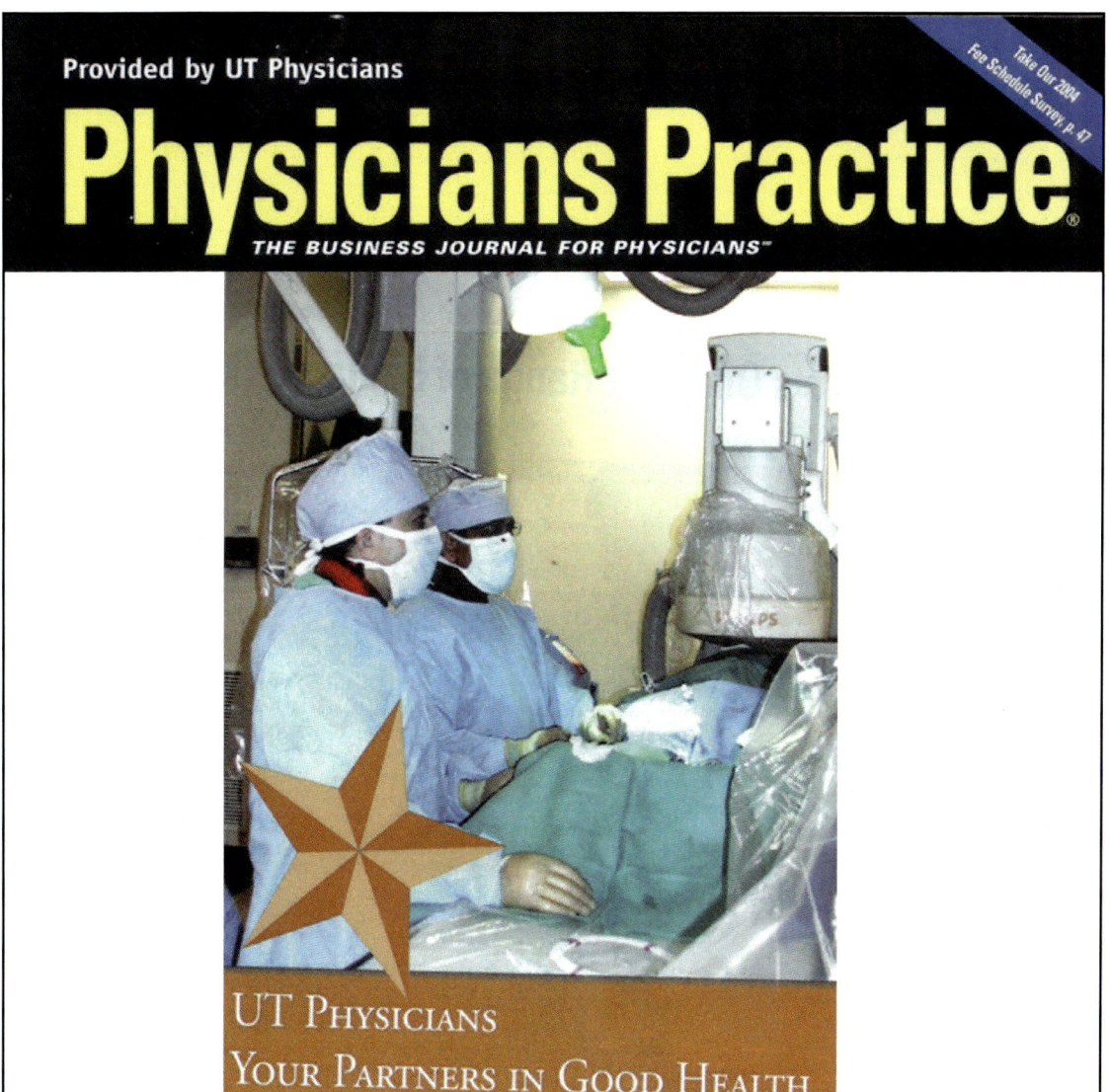

Provided by UT Physicians

Physicians Practice®

THE BUSINESS JOURNAL FOR PHYSICIANS™

Take Our 2004
Fee Schedule Survey, p. 47

UT PHYSICIANS
YOUR PARTNERS IN GOOD HEALTH

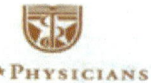

UT Specialists Offer Full Range of Pediatric Cardiology

By Darla Brown

Patients with congenital heart defects require dedicated specialists who, with the latest techniques and advances, can care for the broad range of problems such patients present. UT Physicians recently expanded the pediatric cardiology division, featuring teams of specialists who can effectively treat patients spanning in age from fetus to adults who have newly discovered congenital heart defects or who have been treated for congenital heart problems since they were children.

Under the leadership of John Sparks, M.D., chairman of the Department of Pediatrics at The University of Texas Medical School at Houston, and Hazim Safi, M.D., chairman of the Department of Cardiothoracic Surgery, the program has blossomed over the last two years to include in addition to general pediatric cardiologists, pediatric cardiologists who specialize in interventional procedures, a pediatric cardiovascular surgeon, and cardiologists who specialize in echocardiography. Also central to the team are perfusionists, intensive care nurses, pediatric sonographers, pediatric catheterization technologists, nurse practitioners, anesthesiologists, pediatric cardiac intensivists, and operating room nurses, all of whom are experienced in caring for pediatric patients.

"We can now really offer a full range of pediatric cardiac services," Dr. Sparks said. "And the addition of a pediatric cardiac surgical program has given us a new dimension. We can treat all ages and problems, from routine to complex and from diagnostic to interventional procedures."

Because the physicians are faculty members and researchers at the UT Medical School at

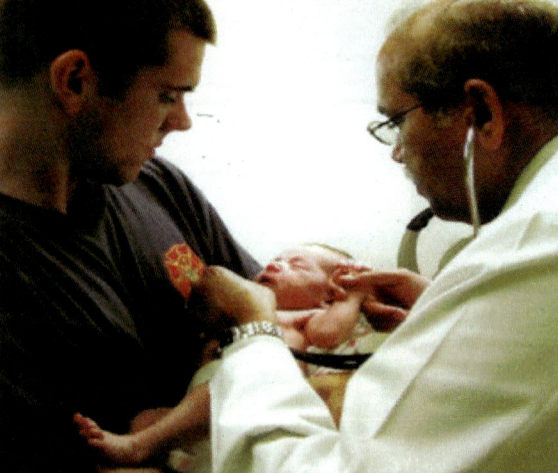

Dr. Syamasundar Rao examines a very young patient held by his father.

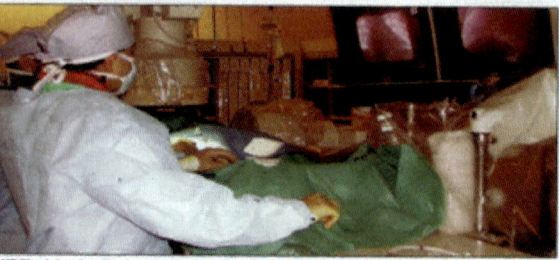

A UT Physicians' pediatric cardiologist performs a cardiac catheterization on a teenage patient

Houston, patients have the benefit of being cared for by physicians who are making the latest advances in this specialty through research.

Dr. Sparks' first step in growing the program was recruiting P. Syamasundar Rao, M.D., as director of the Division of Pediatric Cardiology. "Dr. Rao is a senior interventional cardiologist

who has developed new procedures to help children who have not been able to be helped before," Dr. Sparks said.

About 1 percent of live-born babies have congenital structural defects. In about a fourth of those cases, doctors can use catheter-based interventions rather than an invasive heart surgery to correct the problem. These less-invasive procedures require just a 23-hour hospital stay, no general anesthesia is necessary, less blood for transfusion is needed, and there is no scar on the chest, Dr. Rao said.

"The practice of interventional cardiology is 15 years old, and I've been doing it for 20 years," Dr. Rao said, smiling. He literally wrote the book on the subject, "Catheter-Based Devices."

"This level of experience in the interventional side is important and unique in the country," Dr. Sparks said.

In additional to his clinical practice, Dr. Rao is leading research to develop tomorrow's pediatric cardiology procedures. He is working on devices to close atrial septal defects and other types of holes in the heart. He also is using new flexible stents to open narrowed blood vessels, and he is in the planning phases of a trial that would explore whether it is possible to insert artificial heart valves through a catheter, thus eliminating the need for open-heart surgery.

Recently E.B. Sideris, M.D., the inventor of the buttoned device, was recruited to the faculty. He will not only perform routine interventional pediatric cardiology procedures, but he also will devote time to develop a number of new devices that may be useful in treating children with heart defects.

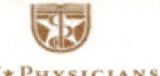

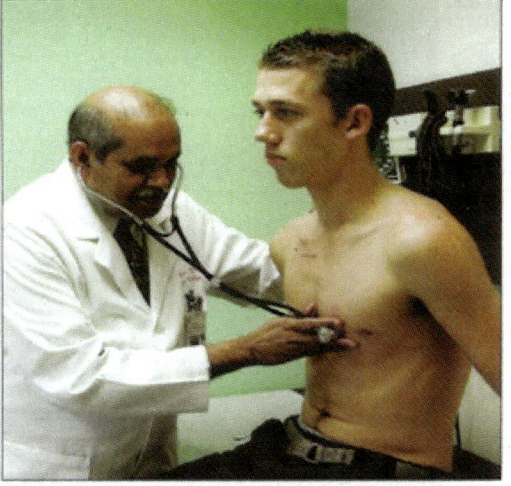

Transcatheter methods have replaced many traditional surgeries and through research such as Dr. Rao's, they are poised to be the preferred method of treatment for other current surgical procedures.

But not all pediatric heart problems can be treated interventionally – the surgical component is an equally important part of the program.

The surgery side is headed up by Bradley Allen, M.D., who came to the program from the Heart Institute for Children in Chicago, which he said is the busiest pediatric heart program in the Midwest.

"We performed 600 pediatric heart surgeries a year there, and I expect we'll have at least 150 here our first year," he said.

Over the last 10 years, Dr. Allen's research has focused on protecting the pediatric heart during surgery.

"These advances have allowed us to do more complex surgeries and have reduced the mortality and morbidity rates of surgery," he said. "We're also doing more newborn surgeries because many congenital defects can be repaired at a younger and younger age."

Another area of Dr. Allen's research involves blue babies who are hypoxic and often get worse after surgery. But by slowing returning oxygen to these patients, Dr. Allen and his colleagues have been able to limit the reoxygenation injury by limiting the oxygen-free radicals that are formed.

Until now, Houston has been the only major city with just one pediatric heart program. Two programs in town means a reduction in the time waiting for an appointment, catheter intervention, or surgery; the means for an accessible second opinion; and the promotion of healthy competition, which is in the best interest of the patients and the community.

"It is our intent to further the notion that Houston is a place you

come to for heart disease," Dr. Sparks said. "Texas Childrens Hospital is a well-known heart center, and I hope that we'll complement that program."

Patients of UT Physicians who require surgery or hospital-based procedures are cared for at Memorial Hermann Children's Hospital, a modern facility recently outfitted with a special unit to take care of pediatric cardiology patients postoperation.

Outpatients are seen primarily at the UT Physicians' main offices in the Texas Medical Center's Hermann Professional Building. The remodeled office, which is specifically designed for pediatric cardiology, allows the pediatric cardiology team to see patients five days a week, with the average wait of two weeks for an appointment.

"But, we always make exceptions for those patients who need to be seen more urgently," Dr. Rao added.

The UT Physicians pediatric cardiology division is committed to being service friendly to its patients and their referring physicians, who play an integral part of the decision-making process.

"We want the child to return to their referring physician, so the goal is to communicate with the family and physician – we want to make sure they are kept in the loop," Dr. Allen said. To this end, the admissions process has been streamlined and more nurses have been hired to involve the family in the patient's care.

Dr. Rao said that the group also is dedicated to the continuity of care – the patients see their same doctor during their visits, which builds the doctor-patient relationship and provides a personal touch.

Another aspect of the patient-friendly mission is establishing satellite clinics, taking the doctor to the patient. Patients are currently seen at The Woodlands satellite clinic and UT Physicians plan to open more satellite offices to meet patients' needs.

"When I go to the patients, it's easier for just me to make the drive instead of having 10 patients drive back and forth to me at my Texas Medical Center office," Dr. Rao said.

The Division of Pediatric Cardiology works in concert with the high-risk maternal fetal program of UT Physicians and also the UT Physicians obstetricians.

"A fetal echocardiogram can pick up problems before birth, which allows us to work together with the neonatologists and obstetricians to diagnose and treat these problems earlier," Dr. Allen said. Two of our cardiologists, Regina Lantin, M.D., and Monesha Gupta, M.D., are experts in this domain.

Memorial Hermann Hospital also has the unique benefit of LifeFlight, the ambulance helicopter, which transports patients from the Houston area and beyond.

"Presently, one-quarter of LifeFlight transports are babies and children, so having such a specialized transport team is a huge asset," Dr. Sparks said.

For more information or to refer a patient, call 1-877-4UT-DOCS, or 713-70-HEART. ★

Dr. Syamasundar Rao examines a young patient in the newly-expanded UT Physicians pediatric cardiology offices. The UT pediatric cardiology team treats patients from in utero to young adults, for all types of cardiac problems.

Figures 84, 85 and 86. A copy of the review of Pediatric Cardiology program published by the Physicians Practice of UT Physicians in 2004.

When I was conferred the Dr. K. C. Chaudhuri Lifetime Achievement Award, it was publicized in the Scoop, a publication of the University of Texas McGovern Medical School at Houston (Figures 87 and 88).

Rao honored with lifetime achievement award

SCOOP
August 2017

☑ WRITTEN BY
Darla Brown, Office of Communications
m.darla.brown@uth.tmc.edu (mailto:m.darla.brown@uth.tmc.edu)

⊙ POSTED ON
August 16, 2017

P. Syamasundar Rao, M.D., professor of pediatrics
(https://med.uth.edu/pediatrics/), Division of Pediatric Cardiology
(https://med.uth.edu/pediatrics/divisions/cardiology/), is the
recipient of the Xth Dr. K.C. Chaudhuri Lifetime Achievement Award
2017.

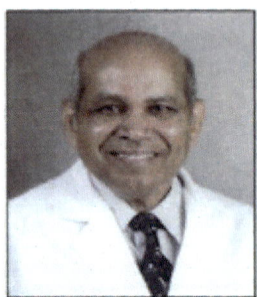

Presented by the Indian Journal of Pediatrics (IJP), the award is
bestowed by the Trustees of Dr. K. C. Chaudhuri Foundation and
recognizes and honors Rao's outstanding contributions in the field
of academics, research, and patient care in pediatrics.

P. Syamasundar Rao,
M.D.

Rao will receive the award in Delhi, India, in September at Xth Dr. K.C. Chaudhuri Oration and
IJP Annual Day, where he will deliver a speech reflecting his lifetime accomplishments, which
also will be published in IJP.

Rao joined McGovern Medical School in 2002 as director of the Division of Pediatric
Cardiology. "I was recruited to start the division, and we started with two pediatric
cardiologists, and now we have 11," he said. The division is currently led by **John Breinholt,
M.D.**, associate professor of pediatrics.

Rao recently retired from full-time faculty status following a 45-year career in academic
medicine, 15 of which were spent at UTHealth.

Before joining McGovern Medical School, Rao was on faculty at Medical College of Georgia, King Faisal Specialist Hospital and Research Center in Saudi Arabia, University of Wisconsin Medical School, and Saint Louis University School of Medicine.

"But this was the place I stayed the longest," he said. "From the beginning I was interested in academic medicine. If you want to do real pediatric cardiology, this is the place."

Rao graduated from Andhra Medical College in India and completed residencies in pediatrics at King George Hospital in India, Mercy Hospital in Des Moines, and Good Samaritan Hospital in Phoenix. He completed his fellowship in pediatric cardiology at Stanford University School of Medicine and at University Hospitals of Cleveland and Case-Western Reserve University School of Medicine. He was a research fellow in pediatric cardiology and cardiovascular physiology at UCLA School of Medicine.

A pioneer in interventional pediatric cardiology, his contributions span the decades: catheterization and angiography in the 1970s, balloon angioplasty/valvuloplasty in the 1980s, transcatheter catheter closure of cardiac defects in the 1990s, new pediatric cardiology/pediatric cardiovascular surgery program in the 2000s and educational programs and teaching material for physicians in the 2010s.

Rao has sponsored more than 45 postdoctoral fellow and been the course director of an annual pediatric cardiology symposium for physicians for more than a decade. His teaching responsibilities include junior medical students and elective third- and fourth-year medical students as well as observers, pediatric residents, and pediatric cardiology fellows.

He has published hundreds of papers and is an invited lecturer and guest professor around the world speaking on pediatric cardiac defects, interventions, and management. He holds membership in many national and international organizations, including the American College of Cardiology, the Society for Pediatric Research, the Indian Medical Association, and the International College of Pediatrics.

His numerous honors include the Outstanding Scientist Award from American Association of Cardiologists of Indian Origin and the Outstanding Scientist Award from American Telugu Association. He delivered John Lind's Lecture at Swedish Pediatric Association, Gothenburg, Sweden, and Kreidberg's Lecture at Tufts University/New England Medical Center, Boston. He is the chief editor of the Pediatric Cardiology Section of Medscape and WebMD.

"I believe my most important contribution has been in interventional pediatric cardiology. Most of our patients require open heart surgery, and one of the things I have done is to try to determine how to treat these children without surgery," he said.

Figures 87 and 88. A copy of the story published in the Scoop, a publication of the University of Texas McGovern Medical School at Houston when I was conferred with the Dr. K. C. Chaudhuri Lifetime Achievement Award.

Following acceptance of the award in New Delhi, we travelled to our native state of Andhra Pradesh, as detailed in the first chapter. An extensive write-up of more than four pages was published in Kalingakomati Jathiya Pathrika in the August/September 2017 issue. Sample half-pages are shown in figures 89 through 91; this publication uses our native language, Telugu.

తెలుగుజాతి ముద్దుబిడ్డ

డాక్టర్ పట్నాన శ్యామసుందరరావు

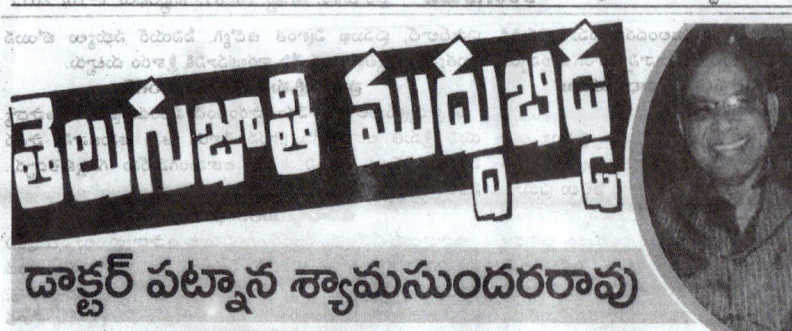

ప్రస్తుత సమాజంలో పిల్లలకు ఉన్నత విద్యాభ్యాసానికి కృషి చేస్తూ డాక్టరుగానో, ఇంజనీరుగానో కొడుకుని చూడాలని తల్లిదండ్రులు ఎంతగానో కృషి చేస్తుంటారు. కొడుకును ఇంజనీరుగానో, డాక్టరుగానో తయారు చేసిన తర్వాత ఎంతగానో ఆనందభరిత గర్వాన్ని అనుభవిస్తారు. అలాంటి ఒక వ్యక్తి ప్రముఖ డాక్టరుగాను, రాష్ట్ర, జాతీయ స్థాయిలో గుర్తింపు తెచ్చుకొని దేశ విదేశాల్లో పేరు ప్రఖ్యాతులు సంపాదించి తెలుగు రాష్ట్రాలకు, భారతదేశానికి గర్వకారణంగా నిలబడితే ఆయన గొప్పతనానికి తల్లిదండ్రులు, బంధువులే కాదు.. తెలుగు ప్రజలందరూ ఆనందించి అభినందిస్తారు. అదే జాతీయంలో గుర్తింపు పొందితే .. దానివలన కలిగే ఆనందానికి అవధులుండవు.

విజయనగరం జిల్లా పార్వతీపురం మండలం ఉల్లిభద్ర గ్రామంలో 1941 సెప్టెంబరు 21న పివిబి కృష్ణారావు, శ్రీమతి సావిత్రమ్మలకు తొలి సంతానంగా జన్మించి, దేశ విదేశాలలో ప్రముఖ వైద్యుడుగా గుర్తింపుపొందింది, ప్రస్తుతం అమెరికాలో స్థిరపడి 2017 సెప్టెంబరు 10న ఢిల్లీలో గల ఎయిమ్స్ ఆసుపత్రిలో డాక్టర్ కె.సి.చౌదరి లైఫ్ టైమ్ అచీవ్మెంట్ అవార్డు 2017ని అందుకున్నారు. ఆయనే ప్రముఖ చిన్న పిల్లల వైద్యనిపుణుడు, ప్రొఫెసర్ అయిన డాక్టర్ పట్నాన శ్యామసుందరరావు. ఈ విధంగా పేరు ప్రభ్యాతులు సంపాదించినవారు తెలుగువారిలో కొద్దిమందే ఉంటారు. వారిలో ఆయన ఒకరు. దేశానికి, తెలుగు రాష్ట్రాలకు ఇంతటి ఘనకీర్తి సాధించిన ఆయన జీవిత చరిత్రను ఒకసారి పరిశీలించి, నేటి యువతకు ఆదర్శమూర్తిగా సమాజానికి పరిచయం చేద్దాం. ఇది మనందరి బాధ్యతగా భావించి, ఆశీర్వదించి, అభినందిద్దాం. వివరాలలోకి వెళ్దాం.

శ్యామసుందర చరితం.. సుమధుర భరితం

గెలుపు మాత్రమే మాట్లాడుతుంది. ఓ మనిషి విజయం మాత్రమే లోకం అతడి వైపు చూసే అవకాశం ఇస్తుంది. సంకల్ప బలంతో అంచెలంచెలుగా ఎదిగిన డాక్టరు శ్యామసుందరరావు జీవితం అందుకు ప్రబల నిదర్శనం. దేశ విదేశాలలో చిన్న పిల్లల హృదయ నిపుణుడిగా పేరు తెచ్చుకున్న వైనం ఎందరికో ఆదర్శం.

పార్వతీపురం మండలం ఉల్లిభద్ర గ్రామంలో 1941 సెప్టెంబరు 21న శ్రీ ఎవిబి కృష్ణారావు, శ్రీమతి సావిత్రమ్మలకు తొలి సంతానంగా జన్మించిన ఆయన ప్రాథమిక విద్య నుంచి డాక్టరు విద్య అకుంఠిత దీక్షతో ముందుకు సాగిన విధానం అమోఘం.. ఆదర్శనీయం.. అభినందనీయం.. ఆయన విద్యార్థి దశ నుండి విరామం లేకుండా ఎదిగిన విధానాన్ని పరిశీలిద్దాం.

పదకొండో తరగతి వరకు పార్వతీపురం బోర్డు హైస్కూల్ లో చదివి, ఆపైపై విశాఖ ఏవీఎస్ కళాశాలలో ఇంటర్ విద్య అభ్యసించి, ఆంధ్రా మెడికల్ కళాశాలలో వైద్య విద్య పట్టాను 1964లో అందుకున్నారు. 1965 నుంచి 69 విశాఖ కింగ్జహస్పిటల్లోను, యూఎస్ఎ మెర్సీ హాస్పిటల్ (IOWA), గుడ్ సమారిటాన్ హాస్పిటల్ (ARIZONA)లో ఇంటర్న్షిప్ పూర్తిచేశారు. 1969-72 మధ్య పీడియాట్రిక్ కార్డియాలజీ ట్రెయినింగ్ను స్టాన్ ఫర్డ్ యూనివర్సిటీ (కాలిఫోర్నియా), కేస్ వెస్టర్న్ రిజర్వ్ యూనివర్సిటీ (ఓహియో), యూనివర్సిటీ ఆఫ్ కాలిఫోర్నియా (లాస్ ఏంజెల్స్) పొందారు.

ఓ చిన్న అభిలాష ఎందరికో ఊపిరి.. మరెందరికో ప్రాణ ప్రదాయిని

నాలుగు దశాబ్దాలకు పైగా వైద్యునిగా ఆయన ప్రస్థానం అప్రతిహతం.. అనితర సాధ్యం. కన్నవారి దీవెనలతో ఎందరెందరో మన్ననలతో సాగిన ఆయన జీవితం అతి మధురం.

చిన్న పిల్లల హృద్రోగ నివారణకు బెలూన్ సర్జరీలో పేరొందిన ఆయన తెలుగు జాతి గర్వించదగ్గ ఆణిముత్యం.

గెలిచేందుకు దాటివచ్చిన మలుపులు, చదువుతునేందుకు అపహరణ శ్రమించిన క్షణాలు ఇప్పటికీ గుర్తే అంటారాయన.

తన జీవితానికి ఓ గొప్ప అండగా నిలిచిన జీవన సహచరి హైమవతి సహకారం మరువలేనిదని చెబుతారాయన.

సిక్కోలు అల్లుడిగా పేరుగాంచిన ఆయన హరిశ్చంద్రపురం గ్రామానికి చెందిన హైమావతి (డాక్టరు లక్ష్మణమూర్తి, అమ్మడమ్మ పుణ్యదంపతుల కనిష్ఠ పుత్రిక)ని 1966 మార్చి 27న మనువాడారు.

శ్యామసుందరరావు బయోగ్రఫీ (క్లుప్తంగా..)

డాక్టర్ ఎ.శ్యామసుందరరావు యూనివర్సిటీ ఆఫ్ టెక్సాస్ హూస్టన్ మెడికల్ స్కూల్ పీడియాట్రిక్స్, మెడిసిన్ విభాగంలో ప్రొఫెసర్. యూనివర్సిటీ పీడియాట్రిక్ కార్డియాలజీ విభాగానికి అధిపతి. యూనివర్సిటీ ఆఫ్ టెక్సాస్ లోని ఎండి ఆండర్సన్ క్యాన్సర్ సెంటర్ల గల పీడియాట్రిక్స్ విభాగంలో ప్రొఫెసర్ గాను ఉన్నారు. డాక్టరు రావు ఆంధ్ర మెడికల్ కాలేజ్/యూనివర్సిటీ, విశాఖపట్టణం నుంచి వైద్య పట్టా పొందారు. తదనంతరం అక్కడే ఇంటర్న్ షిప్ చేశారు. తర్వాత అమెరికాలోని స్టాన్ ఫర్డ్ యూనివర్సిటీ, కేస్ వెస్టర్న్ రిజర్వ్ యూనివర్సిటీ, యూనివర్సిటీ ఆఫ్ కాలిఫోర్నియా, లాస్ ఏంజెల్స్ నుంచి పీడియాట్రిక్ కార్డియాలజీ ట్రెయినింగ్ పూర్తి చేసుకున్నారు. ట్రెయినింగ్ పూర్తయిన తర్వాత అమెరికాలోని మెడికల్ కాలేజ్ ఆఫ్ జార్జియాలో ఫ్యాకల్టీగా చేరారు. పీడియాట్రిక్స్ ప్రొఫెసర్గా, పీడియాట్రిక్ కార్డియాలజీ విభాగ అసోసియేట్ డైరెక్టర్గా పదోన్నతి పొందారు. తర్వాత సౌదీ అరేబియాలోని రియాద్లో గల కింగ్ ఫైసల్ స్పెషలిస్ట్ హాస్పిటల్ అండ్ రీసెర్చ్ సెంటర్ల పీడియా ట్రిక్స్ విభాగానికి

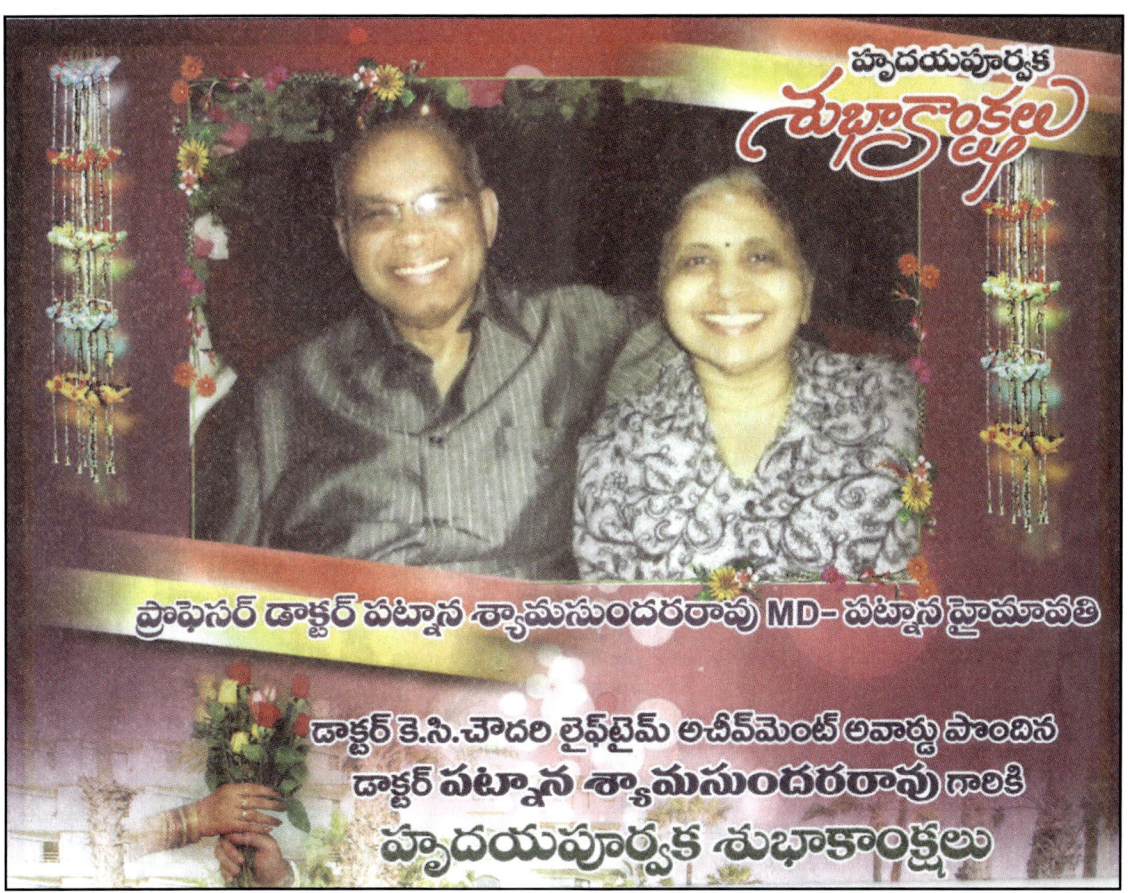

Figures 89 through 91. Sample half pages of the write-up published in Kalingakomati Jathiya Pathrika in the August/September 2017 issue.

REFERENCES

1. Rao PS, Mardini MK, "Pulmonary valvotomy without thoracotomy: The experience with percutaneous balloon pulmonary valvuloplasty," *Ann Saudi Med 1985*; 5:149-55.

2. Rao PS, "Transcatheter treatment of pulmonic stenosis and coarctation of the aorta: The experience with percutaneous balloon dilatation," *Brit Heart J 1986*; 56:250-8.

3. Rao PS, Thapar MK, Wilson AD, "Balloon Angioplasty of native aortic coarctations in neonates and infants < 1 year: Follow-up results." Presented at the Sixty-Third Scientific Sessions of the American Heart Association, Dallas, Texas, November 12-15, 1990, *Circulation 1990*; 82 (Suppl. III):584.

4. Rao PS, "Should balloon angioplasty be used instead of surgery for native aortic coarctation? (Editorial)." *Br Heart J 1995*; 74:578-9.

5. Rao PS, "Should balloon angioplasty be used as a treatment of choice for native aortic coarctations?" *J Invasive Cardiol 1996*; 8:301-13.

6. Rao PS, "Current status of balloon angioplasty for neonatal and infant aortic coarctation." *Progress Pediat Cardiol 2001*; 14:35-44.

7. Rao PS, Jureidini SB, Balfour IC, et al, "Severe aortic coarctation in infants less than 3 months: Successful palliation by balloon angioplasty," *J Intervent Cardiol 2003*; 15:203-8.

8. Doshi AR, Rao PS, "Coarctation of aorta-management options and decision making," *Pediatr Therapeut 2012*; S5:006. DOI: 10.4172/2161-0665.S5-006

9. Rao PS, Wilson AD, Sideris EB, Chopra PS, "Transcatheter closure of patent ductus arteriosus with buttoned device: First successful clinical application in a child," *Am Heart J 1991*; 121:1799-1802.

10. Rao PS, Sideris EB, Haddad J, et al, "Transcatheter occlusion of patent ductus arteriosus with adjustable buttoned device: Initial clinical experience," *Circulation 1993*; 88:1119-26.

11. Rao PS, Sideris EB, Chopra PS. "Catheter closure of atrial septal defect: Successful use in a 3.6 kg infant," *Am Heart J 1991*; 121:1826-9.

12. Rao PS, Wilson AD, Levy JM, Chopra PS, "Role of 'buttoned' double-disk device in the management of atrial septal defects," *Am Heart J 1992*; 123:191-200.

13. Rao PS, Wilson AD, Chopra PS, "Transcatheter closure of atrial septal defect by 'buttoned' devices," *Am J Cardiol 1992*; 69:1056-61.

14. Rao PS, Kim SH, Choi J, et al, "Follow-up results of transvenous occlusion of patent ductus arteriosus with buttoned device," *J Am Coll Cardiol 1999*; 33:820-6.

CHAPTER 5

CLINICAL AND RESEARCH ENDEAVORS

All my, more than 50 years of, pediatric cardiology practice was at academic medical centers. In addition to taking care of patients with heart disease, I had substantial interest in the development of new knowledge. Initially, I established an animal research laboratory at the Medical College of Georgia with funding from the American Heart Association. While acute experiments were successful,[1] chronic experimental model was difficult to sustain. In addition, the pulmonary vascular impedance studies required Fourier analysis, which was laborious in the 1970s, resulting a rather slow progress of research productivity. I then stumbled into investigating a rare form of a congenital heart defect, tricuspid atresia, which resulted in multiple publications including two text books.[2,3] Slowly, I began organizing multiple clinical studies. In addition, my initial interest in cardiac catheterization and selective cine-angiography mushroomed with the advent of transcatheter interventions. Then, I began organizing a number of single institutional, US multi-institutional and international multi-institutional research projects. The interest in clinical research resulted in publication of 390 papers in journals (as first or senior author), 230 abstract presentations, 14 monographs, and books and 150 book chapters as well as 160 invited presentations and lectureships. These clinical research endeavors resulted in a greater understanding of some of the scientific aspects of pediatric heart disease, which may be discussed under the following categories: 1. Physiologically advantageous ventricular septal defects (VSDs); 2. Tricuspid atresia; 3. Electrocardiography; 4. Echocardiography; 5. Cardiac catheterization, angiography; 6. Transcatheter interventions; 7. Miscellaneous. These items were the subject of the book titled "Pediatric Cardiology: How It Has Evolved Over the last 50 Years," which is concurrently published along with this memoir. The scientific contributions that do not fall into the evolution of pediatric cardiology during the last fifty years will be reviewed in the ensuing chapters of this memoir.

REFERENCES

1. Rao PS, "Effect of acute increase in stroke volume on pulmonary vascular impedance," *Pediatr Res 1980*; 14:449.

2. Rao PS (ed.), "Tricuspid Atresia," *Mount Kisco: Futura Publishing Co.*, 1982.

3. Rao PS, "Tricuspid Atresia," 2nd Edition, *Futura Publishing Co.*, Mt. Kisco, NY, 1992

CHAPTER 6

SKILL ACQUISITION

INTRODUCTION

As alluded to in Chapters 1 and 3, I began postgraduate education immediately after completion of medical school. The training began at the King George Hospital/ Andhra Medical College, Visakhapatnam, India and continued through the Mercy Hospital, Des Moines, Iowa; the Good Samaritan Hospital, Phoenix, Arizona; the Stanford University, Palo Alto, California; the Babies and Children's Hospital/Case-Western-Reserve University, Cleveland, Ohio; and the University of California at Los Angeles, California. These experiences were very valuable and useful during rest of my career. Subsequent skill acquisition in multiple specific subjects within pediatric cardiology discipline will be reviewed in this chapter.

ELECTROCARDIOGRAPHY

My fellowship training under the tutelage of Dr. Jerome Liebman, one of the best teachers and an outstanding electrocardiographer of the 1970s at the Babies' and Children's Hospital of Cleveland/Case-Western Reserve University, Cleveland, Ohio, resulted in exposing me to clinical electrocardiography and research on electrovectorcardiography. This training was of enormous help not only in the interpretation of electrocardiograms (ECGs) during routine care of patients suspected of having cardiac problems, but also for conducting multiple studies[1-11] in this field. These can be found in the chapter on "Electrocardiography" in the book titled "Pediatric Cardiology: How It Has Evolved Over the last 50 Years."

ECHOCARDIOGRAPHY

At the time of my fellowship training in 1969/1970 at Stanford University Medical Center, Palo Alto, California, there were only two echocardiography recording machines in the entire United States, one was at the University of Indiana, Indianapolis, Indiana and the other at the Stanford University. I was exposed to echocardiography to evaluate mitral valve motion and pericardial effusion on M-mode tracings. During subsequent fellowship training at the Case-Western Reserve University and the University of California at Los Angeles, echo machines had not yet arrived at the respective institutions. By 1972, when I joined the Faculty at the Medical College of Georgia, Augusta, Georgia, there were indeed echocardiography facilities at Georgia. Shortly thereafter, Dr. Wesley Covitz (who was trained with Richard Meyer, one of premier pediatric echocardiographers of that time) joined our faculty at Georgia and he has provided me additional understanding on principles and practice of M-mode echocardiography, adding to my knowledge base. This resulted in my active participation in echocardiography research at that time.[12-16] Two-dimensional (2D) echocardiography was coming to vogue as I was leaving the Medical College of Georgia to take a position at the King Faisal Specialist Hospital & Research Center in Riyadh, Saudi Arabia. There were portable echocardiography machines (Apagee) at that institution, which I could use in the clinic setting and perform 2D studies of children following their formal evaluation by history, physical examination, ECG and chest x-ray (norms at that time). This has provided me with experience and expertise to teach sonographers and other trainees. As I gained expertise in 2D, suddenly, Doppler echocardiography surfaced. I then, had to learn this modality as well. Then, as I was leaving Riyadh to join the Faculty at University of Wisconsin, Madison, Wisconsin, color Doppler technique was introduced and again, I had to learn this new technique. Subsequently, introduced echo techniques were also learned as they surfaced.

A strange occurrence is worthy of mention in this memoir. When I was named as the Interim Director of Pediatric Echocardiography Laboratory at the Children's Memorial Hermann Hospital/University of Texas-Houston Medical School, Houston, Texas in 2006, some of the staff critiqued this appointment since I was considered to be an interventional pediatric cardiologist. I responded to this critique by sending them a list of my publications[12-44] as of that date; this number of publications was more than the combined echo publications of the other faculty members who could be appointed to such a position.

Suffices to say, I have been involved in conducting multiple studies employing echocardiography throughout my career and these can be found in the chapter on "Echocardiography" in the book titled "Pediatric Cardiology: How It Has Evolved Over the last 50 Years."

CARDIAC CATHETERIZATION AND CINEANGIOGRAPHY

It is generally known that cardiac catheterization and angiography were indeed the major focus of fellowship training in pediatric cardiology in the late 1960s and early 1970s. Because of this reason, I availed the opportunity of taking several months of pediatric cardiology elective during pediatric residency training and spent a substantial proportion of that elective time in the cardiac catheterization laboratory under the tutelage of Dr. Marian Molthan, Director of Pediatric Cardiology at the Good Samaritan Hospital in Phoenix, Arizona, which helped me immensely during subsequent fellowship training at the Stanford University Medical Center in Palo Alto, California. In addition to performing catheterization studies under the direction of Drs. Norman Sissman and Emmanuel Mesel at the Stanford University Hospital during the fellowship, I had the privilege of performing cardiac catheterizations at Santa Clara Valley Medical Center (an affiliate of the Stanford University) under the direction of Dr. Philip Benaron. The experience with catheterizations continued at the Case-Western University/ Babies' and the Children's Hospital of Cleveland, Cleveland, Ohio, under the direction of Drs. Jerome Liebman and Daniel Silbert and at the UCLA Medical Center in Los Angeles, California, under the direction of Dr. William Vincent. This background helped my conducting multiple studies in matters related to cardiac catheterization and angiography. The results of these studies were reviewed in the chapter on "Cardiac Catheterization and Cineangiography" in the book titled "Pediatric Cardiology: How It Has Evolved Over the last 50 Years."

PERCUTANEOUS CATHETER INTERVENTIONS

Because of my interest in cardiac catheterization as reviewed in the preceding section and in the chapter on "Cardiac Catheterization and Cineangiography," in the book titled "Pediatric Cardiology: How It Has Evolved Over the last 50 Years," I was attracted to catheter interventions as soon as the balloon valvuloplasty/angioplasty techniques became available in early 1980s. Furthermore, the availability of catheter technology, both from Europe and North America, at the King Faisal Specialist Hospital and Research Center in Riyadh, Saudi Arabia, where I was stationed at that time, facilitated my work in this arena. However, it should be mentioned that I was privileged to take a mini-sabbatical with Dr. William Rashkind (considered the father of interventional pediatric cardiology) in mid-1979, when I learned performing atrial septal defect (ASD) and patent ductus arteriosus (PDA) device closures with the Rashkind's hooked device in the calf model and in patients under the tutelage of Dr. Rashkind.[45]

I have also taken every available opportunity to learn new techniques, as and when they become available. Such training with Dr. E. B. Sideris in his Laboratory in Amarillo, Texas, with the use of buttoned device to occlude ASDs and PDAs, with Dr. Lee Benson in Children's Hospital of Toronto, Canada, with the use of USCI PDA Occluding Device and with Dr. R. M. Smalling at the Memorial Hermann Hospital with Amplatzer device are worth mentioning in this memoir. A large number of studies were undertaken and the results of percutaneous catheter interventions were reviewed in multiple chapters in the book titled "Pediatric Cardiology: How It Has Evolved Over the last 50 Years."

REFERENCES

1. Liebman J, Lee MH, Rao PS and Mackay W, "Quantitation of the normal Frank and McFee Parungao orthogonal electrocardiogram in the adolescent," *Circulation 1973*; 48:735-52.

2. Rogers JH, Jr, Rao PS, "Ebstein's Anomaly of the left atrioventricular valve with congenital corrected transposition of the great arteries: Diagnosis by intracavitary electrocardiography," *Chest 1977*; 72:253-6.

3. Rao PS, Monarrez CN, "Electrocardiographic differentiation of posterobasal left ventricular hypertrophy from right ventricular hypertrophy," *J Electrocardiol 1981*; 14:25-30.

4. Kulangara RJ, Boineau JP, Rao PS, "Electrovectorcardiographic features of tricuspid atresia," In. Rao PS (ed.), Tricuspid Atresia, *Futura Publishing Co.*, Mount Kisco, New York, 1982, Chapter 9.

5. Rao PS. Kulangara RJ, Boineau JP, Moore HV, "Electrovectorcardiographic features of tricuspid atresia," In. Rao PS (ed.), Tricuspid Atresia, 2nd Edition, *Futura Publishing Co.,* Mt. Kisco, NY, 1992, Chapter 9.

6. Kulangara RJ, Boineau JP, Moore HV, Rao PS, "Ventricular activation and genesis of QRS in tricuspid atresia," *Circulation 1981*; 64:VI-225.

7. Rao PS, Thapar MK, "The AFORMED phenomenon: A proposed etiology," *Am J Cardiol 1983*; 52:655.

8. Rao PS, Thapar MK, Harp RJ, "Racial variations in electrocardiograms and vectorcardiograms between black and white children and their genesis," *J Electrocardiol 1984*; 17:239-52.

9. Rao PS, "Racial differences in electrocardiograms and vectorcardiograms between black and white adolescents," *J Electrocardiol 1985*; 18:309-13.

10. Rao PS, Najjar HN, "Congestive cardiomyopathy due to chronic tachycardia: resolution of cardiomyopathy with antiarrhythmic drugs," *International J Cardiol 1987*; 17:216-20.

11. Rao PS, Solymar L, "Electrocardiographic changes following balloon dilatation of valvar pulmonic stenosis," *J Interventional Cardiol 1988*; 1:189-97.

12. Rees AH, Rao PS, Rigby JJ, Miller MD, "Echocardiographic estimation of left-to-right shunt in isolated ventricular septal defects," *European J Cardiol 1978*; 7:25-33.

13. Truman TA, Rao PS, Kulangara RJ, "Use of contrast echocardiography in the diagnosis of anomalous connection of the right superior vena cava to the left atrium," *Brit Heart J 1980*; 44:718-723.

14. Alpert BS, Rao PS, Moore HV and Covitz W, "Surgical correction of anomalous right superior vena cava to the left atrium: Post-operative contrast echo evaluation," *J Thorac Cardiovasc Surg 1981*; 82:301-305.

15. Covitz W, Rao PS, Strong WB and Reyes L, "Echocardiographic assessment of the aortic root in syndromes with left ventricular hypoplasia," *Pediat Cardiol 1982*; 2:19-23.

16. Rao PS and Kulangara RJ, "Echocardiographic evaluation of global left ventricular performance in infants and children," *Indian Pediat 1982*; 19:21-32.

17. Rao PS, "Non-invasive evaluation of left ventricular function in infants and children," *Saudi Med J 1983*; 4:195-209.

18. Covitz W, Rao PS, "Non-invasive evaluation of patients with tricuspid atresia (Roentgenography, Echocardiography, and Nuclear Angiography)," In. Rao PS. "Tricuspid Atresia," *Futura Publishing Co.,* Mount Kisco, New York, 1982:127-145

19. Rao PS, Andaya WG and Whisennand HW, "Contrast echocardiography in the differential diagnosis of hypoxemia following open heart surgery," *King Faisal Specialist Hospital Medical Journal 1983*; 3:121-4.

20. Rao PS, Thapar MK, Haggard RJ and Strong WB, "Left ventricular muscle mass by m-mode echocardiography in children," *J Cardiovasc Ultrasonography 1983*; 2:381-9.

21. Rao PS, Thapar MK, "Influence of race and sex on echocardiographic measurements in children," *J Cardiovasc Ultrasonography 1984*; 3:75-82.

22. Balfour IC, Covitz W, Davis H, Rao PS, Strong WB, Alpert BS, "Cardiac size and function in Children with Sickle Cell Anemia," *Am Heart J 1984*; 108:345-350.

23. Rao PS, Andaya WG, "Chronic afterload reduction in infants and children with primary myocardial disease," *J Pediat 1986*; 108:530-4.

24. Rao PS, "Value of echo-Doppler studies in the evaluation of the results of balloon pulmonary valvuloplasty," *J Cardiovasc Ultrasonography 1986*; 5:309-14.

25. Rao PS, "Doppler ultrasound in the prediction of transvalvar pressure gradients in patients with valvar pulmonic stenosis," *International J Cardiol 1987*; 15:195-203.

26. Rao PS, "Atrioventricular canal mimicking tricuspid atresia: echocardiographic & angiographic features," *Brit Heart J 1987*; 58:409-412.

27. Rao PS, "Doppler echocardiography in non-invasive diagnosis of heart disease in infants and children," *Indian J Pediatr 1988*; 55:80-95.

28. Rao PS, "Value of echo-Doppler studies in the evaluation of the results of balloon angioplasty of aortic coarctation," *J Cardiovasc Ultrasonography 1988*; 7:215-20.

29. Rao PS, Carey P, "Doppler ultrasound in the prediction of pressure gradients across aortic coarctation," *Am Heart J 1989*; 118:299-301.

30. Wilson AD, Rao PS, Aeschlimann S, "Normal fetal foramen flap and transatrial Doppler velocity pattern," *J Am Soc Echocard 1990*; 3:491-4.

31. Rao PS, Langhough R, "Relationship of echocardiographic, shunt flow, and angiographic size to the stretched diameter of the atrial septal defect," *Am Heart J 1991*; 122:505-8.

32. Rao PS, Langhough R, Beekman RH, Lloyd TR, Sideris EB, "Echocardiographic estimation of balloon-stretched diameter of secundum atrial septal defects for transcatheter occlusion," *Am Heart J 1992*; 124:172-5.

33. Rao PS, Levy J, Nikicicz E, Gilbert-Barness EF, "Tricuspid atresia: Association with persistent truncus arteriosus - A review," *Am Heart J 1991*; 122:829-835.

34. Reddy SCB, Rao PS, Ewenko J, et al, "Echocardiographic predictors of success of catheter closure of atrial septal defect with the buttoned device," *Am Heart J 1995*; 129:76-82.

35. Reddy SCB, Chopra PS, Rao PS, "Mixed type of total anomalous pulmonary venous connection: echocardiographic limitations and angiographic advantages," *Am Heart J 1995*; 129:1034-8.

36. Rao PS, Ende DJ, Wilson AD, et al, "Follow-up results of transcatheter occlusion of atrial septal defect with buttoned device," *Canad J Cardiol 1995*; 11:695-701.

37. Singh GK, Marino CJ, Rao PS, "Left heart outflow obstruction, aortic stenosis and coarctation of the aorta: An echocardiographic assessment," *Pediat Ultrasound Today 1996*; 1:61-76.

38. Singh GK, Marino C, Rao PS, "Ultrasound as an adjunct to cardiac intervention in the pediatric patient," *J Invasive Cardiol 1996*; 8:341-9.

39. Singh GK, Marino CJ, Rao PS, "Echocardiographic evaluation of coarctation of the aorta in adults," *Cardiac Ultrasound Today 1997*; 3:111-24.

40. Jureidini SB, Hormann JW, Williams J, Ferdman B, Rao PS, "Morphometric assessment of the innominate vein in the prediction of persistent left superior vena cava," *J Am Soc Echocard 1998*; 11:372-6.

41. Jureidini SJ, Marino C, Rao PS, et al, "Transthoracic color and pulsed Doppler echocardiographic assessment of normal coronary artery flow in children," *J Am Soc Echocard 1998*; 11:409-20.

42. Rao PS, Galal O, Patnana M, et al, "Results of three-to-ten-year follow-up of balloon dilatation of the pulmonary valve," *Heart 1998*; 80:591-5.

43. Jureidini SB, Marino CJ, Singh GK, Balfour IC, Rao PS, "Aberrant coronary arteries: A reliable echocardiographic screening method, *J Am Society of Echocard 2003*; 16:756-63.

44. Gupta M, Rao PS, "Cardiac function in juvenile rheumatoid arthritis," *J Postgrad Med 2004*; 50:266-7.

45. Rao PS, "History of transcatheter interventions in pediatric cardiology," In. Vijayalakshmi IB, (ed.), Cardiac Catheterization and Imaging (From Pediatrics to Geriatrics), *Jaypee Publications*, New Delhi, India, 2015:3-20.

CHAPTER 7

CASE REPORTS

INTRODUCTION

My contributions to clinical research literature began with single case reoprts[1-16] and case series with small numbers[17-32] and was extended to single institutional,[33-76] Food and Drug Administration (FDA)-approved multi-institutional,[77-79] and international multi-institutional[80-83] clinical studies. In this chapter, contribution to literature with single case reports[1-16,84-118] will be reviewed. Each of these case reports, while rare and important clinical observations, do demonstrate a clinical point that is useful to the pediatricians, pediatric cardiologists and/or other physicians. This review will also include reports in which small number ($\leq$ 5 cases) of cases were examined.

CONGENITAL PULMONARY CYST

Case Report

A female infant with a birth weight of 6 lb 7 oz, born after a full-term, normal pregnancy and delivery with an Apgar score of 9 presented at three weeks of age with a two-week history of tachypnea. There were no other symptoms and the infant's physical examination was normal with the exception of tachypnea (respiratory rate of 50 per minute) and mild inter-costal and sub-costal retractions. A chest roentgenogram was obtained (Figure 1), which was interpreted as a pulmonary cyst. The heart was pushed to the right by the cyst (dextroposition of the heart). At thoracotomy, a huge lung cyst, involving the lower lobe of the left lung, was found and was resected and the patient made an uneventful recovery.

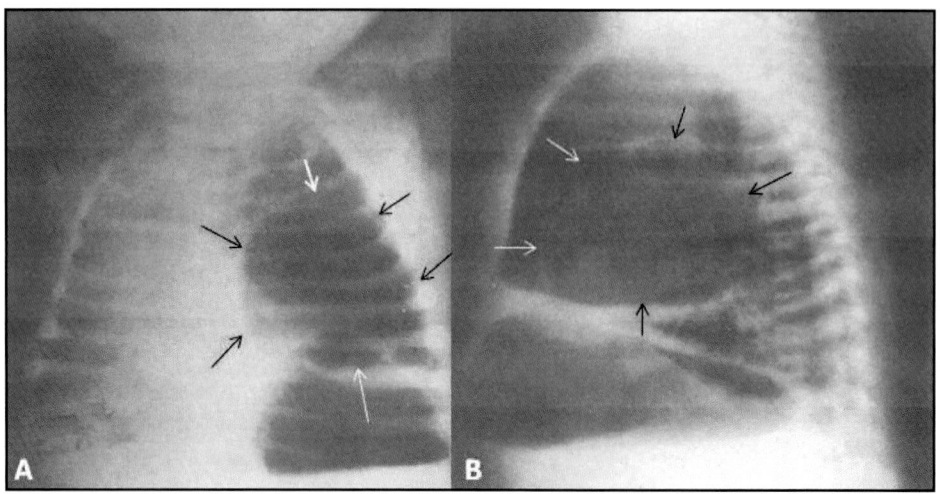

Figure 1. Chest x-ray in posterio-anterior (A) and lateral (B) views demonstrating a large pulmonary cyst, marked with arrows. Note that the heart is pushed to the right, dextroposition of the heart. Reproduced from Rao PS, *Amer J Dis Child 1970*; 119:341-2.

Discussion

Congenital pulmonary cysts in the neonate are uncommon and are considered as errors in embryological development. They are of several categories namely, bronchogenic cell, alveolar cell, and combined cell types, on the basis of the cellular component of the cell wall of the cyst. The symptoms depend largely upon the size of the cyst. These patients may not be discovered until a chest x-ray is performed for other reasons or may present with symptoms of tachypnea, dyspnea, and cyanosis in the neonatal period secondary to compression of lung tissue. The findings depend upon the size and location of the cyst. Dextroposition of the heart or tracheal shift and hyper-resonance, diminished breath sounds, and rales may be detected on physical examination. The chest x-ray findings may demonstrate a cyst, as in our case (Figure 1) or may be misinterpreted as pneumothorax. Other conditions simulating the cyst are staphylococcal pneumonia, diaphragmatic hernia, congenital lobar emphysema, sequestrated lobe, and hydro-pneumothorax or pyo-pneumothorax. In symptomatic cases, cystectomy, segmentectomy, lobectomy, or pneumonectomy, depending upon the size and location of the cyst is suggested. Percutaneous aspiration of the cyst is not recommended, except as an emergency measure to relieve the tension. Some authorities advocate no surgical intervention because of the possibility of spontaneous regression of the pulmonary cysts, but most authorities recommend surgical excision of the cysts.[1]

LATE RESPIRATORY DISTRESS IN A PREMATURE INFANT

Case Report

A premature male infant was born at twenty-five weeks of gestation and weighed 2 lb 12 oz at birth. Abruptio placenta and prolapse of the umbilical cord complicated the delivery and required resuscitation with oxygen. The chest x-ray was normal at that time. The baby was placed in an incubator in thirty-five percent oxygen, which was discontinued within twenty-four hours. At the age of thirty-one days, tachypnea and recurrent apnea with cyanosis developed. Auscultation revealed bilateral rales in the chest, again necessitating resuscitation with O_2, administered by bag and mask. Chest x-ray (Figure 2) revealed a diffuse parenchymal reticular pattern with multifocal areas of radiolucency. This roentgenographic pattern, along with the clinical findings, is essentially diagnostic of the Wilson-Mikity syndrome.

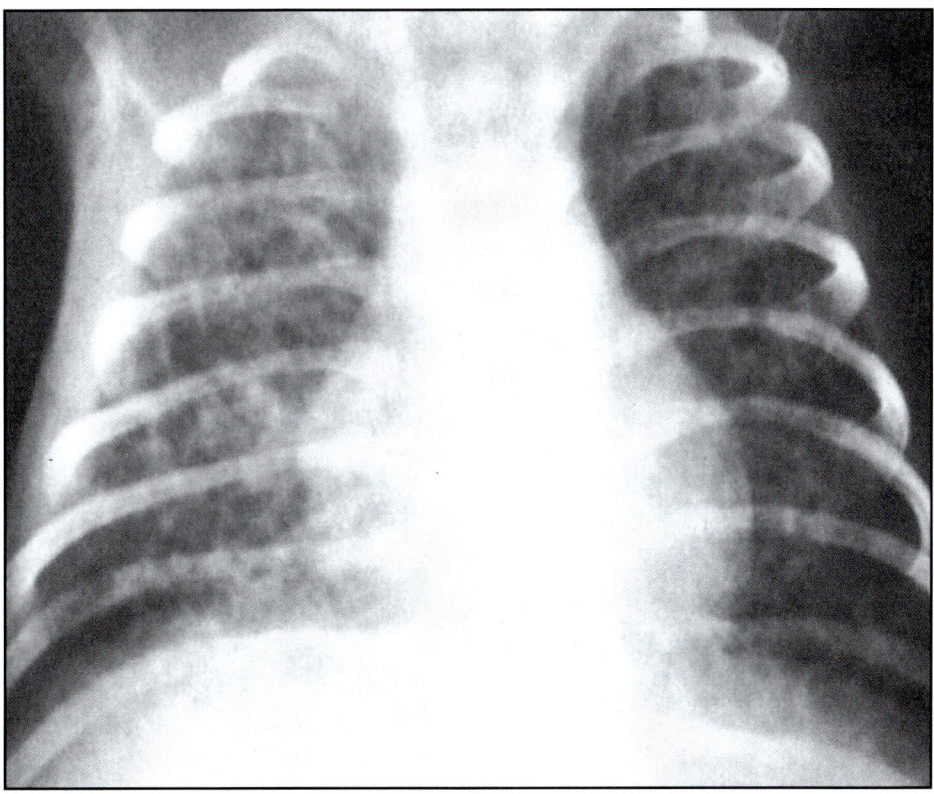

Figure 2. Chest x-ray in posterio-anterior view demonstrating a diffuse parenchymal reticular pattern with multifocal areas of radiolucency. This roentgenographic pattern, along with the clinical findings, is essentially diagnostic of the Wilson-Mikity syndrome. Reproduced from Rao PS, *Chest 1970*; 57:495-6.

Discussion

Wilson and Mikity originally described this condition in 1960, and is now called Wilson-Mikity syndrome.[2] The etiology is not clearly understood, but is considered to be due to pulmonary dysmaturity with uneven postnatal development of pulmonary alveoli in the premature infants.[2] No consistent relationship with O_2 therapy has been established. Bronchopulmonary dysplasia is another condition seen in the neonatal period and should be distinguished from Wilson-Mikity syndrome. The cystic appearance on the chest x-ray in the third stage of bronchopulmonary dysplasia resemble those of Wilson-Mikity syndrome; however, it follows treatment of severe hyaline membrane disease with high concentrations of O_2 and artificial ventilation.[2] The clinical presentation of Wilson-Mikity syndrome is characteristic in that the infant is premature with minimal or no respiratory distress at birth but, develops progressive respiratory distress, with dyspnea, tachypnea, cough, cyanosis, and rales in a few days to weeks. Diffuse reticular pattern of both lungs with areas of multifocal radiolucency are usually seen, similar to those seen in figure 2. Progressive pulmonary insufficiency with signs of right heart failure develop in patients with fatal outcome. But, about half of the patients eventually recover from their pulmonary disease. Pulmonary function studies are abnormal with decreased lung compliance, increased expiratory flow resistance, and increased breathing effort. Respiratory acidosis develops in spite of increased minute volume. Arterial O_2 desaturation is thought to be secondary to intrapulmonary right-to-left shunting.[2] The treatment is largely supportive.[2]

FEVER, VOMITING AND DOME-SHAPED DENSITY IN RIGHT THORAX

Case Report

A four-month-old boy presented with a history of fever, poor feeding, vomiting, and slight cough for two days. Past history is essentially normal except for an Apgar score of six at birth. Breath sounds were diminished at the right base. Laboratory studies were normal. Chest x-ray (Figure 3) was performed, which revealed a dome-shaped density in the right thorax that did not coincide with any pulmonary lobe or segment. The elevation of the inferior liver margin in the abdomen indicated that the abnormal shadow was the liver. On the basis of these findings eventration of the right hemi-diaphragm was suspected. To confirm the diagnosis, a diagnostic pneumoperitonium was performed (Figure 4), which confirmed the diagnosis.

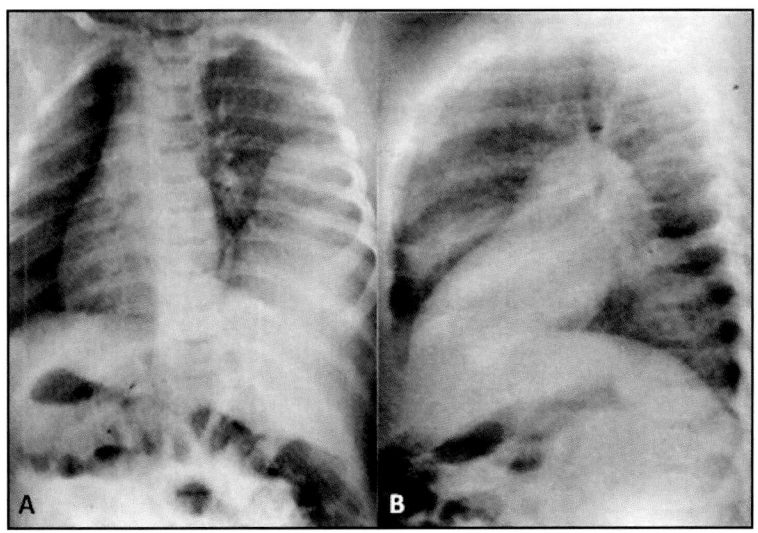

Figure 3. Chest x-ray in posterio-anterior (A) and lateral (B) views showing a dome-shaped density in the right thorax (the x-ray was reversed by the printer). The distribution of the density did not coincide with any pulmonary lobe or segment. The elevation of the inferior hepatic margin in the abdomen indicated that the abnormal shadow was the liver. Reproduced from Rao PS and Patel JK, *Chest 1970*; 58:89-90.

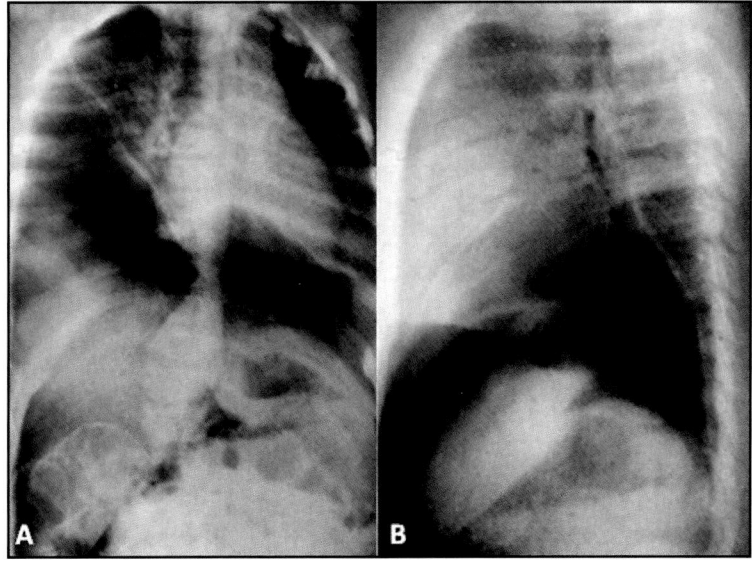

Figure 4. Diagnostic pneumoperitonium with chest x-ray in posterio-anterior (A) and lateral (B) views. This demonstrated air below the diaphragm suggesting eventration of the diaphragm instead of pneumonia or other lung pathology. Reproduced from Rao PS, Patel JK, *Chest 1970*; 58:89-90.

Discussion

Eventration of the diaphragm is classified into adult and infantile types.[3] It is generally thought to be the result of congenital mal-development of the diaphragmatic musculature. However, such an abnormality may occasionally be caused by phrenic nerve injury during birth. The true incidence of eventration is not known, but in mass x-ray surveys of adults, it was found to be one in 10,000 people.[3] Total eventration is thought to be more common on the left side and partial eventration on the right.[3]

Clinical findings largely depend on the extent of eventration. There may be no symptoms or the patient may present with dyspnea, tachypnea, and cyanosis in the newborn period, requiring immediate treatment. Seesaw cyclic motions of the epigastrium with respiration and Hoover's sign (uninhibited divergence of costal margin from midline on inspiration), if present, are helpful in making the diagnosis. Percussion on the affected side may be dull or tympanic depending on the organs migrated under the diaphragm.

Fluoroscopy and chest x-rays are generally useful in arriving at the diagnosis. In right-sided eventrations, the lesser amount of liver shadow in the abdomen, i.e., elevation of the inferior margin of the liver helps to distinguish eventration from the other conditions.[3] Diagnostic pneumoperitonium is likely to establish the diagnosis, but the current availability of ultrasound technology, diagnostic pneumoperitoneum may not be necessary at the present time.

Symptomatic newborns with diaphragmatic eventration should be treated surgically; plication of the eventrated diaphragm is successful in relieving the symptoms with good long-term results. Some authorities suggest that asymptomatic patients also should be addressed surgically.[3]

FOREIGN BODY (PEANUT) IN THE LEFT MAIN STEM BRONCHUS

Case Report

A thirteen-month-old girl with a history of poor appetite, loss of weight, cough, and intermittent low grade fever was admitted to the hospital for evaluation and treatment. No history of choking episodes was elicited. Past history revealed that a relative who had active pulmonary tuberculosis lived with the infant's family for a short period of time, four months prior to the current admission. Because of this reason, the local health department performed tuberculin skin test, which was positive and treatment with isoniazid was initiated. On examination, her weight and height were between the third and tenth percentile. Decreased breath sounds on auscultation and hyper tympanic note on percussion were noted over the left side of the chest.

Intermediate strength purified protein derivative (PPD) test was positive. Chest roentgenograms were obtained (Figure 5). On the basis of the history, physical examination, and chest x-ray findings, a diagnosis of endobronchial tuberculosis was entertained. However, prior to beginning treatment, bronchoscopy was performed to appraise the extent of airway encroachment.

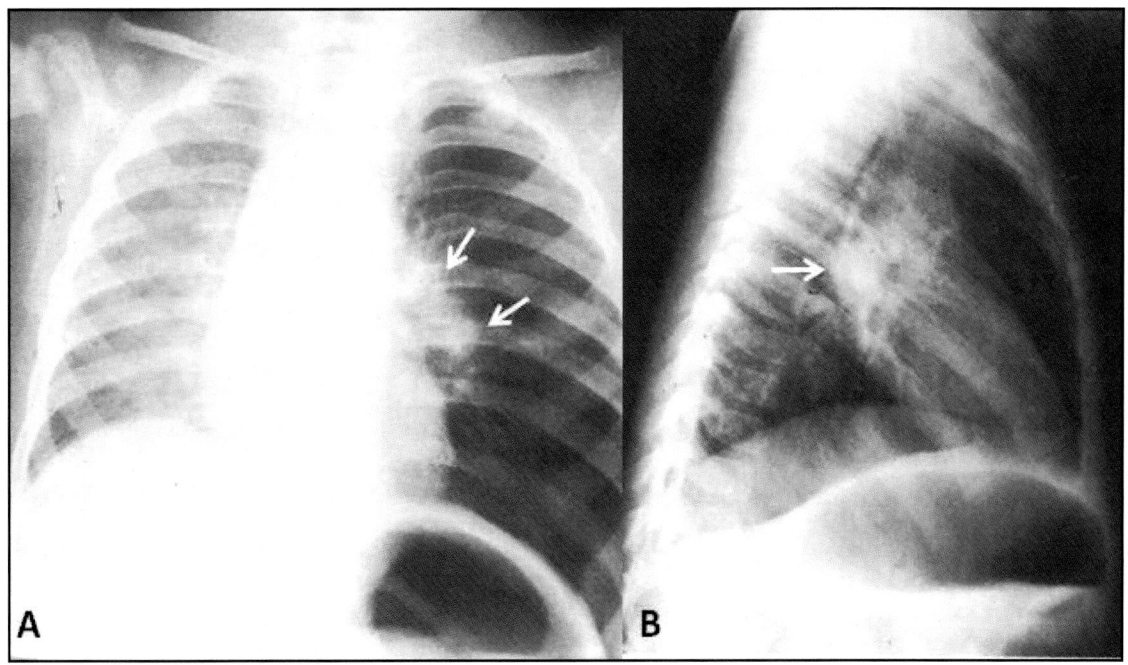

Figure 5. Chest x-ray in posterio-anterior (A) and lateral (B) views showing hyper-aeration of the left lung and a slight shift of the heart and mediastinum to the right. The left diaphragm is also flattened. There are no areas of infiltration or consolidation in the lung, but prominent densities (arrows in A and B) suggestive of enlarged lymph nodes were also seen. Modified from Rao PS, et al, *Amer J Dis Child 1970*; 120:51-52.

Positive PPD in an infant with poor appetite, loss of weight, and fever is suggestive of primary tuberculosis. This is particularly so given the patient's exposure to a subject with active pulmonary tuberculosis. The x-rays show hyper aeration of the left lung with a shift of the heart and mediastinum to the right. The left leaf of the diaphragm is also flattened. While no areas of infiltration or consolidation were seen, prominent shadows suggestive of enlarged lymph nodes were seen (arrows in Figure 5). Endobronchial tuberculosis with compression of the bronchus by adenopathy may produce changes seen in figure 5.

Discussion

Even though there was no history of choking or aspiration, the possibility of foreign body aspiration should be considered in this age group. Consequently, bronchoscopy was performed that revealed a peanut in the left main stem bronchus and was extracted during bronchoscopy. The peanut and the adjacent edema of the bronchus caused partial bronchial obstruction and acted as a check valve so the air entered the left lung, but was unable to leave the left lung since the bronchus becomes smaller during expiration, producing the roentgenographic appearance shown in figure 5. The baby improved and the treatment with isoniazid was continued because of the positive PPD.

COR PULMONALE AS A COMPLICATION OF VENTRICULOATRIAL SHUNTS

Introduction

Cerebral ventricle-to-right atrial shunts with Pudenz-Heyer or Spitz-Holter valves were widely used to treat hydrocephalus in the 1960s. Development of pulmonary hypertension with chronic cor pulmonale is rare with these shunts. We reported a patient who developed such a complication along with description of specialized pulmonary function studies in the early detection of such complication.[5]

Case Report

An eleven-year-old white boy was hospitalized in April 1969 with a history of progressive weakness, dyspnea, and pedal edema. He was diagnosed to have hydrocephalus and had a ventriculo-atrial shunt with a Pudenz-Heyer valve implanted at the age of six months. The shunt was thought to be functioning well when he was evaluated at the age of two years. He was asymptomatic until he was nine-and-a-half years old, when he developed signs of congestive heart failure (CHF) and was treated at another hospital with digitalis and diuretics with some improvement. Right heart catheterization at the same institution revealed a mean right atrial pressure of 35 mmHg and right atrial angiography revealed slow emptying of the contrast, filling defects on the right lateral atrial wall and in the right and left pulmonary arteries. The ventriculo-atrial shunt was removed shortly thereafter. The patient was referred to our group for further evaluation and management.[5]

Pertinent findings on examination included height and weight below the third percentile, head circumference above the ninety-seventh percentile, pretibial edema, prominent "a" wave in the left side of the neck, no venous pulsations on the right side, palpable right ventricular heave, markedly accentuated single second heart sound, an audible fourth heart sound at left lower sternal border, a Grade I/VI ejection systolic murmur at the mid-left sternal border, liver edge palpable five centimeter below the right costal margin, clear lung fields on auscultation, and normal neurological examination.

Electrocardiogram (ECG) (Figure 6) and the vectorcardiogram (not shown) revealed right atrial and ventricular hypertrophy. Chest roentgenogram (Figure 7) showed moderate cardiomegaly and prominent main pulmonary artery (PA) segment and clear lung fields. Lung scan131 with I-labeled macro-aggregated albumin was suggestive of multiple pulmonary emboli. Blood gas analysis showed pH 7.56; PaO_2 80 mmHg, $PaCO_2$ 23 mmHg and bicarbonate 24 mEq/liter. Routine pulmonary function studies revealed restrictive lung disease. The ratio of wasted ventilatory volume (physiological dead space) to tidal volume (VD:VT) using Bohr's equation was 0.58 (normal is 0.3 or less).

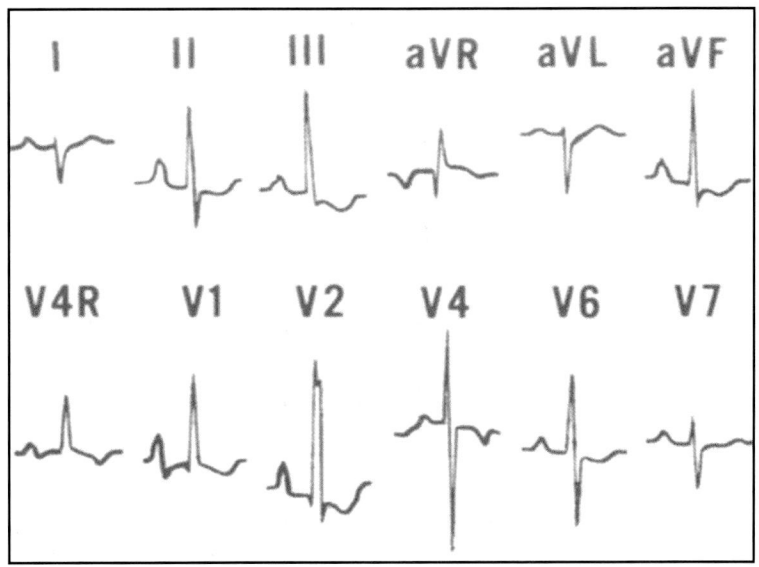

Figure 6. Electrocardiogram shows right axis deviation with right atrial hypertrophy and marked right ventricular hypertrophy. Reproduced from Rao PS, et al, *J Neurosurg 1970*; 33:221-225.

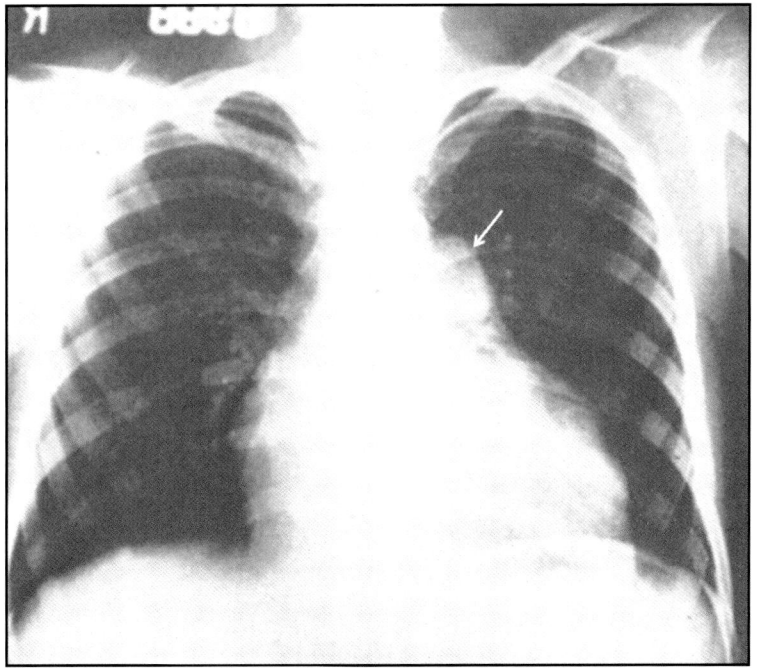

Figure 7. Chest x-ray in posteroanterior view demonstrating cardiomegaly and prominent main pulmonary artery segment (arrow). The peripheral pulmonary vasculature is diminished. Modified from Rao PS, et al, *J Neurosurg 1970*; 33:221-225.

Vigorous treatment with digitalis and diuretics resulted in only temporary relief. During the next year, he continued to deteriorate and died of intractable right ventricular failure. Postmortem revealed right atrial thrombosis, severe right ventricular hypertrophy, multiple thrombo-emboli in the large and medium-sized pulmonary arteries, and intimal proliferation of the pulmonary arterioles.

Discussion

The case presented demonstrated development of cor pulmonale secondary to pulmonary thrombo-embolism, which was produced by thrombi that arose following a ventriculo-atrial shunt with a Pudenz-Heyer valve for treatment of hydrocephalus. The causes of thrombo-embolic complications were not well understood, but the hypotheses, as reviewed by us,[5] include infection, periarteritis due to autoimmune reaction of the pulmonary vessels to protein of cerebrospinal fluid, release of brain thromboplastin resulting in thrombosis at the point of contact with plasma coagulation factors, and simply the presence of a foreign body in the cardiovascular system for prolonged periods of time.

Early detection of pulmonary hypertension by periodic (every six months) evaluation by chest x-ray and ECG studies was suggested by some investigators, but early detection of pulmonary hypertension is of limited value since obstruction of sixty percent of the pulmonary vascular bed occurs by the time pulmonary hypertension develops.[5] Detection of multiple filling defects on radioisotope scanning in a child with a ventriculo-atrial shunt would be suggestive of pulmonary embolization and might be useful in early identification. Based on the observations of Nadel and associates[119] and those of ours,[5] we suggested that specialized pulmonary function studies such as $V_D:V_T$, pulmonary diffusing capacity, pulmonary capillary blood volume, blood gas, and pH be performed periodically to detect obstruction of pulmonary vasculature prior to the development of pulmonary hypertension and cor pulmonale.[5] However, it should be noted that ventriculo-atrial shunts are no longer performed to treat hydrocephalus, but instead ventriculo-peritoneal shunts are used at the present time.

In summary, a rare case of pulmonary thrombo-embolism with resultant pulmonary hypertension and cor pulmonale following ventriculo-atrial shunt for hydrocephalus was presented with the recommendation to use of special pulmonary function studies for early detection and if found to be positive, immediate removal of the shunt system may eliminate further embolization into the lungs and prevent irreversible pulmonary vascular disease.

CONGENITAL HEART DISEASE IN THE DE LANGE SYNDROME

Introduction

The prevalence of congenital heart disease (CHD) in de Lange syndrome has not been systematically studied as of early 1970s. The objective of our report[6] was to present a patient with classic manifestations of de Lange syndrome with pulmonary stenosis and to examine the literature to determine the incidence and types of CHD present in this syndrome.

Case Report

A baby boy weighing 3 pounds 14 ounces was born at thirty-six weeks of a normal gestation. Physical examination revealed wide upper lip, upturned nose, horizontal cleft in the chin, hairy eyebrows, and low-set ears (Figure 8), features typical for de Lange syndrome. Cutis marmorata, hypertrichosis, hypoplastic and widely spaced nipples, bilateral hemi-melia with a single digit, and rocker-bottom feet were also obvious. Physical examination at two week of age revealed right ventricular heave, normal first heart sound, split second heart sound with diminished pulmonary component, a grade 3/6 ejection systolic murmur heard best at the upper left sternal border with radiation into the back bilaterally, no diastolic murmurs, and no signs of CHF.

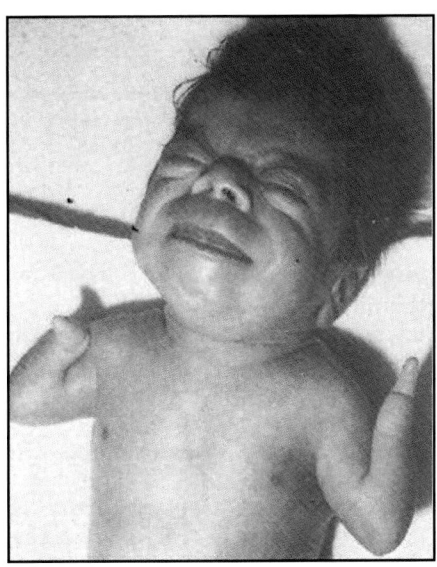

Figure 8. Photograph of a baby with de Lange syndrome.
Reproduced from Rao PS, Sissman NJ, *J Pediatr 1971*; 79:674-7.

Chest x-ray revealed thirteen ribs on both sides, two mid-thoracic hemi-vertebrae, and an odd segmental pattern of the sternum, mild cardiac enlargement, and normal pulmonary vascular markings. Upper extremity radiographs revealed short humerus and a single forearm bone, probably radius, on both sides. The ECG indicated right axis deviation and right atrial (RA) and right ventricular (RV) hypertrophy. Normal male karyotype was found on chromosomal analysis. Cardiac catheterization and cineangiography performed at three weeks of age confirmed the diagnosis of severe valvar pulmonary stenosis with intact ventricular septum, a small patent ductus arteriosus (PDA) and a patent foramen ovale (PFO). The baby was transferred to another hospital for palliative care.

Literature Review

Detailed review of the literature identified 250 cases of de Lange syndrome from 117 papers.[6] These papers were examined for the presence or absence of CHD and if present, the type of CHD. Three groups were identified. Group I was made up of patients with a definitive diagnosis of CHD - 37 of 250 (15 percent). Group II consisted of 30 (12 percent) cases in whom physical findings, usually a cardiac murmur, suggestive of CHD were present, but no additional finding to confirm CHD were presented by the respective authors. Group III patients had no CHD. The type of heart defect identified is listed in Table I; VSD appears to be the most common defect.

Table I. Relative incidence of various known types of congenital heart defects in De Lange Syndrome (Thirty-seven cases).

Nature of Heart Defect	Number
Ventricular septal defect	10
Patent ductus arteriosus	7
Pulmonary stenosis*	6
Patent foramen ovale	5
Anomalous systemic venous drainage	3
Atrial septal defect	3
Tetralogy of Fallot	2
Miscellaneous**	18
Total	54#

*Includes one case with infundibular pulmonary stenosis and one with a bicuspid pulmonary valve.

**One case each of truncus arteriosus, aortic stenosis, hypoplasia of one of the cusps of aortic valve, coarctation of aorta, right aortic arch, separate origin of the right subclavian and carotid arteries from aortic arch, hypoplastic left heart syndrome, and high origin of right coronary artery. Two cases each of abnormal insertion of chordae tendineae and endocardial fibroelastosis in association with other defects. In six cases the defect was not clearly stated or not stated.

#The discrepancy between totals is due to the occurrence of more than one defect in some patients.

Discussion

The baby presented had typical features of de Lange syndrome. Cardiac findings were those of valvar pulmonary stenosis, confirmed by cardiac catheterization and cineangiography. Extensive review of previously published reports indicated at least 15 percent prevalence of CHD, significantly higher than 0.8% incidence in normal population. The incidence of CHD is lower than that seen with Down Syndrome and we concluded that CHD is not an integral part of de Lange syndreome.[6] However, it should be noted that many children (at least 12 percent) had not been adequately studied to determine the presence and type of CHD. Consequently, the true incidence of CHD may be higher. The most common defect in de Lange syndrome in this survey was VSD, similar to that seen in normal population.

Because of invariably severe mental retardation associated with this syndrome, no open-heart surgery to treat pulmonary stenosis was undertaken, in keeping with thinking in 1970s. However, more recent de Lange syndrome cases seen and cared by me did undergo transcatheter intervention to treat valvar pulmonary stenosis.

GROWTH RETARDATION IN STEROID DEPENDENT ASTHMA - MANAGEMENT WITH CORTICOTROPHIN (ACTH)

Introduction

A number of complications have been reported with long-term therapy with steroids in children. More common among these complications are adrenal atrophy with failure to react in stressful situations, suppression of obvious signs of infection, and growth failure.[7] The purpose of our paper was to document growth retardation in a patient who was on long-term prednisone treatment who was switched to corticotrophin (ACTH) in an attempt restore his growth.[7]

Case Report

A twelve-and-a-half year old young man was seen for evaluation and management of his asthma. He had a perennial asthma from early infancy. He was skin tested and desensitized for house-dust, molds, pollens, and bacteria multiple times with only transient improvement with each of these regimens. In addition to conventional bronchodilator therapy available at that time, he required oral prednisone, 5 to 10 mg daily for control of his asthma. When evaluated by us at the age of twelve-and-a-half years, his heart and respiratory rates were normal, the antero-posterior diameter of the chest was markedly increased and auscultation revealed moderate expiratory wheezes and many scattered rhonchi bilaterally. Chest roentgenogram revealed marked hyperinflation with flattened diaphragms. Pulmonary function studies were consistent with striking obstructive airway disease, which reversed partially following bronchodilators. He was managed with a program that included environmental control, oral and aerosol bronchodilators, and maintenance doses of 5 to 10 mg of prednisone per day. His symptoms were under good control, with an infrequent need for subcutaneous sympathomimetic medications. Efforts to modify prednisone therapy to an alternate day regimen failed. The most important problem was the absence of growth (Figure 9). During the two and a half years of treatment he had grown only three centimeters (3.0 cm), an obviously decreased growth velocity (Figure 9A) and remarkably reduced standing height (Figure 9B).

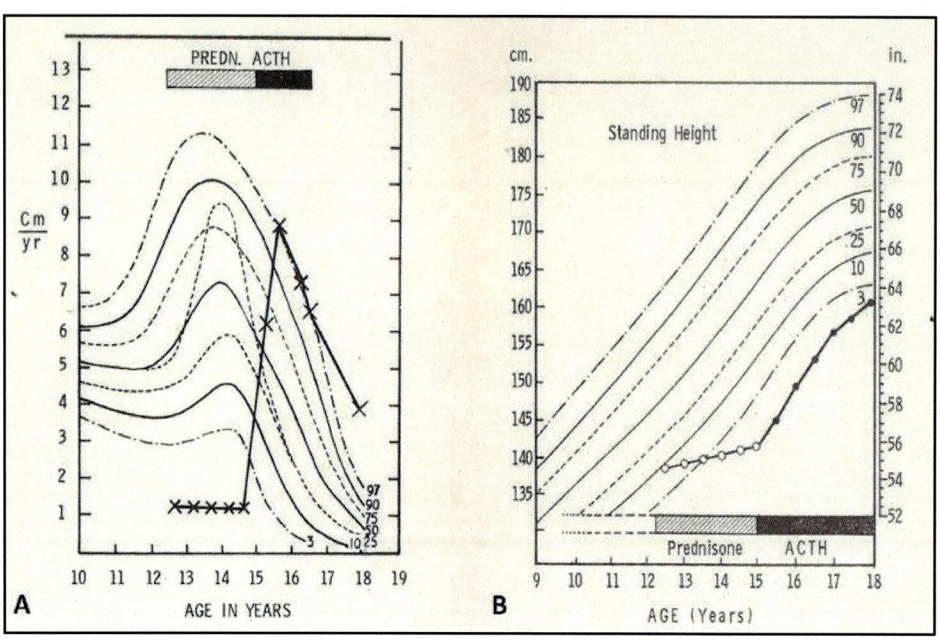

Figure 9. A. Patient's height velocity was plotted on height velocity curve from Tanner et al.[120] Normal percentiles (third through ninety-seventh) of height velocity are marked. The patient's height velocity was calculated as cm/yr per each six-month period of observation. Prednisone (hashed bar) and ACTH (solid bar) periods are shown. The height velocity was below third percentile during the prednisone treated period, while the height velocity varied from fiftieth to above ninety-seventh percentile during ACTH treatment, a remarkable improvement.

B. This is similar to A, but patient's standing height was plotted on curve from Tanner et al.[120] Normal standing height percentiles (third through ninety-seventh) for age are drawn. Again, prednisone and ACTH period are indicated. Growth failure while on prednisone therapy and improvement with ACTH was clearly noted. Reproduced from Rao PS, Lipow HW, *Clin Pediat 1972*; 11:93-7.

To address this growth problem, his treatment was switched to daily subcutaneous injections of 40 units of ACTH at fifteen years of age. During the following year-and-a-half he grew 11.5 cm. His height velocity has improved and normalized (Figure 9A) and his standing height increased (Figure 9B). The bone age was 11.5 years prior to starting ACTH treatment and advanced to fourteen years after the one-and-a-half years of ACTH therapy. Prior to ACTH, he had no secondary sexual characteristics, but the growth of pubic hair started after year-and-a-half treatment with ACTH. During the period of ACTH therapy, the control of the asthma was similar to the time of prednisone treatment with regard to the need for bronchodilators, hospitalizations, and number of days absent from the school. Pulmonary function tests after a year-and-a-half of ACTH therapy showed mild obstruction with hyperinflation. After one-and-a-half years, his ACTH administration was reduced to 40 units on alternate days. By the end of the period of observation when he was eighteen-years-old, his linear growth was satisfactory (Figure 9) with a height of 63-1/4 inches placing him out of the significantly dwarfed range.

Discussion

Inhibition of growth with long-term treatment with steroids is well recognized[7] and our patient is a good example of such a phenomenon. Growth retardation associated with steroid treatment of asthma, nephrotic syndrome and rheumatoid arthritis appears to improve by substitution of prednisone with ACTH or a combination of ACTH and steroids,[121] as demonstrated in our patient. The mechanism for growth retardation with steroids is not clearly understood, but is likely to be suppression of endogenous ACTH by prednisone. When ACTH is administered, it may stimulate adrenals to produce growth-promoting factors. Several practical tips with regard to the usage of steroids in children were reviewed for the interested reader.[7]

In summary, when long-term steroid treatment is necessary in children during the growth period, their height should be closely monitored. If growth retardation is documented, switching to ACTH should be entertained.

SYSTEMIC VENOUS ANOMALIES AND PARTIAL HETEROTAXIA WITH NORMAL HEART[8]

These findings were reviewed in the chapter on "Cardiac Catheterization and Cineangiography" in the book titled "Pediatric Cardiology: How It Has Evolved Over the last 50 Years" and will not be repeated.

EBSTEIN'S MALFORMATION OF THE TRICUSPID VALVE WITH ATRESIA[9]

This was discussed in the chapter on "Tricuspid Atresia" in the book titled "Pediatric Cardiology: How It Has Evolved Over the last 50 Years" and will not be reviewed here.

SUPERIOR VENA CAVAL OBSTRUCTION IN TOTAL ANOMALOUS PULMONARY VENOUS CONNECTION

Introduction

Total anomalous pulmonary venous connection (TAPVC) is generally classified into supra-diaphragmatic and infra-diaphragmatic types. Infra-diaphragmatic type is typically associated with obstruction to pulmonary venous return while the supra-diaphragmatic type is rarely associated with pulmonary venous obstruction. The objective of this report was to present an atypical type of obstruction to pulmonary venous return in a case of supra-diaphragmatic TAPVC and to review the literature to determine types of obstruction seen in the supra-diaphragmatic TAPVC.[10]

Case Report

A male infant, a product of a full-term normal pregnancy and delivery, presented with signs of CHF at the age of two months. Examination revealed tachypnea, mild to moderate cyanosis, a heart rate of 180/minute, normal blood pressure, and an enlarged liver, palpable 5 cm below the right costal margin. The precordium was hyper-dynamic with a prominent right ventricular impulse. The second heart sound was narrowly split. A grade 2/6 ejection systolic murmur at the left upper stenal border, and a grade 2/6 mid-diastolic flow rumble at the left lower sternal border were heard. Chest roentgenogram showed moderate cardiomegaly with increased pulmonary vascular markings (Figure 10). The ECG showed RA and RV hypertrophy (Figure 11).

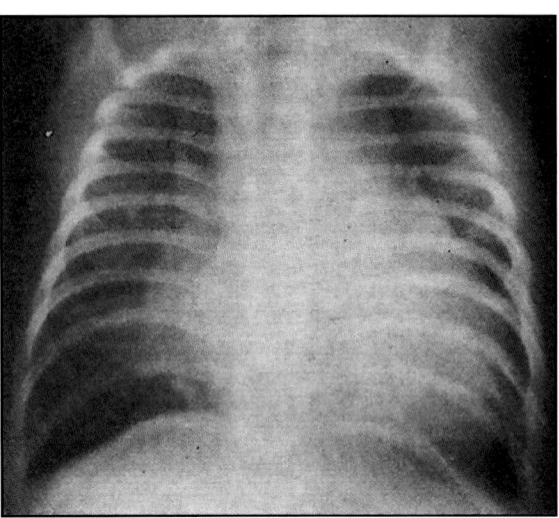

Figure 10. Posteroanterior view of the chest x-ray showing moderate cardiomegaly and increased pulmonary vasculature. Reproduced from Rao PS, Silbert DR, *Brit Heart J 1974*; 36:228-32.

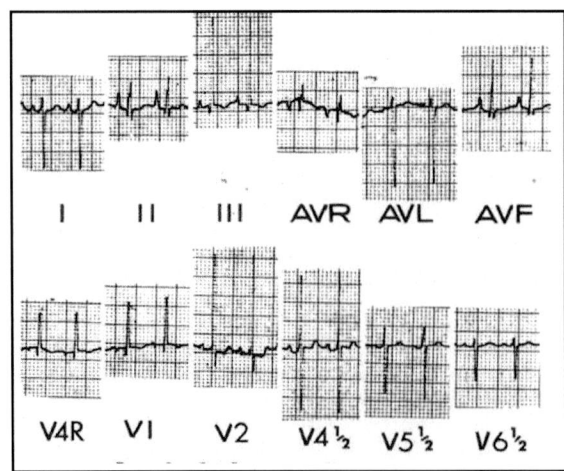

Figure 11. Electrocardiogram showing right atrial and right ventricular hypertrophy. Reproduced from Rao PS, Silbert DR, *Brit Heart J 1974*; 36:228-32.

Following treatment of CHF, cardiac catheterization and selective cineangiography were carried out. The RV and PA pressures were at systemic level. There was a 12 mmHg mean pressure difference between the right atrium and the superior vena cava (SVC). Levophase of the main PA cineangiogram was faint without opacification of a common pulmonary vein. But the SVC was opacified faintly with subsequent right atrial opacification. SVC cineangiogram (Figure 12) showed retrograde filling of the azygos vein with subsequent opacification of inferior vena cava and right atrium. Only a tiny amount of contrast passed from the SVC into the right atrium. Attempts to catheterize the common pulmonary vein from the SVC failed, and therefore, additional pressure gradient from the common pulmonary vein to the SVC could not be excluded. Balloon atrial septostomy was performed, which abolished the interatrial pressure gradient (2.0 mmHg vs. 0.5 mmHg). Treatment of CHF was continued. Since there was persistent CHF and failure to gain weight, surgical relief of the SVC obstruction was undertaken at the age of five months. At surgery, the SVC appears to be inserted into the right atrium in a more posterior position than is normally seen. A linear vertical incision was made at the RA and SVC junction, which was closed in a transverse fashion. The pressures in the SVC and right atrium were equalized after the procedure. The infant seemed to improve, but the next morning the baby suddenly deteriorated and died.

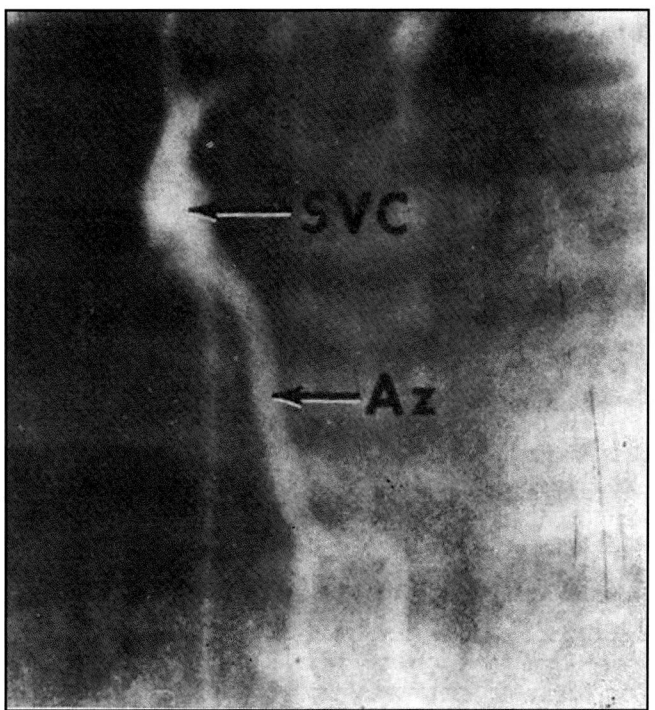

Figure 12. Selected frame from superior vena caval (SVC) cineangiogram in posteroanterior view showing prompt opacification of the azygos vein (Az). Note absence of opacification of the right atrium. In the cineangiographic frames that followed the inferior vena cava was filled with contrast subsequent to Az opacification and then the right atrium. Reproduced from Rao PS, Silbert DR, *Brit Heart J 1974*; 36:228-32.

Autopsy findings revealed RV and PA enlargement. The left atrium (LA) and the left ventricle (LV) were of normal size. The pulmonary venous drainage is diagrammatically portrayed in Figure 13. Two pulmonary veins drain the left lung, which joined each other behind the heart. This common pulmonary vein coursed across the midline and ascended superiorly to join the postero-lateral aspect of the SVC. Four pulmonary veins from the right lung joined the lateral convexity of the common pulmonary vein (Figure 13). The common pulmonary vein emptied into the SVC; its orifice was located slightly inferior to the opening of the azygos vein. The SVC was of adequate size, but there was a ring-like fibrous constriction at the junction of the SVC with the RA, which was partially enlarged during surgery. On histological examination grade II changes (Heath-Edwards) of the pulmonary vasculature were seen.

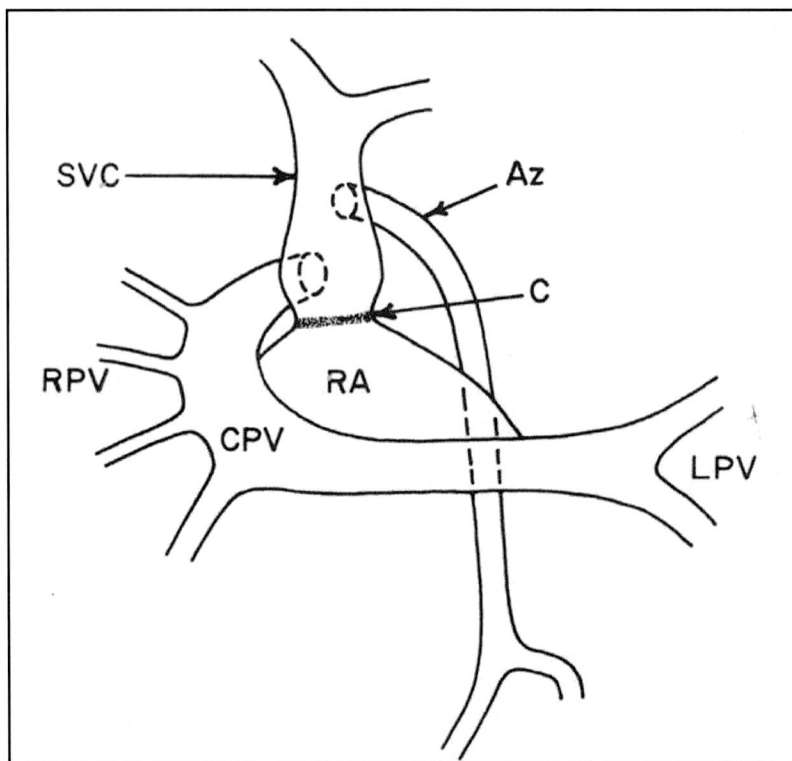

Figure 13. Diagrammatic sketch of the pulmonary venous return found on postmortem examination. Two pulmonary veins draining the left lung fuse and form a common pulmonary vein (CPV) which traverses to the right and then ascends to empty into the postero-lateral aspect of the superior vena cava (SVC). Four right pulmonary veins (RPVs) join the lateral convexity of the CPV. The position of the azygos vein (Az) opening into the SVC and the constricted site of the SVC (arrow) are also shown. C, constricted area of the SVC; LPV, left pulmonary veins; RA, right atrium. Reproduced from Rao PS, Silbert DR, *Brit Heart J* 1974; 36:228-32.

Literature Review

A detailed review of the literature was performed to discern the types of obstruction seen in supra-diaphragmatic TAPVC.[10] This review indicated that pulmonary venous obstruction occurs in all types of supra-diaphragmatic TAPVC and each of these was referenced in our publication.[10] In the most common type of TAPVC, connection to the left innominate vein, the obstruction of the vertical vein may be intrinsic or extrinsic. The intrinsic obstruction can result from narrowing of the anomalous vertical vein at its junction with the common pulmonary vein or at its junction with the left innominate vein or it may be due to narrowing of the left innominate vein. The extrinsic obstruction is secondary to compression of the vertical vein as it passes between left pulmonary artery and left bronchus. In cases with connection of common pulmonary vein with the azygos vein, the connecting vessel was small causing obstruction in one case and in another case the nature of the obstruction was not described.[10] In cases with connection to the right atrium, atresia or stenosis of the vessel connecting the common pulmonary vein to the right atrium can occur. In subjects with connection to the coronary sinus, stenosis at the junction of the pulmonary venous confluence with the coronary sinus and stenosis of the individual pulmonary veins as they enter the coronary sinus has been reported. In patients with connection to the azygos vein, small or narrow connecting vessel was present causing obstruction. Obstruction may occur at the level of the atrial septum, which could be treated with balloon atrial septostomy. Rarely, the common pulmonary vein may not have any connection with the systemic veins; such cases are not truly TAPVCs.[10]

In summary, our review indicated that pulmonary venous obstruction occurs more frequently in supra-diaphragmatic types of TAPVC than was thought prior to the review. The obstruction to pulmonary venous return in cases with TAPVC may be classified into: 1. Intrinsic stenosis or atresia of the vessel connecting the common pulmonary vein with systemic venous system; 2. Extrinsic compression of the connecting vessel; and 3. Obstruction at the atrial septal level.[10]

Discussion

Our case is a rare instance of obstruction in supra-diaphragmatic TAPVC with physiologically and anatomically confirmed obstruction at the junction of the SVC with the RA. At the time of that report, only few other similar cases were reported in the literature, one had stenotic ring in the SVC similar to our case and the other cases had stenosis of the common pulmonary vein at its entrance into the SVC.[10] The other types of obstructed supra-diaphragmatic TAPVC were described as of the time our report were reviewed in the preceding literature review section.

The embryology of TAPVC with particular attention to the development of circular constriction of the SVC was reviewed[10] for the interested reader.

In summary, we presented an unusual case of supra-diaphragmatic TAPVC in which physiologically and anatomically proven stenosis in the SVC was documented. Extensive review of the literature indicated that pulmonary venous obstruction occurs in supra-diaphragmatic TAPVC more often than previously recognized.[10]

GROWTH OF HYPOPLASTIC RIGHT VENTRICLE FOLLOWING PULMONARY VALVOTOMY[11]

This subject was reviewed in the chapter on "Cardiac Catheterization and Cineangiography" in the book titled "Pediatric Cardiology: How It Has Evolved Over the last 50 Years" and will not be repeated.

DIAGNOSIS OF EBSTEIN'S ANOMALY OF THE LEFT ATRIOVENTRICULAR VALVE WITH CONGENITAL CORRECTED TRANSPOSITION OF THE GREAT ARTERIES BY INTRACAVITARY ELECTROCARDIOGRAPHY[12]

This was also discussed in the chapter on "Cardiac Catheterization and Cineangiography" in the book titled "Pediatric Cardiology: How It Has Evolved Over the last 50 Years" and will not be reviewed here.

GROWTH PHENOMENON AS A CAUSE OF KINKING OF THE RIGHT PULMONARY ARTERY IN WATERSTON ANASTOMOSIS[13]

This subject was also reviewed in the chapter on "Cardiac Catheterization and Cineangiography" in the book titled "Pediatric Cardiology: How It Has Evolved Over the last 50 Years" and will not be repeated here.

USEFULNESS OF PULMONARY VEIN WEDGE ANGIOGRAPHY IN VISUALIZATION OF OBSTRUCTED PULMONARY ARTERY[14]

This matter was discussed in the chapter on "Cardiac Catheterization and Cineangiography" in the book titled "Pediatric Cardiology: How It Has Evolved Over the last 50 Years" and will not be reviewed here.

FALSE ANEURYSM OF THE RIGHT PULMONARY ARTERY: A NEW COMPLICATION OF THE WATERSTON ANASTOMOSIS[15]

This was reviewed in the chapter on "Cardiac Catheterization and Cineangiography" in the book titled "Pediatric Cardiology: How It Has Evolved Over the last 50 Years" and will not be discussed here.

CONTRAST ECHOCARDIOGRAPHY IN THE DIAGNOSIS OF ANOMALOUS CONNECTION OF THE RIGHT SUPERIOR VENA CAVA TO THE LEFT ATRIUM[16]

This was reviewed in the chapter on "Echocardiography" in the book titled "Pediatric Cardiology: How It Has Evolved Over the last 50 Years" and will not be discussed here.

SPONTANEOUS CLOSURE OF PHYSIOLOGICALLY ADVANTAGEOUS VENTRICULAR SEPTAL DEFECTS

Spontaneous closure of physiologically advantageous ventricular septal defects (VSDs) in tricuspid atresia and double-outlet RV[17] and functional closure of VSDs in tricuspid atresia[19] was discussed in the chapter on "Physiologically Advantageous VSDs" in the book titled "Pediatric Cardiology: How It Has Evolved Over the last 50 Years" and will not be reviewed here.

CONTRAST ECHOCARDIOGRAPHY IN THE DIFFERENTIAL DIAGNOSIS OF HYPOXEMIA FOLLOWING OPEN HEART SURGERY[84]

This was discussed in the chapter on "Echocardiography" in the book titled "Pediatric Cardiology: How It Has Evolved Over the last 50 Years" and will not be reviewed here.

CHANGING MURMUR OF PATENT DUCTUS ARTERIOSUS[21]

This was discussed in the chapter on "Patent Ductus Arteriosus" in the book titled "Pediatric Cardiology: How It Has Evolved Over the last 50 Years" and will not be reviewed here.

SYNDROME OF SINGLE VENTRICLE WITH LEFT ATRIOVENTRICULAR VALVE ATRESIA AND INTERATRIAL OBSTRUCTION: PALLIATIVE MANAGEMENT WITH SIMULTANEOUS ATRIAL SEPTOSTOMY AND PULMONARY ARTERY BANDING

Four infants between the ages of two days and four months were referred to us for evaluation of cyanosis.[25,122] Clinical, chest x-ray, ECG, cardiac catheterization, and selective cineangiography data revealed diagnoses of single ventricle, left atrioventricular (AV) valve atresia, and interatrial obstruction, but without pulmonary stenosis in each case. Relief of interatrial obstruction by balloon atrial septostomy in two infants produced marked fall in the left atrial and PA mean pressures and pulmonary vascular resistance (PVR) along with marked increase in the left-to-right interatrial shunt, pulmonary blood flow, and systemic arterial oxygen saturation (See Tables I and II of Reference 25). The other two infants have surgical atrial septostomy. Because of this predictable fall in PVR, banding of the PA was performed in each case with good results, both immediately after the procedure and at follow-up. There were only a few reported cases of single ventricle with left AV valve atresia as of that time.[25,122] Obstruction at the atrial level appears to be common in this lesion. The concept that relieving the interatrial obstruction results in rapid and predictable decrease in the PVR was emphasized and concomitant PA banding at the time of atrial septostomy (surgical or balloon) is recommended for the infants with this type of anatomy.[25,122] At that time, we have also theorized that modified Fontan type procedure may eventually be applicable to this type of anatomy and that it is important to keep PA pressures and PVR within normal range.[25]

CHYLOPERICARDIUM: A NEW COMPLICATION OF BLALOCK-TAUSSIG ANASTOMOSIS

Introduction

Chylopericardium following Blalock-Taussig (BT) shunt is extremely rare, especially in those patients in whom the pericardial cavity is not opened during surgery. The purpose of our report was to document a case of chylopericardium, which developed after a BT shunt, to point out its rarity, and to discuss management strategies.[85]

Case Report

A three-month-old infant weighing 2.4 kg with cyanosis was referred to us for evaluation and treatment. Evaluation including cardiac catheterization revealed a diagnosis of tricuspid atresia with normally related great arteries and a small VSD resulting in severe pulmonary oligemia.[85] A right BT shunt was performed. The surgery did not require entering into the pericardial cavity. The infant improved and was discharged home a few days after the procedure. Because of the development dyspnea, tachycardia and diaphoresis four weeks after the surgery, anticongestive measures were instituted. Cardiomegaly was present on chest x-ray. Echocardiogram revealed a large pericardial effusion. Pericardiocentesis was performed resulting in drainage of 110 ml of chylous fluid. Analysis of the drained fluid revealed albumin - 2.8 gm/100 ml (simultaneous serum albumin - 3.4 gm), electrolytes - same as serum values, and triglycerides - 1,210 mg/100 ml. Microscopic examination showed lymphocytes and no bacteria. These findings were thought to be consistent with chylous effusion. Two additional pericardiocentesis procedures were required twenty-four hours apart, each time draining 65 ml of chylous fluid and therefore, pericardial window via left lateral thoracotomy was performed and drainage tubes were placed. The infant was started on medium-chain triglyceride (MCT) formula (Portagen, Mead Johnson, Evansville, IN). Within a few days, the pericardial drainage ceased and the chest tubes removed. The infant was continued on MCT formula. Revaluation in the outpatient department a month later did not show evidence for recurrence of pericardial effusion and functioning BT shut with satisfactory O$_2$ saturations.

Discussion

We stated that post-operative chylopericardium was first reported in early 1970s[123] following surgical repair of pulmonary atresia with VSD. Subsequently, a number of other investigators reported chylopericardium following a number of other surgical procedures, as reviewed and referenced in our publication.[85] The causation of chylopericardium was not well understood and several hypotheses have been advanced and include obstruction of thoracic duct secondary to thrombosis of the jugular and/or subclavian veins, transection of cardiac lymphatics in the pericardial cavity, injury to the thoracic duct, obstruction to normal flow through the thoracic duct, and/or a combination thereof. High prevalence of variations of the thoracic duct system was pointed out, which may predispose to inadvertent injury to the thoracic duct system during surgery.

We have also suggested that this complication, though rare, should be added to the list of complications associated with BT shunts.[85]

Extensive literature search with the help of an experienced librarian in 1983 prior to submitting the paper for publication did not reveal any reports of chylopericardium following BT shunt without violating the pericardium. Consequently, we stated that chylopericardium following surgery was first reported in early 1970s.[123] Unfortunately, this was incorrect, as pointed out by Dr. Louchimo;[124] these authors from Helsinki, Finland were indeed the first to report chylopericardium following BT shunt in a twenty-one-month-old in German literature (Z Kinderchurgie) in 1966. We did convey our regret for this oversight,[124] but PubMed search even in 2019 did not show this citation.

The management of patients with postoperative chylopericardium consists of performing pericardiocentesis to relieve cardiac tamponade and then starting a medium-chain triglyceride diet.[85,125] Repeat echocardiograms to detect any fluid in the pericardial sac should be performed. If need for repeated pericardiocentesis arises, tube pericardiostomy (or per-catheter drainage) should be undertaken. The MCT diet should be followed for at least four weeks and then switched to a normal, fat-containing diet. Again, the patient should be monitored to ensure that no re-accumulation of pericardial fluid ensues. We think that this regimen is likely to be successful in most cases of postoperative chylopericardium. In the uncommon patient, resistant to this type of therapy, thoracic duct ligation may have to be performed. We are somewhat opposed[125] to the approach of partial pericardiectomy with or without ligation of the thoracic duct in all patients advocated by Rose and associates.[126]

In summary, we reported a rare case of chylopericardium following BT shunt, reviewed the possible causation and offered management strategies. We suggested that this complication should not deter performing BT shunt in babies requiring palliation for cyanotic CHD with pulmonary oligemia.[85,125]

TRANSCATHETER KNIFE (BLADE) ATRIAL SEPTOSTOMY

Four infants aged twelve hours to seven months with diagnoses of transposition of the great arteries (TGA) (N=3) and mitral atresia with single ventricle (N =1) had balloon atrial septostomy. The O_2 saturations did not improve in the infants with TGA and in the baby with mitral atresia the interatrial mean pressure difference did not fall. All four infants underwent blade atrial septostomy, three during the same study and one, two days later, with resultant improvement in systemic arterial O_2 saturation in the TGA patients (immediate improvement in two and delayed improvement in one patient) and decrease in mean interatrial pressure difference in the mitral atresia patient. In the mitral atresia patient, there was also fall in PVR and increase in left to right shunt with a higher pulmonary to systemic flow ratio (Qp:Qs).[30,32] Equally impressive was the improvement in symptomatology (cough and tachypnea) and pulmonary venous congestion on chest x-ray film. Each of these infants underwent successful corrective (Senning operation in TGA patients) or palliative (PA banding in the mitral atresia patient) surgery later. It was concluded that blade atrial septostomy is safe and effective in non-surgical palliation of CHD to increase a restrictive interatrial defect, especially if balloon atrial septostomy was not successful.[30,32]

SCIMITAR SYNDROME

Introduction

Scimitar syndrome, as described by Neill and her colleagues,[127] consists of a triad of anomalies, namely hypoplastic right lung, dextroposition of the heart (a rightward shift of the heart), and anomalous pulmonary venous connection of the right lung to the inferior vena cava (IVC). The anomalously draining pulmonary vein becomes larger as it descends into IVC and appears as a scimitar-shaped shadow on chest x-ray, justifying the name, Scimitar syndrome. In addition to the three abnormalities described above, there is usually an abnormal tracheobronchial tree on the right side, and an anomalous systemic arterial supply from below the diaphragm to the lower lobe of the right lung.[31,127] The purpose of our report was to present findings of scimitar syndrome in four patients, including a rare type of left-sided scimitar.[31]

Case Reports

Four patients aged six months to three years were presented[31] with typical features of Scimitar syndrome; one of them however, had left lung hypoplasia with a left sided scimitar-shaped shadow on the left side. Three of these patients had hypoplastic right lung with dextroposition of the heart (Figure 14A), while the fourth patient had hypoplastic left lung with displacement of the heart more to the left than usual position (Figure 14B). Scimitar sign was present, which was more clearly seen on tomography (Figure 15). Pulmonary perfusion scans revealed hypoplastic right or left lung (Figure 16). Cardiac catheterization revealed normal PA pressure in one, mild elevation in two and severe increase in one patient. Definitive step in O_2 saturation in the IVC was demonstrated in one patient. Evidence for atrial septal defect (ASD) was found in one patient. Levophase of the PA cineangiograms indicated anomalous drainage of pulmonary veins into the IVC (Figure 17). Angiograms from the left heart revealed arteries from the descending aorta or celiac axis supplying right lower lobe of the lung in three cases and the left lung in one patient.

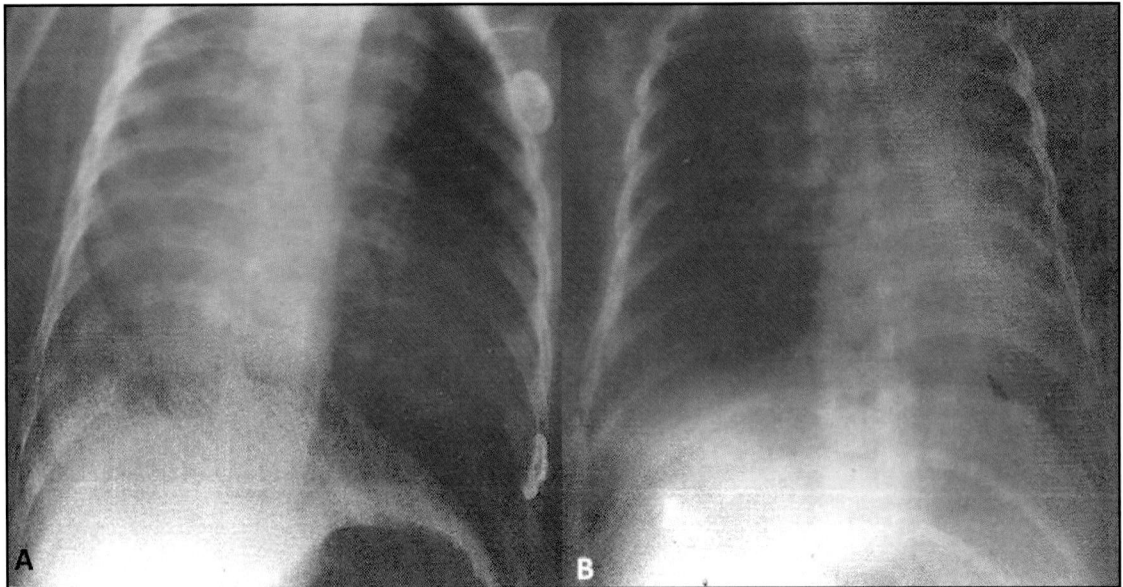

Figure 14. Chest x-rays in posterio-anterior view of two infants with Scimitar syndrome demonstrating rightward (A) or leftward (B) shift of the heart secondary to hypoplasia of the right or left lungs, respectively. Reproduced from Mardini MK, Rao PS, *Arab J Med 1984*; 3:13-23.

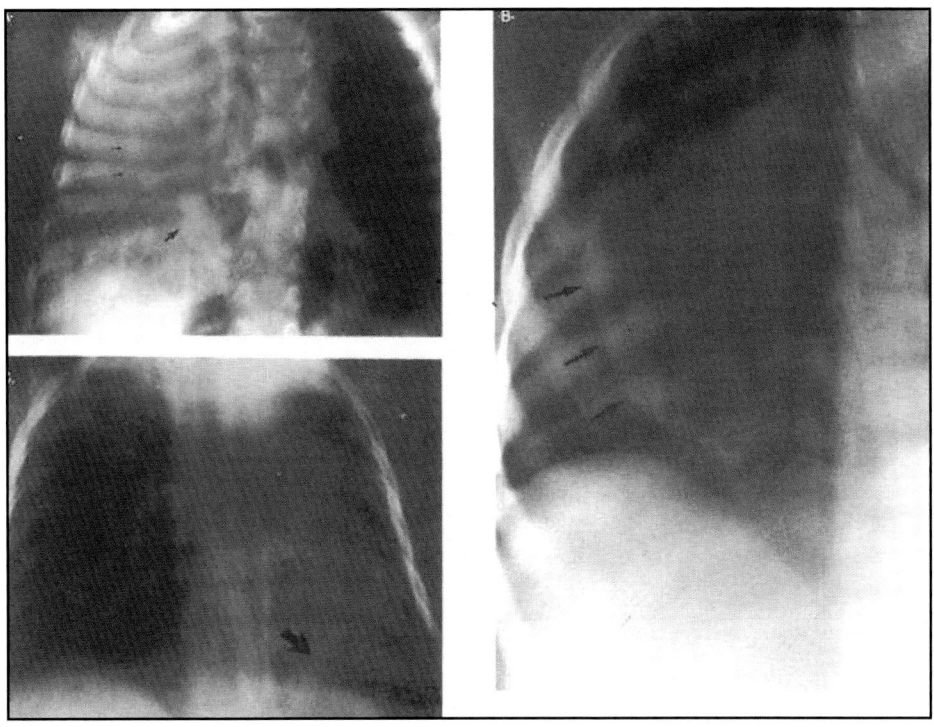

Figure 15. Tomograms demonstrating scimitar sign indicating anomalous pulmonary venous drainage in patients with right (A and B) or left (C) Scimitar syndromes. Reproduced from Mardini MK, Rao PS, *Arab J Med 1984*; 3:13-23.

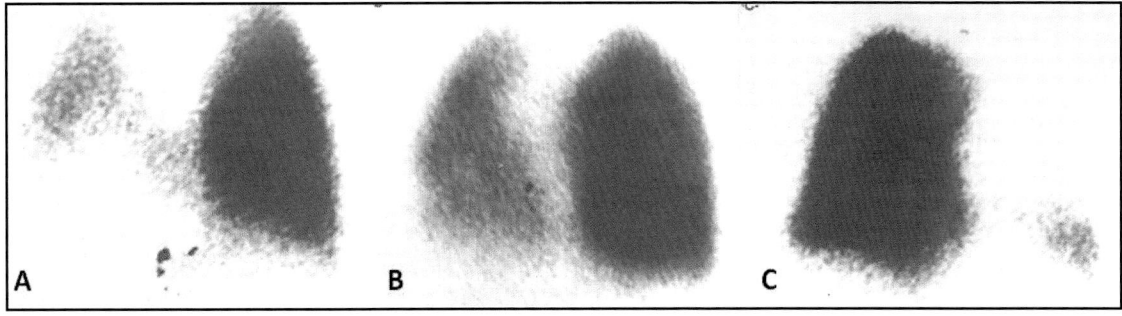

Figure 16. Pulmonary perfusion scans demonstrating decreased perfusion to the right (A and B) or left (C) lungs in patients with right (A and B) or left (C) Scimitar syndromes. Reproduced from Mardini MK, Rao PS, *Arab J Med 1984*; 3:13-23.

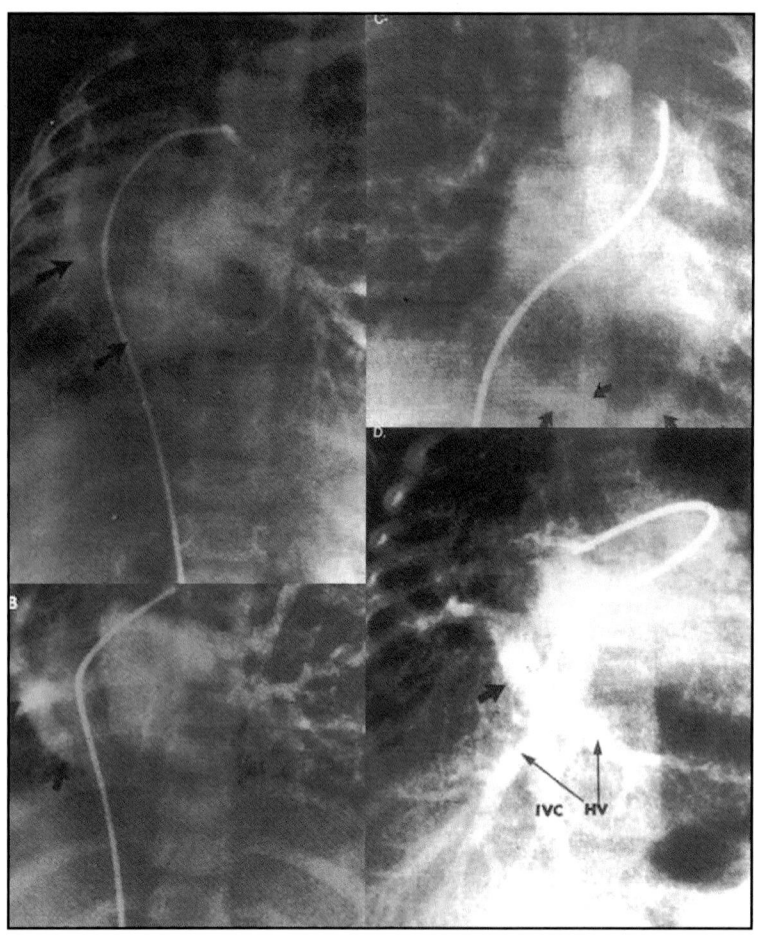

Figure 17. Selected frames from levo-angiographic phases of pulmonary artery cineangiograms in posteroanterior view showing drainage of anomalous pulmonary veins (arrows) in four patients with right (A, B and D) or left (C) Scimitar Syndromes. Reproduced from Mardini MK, Rao PS, *Arab J Med 1984*; 3:13-23.

Discussion

Although, the autopsy findings of this syndrome were described in 1836, clinical findings in 1912 and angiographic documentation in 1949,[31] it was not a well-known clinical entity until Neill coined the term "Scimitar Syndrome."[127] Detailed review of the literature published as of the time of our publication was performed and the results tabulated (Table 2 of Reference 31). In general, it is a right-sided syndrome. Our report included one case of left-sided Scimitar syndrome; this was only the second such case documented, the first one is that reported by D'Cruz and Arcilla.[128] The prevalence of this syndrome is low, four out of 596 patients (less than one percent) catheterized during the period of observation. The etiology, clinical manifestations, and management was reviewed for the interested reader.[31]

CONTRAST ECHOCARDIOGRAPHY IN THE DIFFERENTIAL DIAGNOSIS OF HYPOXEMIA FOLLOWING OPEN HEART SURGERY[84]

This was discussed in the chapter on "Echocardiography" in the book titled "Pediatric Cardiology: How It Has Evolved Over the last 50 Years" and will not be reviewed here.

SYNDROME OF ABSENT PULMONARY VALVE: SURGICAL CORRECTION WITH PULMONARY ARTERIOPLASTY

Introduction

Syndrome of absent pulmonary valve with tetralogy of Fallot (TOF) is a rare variant of TOF. In this publication we report successful surgical correction in an infant with this syndrome.[86]

Case Report

A thirteen-month old baby with classic features of syndrome of absent pulmonary valve (Figures 18A and 19A) with TOF had successful surgical repair by the closure of the VSD and relief of the pulmonary valve obstruction. At the same time, partial resection and plastic repair of the aneurysmally dilated main and branch PAs was performed.[86] Clinical, chest x-ray (Figure 18B), cardiac catheterization (See Table of Reference 86) and angiographic (Figure 19 B) data following surgery suggested excellent results.

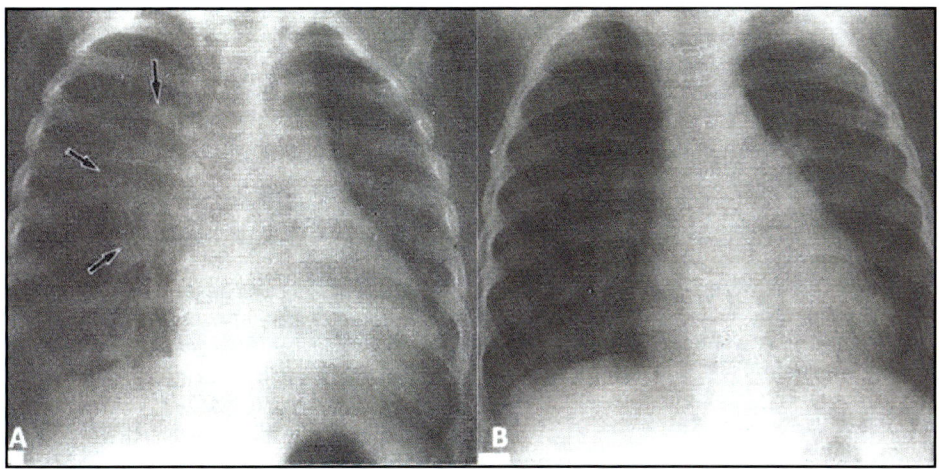

Figure 18. A. Chest x-ray in posteroanterior view performed prior to surgery demonstrating moderate cardiomegaly with dilated right pulmonary artery (arrows). B. Repeat chest x-ray twelve months following surgery showing near normal sized heart and no prominent pulmonary arteries. Reproduced from Rao PS and Lawrie GM, *Brit Heart J* 1983; 50:586-9.

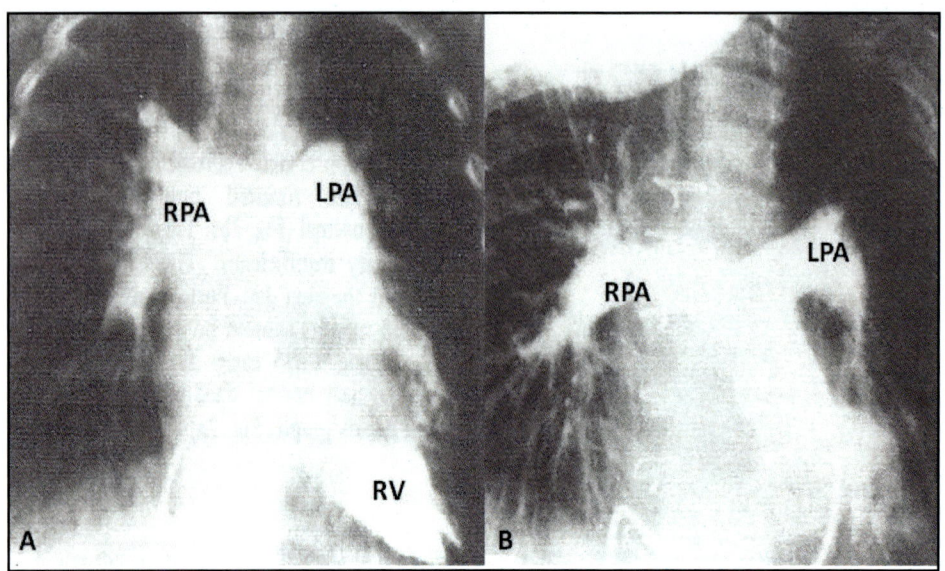

Figure 19. A. Selected cine frame from right ventricular (RV) cineangiogram demonstrating markedly dilated main, right (RPA) and left (LPA) pulmonary arteries prior to surgery. B. Repeat cineangiogram performed following surgery demonstrating marked improvement of the branch pulmonary arteries. Modified from Rao PS and Lawrie GM, *Brit Heart J 1983*; 50:586-9.

Discussion

Two types of clinical presentations are known: Group I, neonates with severe respiratory distress and Group II, patients presenting beyond six months of life with no significant respiratory symptoms. Our patient belongs to group II. It is recommended that plastic repair of the aneurysmally dilated PAs and closure of the VSD, and surgical relief of RV outflow tract obstruction should be performed early, probably at the age of one to two years for the group II patients. While some surgeons recommend prosthetic replacement of the pulmonary valve at the time of primary repair,[129] our view[86] is that valve replacement is not needed in all cases at the time of primary surgery.

TRANSIENT EOSINOPHILIC PULMONARY INFILTRATION WITH INTESTINAL SCHISTOSOMIASIS AND MITRAL STENOSIS

Introduction

Pulmonary infiltration with eosinophelia (PIE) is rare, but a well recognized entity.[130] The association of PIE is even less common with *Schistosomia Mansoni* infestation.[87] We reported the association PIE in a child with mitral stenosis and its successful management.[87]

Case Report

A ten-year-old child presented with a history of cough and moderate dyspnea. Pertinent clinical findings were palpable liver and spleen and widespread rhonchi and wheezes in both lungs. He also had soft ejection systolic murmur at the left sternal border and a mid-diastolic murmur at the apex with presystolic accentuation. Chest roentgenogram revealed mild cardiomegaly, left atrial enlargement, prominent main PA segment and widespread fluffy pulmonary infiltrates (Figure 20A). Differential count: Eosinophils – 19 percent; Neutrophils – 64 percent; lymphocytes – 11 percent; Erythrocyte sedimentation rate - 35 mm/hr; Sputum – 40 percent eosinophils; Bone marrow - marked eosinophilic hyperplasia; Stool - positive for ova of *Schistosomia Mansoni* and occult blood; Serum immunoglobulins: IgG - 1420 mg/dl, IgA - 205 mg/dl, IgM - 220 mg//dl, and IgD - 1 mg/dl. M-mode echocardiogram showed severely decreased E-F slope of the mitral valve consistent with mitral stenosis. Cardiac catheterization and selective cineangiography revealed moderate elevation of PA (56/27 mmHg) and PA wedge (mean of 20 mmHg) pressures indicative of significant mitral stenosis. Anti-congestive measures were instituted and treatment with anti-bilharzias (Ambilhar) medication was started. However, the respiratory distress and pulmonary infiltrates (Figure 20B) improved prior to initiation of antibilharzia (Ambilhar) treatment. Three months later, he had successful open mitral commisurotomy.

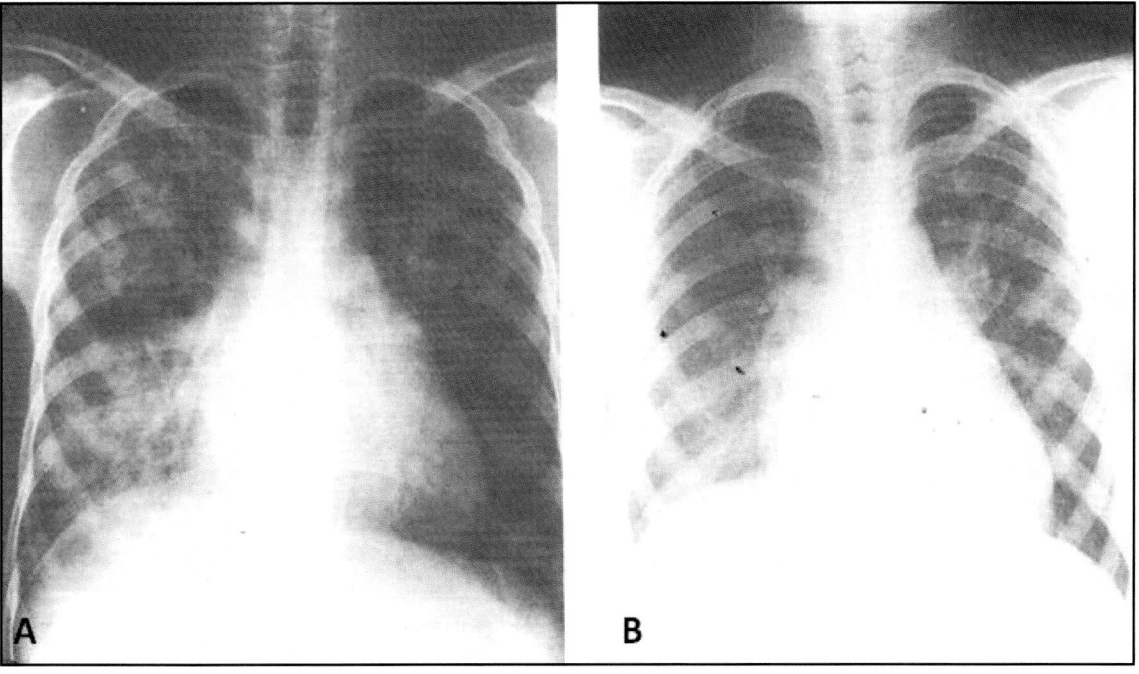

Figure 20. A. Chest x-ray in posterio-anterior view at the time of initial presentation showing puffy infiltrations, particularly noticeable in the right lung. B. Repeat chest x-ray five days later demonstrating almost complete clearance of the lung. Reproduced from Rao PS, et al, *King Faisal Specialist Hospital Med J 1984*; 4:355-8.

Discussion

The pulmonary infiltrates appear to be due to hyper-eosinophilia of *Schistosomia Mansoni* and not secondary to mitral stenosis in that there were no kerly B lines, cephalization of pulmonary flow or symmetric central haziness, typical for mitral stenosis. The unusual association of PIE and mitral stenosis was recognized and both were treated successfully.[87]

ATRIOVENTRICULAR CANAL MIMICKING TRICUSPID ATRESIA[88]

This was reviewed in the chapter on "Tricuspid Atresia" in the book titled "Pediatric Cardiology: How It Has Evolved Over the last 50 Years" and will not be reviewed here.

CONGESTIVE CARDIOMYOPATHY DUE TO CHRONIC TACHYCARDIA[89]

This case was reviewed in the chapter on "Electrocardiography" in the book titled "Pediatric Cardiology: How It Has Evolved Over the last 50 Years" and will not be reviewed here.

USE OF PROPRANOLOL FOR SEVERE DYNAMIC INFUNDIBULAR OBSTRUCTION PRIOR TO BALLOON PULMONARY VALVULOPLASTY

The prevalence of dynamic infundibular obstruction in association with severe pulmonary stenosis and balloon pulmonary valvuloplasty[131] was reviewed in the chapter on "Pulmonary Stenosis" in the book entitled "Pediatric Cardiology: How It Has Evolved Over the last 50 Years." This particular case[90] describes a ten-year-old girl with severe pulmonary valvar stenosis with associated infundibular obstruction. This infundibular obstruction was very severe and consequently we were unable to advance any catheter into the PA. Administration of 0.5 mg of Propranolol intravenously resulted in reduction of the obstruction, which allowed passage of catheters and balloon pulmonary valvuloplasty could be performed without any complications. Following the procedure, oral propranolol treatment was initiated which helped to resolve the infundibular obstruction during follow-up. We have therefore recommended the use of propranolol in patients with severe infundibular obstruction so that balloon pulmonary valvuloplasty can be performed.[90]

In response to the letter to the editor following our publications on infundibular stenosis,[90,131] we have detailed step by step description of the management of infundibular stenosis associated with pulmonary stenosis and balloon pulmonary valvuloplasty,[132] which may be reviewed by the interested reader.

CATHETER CLOSURE OF ATRIAL SEPTAL DEFECT: SUCCESSFUL USE IN A 3.6 KG INFANT[91]

This case was reviewed in the chapter on "Atrial Septal Defect" in the book titled "Pediatric Cardiology: How It Has Evolved Over the last 50 Years" and will not be repeated here.

TRANSCATHETER CLOSURE OF PATENT DUCTUS ARTERIOSUS WITH BUTTONED DEVICE: FIRST SUCCESSFUL CLINICAL APPLICATION IN A CHILD[92]

This case was reviewed in the chapter on "Patent Ductus Arteriosus" in the book titled "Pediatric Cardiology: How It Has Evolved Over the last 50 Years" and will not be repeated here.

TRICUSPID ATRESIA: ASSOCIATION WITH PERSISTENT TRUNCUS ARTERIOSUS - A REVIEW[93]

This case was reviewed in the chapter on "Tricuspid Atresia" in the book titled "Pediatric Cardiology: How It Has Evolved Over the last 50 Years" and will not be repeated here.

AN UNUSUAL PRESENTATION OF COARCTATION OF THE AORTA IN INFANCY: ROLE OF BALLOON ANGIOPLASTY IN THE CRITICALLY ILL INFANT[94]

Introduction

This case[94] was mentioned in the chapter on "Coarctation of the Aorta" in the book entitled "Pediatric Cardiology: How It Has Evolved Over the last 50 Years" and will only be briefly reviewed here.

Case Report

A three-month-old infant was referred to our practice in March 1989 for evaluation of his failure to thrive and CHF. Examination revealed a bay weighing of four kilograms (4.0 kg) with tachycardia, tachypnea, a loud third heart sound with a gallop, no cardiac murmur, hepatomegaly, and barely palpable brachial and femoral pulses. Arm blood pressure was 90 mmHg and leg pressure was not recorded by the admitting house-officer. Chest x-rays showed severe cardiomegaly (Figure 21A) and pulmonary venous congestion. ECG indicated LV hypertrophy with ST segment depression and biphasic T waves in the left chest leads. Echocardiogram demonstrated a severely dilated LV with decreased LV shortening fraction (Figure 22A). Anti-congestive treatment including digoxin, furosemide, and afterload reduction with hydralazine was initiated. The infant improved with respect to the signs of CHF. Revaluation, the following day, revealed good brachial pulses with poorly palpable femoral pulses. The right arm blood pressure was 140/80 mm Hg and the right leg blood pressure was 86/54 mm Hg. Echo-Doppler studies were repeated which showed aortic coarctation with a descending aortic Doppler flow velocity of 4 m/sec. The LV function continued to be poor. Because of poor LV function and my past experience, balloon angioplasty was preferred to surgical management.

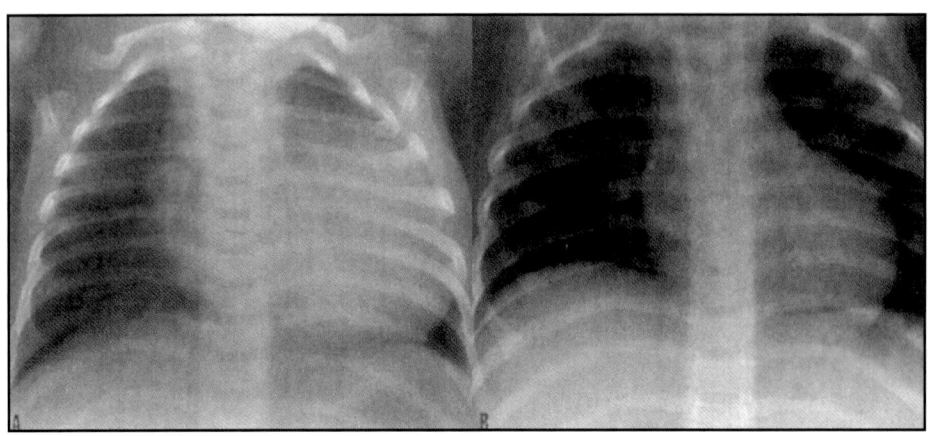

Figure 21. A. Chest x-ray in postero-anterior view at presentation showing marked cardiomegaly and pulmonary venous congestion. B. Dramatic improvement of the cardiac size and pulmonary venous congestion on a chest x-ray obtained twelve months following balloon angioplasty. Reproduced from Saluhuddin N, Wilson AD, Rao PS, *Am Heart J 1991*; 122:1772-5.

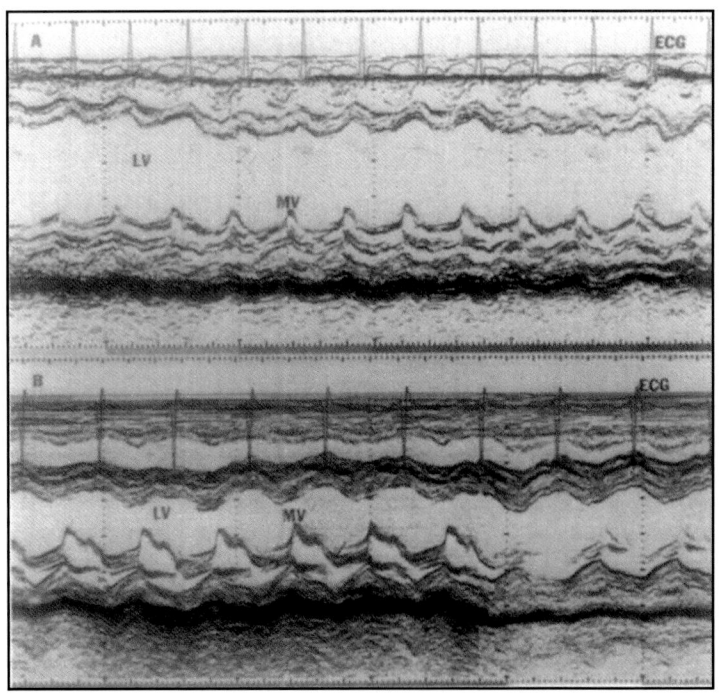

Figure 22. A. M-mode echocardiogram of the left ventricle (LV) at the time of initial presentation. Marked enlargement of the LV and poor LV function are shown. B. A similar echogram of the LV twelve months following balloon angioplasty shows remarkable improvement in LV size and function. ECG, Electrocardiogram; MV, mitral valve. Reproduced from Saluhuddin N, Wilson AD, Rao PS, *Am Heart J 1991*; 122:1772-5.

Cardiac catheterization and cineangiography revealed discrete aortic coarctation measuring 2.7 mm with a peak systolic pressure gradient of 45 mmHg across the coarctation. Balloon angioplasty catheter carrying an 8 mm diameter balloon was used to dilate the coarctation segment with resultant reduction of the gradient to 15 mmHg and increase in coarctation segment size to 6.0 mm.[94] Anti-congestive measures (digitalis, furosemide, and hydralazine) were continued and the baby was periodically evaluated. Gradual but consistent improvement was observed and by twelve months, the chest x-ray (Figure 21B) and echocardiogram (Figure 22B) normalized. Repeat cardiac catheterization and angiography revealed a residual gradient of 10 mmHg and continued angiographic improvement.

Discussion

Discussion of the unusual appearance of "hypertensive cardiomyopathy" in an infant with aortic coarctation, issues related to the diagnosis at the time of presentation, and the choice of therapy were reviewed[94] for the interested reader.

CHYLOTHORAX, AN UNUSUAL COMPLICATION OF BAFFLE OBSTRUCTION FOLLOWING MUSTARD OPERATION: SUCCESSFUL TREATMENT WITH BALLOON ANGIOPLASTY[95]

This case was reviewed in the chapter on "Miscellaneous Obstructive Lesions" in the book titled "Pediatric Cardiology: How It Has Evolved Over the last 50 Years" and will not be repeated here.

TRANSUMBILICAL BALLOON COARCTATION ANGIOPLASTY IN A NEONATE WITH CRITICAL AORTIC COARCTATION

Introduction

This case[96] was mentioned in the chapter on "Coarctation of the Aorta" in the book entitled "Pediatric Cardiology: How It Has Evolved Over the last 50 Years" and will only be briefly reviewed here. We reported feasibility of balloon angioplasty for native coarctation via an umbilical artery, sparing the femoral arteries.[96]

Case Report

An eleven-day-old infant with cyanosis, grunting, and poor perfusion with an initial pH of 7.1 and a base deficit of 12.8 was initially resuscitated with volume expansion, endotracheal ventilation, and vasopressor agents. Pediatric cardiology consultation along with echo-Doppler studies revealed severe aortic coarctation and poor LV function. Intravenous prostaglandin E1 (PGE1) infusion was started, which showed improvement. After arrival at our institution and further stabilization in the pediatric intensive care unit was followed by cardiac catheterization with selective cineangiography, which revealed mild aortic stenosis and severe coarctation of the aorta with a peak-to-peak gradient of 35 mm Hg. The coarctation segment measured 2 mm. Balloon angioplasty of aortic coarctation was performed via the umbilical artery with a #5.3F Proflex 5 balloon dilatation catheter (*Peripheral Systems Group*, Mountain View, Calif.) carrying a 6 mm diameter balloon. The procedure resulted in a decrease of the gradient from 35 mmHg to 3 mmHg and an increase in the coarcted aortic segment from 2 mm to 5.5 mm.[96] The PGE1 infusion was discontinued in the catheterization laboratory and the baby was weaned off the respirator over the next several hours, extubated twenty hours later, and discharged home two days after balloon angioplasty. Reevaluation, two weeks following discharge, revealed adequate weight gain, no signs of CHF, and no arm-to-leg blood pressure difference. Since the submission of this paper for publication, another infant, aged ten days with severe aortic coarctation associated with common AV septal defect also underwent transumbilical balloon angioplasty with a #5.3F Proflex 5 balloon dilation catheter carrying a 6 mm balloon with remarkable improvement (Figure 1 of Reference 96).

Discussion

On the basis of these experiences, we concluded that transumbilical arterial approach to balloon angioplasty of aortic coarctation is feasible and recommend the umbilical artery route for this procedure.[96]

TRANSCATHETER CLOSURE OF PATENT DUCTUS ARTERIOSUS WITH AN ADJUSTABLE BUTTONED DEVICE IN AN ADULT PATIENT[97]

This case was reviewed in the chapter on "Patent Ductus Arteriosus" in the book titled "Pediatric Cardiology: How It Has Evolved Over the last 50 Years" and will not be repeated here.

DELAYED PRESENTATION OF ANOMALOUS CIRCUMFLEX CORONARY ARTERY ARISING FROM PULMONARY ARTERY FOLLOWING REPAIR OF AORTOPULMONARY WINDOW IN INFANCY

Introduction

Anomalous origin of the circumflex coronary artery from the PA is an extremely rare condition and may coexist with other CHD. We reported such a rare case in association with aortopulmonary (AP) window, which was detected several years following repair of the AP window.[98]

Case Report

Initial presentation was at the age of thirteen days with cyanosis and a cardiac murmur. Clinical and cardiac catheterization findings demonstrated AP window. Because of associated CHF, anti-congestive measures with digoxin and furosemide were instituted, which achieved good control of CHF. Surgical correction of AP window was performed at the age of thirteen months; aortic side of the AP window was repaired primarily and the PA side was closed with a pericardial patch. She made an uneventful recovery and was discharged home. She was subsequently followed intermittently in the clinic. At the age of fifteen years, she presented with symptoms of exercise-induced chest pain. Physical examination was non-contributory. ECG showed right axis deviation and an incomplete right bundle branch block pattern. Echocardiogram did not demonstrate any significant abnormalities. Exercise test with thallium showed stress-induced reversible ischemia of the anterolateral wall of the LV. Cardiac catheterization demonstrated a step-up in oxygen saturation in the PA, and normal pressures. Selective angiography demonstrated paradoxical motion in the posterior wall of the LV, no mitral insufficiency, and no residual AP window. Selective coronary angiography revealed normal right, left main, and left anterior (LAD) descending (Figure 23) coronary arteries. The circumflex coronary artery opacified late in a retrograde fashion via collateral vessels from the LAD (Figure 24) and emptied into the posterior wall of the PA. She underwent reoperation. At surgery, a bypass graft (segment of autologous saphenous vein) was inserted connecting the aorta to the second obtuse marginal branch of the circumflex coronary artery. The ostium of the anomalous circumflex coronary artery was suture ligated to prevent coronary steal. She was discharged home five days after surgery. Follow-up, four months later, revealed no evidence for any symptoms and well-healed scar of the surgery.[98]

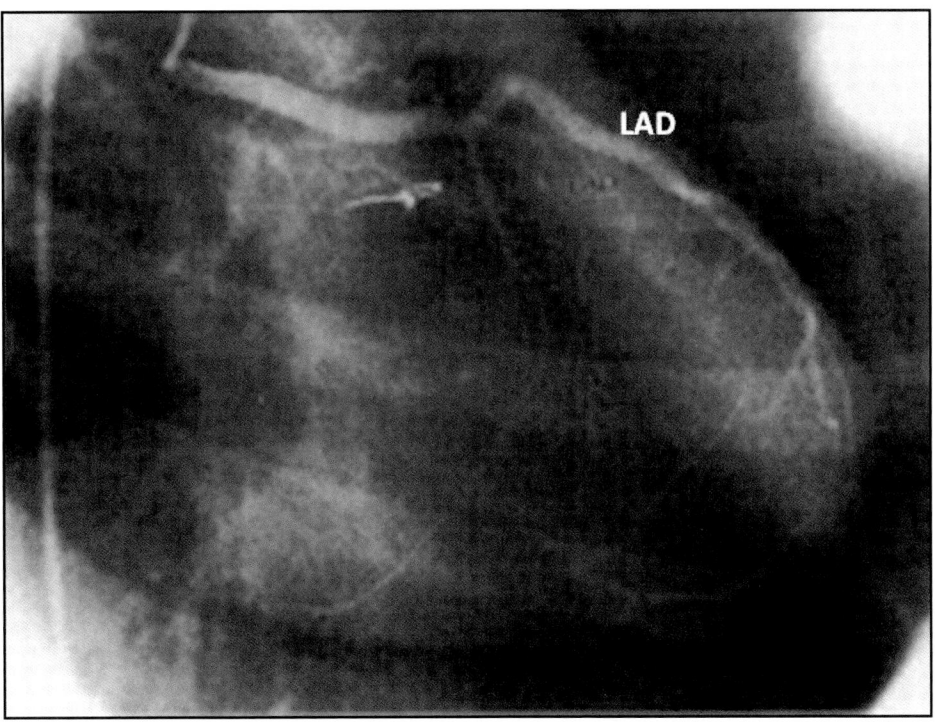

Figure 23. Coronary angiogram of the left main coronary artery demonstrating a normal left anterior descending artery (LAD) with an absence of the circumflex vessel. Reproduced from Chopra PS, Reed WH, Wilson AD, Rao PS, *Chest 1994*; 106:1920-2.

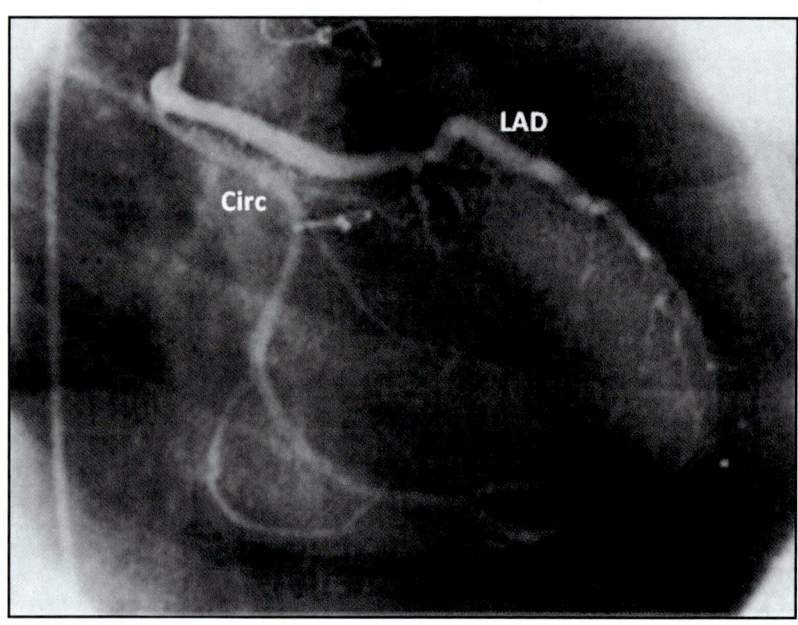

Figure 24. The distal circumflex is seen filling in a retrograde fashion from the LAD. Reproduced from Chopra PS, Reed WH, Wilson AD, Rao PS, *Chest 1994*; 106:1920-2.

Discussion

As mentioned earlier, anomalous circumflex coronary artery from the PA is extremely rare and extensive literature search at the time publication of our paper showed only five published cases.[98] Once identified, surgical correction is recommended to eliminate coronary steal and to restore myocardial perfusion pressure to normal. Of many surgical options (ligation of the anomalous coronary artery, aortic re-implantation, Blalock-Taussig type of shunt, aorto-coronary bypass graft, or transpulmonary artery aortocoronary reconnection) reviewed in our publication,[98] our preference is to re-implant the anomalous coronary artery into the aorta, but because of extensive fibrosis in this region secondary to prior surgery, we have performed bypass graft to address this anomaly.[98]

MIXED TYPE OF TOTAL ANOMALOUS PULMONARY VENOUS CONNECTION: ECHOCARDIOGRAPHIC LIMITATIONS AND ANGIOGRAPHIC ADVANTAGES[99]

Two cases of mixed type of total anomalous pulmonary venous connection were reviewed in the chapter on "Echocardiography" in the book titled "Pediatric Cardiology: How It Has Evolved Over the last 50 Years" and will not be repeated here.

PERCUTANEOUS TRANSLUMINAL CORONARY ANGIOPLASTY FOR TAKAYASU'S ARTERITIS[100]

This case was reviewed in the chapter on "Miscellaneous Obstructive Lesions" in the book titled "Pediatric Cardiology: How It Has Evolved Over the last 50 Years" and will not be repeated here.

ANEURYSM OF THE MEMBRANOUS VENTRICULAR SEPTUM RESULTING IN PULMONARY OUTFLOW TRACT OBSTRUCTION IN CONGENITALLY CORRECTED TRANSPOSITION OF THE GREAT ARTERIES[101]

This case was reviewed in the chapter on "Cardiac Catheterization and Cineangiography" in the book titled "Pediatric Cardiology: How It Has Evolved Over the last 50 Years" and will not be repeated here.

TRANSCATHETER MANAGEMENT OF NEONATES WITH PULMONARY ATRESIA AND INTACT VENTRICULAR SEPTUM[102]

This case was reviewed in the chapters on "Stents" and "Neonatal Interventions" in the book titled "Pediatric Cardiology: How It Has Evolved Over the last 50 Years" and will not be repeated here.

AORTOPULMONARY WINDOW: SUCCESSFUL TRANSCATHETER CLOSURE WITH BUTTONED DEVICE IN AN ADULT[103]

This case was reviewed in the chapter on "Miscellaneous Transcatheter Occlusions" in the book titled "Pediatric Cardiology: How It Has Evolved Over the last 50 Years" and will not be repeated here.

TRANSUMBILICAL VENOUS ANTEROGRADE, SNARE-ASSISTED BALLOON AORTIC VALVULOPLASTY IN A NEONATE WITH CRITICAL AORTIC STENOSIS

Introduction

Management of critical aortic valve stenosis in the neonate by balloon aortic valvuloplasty as an alternative to surgery is generally accepted. The procedure is generally performed by percutaneous femoral artery puncture. However, the possibility for femoral artery injury exists. Therefore, alternative approaches using umbilical, carotid, subscapular, or axillary arteries and anterograde (transvenous) femoral venous methods, as referenced in our paper[104] were entertained. In this report, we presented an anterograde transumbilical venous approach to accomplish balloon aortic valvuloplasty in a one-day-old infant with critical aortic valve stenosis.

Case Report

A twelve-hour-old male infant, with a birth weight of 3.3 kg, presented with signs of shock (tachypnea, tachycardia, and poor peripheral pulses). Echocardiography revealed critical aortic stenosis and PGE_1 infusion was started and transported to our institution. Repeat echo-Doppler study demonstrated a dilated, poorly contractile LV, thickened, domed aortic valve leaflets with a tiny Doppler jet across the aortic valve with a peak velocity of 3.5 m/sec. PGE_1 infusion was continued, and dopamine (5 mcg/kg/min) and dobutamine (8 mcg/kg/min) infusions begun following placement of umbilical arterial and venous lines. Initially transumbilical artery balloon dilatation similar to that used for coarctation of aorta[96] was attempted, but balloon dilatation catheter (5F ultrathin carrying 6-mm-diameter balloon [Meditech, Watertown, MA]) could not be positioned across the aortic valve. At this juncture, anterograde aortic valve dilatation via the umbilical vein was contemplated. The umbilical venous catheter was exchanged with a 5F sheath. Through this sheath, a 4F multi-A2 catheter (Cordis) was placed into the left atrium across the PFO and from there into the LV across the mitral valve. A J-shaped, soft-tipped 0.035" Benston guide wire (Cook) was used to advance the catheter from the LV into the aorta. This guide wire was exchanged with a 0.025" J-tipped Amplatz extra-stiff wire (Cook). An ultrathin balloon dilatation catheter (6-mm-diameter) (Meditech) was advanced over this guide wire anterogradely from the umbilical vein into the IVC, right atrium, left atrium, and LV, while maintaining a wide loop of the wire in the LV. Because of difficulty in advancing the balloon catheter across the aortic valve, a gooseneck micro-snare (Microvena, White Bear Lake, MN) was introduced through the 4F multi-A2 catheter (Cordis) in the descending aorta via the umbilical artery to capture the 0.025" J-tipped Amplatz extra-stiff wire forming a guide-wire loop (Figure 25); this facilitated advancing balloon catheter across the aortic valve (Figure 26). This is followed balloon valvuloplasty (Figure 26). At the conclusion of the procedure, there was no significant residual gradient across the aortic valve. LV angiography showed an enlarged LV with poor function, but with broader jet contrast across the aortic valve than that seen prior to balloon valvuloplasty (Figure 27). The baby was gradually weaned off PGE_1, dobutamine, and dopamine drips and the ventilator and was discharged one week following balloon valvuloplasty. At the time of discharge, echocardiogram revealed remarkable improvement in LV size and function with a Doppler peak instantaneous gradient of 25 mm Hg across the aortic valve.[104]

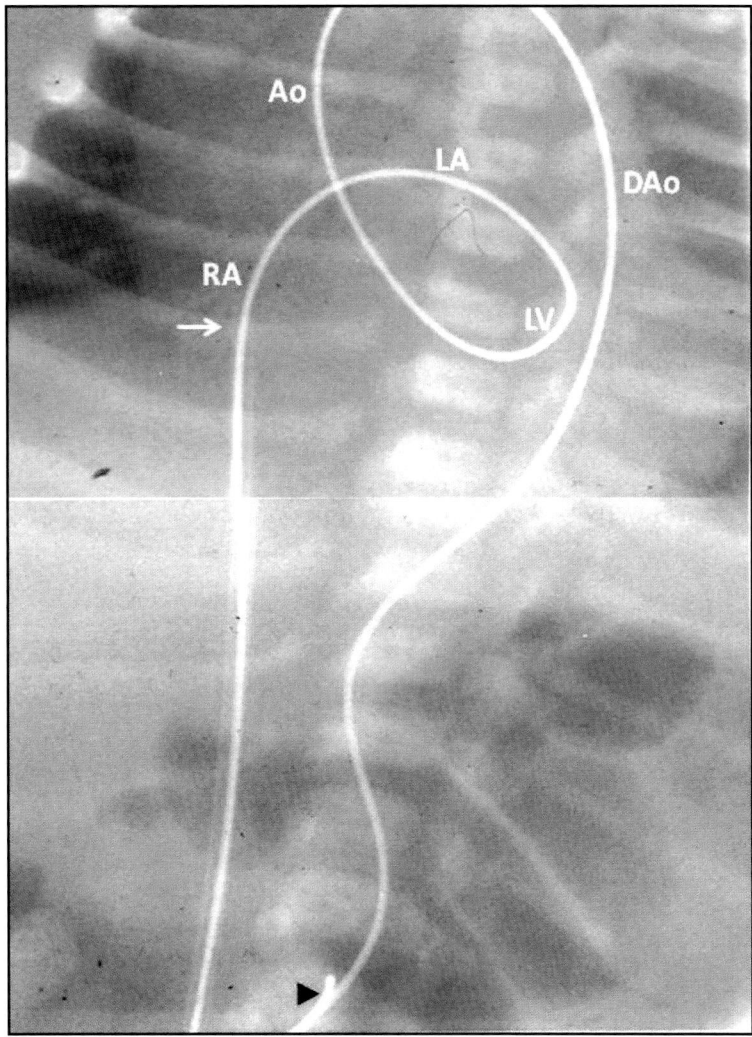

Figure 25. The course of the guide wire "rail" from the umbilical vein-to-umbilical artery for positioning the catheter across the aortic valve is demonstrated. Filled arrow-head shows the tip of the snare holding the wire. The tip of the umbilical venous sheath (arrow) is also shown. The wire "rail" courses through the right atrium (RA), left atrium (LA), left ventricle (LV), ascending aorta (Ao) and descending aorta (DAo). Reproduced from Rao PS, Jureidini SB, *Cathet Cardiovasc Diagn 1998*; 45:144-8.

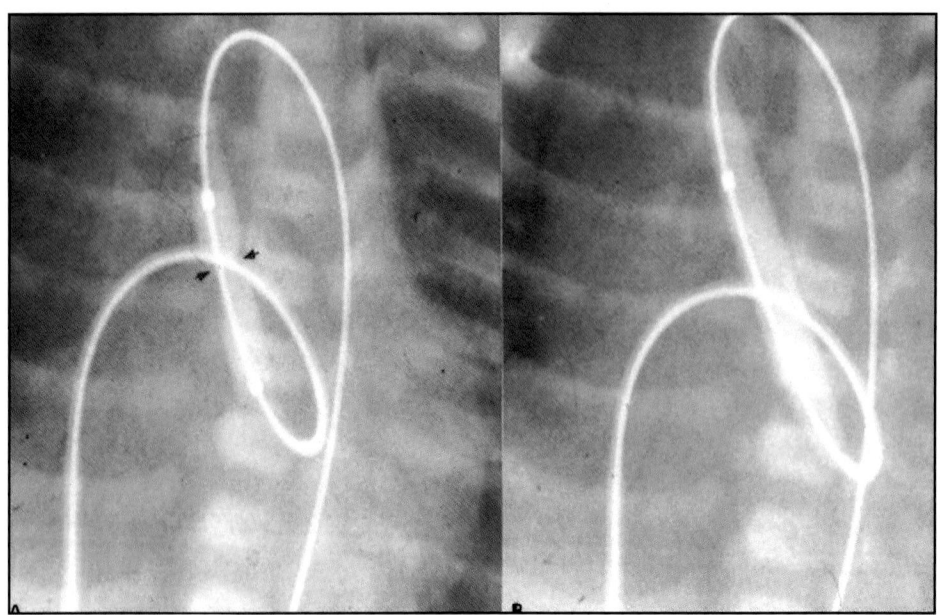

Figure 26. Selected cineradiographic frames demonstrating the position of the balloon across the aortic valve, introduced anterogradely. Note the waisting (arrows) of the balloon during the initial phases of balloon inflation (a), which was completely abolished after full inflation of the balloon (b). Reproduced from Rao PS, Jureidini SB, *Cathet Cardiovasc Diagn 1998*; 45:144-8.

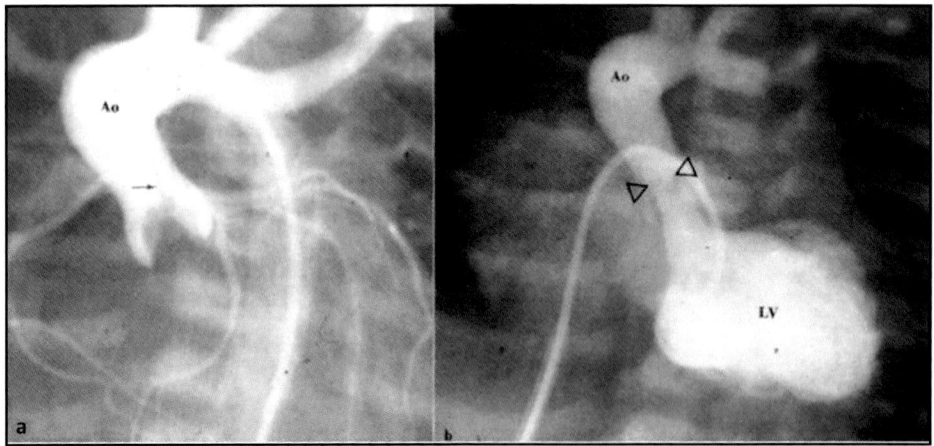

Figure 27. A. Selected frame from the ascending aorta (Ao) cineangiogram prior to balloon aortic valvuloplasty showing a domed aortic valve and a very narrow jet (arrow) of unopacified blood from the left ventricle (LV) to the Ao. Post-stenotic dilatation of the Ao is also seen. B. LV cine-angiographic frame following balloon valvuloplasty demonstrating dilated LV and wide jet of contrast material (arrow-heads) across the aortic valve. Reproduced from Rao PS, Jureidini SB, *Cathet Cardiovasc Diagn 1998*; 45:144-8.

Discussion

We have adopted the anterograde transvenous approach previously used by Hausdorf,[133] and O'Laughlin,[134] and their associates, but employed the umbilical instead of the femoral vein. A guide wire "rail" was created by snaring the wire from the umbilical artery (Figure 26) to stabilize the guide wire in order to position the balloon valvuloplasty catheter across the aortic valve and facilitate successful balloon aortic valvuloplasty. On the basis of this experience, we suggested transumbilical venous anterograde route with transumbilical arterial guide wire snaring, if necessary, for balloon aortic valvuloplasty in the newborn as an alternative to the other routes mentioned earlier. Obviously, successful umbilical venous entry past the ductus venosus and the existence of a PFO are necessary prerequisites for performing this procedure.[104]

In summary, anterograde transumbilical venous route for performing balloon aortic valvuloplasty in the neonate is a feasible and effective alternative method to retrograde femoral, carotid, or umbilical arterial and transfemoral venous anterograde techniques.[104]

Additional Observations

Subsequent to the report just described,[104] the technique was attempted in five additional neonates.[135,136] The procedure was successful in four (80 percent) of these five babies, with good relief of obstruction. No complications were encountered. The single patient in whom we could not accomplish the procedure was due to a very small left ventricle and a guide-wire could not be passed across the aortic valve. We have modified the technique using regular 0.021" guide wires (Cook, Bloomington, IN) instead of extra-stiff Amplatz wires (Cook) and Tyshak-II catheters (Braun, Bethlehem, PA) (Figure 28) and instead of ultrathin balloon valvuoloplasty catheters (Meditech, Natick, MA). In addition, presumably because of the use of these modifications, it was not necessary to use snare, nor to establish a guide wire loop. It was also noted that there was less arrhythmia during the procedure, presumably related use of less stiffer wires and better tracking of the Tyshak-II catheters.[135]

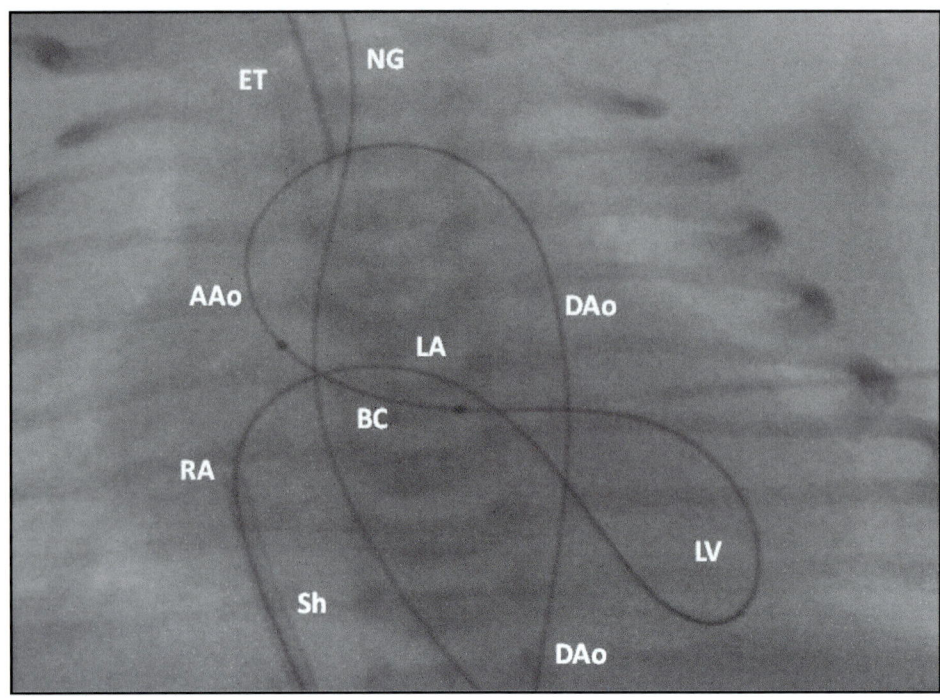

Figure 28. Selected cineradiographic frame demonstrating the course of the guide wire from the umbilical vein (not shown) to the right atrium (RA), left atrium (LA), left ventricle (LV), ascending aorta (AAo) and descending aorta (DAo). The balloon catheter (BC) is positioned across the aortic valve without the use of a snare as shown in figure 25 because of easy tackability of the Tyshak-II catheter used in this case. The sheath (Sh) is seen in the RA positioned via the umbilical vein. ET, endo-tracheal tube; NG, naso-gastric tube.

These experiences further support our advocacy and recommendation to use the transumbilical venous anterograde approach as initial choice in the transcatheter treatment of critical aortic stenosis in the neonate.[135,136]

COIL OCCLUSION OF PATENT DUCTUS ARTERIOSUS WITH RIGHT AORTIC ARCH[105]

Two cases of coil occlusion of PDA in patients with right aortic arch were reviewed in the chapter on "Patent Ductus Arteriosus" in the book titled "Pediatric Cardiology: How It Has Evolved Over the last 50 Years" and will not be repeated here.

SUCCESSFUL THROMBOLYTIC THERAPY OF PULMONARY EMBOLISM ASSOCIATED WITH UROSEPSIS IN AN INFANT

Introduction

Pulmonary embolism (PE), while rare in the pediatric population, can be fatal and carries a high mortality rate. The morbidity and mortality are secondary to hypoxemia and shock complicating severe right heart failure. We reported an infant who developed PE associated with urosepsis who was successfully treated with recombinant tissue plasminogen activator (rt-PA).[106]

Case Report

A thirty-four-day-old male infant presented with symptoms of lethargy, poor feeding, vomiting, and fever. Laboratory tests showed an elevated white blood cell count (22,300/mm2), positive for leukocytes on urine analysis, and positive blood cultures for *Escherichia coli*. Antibiotic therapy with Cefotaxime (150 mg/kg/day) and Gentamycin (8 mg/kg/day) was started to treat urosepsis. Two days later, the patient became dusky with O2 saturation of 92 percent in room air. Arterial blood gases in 100 percent O2 revealed: pH - 7.21, PaCO2 - 37 mmHg, PaO2 - 61 mmHg, and base deficit - 13 mmol/L. The patient was transferred to our institution. Examination revealed tachycardia (142 beats per minute), tachypnea (respiratory rate of 50), hepatomegaly, and a grade 3/6 holosystolic murmur at the lower left sternal border suggestive of tricuspid regurgitation. Echocardiogram revealed dilated RA, RV and PA, and severe tricuspid regurgitation. Based on the tricuspid regurgitation Doppler velocity the RV/PA pressures were estimated to be 60 mmHg. A large pulmonary embolus was seen extending from the distal main to proximal right PA and measured 15 x 5 mm (Figure 29A). There were no other echocardiographic abnormalities.

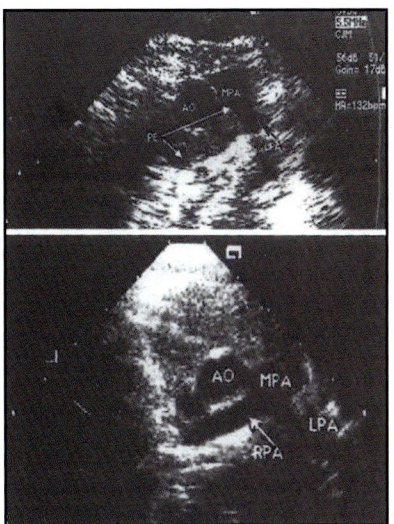

Figure 29. A. Selected video frame from two-dimensional echocardiogram in short-axis view at the level of the great arteries demonstrating a large (15 x 5 mm) pulmonary embolus (PE, arrows) almost completely occluding the right pulmonary artery (RPA) and extending into the distal main pulmonary artery (MPA). B. Similar echocardiogram following thrombolytic therapy showing complete dissolution of RPA embolus. Ao, aorta; LPA, left pulmonary artery. Reproduced from Pugh KJ, Jureidine SB, Ream R, Rao PS, et al, *Pediat Cardiol 2002*; 23:77-9.

Thrombolysis was initiated with rt-PA; a loading dose of 0.5 mg/kg followed by 0.2 mg/kg/hour was administered via a central venous catheter in the right femoral vein. The rt-PA was given for thirty-five hours. After echocardiographic evidence of complete PE lysis (Figure 29B), the rt-PA was switched to heparin drip (loading dose - 50 U/kg followed by 30 U/kg/hour). Twenty-four hours later, aspirin, 5 mg/day as a single dose was started and heparin drip was discontinued. Serial echocardiograms were performed, which demonstrated partial and then total resolution of the PE (Figure 29B). The PA pressures and right heart structures returned to normal. Multiple coagulation and immunologic tests were negative. Voiding cystourethrogram revealed Grade 4 viscero-ureteral reflux on both sides. Urine and blood cultures became negative by the eighth day. Intravenous antibiotics were continued for ten days followed by oral Cefluroxine for two weeks. Follow-up in the clinic, a month after discharge, reveled no symptoms and normal echocardiogram.[106]

Discussion

PE in children is rare, but a serious disease entity that can produce hypoxemia, shock, pulmonary hypertension, and right heart failure. A rare case of PE associated with urosepsis in a young infant was presented. A number of predisposing factors including prolonged use of indwelling central venous catheters (most common), immobility, cardiomyopathy, antecedent surgery, infection, trauma, inherited hypercoagulable disorders, oral contraceptives (in adolescents), and dehydration have been implicated in the causation of PE.[106] We have demonstrated utility of echocardiography in the diagnosis of PE and in monitoring of progress during therapy. Of the available treatment options, namely, surgical embolectomy, anticoagulation with heparin, and thrombolysis with strepto/urokinase/rt-PA, we opted for thrombolysis with rt-PA because of its rapid action. Extremely limited number of reports of the use of rt-PA as of the time of our report[106] was pointed out. Of the multiple regimens, we chose a combination of bolus infusion followed by continuous infusion of rt-PA. The major risk of rt-PA is bleeding, which fortunately did not occur in our patient.

In summary, a rare case of PE in an infant with urosepsis was documented. Role of echocardiography in the diagnosis and post-treatment follow-up was emphasized. The rapid effectiveness of thrombolysis with rt-PA is pointed out.[106]

TRANSCATHETER OCCLUSION OF RUPTURED SINUS OF VALSALVA ANEURYSM[107]

This case was reviewed in the chapter on "Miscellaneous Transcatheter Occlusions" in the book titled "Pediatric Cardiology: How It Has Evolved Over the last 50 Years" and will not be repeated here.

TOTAL PERCUTANEOUS CORRECTION OF TETRALOGY OF FALLOT WITH DOMINANT PULMONARY VALVE STENOSIS[108]

This case was reviewed in the chapter on "Ventricular Septal Defects" in the book titled "Pediatric Cardiology: How It Has Evolved Over the last 50 Years" and will not be repeated here.

SEVERE INTRAVASCULAR HEMOLYSIS AFTER TRANSCATHETER COIL OCCLUSION OF PATENT DUCTUS ARTERIOSUS[109]

This case was reviewed in the chapter on "Patent Ductus Arteriosus" in the book titled "Pediatric Cardiology: How It Has Evolved Over the last 50 Years" and will not be repeated here.

STENT THERAPY FOR CLOTTED BLALOCK-TAUSSIG SHUNTS[110]

Three cases of stent therapy for clotted Blalock-Taussig shunts were reviewed in the chapter on "Stents" in the book titled "Pediatric Cardiology: How It Has Evolved Over the last 50 Years" and will not be repeated here.

DEVELOPMENT OF SUPRAVALVULAR PULMONARY ARTERY STENOSIS FOLLOWING A NUSS PROCEDURE

Introduction

Deformity of the anterior chest wall producing posterior indentation of the sternum is generally referred to as pectus excavatum (PEx). Indications for surgical intervention are not clearly established. Nuss procedure[137] is one such methods used to address PEx. In this procedure, a steel convex bar with its convexity facing anteriorly is inserted in the chest to help improve the chest deformity. The steel bar is removed two years later. In one of our patients, the Nuss bar produced compression of the heart. The purpose of this report is to document this complication and to review long term complications associated with this approach in the management of PEx.[111]

Case Report

An eleven-year-old female with PEx (Figure 30A) had a Nuss procedure. Shortly before the planned removal of the Nuss bar at the age of thirteen years, a cardiac murmur was heard with resultant referral to Pediatric Cardiology. She did have sharp, pinching pain in the left chest with sneezing and some inability to sleep supine. Pertinent finding on examination were height and weight between twenty-fifth and fiftieth percentile, normal cardiac impulses, no thrills, single second heart sound at the left upper sternal border, and a grade 3/6 ejection systolic murmur at the left mid-sternal border, peaking in late systole and radiating to the infraclavicular regions and axillae. The chest roentgenogram (Figure 31A) demonstrated upper limits of normal cardiac size with slight prominence of the RV outflow tract. This appears to be slightly more prominent than seen on the chest film taken shortly after the Nuss bar placement (Figure 31B). ECG showed normal sinus rhythm, right axis deviation and RSR prime pattern of the QRS in the right chest leads indicative of RV hypertrophy. Echo-Doppler study showed moderate dilatation of the RV, echo-dense structures within and outside the PA (Figure 32A), origin of the flow disturbance in the PA (Figure 32B), no gradient across the pulmonary valve (Figure 32C), and increased Doppler flow velocity across this region with a peak instantaneous gradient of 94 mmHg and a mean of 56 mmHg (Figures 32 D). It was concluded that the Nuss bar was producing compression in the supravalvular PA region and the removal of the bar was suggested. The bar was removed via lateral thoracotomy without any complications. Repeat pediatric cardiology evaluation, five months later, indicated improved symptomatology, no systolic murmur, and a grade 2/6 early diastolic decrescendo murmur best heard at the left upper border. ECG showed increased S-waves in the left chest leads, consistent with mild right RV hypertrophy. Echo-Doppler study revealed mild RV dilatation, trivial residual gradient across the PA (15 mm Hg) and mild to moderate pulmonary insufficiency (Figure 33).

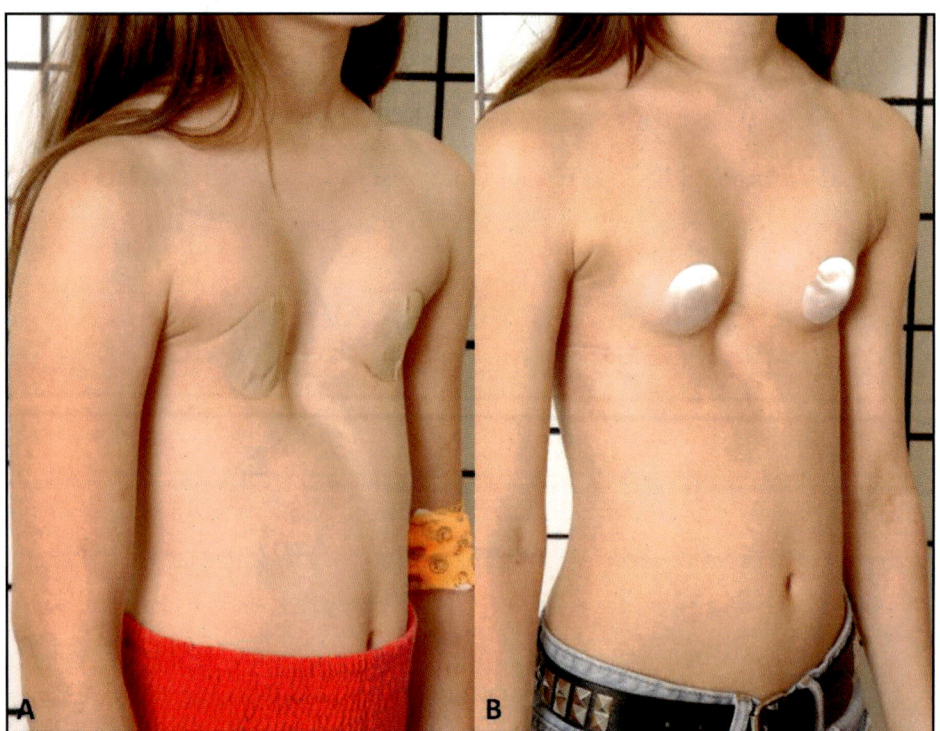

Figure 30. A. Photograph of the chest demonstrating pectus excavatum. B. Photograph of the chest two years following the Nuss procedure.

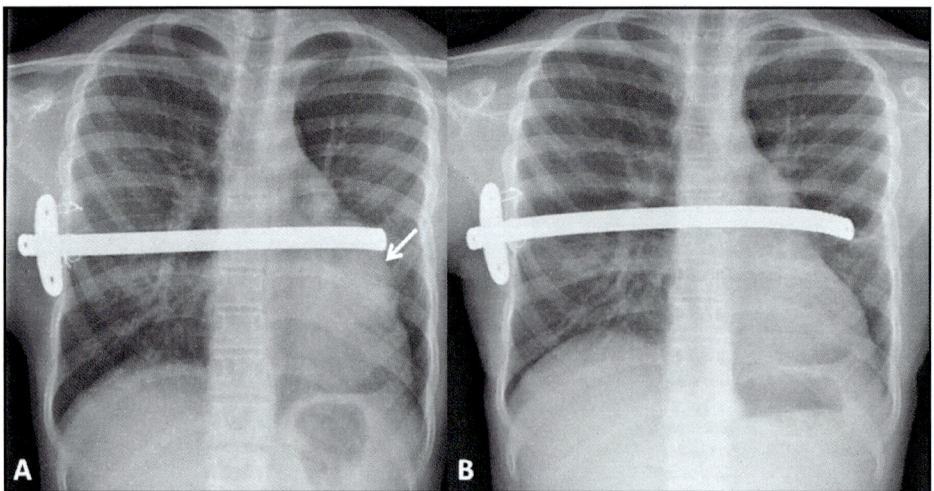

Figure 31. Chest x-rays in posterior–anterior view demonstrating prominent right ventricular outflow tract (arrow in A) which was absent in a chest x-ray obtained on the day of bar placement (B). Reproduced from Mazur L, deYbarrondo L, Pickard L, Rao PS, *J Pediatr Surg 2012*; 47:e61-4.

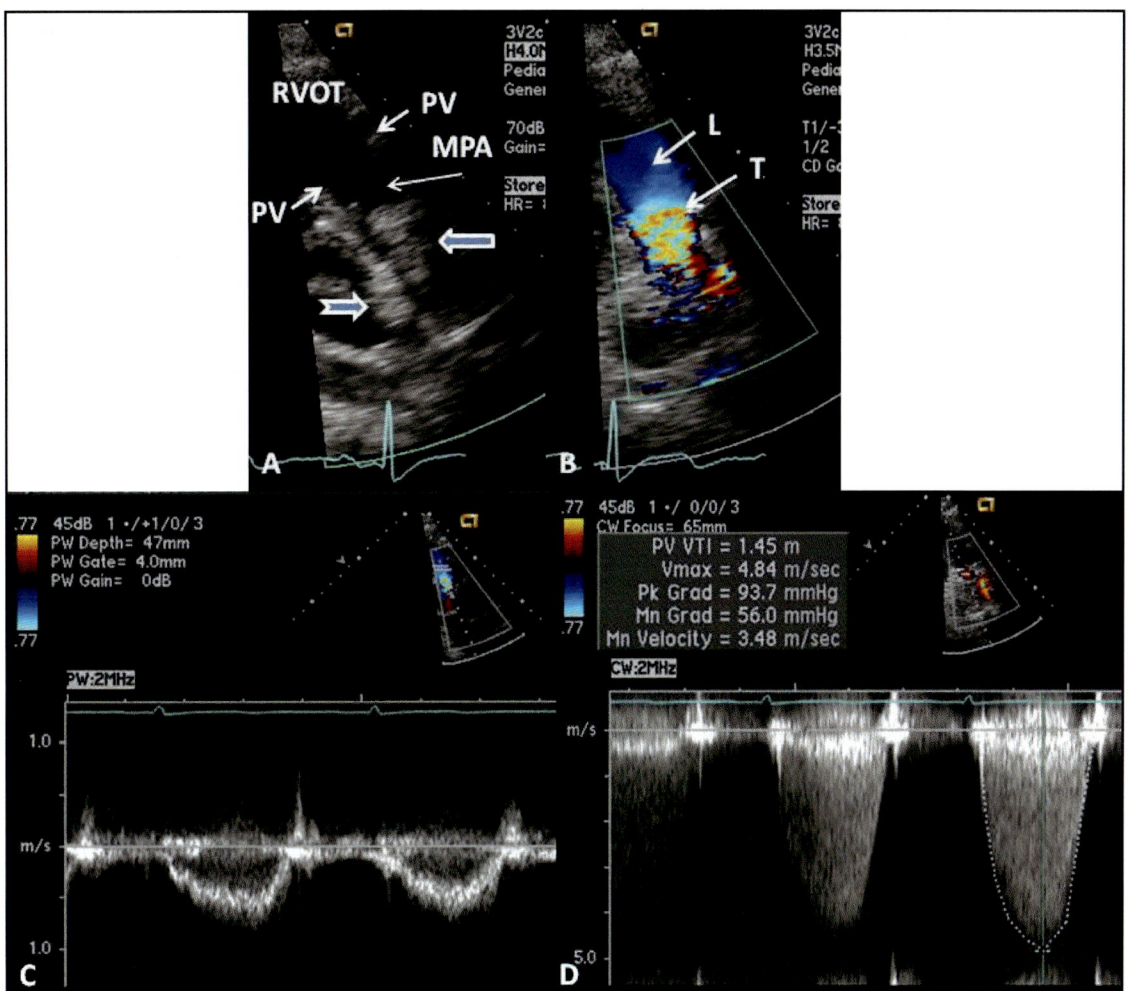

Figure 32. A. Selected video frame from a parasternal short axis view showing echo dense structures (thick blue arrows) within and outside the main pulmonary artery (MPA). Pulmonary valve (PV) leaflets (small arrows) are shown and appear normal. The right ventricular outflow tract (RVOT) and proximal MPA are free of any echo-dense structures. B. Color Doppler mapping of the same structures as in panel A shows normal laminar (L) flow in the RVOT and proximal MPA and turbulent (T) flow starting in the proximal MPA, indicating obstruction. C. Pulse Doppler sampling from the proximal MPA, which shows normal flow velocity. D. Continuous wave Doppler sampling demonstrating high velocity flow across the MPA with a calculated peak instantaneous gradient of 93.7 mmHg and a mean gradient of 56 mmHg, indicating severe obstruction. Reproduced from Mazur L, deYbarrondo L, Pickard L, Rao PS, *J Pediatr Surg 2012*; 47:e61-4.

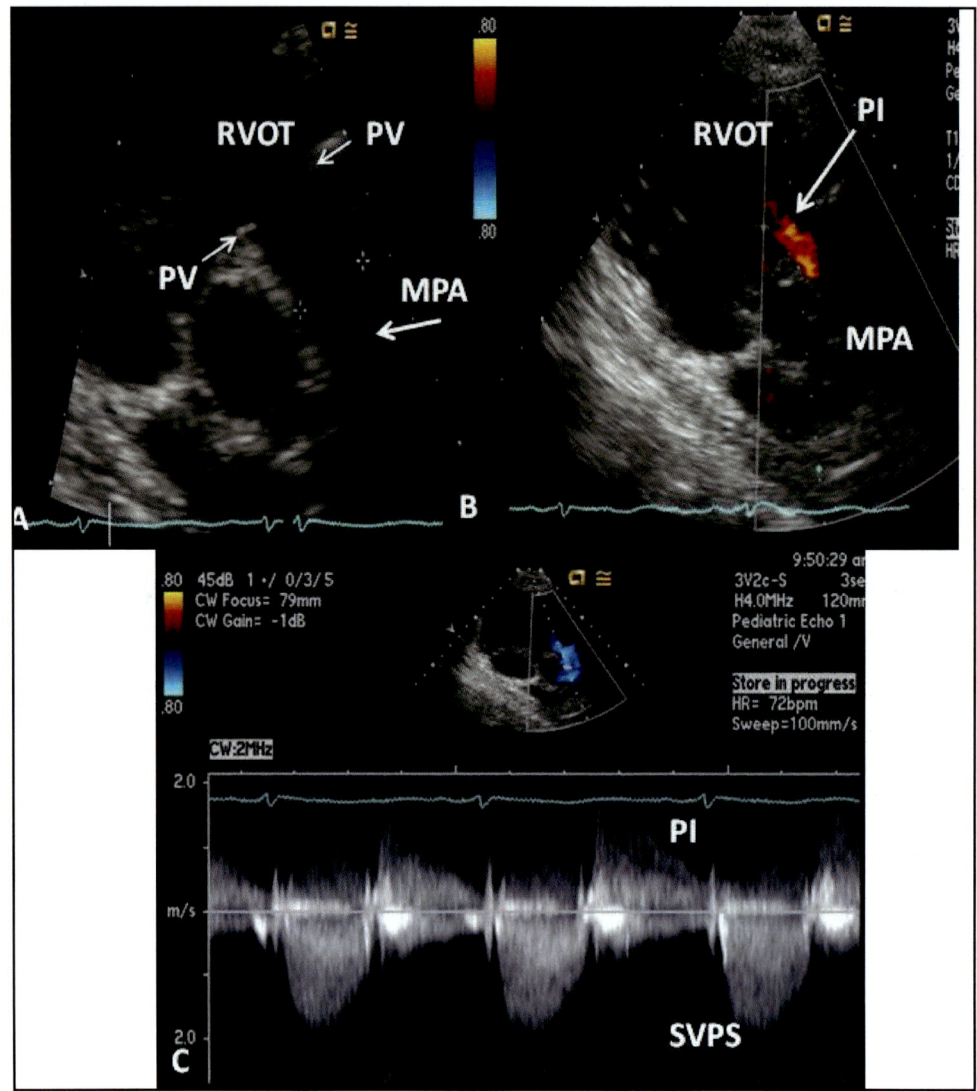

Figure 33. Echo-Doppler studies performed five months after removal of the Nuss bar. A. Selected video frame from a parasternal short axis view demonstrating no echo dense structures in the right ventricular outflow tract (RVOT) and main pulmonary artery (MPA) that was seen prior to removal of the Nuss bar (Figure 32A). Pulmonary valve (PV) leaflets (arrows) are shown. B. Color Doppler mapping of the same structures as in panel A shows mild pulmonary insufficiency (PI) (arrow). C. Continuous wave Doppler sampling demonstrating low Doppler flow velocity across the MPA with a calculated peak instantaneous gradient of 15 mmHg, indicating minimal supravalvular pulmonary stenosis (SVPS) and mild pulmonary insufficiency (PI). Reproduced from Mazur L, deYbarrondo L, Pickard L, Rao PS, *J Pediatr Surg 2012*; 47:e61-4.

Discussion

The Nuss procedure, initially introduced in 1997, is minimally invasive and thought to produce good results.[137] However, a number of complication including bar displacement (prevalence up to 16.6 percent), subcutaneous emphysema, pericardial effusion, cardiac tamponade, erosion of the bar into the internal mammary artery, persistent thoracic outlet syndrome, overcorrection or progression to pectus carinatum, and ossification around the Nuss bar have been reported as referenced in our publication.[111] But, no reports of PA stenosis secondary to the Nuss bar were identified in the literature as of the time of our report. While the reasons for development of this complication are unclear, displacement of the Nuss bar and natural growth of the heart may have resulted in compression of the PA. On the basis of our observation we would suggest careful auscultation by the primary care physician during well child visits and should a new cardiac murmur is found, cardiac evaluation including Echo-Doppler studies should be sought.

In summary, we documented a rare case of development of the supravalvar PA stenosis following the Nuss procedure for PEx. Careful auscultation for any new murmur should help identify such complication.

DEVELOPMENT OF AORTIC COARCTATION FOLLOWING DEVICE CLOSURE OF PATENT DUCTUS ARTERIOSUS[112]

This case was reviewed in the chapter on "Patent Ductus Arteriosus" in the book titled "Pediatric Cardiology: How It Has Evolved Over the last 50 Years" and will not be repeated here.

SUBPULMONARY OBSTRUCTION DUE TO ANEURYSMAL VENTRICULAR SEPTUM IN A PATIENT WITH CONGENITALLY CORRECTED TRANSPOSITION OF THE GREAT ARTERIES IN LEVOCARDIA AND DEXTROCARDIA[113,115]

Both these cases were reviewed in the chapter on "Cardiac Catheterization and Cineangiography" in the book titled "Pediatric Cardiology: How It Has Evolved Over the last 50 Years" and will not be repeated here.

REACTIVE DUCTUS ARTERIOSUS IN A NINETEEN-MONTH-OLD PATIENT[114]

This case was reviewed in the chapter on "Patent Ductus Arteriosus" in the book titled "Pediatric Cardiology: How It Has Evolved Over the last 50 Years" and will not be repeated here.

FLASH PULMONARY EDEMA DURING PULMONARY VASOREACTIVITY TESTING[116]

This case was reviewed in the chapter on "Ventricular Septal Defects" in the book titled "Pediatric Cardiology: How It Has Evolved Over the last 50 Years" and will not be repeated here.

AUSCULTATION IS STILL A VALID TOOL IN THE EVALUATION OF CARDIAC DEFECTS IN CHILDREN[117]

Three cases illustrating the concept that "auscultation is still a valid tool" were reviewed in the chapter on "Ventricular Septal Defects' in the book titled "Pediatric Cardiology: How It Has Evolved Over the last 50 Years" and will not be repeated here.

TRANSCATHETER PERFORATION OF ATRETIC PULMONARY VALVE IN PULMONARY ATRESIA WITH VENTRICULAR SEPTAL DEFECT

Introduction

Percutaneous perforation of atretic pulmonary valve membrane, usually by radio frequency wires and balloon dilatation is a standard method of management of pulmonary atresia with intact ventricular septum.[102,138-140] But, in patients with pulmonary atresia with VSD such an approach is rarely used presumably related to anatomic differences between the two types of pulmonary atresia.[118] The purpose of the report was to document the feasibility of such an approach in pulmonary atresia with VSD (severe tetralogy of Fallot).[118]

Case Report

A three-week-old female infant with a diagnosis of VSD and pulmonary valve atresia underwent central aorto-pulmonary shunt in 1995. Because of increasing cyanosis and polycythemia, cardiac catheterization with selective cineangiography was performed at the age of twenty-two months. The data confirmed the initial diagnosis, a patent aorto-pulmonary shunt, moderate arterial desaturation (77 percent), a Qp:Qs of 1.1, and a normal PVR.

The shunt was entered from the aorta with #4-F Glidecath catheter (Meditech, Inc., Watertown, MA) with the assistance of Benston guide wire (Cook, Bloomington, IN) and a PA cineangiogram was performed (Figure 34a). Then simultaneous injection into the main PA and RV outflow tract was undertaken to visualize the atretic membranous pulmonary valve (Figure 35). Since anterograde perforation of the pulmonary valve was not possible, a retrograde approach was attempted. A Toughy-adapter was connected to the catheter to facilitate injection of the contrast material over the wire. After ensuring that the catheter is in the middle of the pulmonary valve by a test injection through the Toughy-adapter, a 0.021inch straight guide wire was placed at the tip of the catheter and firm, but gentle pressure was applied. This resulted in passing of the guide wire across the atretic pulmonary valve. The catheter was advanced over this guide wire into the RV, and both the guide wire and the catheter were advanced into the right atrium. At this point the guide wire was replaced with an exchange length 0.025 inch "J" shaped extra-stiff Amplatz guide wire (*Cordis Corporation*, Miami, FL). The guide wire in the right atrium was snared with a 15 mm "gooseneck" snare (Microvena, Vadnais Heights, MN) from the femoral vein forming a guide wire loop from the femoral artery, descending and ascending aorta, aorto-pulmonary shunt, main PA, perforated pulmonary valve, RV, RA, IVC, and femoral vein (Figure 36).

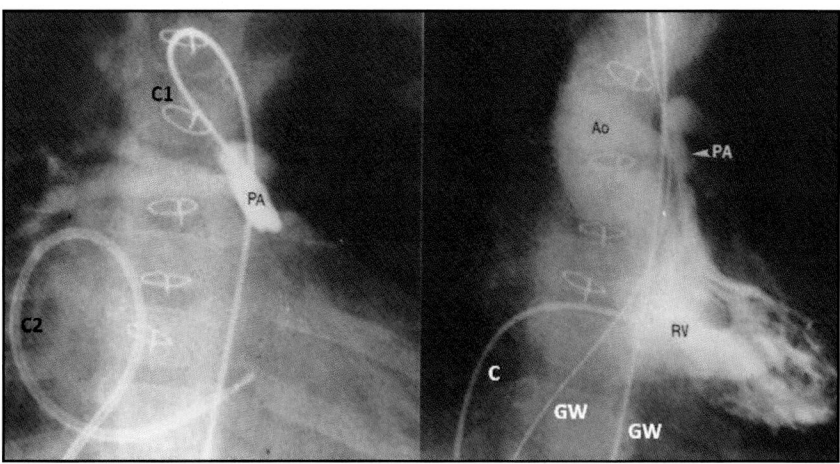

Figure 34. a. Selected frame of main pulmonary artery (PA) cineangiogram in posteroanterior view prior to perforation of the pulmonary valve demonstrating blindly ending PA with opacification of the branch PAs (not labeled). The catheter (C1) was introduced into the PA from the aorta via the central aortopulmonary shunt. C2, catheter in the right atrium. b. Selected frame of right ventricular (RV) cineangiogram in posteroanterior view after pulmonary valve perforation demonstrating forward flow from the RV into the PA. Components of the guide wire (GW) rail are marked. Ao, aorta; C, catheter in the RV. Reproduced from Rao PS, *Congenital Cardiology Today 2018*; 16(11):1-8.

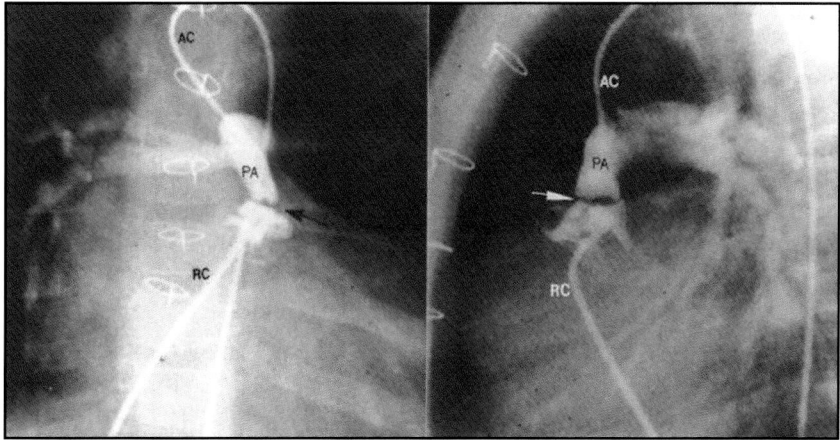

Figure 35. Selected frames in posteroanterior (a) and lateral (b) projections of simultaneous injection of the contrast material into the main pulmonary artery (PA) via a catheter introduced through the central aortopulmonary shunt (AC) and right ventricular outflow tract via a catheter (RC) introduced from the right atrium demonstrating atretic membranous pulmonary valve (black arrow-head in a and white arrow-head in b). Reproduced from Rao PS, *Congenital Cardiology Today 2018*; 16(11):1-8.

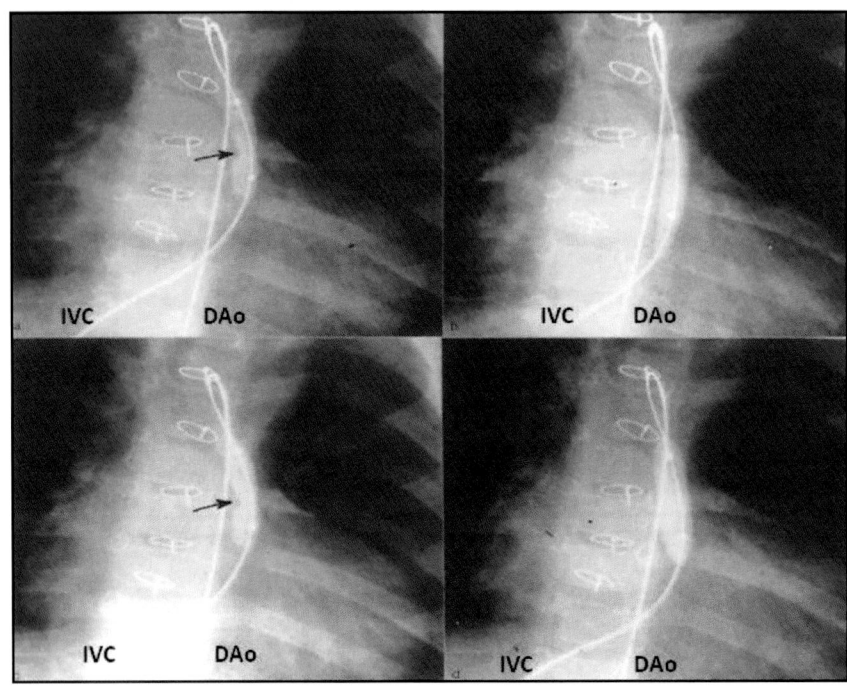

Figure 36. Selected cineradiographic frames in posteroanterior view demonstrating balloon valvuloplasty catheters introduced over the femoral venous end of the guide wire and positioned across the perforated pulmonary valve. Waisting (arrow in a) of the 6 mm balloon is shown, which disappeared on further balloon inflation (b). Similar waisting (arrow in c) of the 8 mm balloon is shown, which also disappeared on further balloon inflation (d). DAo, descending aorta; IVC, inferior vena cava. Reproduced from Rao PS, *Congenital Cardiology Today 2018*; 16(11):1-8.

An Ultrathin balloon angioplasty catheter (Meditech) carrying a 6 mm diameter, 2 cm long balloon was advanced from the femoral vein and positioned across the perforated pulmonary valve (Pulmonary valve annulus measured 7 mm). The balloon was inflated twice with resultant ablation of the waist of the balloon (Figures 36 a and b). The procedure was repeated with an 8 mm diameter, 2 cm long Ultrathin Meditech balloon catheter (Figures 36 c and d). A right ventricular cineangiogram was repeated (Figure 34 b) demonstrating flow across the opened pulmonary valve. The O_2 saturation improved (77 percent vs. 88 percent) and the PA pressure was mildly increased (35/15 mmHg; m-20), but with normal PVR (2 units). No complications were observed during or after the procedure. Echo-Doppler study on the morning after the balloon procedure demonstrated forward flow across the RV outflow tract and pulmonary valve, similar to the angiogram as shown in figure 34b.

Repeat cardiac catheterization one year following the procedure, preparatory to total surgical correction, showed arterial O_2 saturation of 90 percent, normal PA pressure (LPA-26/16; m-18) and normal PVR (2.3 units). Angiography is similar to the prior study. Surgical correction with closure of the VSD, relief of right ventricular infundibular obstruction and enlargement of the main and origins of the branch pulmonary arteries was successfully performed shortly after the cardiac catheterization.[118]

Discussion

While surgical or transcatheter opening of the pulmonary valve is the most commonly used approach in the initial management pulmonary atresia with intact ventricular septum, aortopulmonary shunts are usually utilized for patients with pulmonary atresia with VSD with a plan for subsequent total correction. In this case, an unusual step to transcatheter perforation of the pulmonary valve with the objective to promote growth of the PAs and lessen the risk of total surgical correction was undertaken, given the state of surgery in late 1990s. There were only few reports describing transcatheter perforation of the atretic pulmonary valve in patients with pulmonary atresia and VSD, which were reviewed in our paper.[118]

In summary, percutaneous perforation pulmonary valve and balloon dilatation as an initial palliative procedure to increase pulmonary blood flow may be an effective alternative to palliative shunts in patients with pulmonary atresia with VSD. Establishment of RV-to-PA continuity may produce better surgical results after final corrective surgery.[118]

REFERENCES

1. Rao PS, "Congenital pulmonary cyst," *Amer J Dis Child 1970*; 119:341-2.

2. Rao PS, "Late respiratory distress in a premature infant," *Chest 1970*; 57:495-6. Available at https://doi.org/10.1378/chest.57.5.495

3. Rao PS, Patel JK, "Fever, vomiting and dome shaped density in right thorax," *Chest 1970*; 58:89-90. Available at https://doi.org/10.1378/chest.58.1.89

4. Rao PS, Alva J, Lipow HW, "Foreign body (peanut) in the left main stem bronchus," *Amer J Dis Child 1970*; 120:51-2.

5. Rao PS, Molthan ME, Lipow HW, "Cor pulmonale as a complication of ventriculoatrial shunts," *J Neurosurg 1970*; 33:221-5.

6. Rao PS, Sissman NJ, "Congenital heart disease in the de Lange syndrome," *J Pediatr 1971*; 79:674-7.

7. Rao PS, Lipow HW, "Growth retardation in steroid dependent asthma - Management by corticotrophin (ACTH)," *Clin Pediat 1972*; 11:93-7.

8. Rao PS, Molthan ME, "Systemic venous anomalies and partial heterotaxia with normal heart," *Amer J Dis Child 1973*; 125:749-52.

9. Rao PS, Jue KL, Isabel-Jones J, Ruttenberg HD, "Ebstein's malformation of the tricuspid valve with atresia," *Amer J Cardiol 1973*; 32:1004-9.

10. Rao PS, Silbert DR, "Superior vena caval obstruction in total anomalous pulmonary venous return," *Brit Heart J 1974*; 36:228-32.

11. Rao PS, Liebman J, Borkat G, "Right ventricular growth in a case of pulmonic stenosis with intact ventricular septum and hypoplastic right ventricle," *Circulation 1976*; 53:389-94.

12. Rogers JH Jr. and Rao PS, "Ebstein's anomaly of the left atrioventricular valve with congenital corrected transposition of the great arteries - Diagnosis by intracavitary electrocardiography," *Chest 1977*; 72:253-6.

13. Rao PS and Ellison RG, "The cause of kinking of the right pulmonary artery in Waterston anastomosis: A growth phenomenon," *J Thorac Cardiovasc Surg 1978*; 76:126-9.

14. Rao PS, "Value of pulmonary vein wedge angiography in visualization of obstructed ipsilateral pulmonary artery," *Cardiovasc Radiology 1978*; 1:151-2.

15. Monarrez CN, Rao PS, Moore HV and Strong WB, "False aneurysm of the right pulmonary artery: A new complication of the aorta-right pulmonary artery anastomosis," *J Thorac Cardiovasc Surg 1979*; 77:738-41.

16. Truman TA, Rao PS, Kulangara RJ, "Use of contrast echocardiography in the diagnosis of anomalous connection of the right superior vena cava to the left atrium," *Brit Heart J 1980*; 44:718-23.

17. Rao PS and Sissman NJ, "Spontaneous closure of physiologically advantageous ventricular septal defects," *Circulation 1971*; 43:83-90.

18. Rao PS and Sissman NJ, "The relationship of pulmonary venous wedge to pulmonary arterial pressures," *Circulation 1971*; 44:565-74.

19. Rao PS, Linde LM, Liebman J, Perrin E, "Functional closure of physiologically advantageous ventricular septal defects: Observations in three cases with tricuspid atresia," *Amer J Dis Child 1974*; 127:36-40.

20. Rao PS, "Natural history of the ventricular septal defect in tricuspid atresia and its surgical implications," *Brit Heart J 1977*; 39:276-88.

21. Thapar MK, Rao PS, Rogers JH Jr., et al, "Changing murmur of patent ductus arteriosus," *J Pediatr 1978*; 92:939-41.

22. Rees AH, Rao PS, Rigby JJ, Miller MD, "Echocardiographic estimation of left-to-right shunt in isolated ventricular septal defects," *European J Cardiol 1978*; 7:25-33.

23. Rao PS, Marino BL, Robertson AF, III, "The usefulness of continuous positive airway pressure in the differential diagnosis of cardiac from pulmonary cyanosis in newborn infants.," *Arch Dis Child 1978*; 53:456-60.

24. Rao PS, Thapar MK, Strong WB, "Non-opacification of patent ductus arteriosus in patients with large ventricular septal defects," *Angiology 1978*; 29:888-97.

25. Rao PS, Kulangara RJ, Moore HV, Strong WB, "Syndrome of single ventricle without pulmonic stenosis but with left atrioventricular valve atresia and interatrial obstruction: Palliative management

with simultaneous atrial septostomy and pulmonary artery banding," *J Thorac Cardiovasc Surg 1981*; 81:127-130.

26. Covitz W, Rao PS, Strong WB, Reyes L, "Echocardiographic assessment of the aortic root in syndromes with left ventricular hypoplasia," *Pediat Cardiol 1982*; 2:19-23.

27. Mardini MK and Rao PS, "Left ventricular and aortic catheterization and angiography via a patent ductus arteriosus: A new technique," *Cath Cardiovasc Diag 1983*; 9:89-95.

28. Mardini MK and Rao PS, "A technique of aortic arch angiography in patients with patent ductus arteriosus," *Pediat Cardiol 1983*; 4:53-4.

29. Rao PS, "Left-to-right atrial shunts in tricuspid atresia," *Brit Heart J 1983*; 49:345-9.

30. Rao PS and Mardini MK, "Atrial septostomy without thoracotomy: The experience with transcatheter knife atrial septostomy," *King Faisal Specialist Hospital Medical Journal 1983*; 3:165-71.

31. Mardini MK and Rao PS, "Scimitar Syndrome: Experience with four patients and review of literature," *Arab J Med 1984*; 3:13-23.

32. Rao PS, "Transcatheter blade atrial septostomy," *Cath Cardiovasc Diag 1984*; 10:335-42.

33. Rao PS, "The femoral route for cardiac catheterization in infants and children," *Chest 1973*; 63:239-41.

34. Linde LM and Rao PS, "A modern view of infective endocarditis," *Cardiovasc Clinics 1973*; Vol. 5, No. 2:15-34.

35. Thapar MK, Rao PS, Linde LM, Feldman D, "Infective endocarditis: I. Incidence, etiology, pathology and clinical features," *Paediatrician 1978*; 7:65-84.

36. Rao PS and Monarrez CN, "Electrocardiographic differentiation of posterobasal left ventricular hypertrophy from right ventricular hypertrophy," *J. Electrocardiol 1981*; 14:25-30.

37. Rao PS, Thapar MK, Rogers JH Jr., et al, "Effect of intra-arterial injection of heparin on the complications of percutaneous arterial catheterization in infants and children," *Cath and Cardiovasc Diag 1981*; 7:235-46.

38. Rao PS, Thapar MK, Haggard RJ, Strong WB, "Left ventricular muscle mass by m-mode echocardiography in children," *J Cardiovasc Ultrasonography 1983*; 2:381-9.

39. Rao PS and Thapar MK, "Influence of race and sex on echocardiographic measurements in children," *J Cardiovasc Ultrasonography 1984*; 3:75-82.

40. Rao PS, Thapar MK, Harp RJ, "Racial variations in electrocardiograms and vectorcardiograms between black and white children and their genesis," *J Electrocardiology 1984*; 17:239-52.

41. Balfour IC, Covitz W, Davis H, Rao PS, et al, "Cardiac size and function in children with sickle cell anemia," *Amer Heart J 1984*; 108:345-50.

42. Rao PS, "Racial differences in electrocardiograms and vectocardiograms between black and white adolescents," *J. Electrocardiol 1985*; 18:309-13.

43. Rao PS and Mardini MK, "Pulmonary valvotomy without thoracotomy: The experience with percutaneous balloon pulmonary valvuloplasty," *Ann Saudi Med 1985*; 5:149-55.

44. Rao PS, "Descending aortography with balloon inflation: A technique for evaluation of the size of the patent ductus arteriosus in infants with large proximal left-to-right shunts," *Brit Heart J 1985*; 54:527-32.

45. Rao PS and Andaya WG, "Chronic afterload reduction in infants and children with primary myocardial disease," *J Pediat 1986*; 108:530-4.

46. Rao PS, Mardini MK, Najjar HN, "Relief of coarctation of the aorta without thoracotomy: The experience with percutaneous balloon angioplasty," *Ann Saudi Med 1986*; 6:193-203.

47. Rao PS, "Transcatheter treatment of pulmonic stenosis and coarctation of the aorta: The experience with percutaneous balloon dilatation," *Brit Heart J 1986*; 56:250-8.

48. Rao PS, "Value of Echo-Doppler studies in the evaluation of the results of balloon pulmonary valvuloplasty," *J Cardiovasc Ultrasonography 1986*; 5:309-14.

49. Rao PS, "Balloon angioplasty for coarctation of the aorta in infancy," *J Pediat 1987*; 110:713-8.

50. Rao PS, "Doppler ultrasound in the prediction of transvalvar pressure gradients in patients with valvar pulmonic stenosis," *International J Cardiol 1987*; 15:195-203.

51. Rao PS, "Influence of balloon size on the short-term and long-term results of balloon pulmonary valvuloplasty," *Texas Heart Institute J 1987*; 14:57-61.

52. Rao PS, Najjar HN, Mardini MK, et al, "Balloon angioplasty for coarctation of the aorta: Immediate and long-term results," *Amer Heart J 1988*; 115:657-65.

53. Rao PS, Brais M, "Balloon pulmonary valvuloplasty for congenital cyanotic heart defects," *Amer Heart J 1988*; 115:1105-10.

54. Rao PS, Fawzy ME, Solymar L, Mardini MK, "Long-term results of balloon pulmonary valvuloplasty," *Amer Heart J 1988*; 115:1291-6.

55. Rao PS and Solymar L, "Electrocardiographic changes following balloon dilatation of valvar pulmonic stenosis," *J Interventional Cardiol 1988*; 1:189-97.

56. Rao PS, "Value of Echo-Doppler studies in the evaluation of the results of balloon angioplasty of aortic coarctation," *J Cardiovasc Ultrasonography 1988*; 7:215-20.

57. Rao PS, "Balloon dilatation in infants and children with dysplastic pulmonary valves: Short-term and intermediate-term results," *Am Heart J 1988*; 116:1168-73.

58. Rao PS and Solymar L, "Transductal balloon angioplasty of coarctation of the aorta in the neonate: Preliminary observations," *Am Heart J 1988*; 116:1558-63.

59. Rao PS, Thapar MK, Kutayli F, "Causes of restenosis following balloon valvuloplasty for valvar pulmonic stenosis," *Am J Cardiol 1988*; 62:979-82.

60. Rao PS, "Further observations on the role of balloon size on the short-term and intermediate-term results of balloon pulmonary valvuloplasty," *Brit Heart J 1988*; 60:507-11.

61. Rao PS and Fawzy ME, "Double balloon technique for percutaneous balloon pulmonary valvuloplasty: Comparison with single balloon technique," *J Interventional Cardiol 1988*; 1:257-62.

62. Rao PS, Thapar MK, Kutayli F, Carey P, "Causes of recoarctation following balloon angioplasty of unoperated aortic coarctations," *J Amer Coll Cardiol 1989*; 13:109-15.

63. Rao PS, Solymar L, Mardini MK, et al, "Anticoagulant therapy in children with prosthetic valves," *Ann Thorac Surg 1989*; 47:589-592.

64. Thapar MK, Rao PS, "Significance of infundibular obstruction following balloon valvuloplasty for valvar pulmonic stenosis," *Am Heart J 1989*; 118:99-103.

65. Rao PS, Carey P, "Doppler ultrasound in the prediction of pressure gradients across aortic coarctation," *Am Heart J 1989*; 118:299-301.

66. Rao PS and Carey P, "Remodeling of the aorta following successful balloon coarctation angioplasty," *J Am Coll Cardiol 1989*; 14:1312-7.

67. Rao PS, Thapar MK, Wilson AD, et al, "Intermediate-term follow-up results of balloon aortic valvuloplasty in infants and children with special reference to causes of restenosis," *Am J Cardiol 1989*; 64:1356-60.

68. Rao PS, "Long-term oral diazoxide therapy for pulmonary vascular obstructive disease associated with congenital heart defects," *Am Heart J 1990*; 119:1317-21.

69. Rao PS, Levy JM, Chopra PS, "Balloon angioplasty of stenosed Blalock-Taussig anastomosis: Role of balloon on a wire in dilating occluded shunts," *Am Heart J 1990*; 120:1173-8.

70. Rao PS, Wilson AD, Chopra PS, "Balloon dilatation for discrete subaortic stenosis: Immediate and intermediate-term results," *J Invasive Cardiol 1990*; 2:65-71.

71. Rao PS, Thapar MK, Galal O, Wilson AD, "Follow-up results of balloon angioplasty of native coarctation in neonates and infants," *Am Heart J 1990*; 120:1310-4.

72. Rao PS, Wilson AD, Chopra PS, "Immediate and follow-up results of balloon angioplasty of postoperative recoarctation in infants and children," *Am Heart J 1990*; 120:1315-20.

73. Wilson AD, Rao PS, Aeschlimann S, "Normal fetal foramen flap and transatrial Doppler velocity pattern," *J Am Soc Echocard 1990*; 3:491-4.

74. Solymar L, Rao PS, Mardini MK, et al, "Prosthetic valves in children and adolescents," *Am Heart J 1991*; 121:557-68.

75. Rao PS, Solymar L, Fawzy ME, Guinn G, "Reassessment of usefulness of porcine heterografts in mitral position in children," *Pediat Cardiol 1991*; 12:164-9.

76. Rao PS, Langhough R, "Relationship of echocardiographic, shunt flow, and angiographic size to the stretched diameter of the atrial septal defect," *Am Heart J 1991*; 122:505-8.

77. Rao PS, Sideris EB, Haddad J, et al, "Transcatheter occlusion of patent ductus arteriosus with adjustable buttoned device: Initial clinical experience," *Circulation 1993*; 88:1119-26.

78. Lloyd TR, Rao PS, Beekman RH III, et al, "Atrial septal defect occlusion with the buttoned device: A multi-institutional U.S. Trial," *Am J Cardiol 1994*; 73:286-291.

79. Zamora R, Rao PS, Lloyd TR, et al, "Intermediate-term results of phase I FDA trials of buttoned device occlusion of secundum atrial septal defect," *J Am Coll Cardiol 1998*; 31:674-6.

80. Rao PS, Sideris EB, Hausdorf G, et al, "International experience with secundum atrial septal defect occlusion by the buttoned device," *Am Heart J 1994*; 128:1022-35.

81. Rao PS, Kim SH, Rey C, et al, "Results of transvenous buttoned device occlusion of patent ductus arteriosus in adults," *Am J Cardiol 1998*; 82:827-9.

82. Rao PS, Kim SH, Choi J, et al, "Follow-up results of transvenous occlusion of patent ductus arteriosus with buttoned device," *J Am Coll Cardiol 1999*; 33:820-6.

83. Rao PS, Berger F, Rey C, et al, "Results of transvenous occlusion of secundum atrial septal defects with 4th generation buttoned device: Comparison with 1st, 2nd and 3rd generation devices," *J Am Coll Cardiol 2000*; 36:583-92.

84. Rao PS, Andaya WG, Whisennand HW, "Contrast echocardiography in the differential diagnosis of hypoxemia following open heart surgery," *King Faisal Specialist Hospital Medical Journal 1983*; 3:121-4.

85. Feteih W, Rao PS, Whisennand HW, et al, "Chylopericardium: A new complication of Blalock-Taussig anastomosis," *J Thorac Cardiovasc Surg 1983*; 85:791-4.

86. Rao PS and Lawrie GM, "Syndrome of absent pulmonary valve: Surgical correction with pulmonary arterioplasty," *Brit Heart J 1983*; 50:586-9.

87. Rao PS, Harfi HA, Shebib SM, Guinn G, "Transient eosinophilic pulmonary infiltration with intestinal schistosomiasis and mitral stenosis," *King Faisal Specialist Hospital Med J 1984*; 4:355-8.

88. Rao PS, "Atrioventricular canal mimicking tricuspid atresia: Echocardiographic & angiographic features," *Brit Heart J 1987*; 58:409-12.

89. Rao PS, Najjar HN, "Congestive cardiomyopathy due to chronic tachycardia: Resolution of cardiomyopathy with antiarrhythmic drugs," *International J Cardiol 1987*; 17:216-20.

90. Thapar MK, Rao PS, "Use of propranolol for severe dynamic infundibular obstruction prior to balloon pulmonary valvuloplasty," *Cathet Cardiovasc Diag 1990*; 19:240-1.

91. Rao PS, Sideris EB, Chopra PS, "Catheter closure of atrial septal defect: Successful use in a 3.6 kg Infant," *Am Heart J 1991*; 121:1826-9.

92. Rao PS, Wilson AD, Sideris EB, Chopra PS, "Transcatheter closure of patent ductus arteriosus with buttoned device: First successful clinical application in a child," *Am Heart J 1991*; 121:1799-1802.

93. Rao PS, Levy J, Nikicicz E, Gilbert-Barness EF, "Tricuspid atresia: Association with persistent truncus arteriosus - A review," *Am Heart J 1991*; 122:829-35.

94. Salahuddin N, Wilson AD, Rao PS, "An unusual presentation of coarctation of the aorta in infancy: Role of balloon angioplasty in the critically ill infant," *Am Heart J 1991*; 122:1772-5.

95. Rao PS and Wilson AD, "Chylothorax, an unusual complication of baffle obstruction following Mustard operation: Successful treatment with balloon angioplasty," *Am Heart J 1992*; 123:244-8.

96. Rao PS, Wilson AD, Brazy J, "Transumbilical balloon coarctation angioplasty in a neonate with critical aortic coarctation," *Am Heart J 1992*; 124:1622-4.

97. Lochan R, Rao PS, Samal AK, et al, "Transcatheter closure of patent ductus arteriosus with an adjustable buttoned device in an adult patient," *Am Heart J 1994*; 127:941-3.

98. Chopra PS, Reed WH, Wilson AD, Rao PS, "Delayed presentation of anomalous circumflex coronary artery arising from pulmonary artery following repair of aortopulmonary window in infancy," *Chest 1994*; 106:1920-2.

99. Reddy SCB, Chopra PS, Rao PS, "Mixed type of total anomalous pulmonary venous connection: Echocardiographic limitations and angiographic advantages," *Am Heart J 1995*; 129:1034-8.

100. Lee HY and Rao PS, "Percutaneous transluminal coronary angioplasty for Takayasu's arteritis," *Am Heart J 1996*; 132:1084-6.

101. Reddy SCB, Chopra PS, Rao PS, "Aneurysm of the membranous ventricular septum resulting in pulmonary outflow tract obstruction in congenitally corrected transposition of the great arteries: A review," *Am Heart J 1997*; 133:112-9.

102. Siblini G, Rao PS, Singh GK, et al, "Transcatheter management of neonates with pulmonary atresia and intact ventricular septum," *Cathet Cardiovasc Diag 1997*; 42:395-402.

103. Jureidini SB, Spadaro JJ, Rao PS, "Aortopulmonary window: Successful transcatheter closure with buttoned device in an adult," *Am J Cardiol 1998*; 81:371-2.

104. Rao PS and Jureidini SB, "Transumbilical venous anterograde, snare-assisted balloon aortic valvuloplasty in a neonate with critical aortic stenosis," *Cathet Cardiovasc Diag 1998*; 45:144-8.

105. Rao PS, Wagman AJ, Chen S, "Coil occlusion of patent ductus arteriosus with right aortic arch," *Cathet Cardiovasc Intervent 2001*; 52:79-82.

106. Pugh KJ, Jureidine SB, Ream R, Rao PS, Dossier J, "Successful thrombolytic therapy of pulmonary embolism associated with urosepsis in an infant," *Pediat Cardiol 2002*; 23:77-9.

107. Rao PS, Bromberg BI, Jureidini SB, Fiore AC, "Transcatheter occlusion of ruptured sinus of Valsalva aneurysm: Innovative use of available technology," *Cath Cardiovasc Intervent 2003*; 58:130-4.

108. Sideris EB, Macuil B, Justiniano S, Rao PS, "Total percutaneous correction of tetralogy of Fallot variant with dominant pulmonary valve stenosis," *Heart 2005*; 91:345-7.

109. Gupta K and Rao PS, "Severe intravascular hemolysis after transcatheter coil occlusion of patent ductus arteriosus," *J Invasive Cardiol 2005*; 17(10): E15-E17, ISSN: 1042-393, Vol. 17, Issue 10, October 2005, pp. E15-E17.

110. Tsounias E and Rao PS, "Stent therapy for clotted Blalock-Taussig shunts," *Congenital Cardiol Today 2010*; 8(7):1-9.

111. Mazur L, deYbarrondo L, Pickard L, Rao PS, "Development of supravalvular pulmonary artery stenosis following a Nuss procedure," *J Pediatr Surg 2012*; 47(12):e61-4. PMID:23217921.

112. Doshi AR and Rao PS, "Development of aortic coarctation following device closure of patent ductus arteriosus," *J Invasive Cardiol 2013*; 25:464-7.

113. Yarrabolu TR, Thapar MK, Rao PS, "Subpulmonary obstruction due to aneurismal ventricular septum in a patient with congenitally corrected transposition of the great arteries and dextrocardia," *Congenital Cardiology Today 2014*; 12(7):1-8.

114. Yates MC, Gautam NK, Rao PS, "Reactive ductus arteriosus in a nineteen-month-old patient," *Congenital Cardiology Today 2015*; 13(5):1-7.

115. Yarrabolu TR, Thapar MK, Rao PS, "Subpulmonary obstruction from aneurismal ventricular septum in a child with dextrocardia and congenitally corrected transposition of the great arteries," *Tex Heart Inst J 2015*; 42(6):590-592, eCollection 2015 December.

116. Yarrabolu TR, Naidu DP, Pawelek O, Rao PS, "Flash pulmonary edema during pulmonary vasoreactivity testing," *J J Pulmonol 2016*, 2(3):028.

117. Rao PS, "Auscultation is still a valid tool in the evaluation of cardiac defects in children," *Congenital Cardiology Today 2018*; 16(8):1-6.

118. Rao PS, "Transcatheter perforation of atretic pulmonary valve in pulmonary atresia with ventricular septal defect," *Congenital Cardiology Today 2018*; 16(11):1-8.

119. Nadel JA, Gold WM, Burgess JH, "Early diagnosis of chronic pulmonary vascular obstruction: Value of pulmonary function tests," *Am J Med 1968*; 44:16-25.

120. Tanner JM, Whitehouse RH, Takaishi ML, "Standards from birth to maturity for height, weight, height velocity and weight velocity: British children, 1965 - Part II," *Arch Dis Child 1966*; 41:613-35, PMID: 5927918.

121. Friedman M, Strang LB, "The effects of corticosteroid and ACTH therapy on growth and on the hypothalamic-pituitary adrenal axis of children," *Scand J Respir Dis Suppl. 1969*; 68:58-69.

122. Rao PS, Moore HV, Strong WB, "Surgery for mitral atresia and interatrial obstruction without pulmonic stenosis (Letter)," *Circulation 1980*; 62:201-202.

123. Thomas CS Jr, McGoon DC, "Isolated massive chylopericardium following cardiopulmonary bypass," *J Thorac Cardiovasc Surg. 1971*; 61:945-8.

124. Rao PS, "Chylopericardium following Blalock-Taussig anastomosis (Letter)," *J Thorac Cardiovasc Surg 1984*; 87:642.

125. Rao PS and Whisennand HW, "Chylopericardium (Letter)," *Ann Thorac Surg 1983*; 36:494-5.

126. Rose DM, Colvin SB, Danilowicz D, Isom OW, "Cardiac tamponade secondary to chylopericardium following cardiac surgery: Case report and review of the literature," *Ann Thorac Surg 1982*; 34:333-6.

127. Neill CA, Ferencz C, Sabiston DC, Sheldon H, "The familial occurrence of hypoplastic right lung with systemic arterial supply and venous drainage "scimitar syndrome"," *Bull Johns Hopkins Hosp 1960*; 107:1-21.

128. D Cruz IA, Arcilla RA, "Anomalous venous drainage of the left lung into the inferior vena cava. A case report," *Am Heart J. 1964*; 67:539-44.

129. Ilbawi MN, Idriss FS, Muster AJ, et al, "Tetralogy of Fallot with absent pulmonary valve. Should valve insertion be part of the intracardiac repair?" *J Thorac Cardiovasc Surg 1981*; 81:906-15.

130. Chusid MJ, Dale DC, West BC, Wolff SM, "The hypereosinophilic syndrome: Analysis of fourteen cases with review of the literature," *Medicine (Baltimore) 1975*; 54:1-27.

131. Thapar MK and Rao PS, "Significance of infundibular obstruction following balloon valvuloplasty for valvar pulmonic stenosis," *Am Heart J 1989*; 118:99-103.

132. Rao PS, Thapar MK, "Balloon pulmonary valvuloplasty (Reply to Letter)," *Am Heart J 1991*; 121:1839-40.

133. Hausdorf G, Schneider M, Schrimer KR, et al, "Anterograde balloon valvuloplasty of aortic stenosis in children," *Am J Cardiol 1993*; 71:460-2.

134. O'Laughlin MP, Slack MC, Grifka R, Mullins CE, "Pro-grade double balloon dilatation of congenital aortic valve stenosis: A case report," *Cathet Cardiovasc Diag 1993*; 28:134-6.

135. Rao PS, "Anterograde transumbilical venous balloon aortic valvuloplasty (Letter)," *Cath Cardiovasc Intervent 2002*; 56:439.

136. Rao PS, "Anterograde balloon aortic valvuloplasty in the neonate via the umbilical vein (Letter)," *Cath Cardiovasc Intervent 2003*; 59:291-2.

137. Nuss D, Kelly RE, Croitoru DP, et al, "A 10-year review of a minimally invasive technique for the correction of pectus excavatum," *J Pediatr Surg 1998*; 33:545-52.

138. Rao PS, "Comprehensive management of pulmonary atresia with intact ventricular septum," *Ann Thorac Surg 1985*; 40:409-413.

139. Rao PS, "Pulmonary atresia with intact ventricular septum," *Current Treatment Options in Cardiovasc Med 2002*; 4:321-336.

140. Rao PS, "Role of interventional cardiology in the treatment of neonates: Part III," *Neonatology Today 2007*; 2(11):1-10.

CHAPTER 8

EDITORIAL COMMUNICATIONS

INTRODUCTION

I have contributed to a number of editorials[1-64] and letters to the editor[65-102] over the years. Some of these editorials[1,3,9,16,24,30,35,42,62] were for the purpose of introducing symposia organized by me for the several journals, namely, Paediatrician,[1] The Indian Journal of Pediatrics,[3,9,24,35,42,62] The Journal of Invasive Cardiology,[16,30,49] and The Current Interventional Cardiology Reports. Others[2,4-8,13,50,55,56.58.60,63] were ad hoc editorials written on subjects of importance for those particular times. Most of the editorials, however, were communications[10-12,14,15,17-23,25-29,31-34,36-41,43-48,51-54,57,59,61,64] following concurrently published papers, requested by the Chief Editors of the respective journals.

EDITORIALS INTRODUCING SYMPOSIA

Early in my academic career in the 1970s, I was asked to organize seminars in Pediatric Cardiology by Dr. George Maragos, Chief Editor of the journal *Paediatrician*, a publication of S. Karger, Basel, Switzerland. The topics selected (Figures 1, 2 and 3) ranged from preventive aspects of congenital heart disease (CHD), principles of understanding of electrocardiograms (ECG) and echocardiograms, functional murmurs and management of congestive heart failure (CHF) to surgery for complex CHD. These papers were written by experts in the respective fields around the world, including our group from the Medical College of Georgia in Augusta, Georgia, USA.

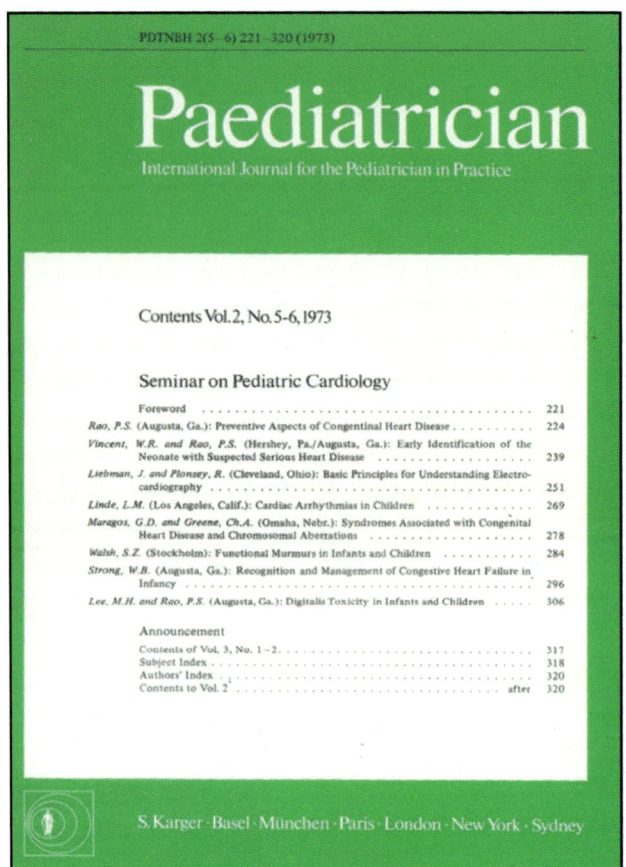

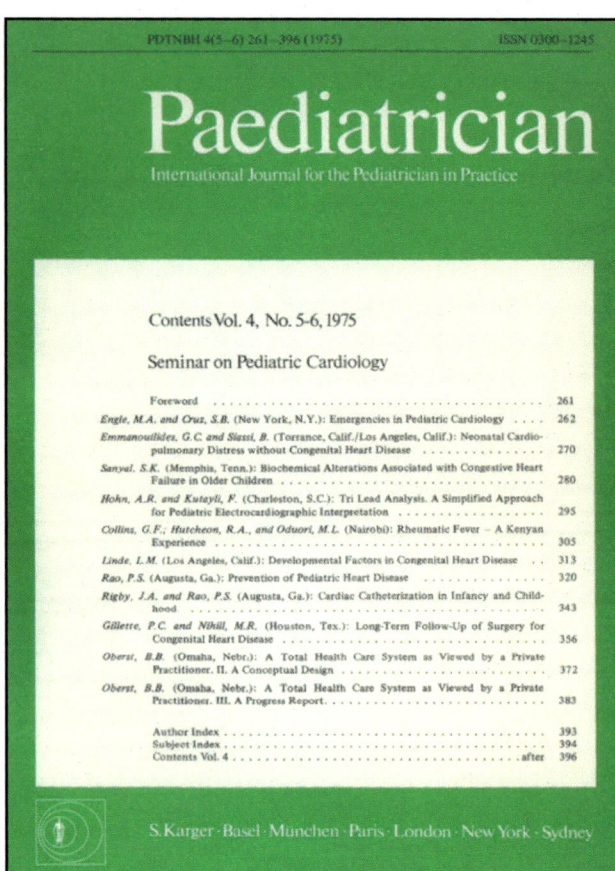

Figure 1. Photograph of the cover page of the journal *Paediatrician* (Vol. 2, No. 5-6, 1973) that I organized and edited

Figure 2. Photograph of the cover page of the journal *Paediatrician* (Vol. 4, No. 5-6, 1975) that I organized and edited.

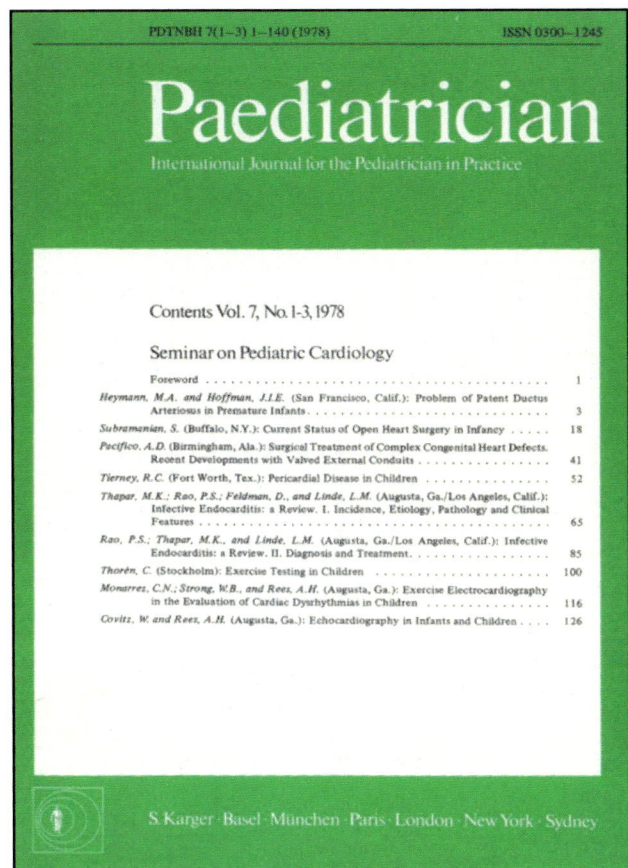

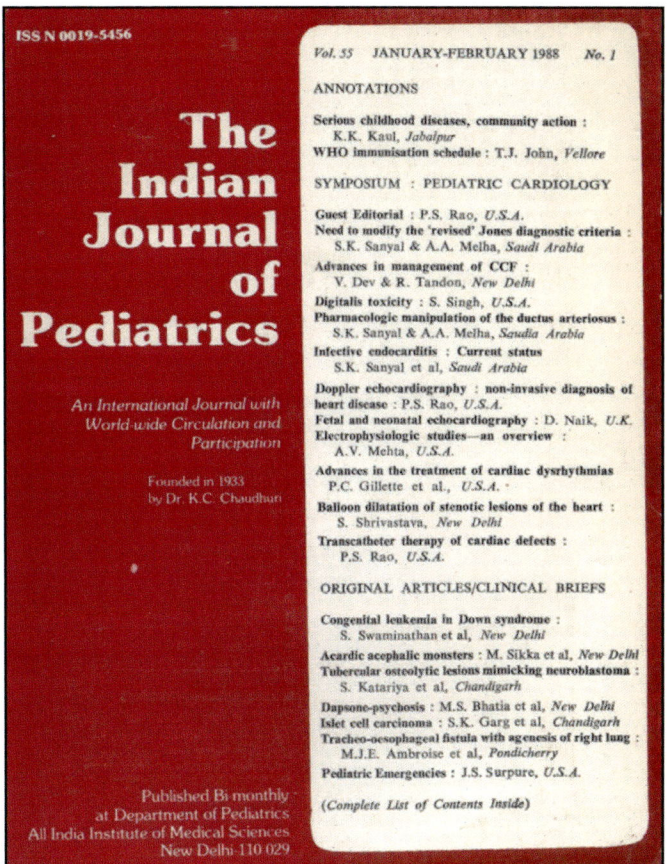

Figure 3. Photograph of the cover page of the journal *Paediatrician* (Vol. 7, No. 1-3, 1978) that I organized and edited.

Figure 4. Photograph of the cover page of *The Indian Journal of Pediatrics* (Vol. 55, No. 1, 1988) that I organized and edited.

In late 1980s, the Editor-in-Chief of *The Indian Journal of Pediatrics*, Dr. I. C. Verma invited me to organize a symposia for the pediatricians in India, which I gladly accepted and the first symposium was published in 1988.[3] As time passed by, additional requests to organize such symposia resulted in publication of symposia in 1991,[9] 1998,[24] 2002,[35] 2005,[42] and most recently in 2015.[62] In 2002, Dr. Anita Saxena of All India Institute of Medical Sciences (AIMS) in New Delhi joined me as a co-editor to organize and edit the symposia published in 2002 and later. Again, the topics included basic issues related to diagnosis and management of common cardiac problems in children, newer diagnostic modalities, and recent advances in transcatheter and surgical therapy. Some of the topics presented in these symposia are shown figures 4 through 7. We (the co-editor and I) invited experts in the respective fields around the world to contribute to these symposia.

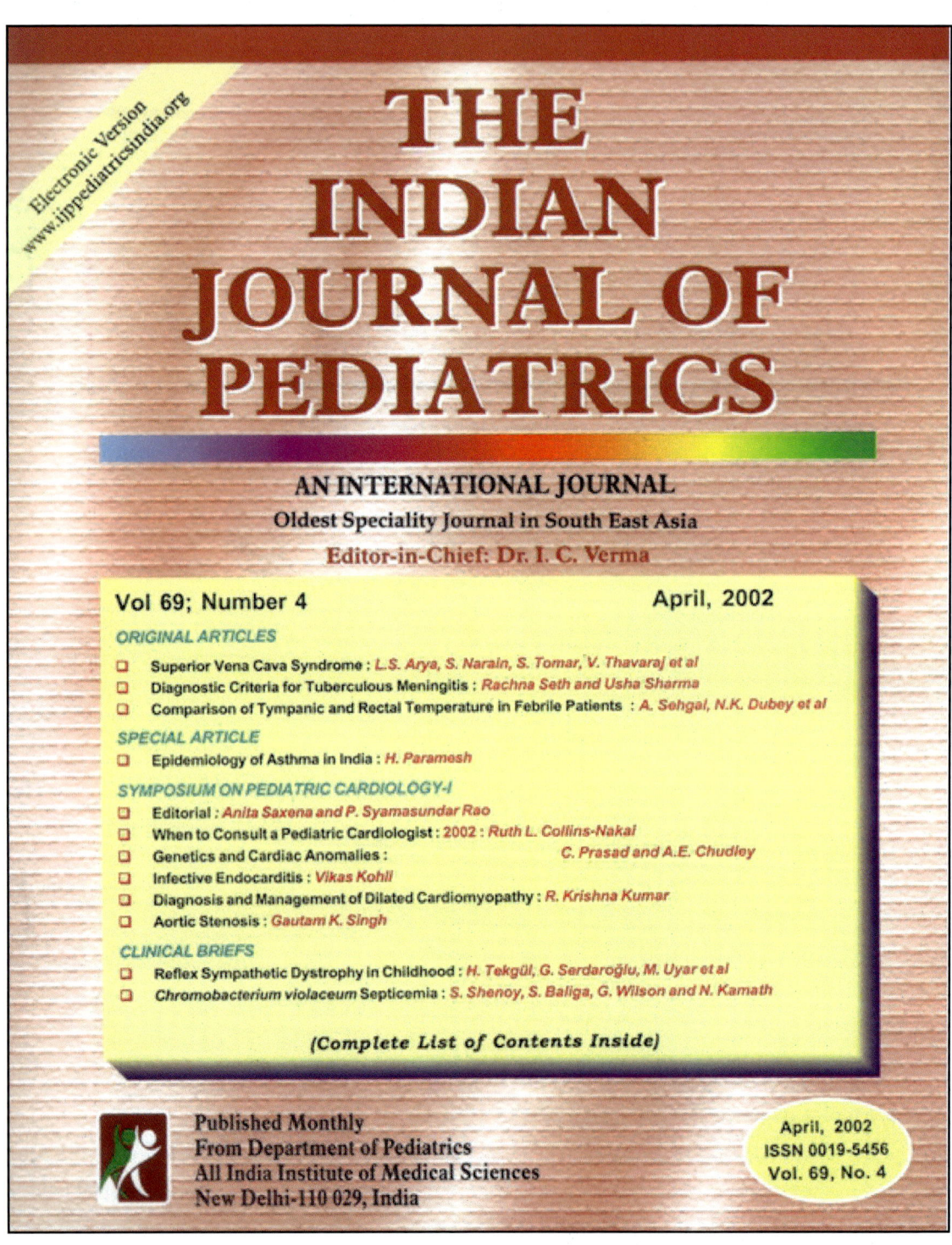

Figure 5. Photograph of the cover page of *The Indian Journal of Pediatrics* (Vol. 69, No. 4, 2002) that Dr. Saxena and I organized and edited.

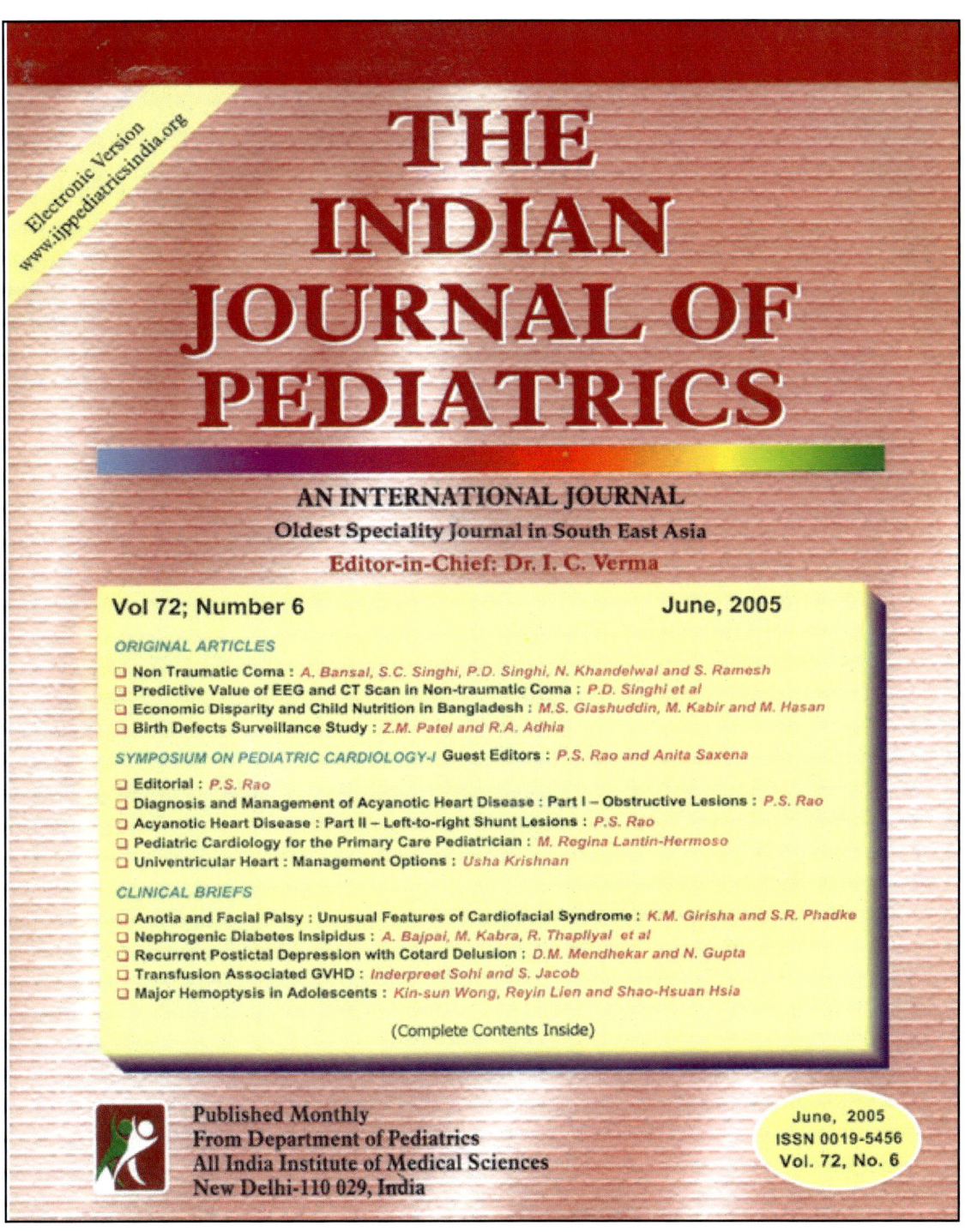

Figure 6. Photograph of the cover page of *The Indian Journal of Pediatrics* (Vol. 72, No. 6, 2005) that Dr. Saxena and I organized and edited.

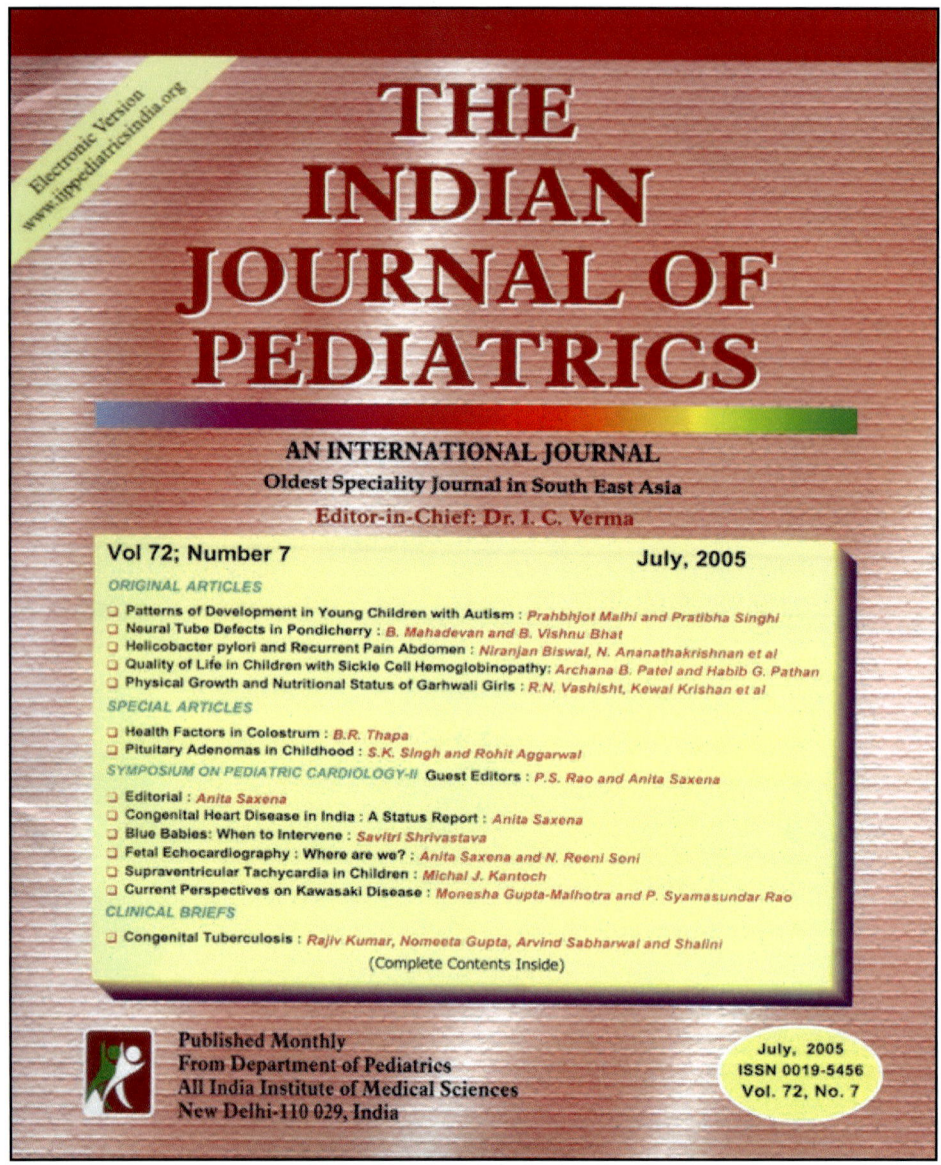

Figure 7. Photograph of the cover page of *The Indian Journal of Pediatrics* (Vol. 72, No. 7, 2005) that Dr. Saxena and I organized and edited.

Dr. Richard Shaw, the Editor-in-Chief of *The Journal of Invasive Cardiology* invited me in mid-1990s to organize an issue on Cardiac (Catheter) Interventions in the Pediatric Patient, which resulted in publication of a special issue[16] in the September of 1996 (Figure 8). These papers addressed several interventional pediatric cardiology topics/techniques. In early 2000, Dr. Shaw requested that I help create a special section in the journal on *Interventional Pediatric Cardiology*, which came to fruition in January 2001 (Figure 9).[30] The section on interventional pediatric cardiology continued thereafter. In late 2008, I was asked by the Chief Editor of *The Journal of Invasive Cardiology* to organize a symposium on "Structural Heart Disease in Adults;" this was successfully accomplished (Figures 10 and 11) in two different issues of the Journal.[49,50] In the second issue,[50] I presented a review on when and how should atrial septal defects be closed in adults.[103]

The Journal of
Invasive Cardiology

September 1996
Volume 8/Number 7

Cardiac Interventions in the Pediatric Patient

Transcatheter Occlusion of Patent Ductus Arteriosus: State of the Art
P. Syamasundar Rao, MD and Eleftherios B. Sideris, MD

Transcatheter Closure of Atrial Septal Defects: Role of Buttoned Devices
Eleftherios B. Sideris, MD and P. Syamasundar Rao, MD

Balloon Dilatation of Discrete Membranous Subaortic Stenosis
Zuhdi Lababidi, MD

Should Balloon Angioplasty be Used as a Treatment of Choice for Native Aortic Coarctations?
P. Syamasundar Rao, MD

Role of Stents in the Management of Congenital Heart Defects
Jay S. Chandar, MD, Steven B. Wolfe, MD, P. Syamasundar Rao, MD

Critical Pulmonary Stenosis in the Neonate: Role of Transcatheter Management
Saadeh B. Jureidini, MB, ChB and P. Syamasundar Rao, MD

Coil Embolization in the Management of Cardiac Problems in Children
Ghassan Siblini, MD and P. Syamasundar Rao, MD

Ultrasound as an Adjunct to Cardiac Interventions in Pediatric Patients
Gautam K. Singh, MD, Cynthia Marino, RDMS, P. Syamasundar Rao, MD

Health Management Publications, Inc.

ISSN 1042-3931

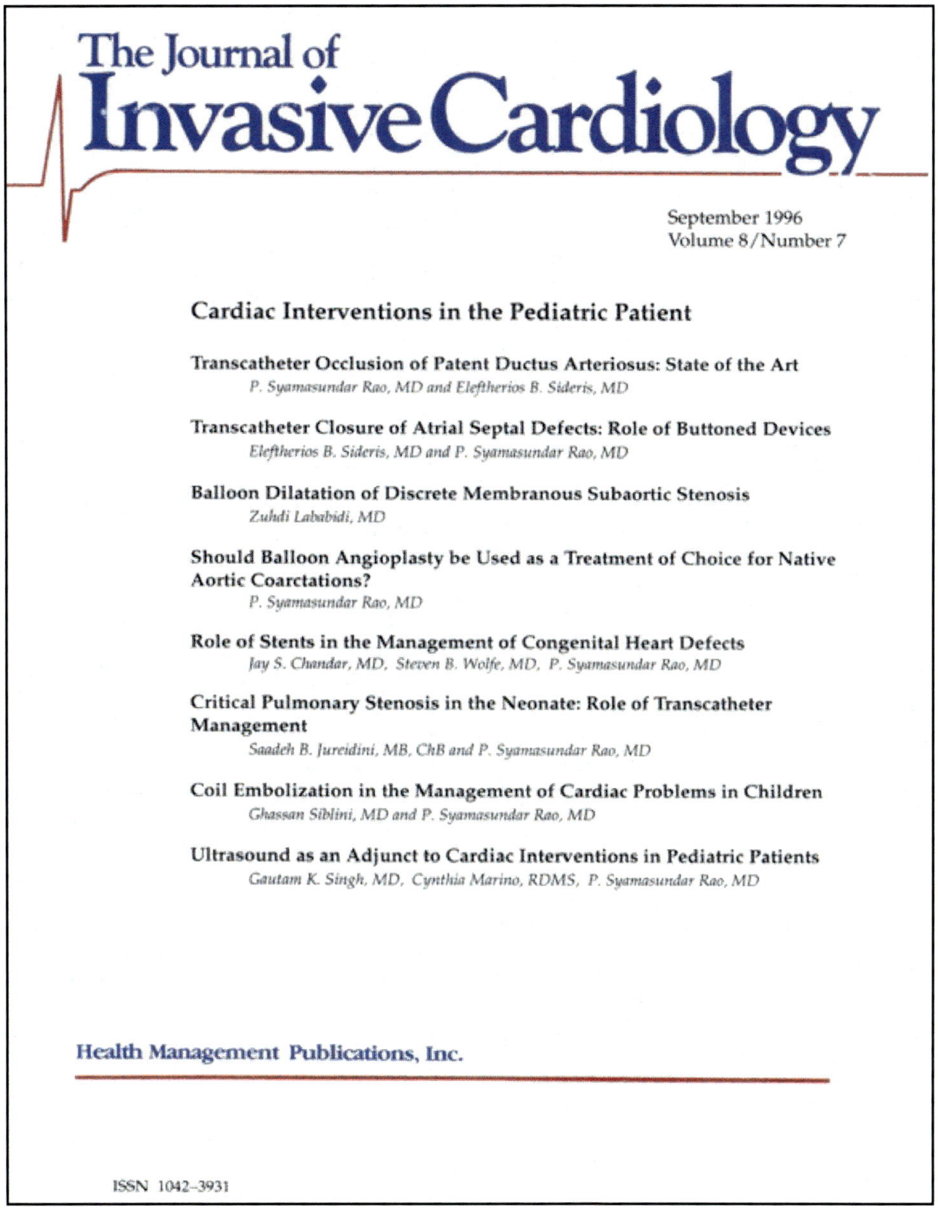

Figure 8. Photograph of the cover page of *The Journal of Invasive Cardiology* (Vol. 8, No. 7, 1996) that I organized and edited.

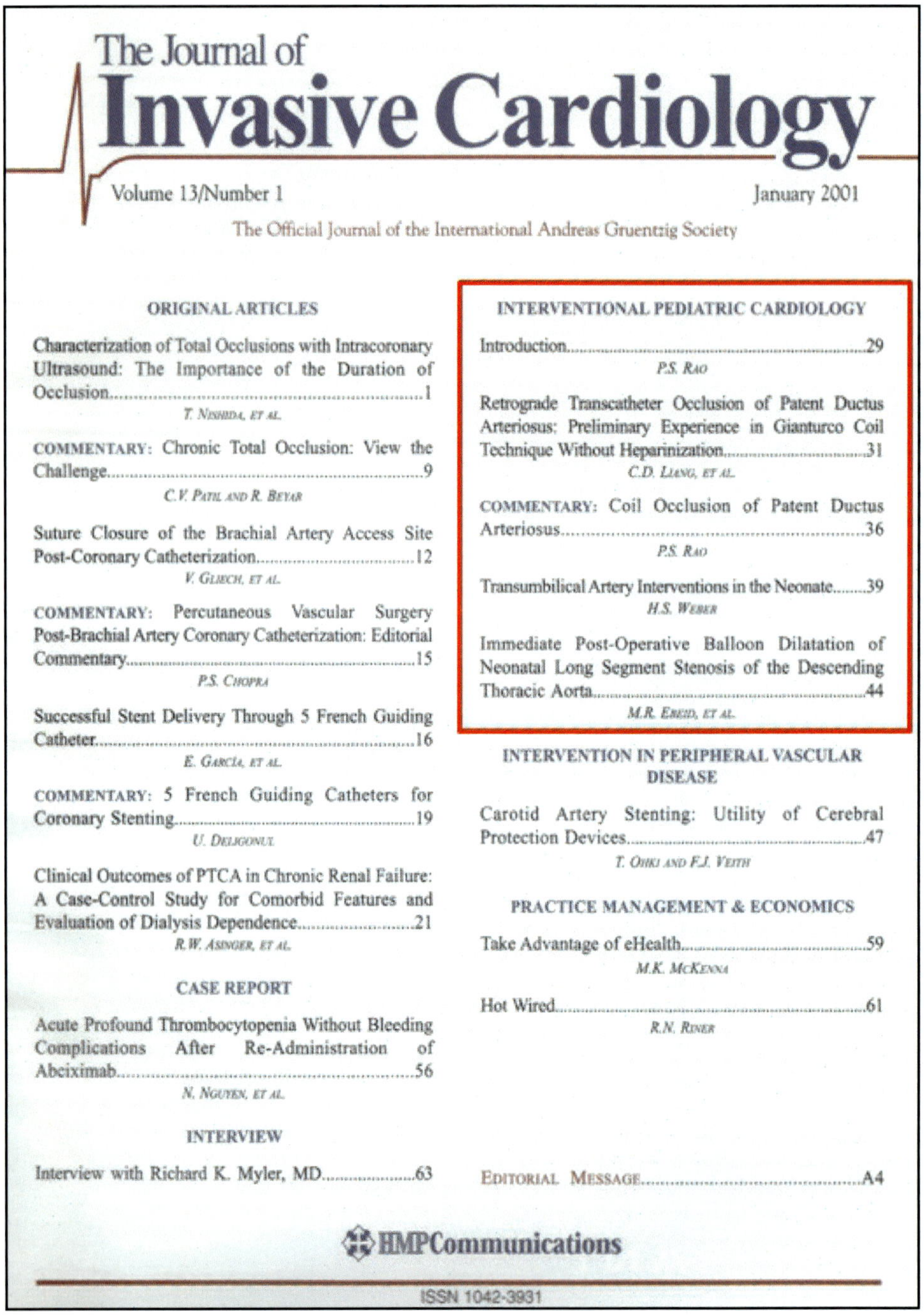
The Journal of
Invasive Cardiology

Volume 13/Number 1 January 2001

The Official Journal of the International Andreas Gruentzig Society

ORIGINAL ARTICLES

CASE REPORT

INTERVIEW

INTERVENTIONAL PEDIATRIC CARDIOLOGY

INTERVENTION IN PERIPHERAL VASCULAR DISEASE

PRACTICE MANAGEMENT & ECONOMICS

HMPCommunications

ISSN 1042-3931

Figure 9. Photograph of the cover page of *The Journal of Invasive Cardiology* (Vol. 13, No. 1, 2001) in which a special section on "Interventional Pediatric Cardiology" (outlined in the red box) that I organized and edited was published.

FOCUS: STEMI Interventions
Structural Heart Disease in Adults

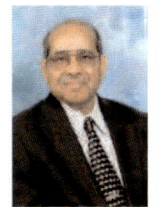

Guest Editor: *P. Syamasundar Rao, MD*

Department of Pediatrics, Division of Pediatric Cardiology, The University of Texas-Houston Medical School/Children's Memorial Hermann Hospital, Houston, Texas
E-mail: p.syamasundar.rao@uth.tmc.edu

The incidence of con- genital heart defects (CHD) is approximately 8 per 1,000 live births. With the advances in the diagnosis and management of CHD, a large number of these children survive into adulthood. The current estimate of adults with CHD is in the order of 1 million in the U.S. alone. Because of the high prevalence of coronary heart disease in adults, the major emphasis in training cardiologists is in the area of adult coronary heart disease. Similarly, most cardiologists' experience is predominantly in adult coronary heart disease. Consequently, there is a relative lack of expertise in the arena of CHD in the adult cardiology community. Therefore, it is important that efforts be made to impart CHD knowledge n the continuing medical education of cardiologists. The symposium on CHD in this and the next issue of the *Journal* is an attempt to fulfill this requirement.

The type of CHD seen in adults is different from that seen n childhood. The type of adult heart disease can best be understood by examining the incidence of the CHD at centers that care for adults with CHD. At one center, the outpatients seen were analyzed and the frequency, in descending order, was as follows: left-to-right shunts, left ventricular (LV) outflow tract obstruction, cyanotic heart defects, arrhythmias and pulmonary stenosis. In another institution, the defects were: left- o-right shunts, tetralogy of Fallot, single ventricle, LV outflow tract obstruction and transposition of the great arteries (TGA). The distribution of the inpatient population was slightly different: single-ventricle lesions including tricuspid atresia, secundum atrial septal defects (ASDs), Eisenmenger syndrome...

Figure 10. A copy of the introduction to a symposium on "Structural Heart Disease in Adults" in *The Journal of Invasive Cardiology* that I organized and edited.

FOCUS: STRUCTURAL HEART DISEASE

Figure 11. A copy of the contents of a symposium on "Structural Heart Disease in Adults" in *The Journal of Invasive Cardiology* that I organized and edited.

I was invited by Dr. David Holmes Jr, Editor-in-Chief of *The Current Interventional Cardiology Reports* to organize and edit the "Pediatric Interventional Cardiology" section. This is a quarterly publication of the *Current Science, Inc.*, Philadelphia, PA. Three sample issues are shown in figures 12, 13, and 14. These papers addressed transcatheter occlusion of atrial septal defects, patent ductus arteriosus and ventricular septal defects by respective experts in the field.

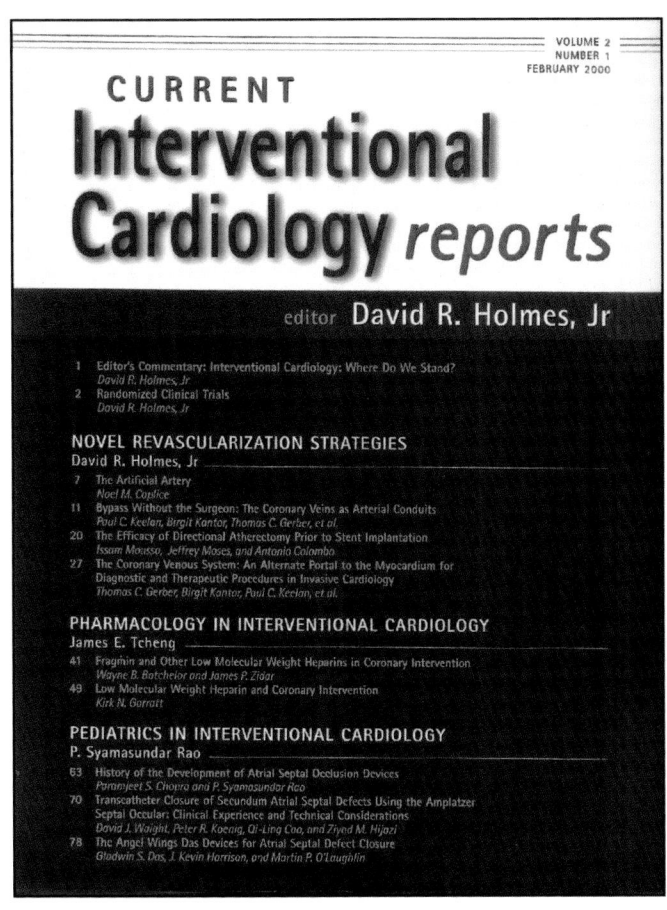

Figure 12. Photograph of the cover page of *The Current Interventional Cardiology Reports* (Vol. 2, No. 1, 2000) in which a section on "Pediatric Interventional Cardiology" that I organized and edited was published.

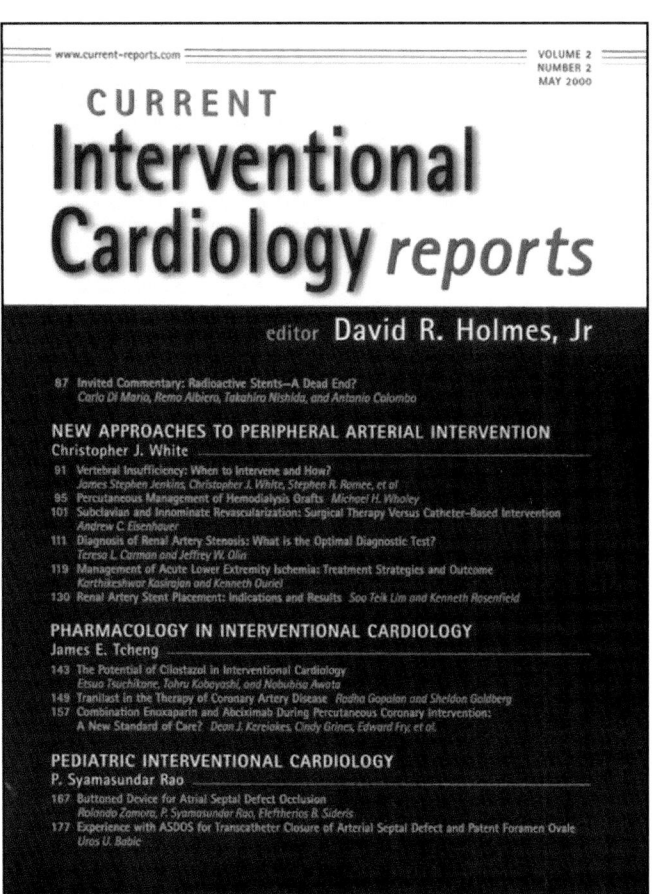

Figure 13. Photograph of the cover page of *The Current Interventional Cardiology Reports* (Vol. 2, No. 2, 2000) in which a section on "Pediatric Interventional Cardiology" that I organized and edited was published.

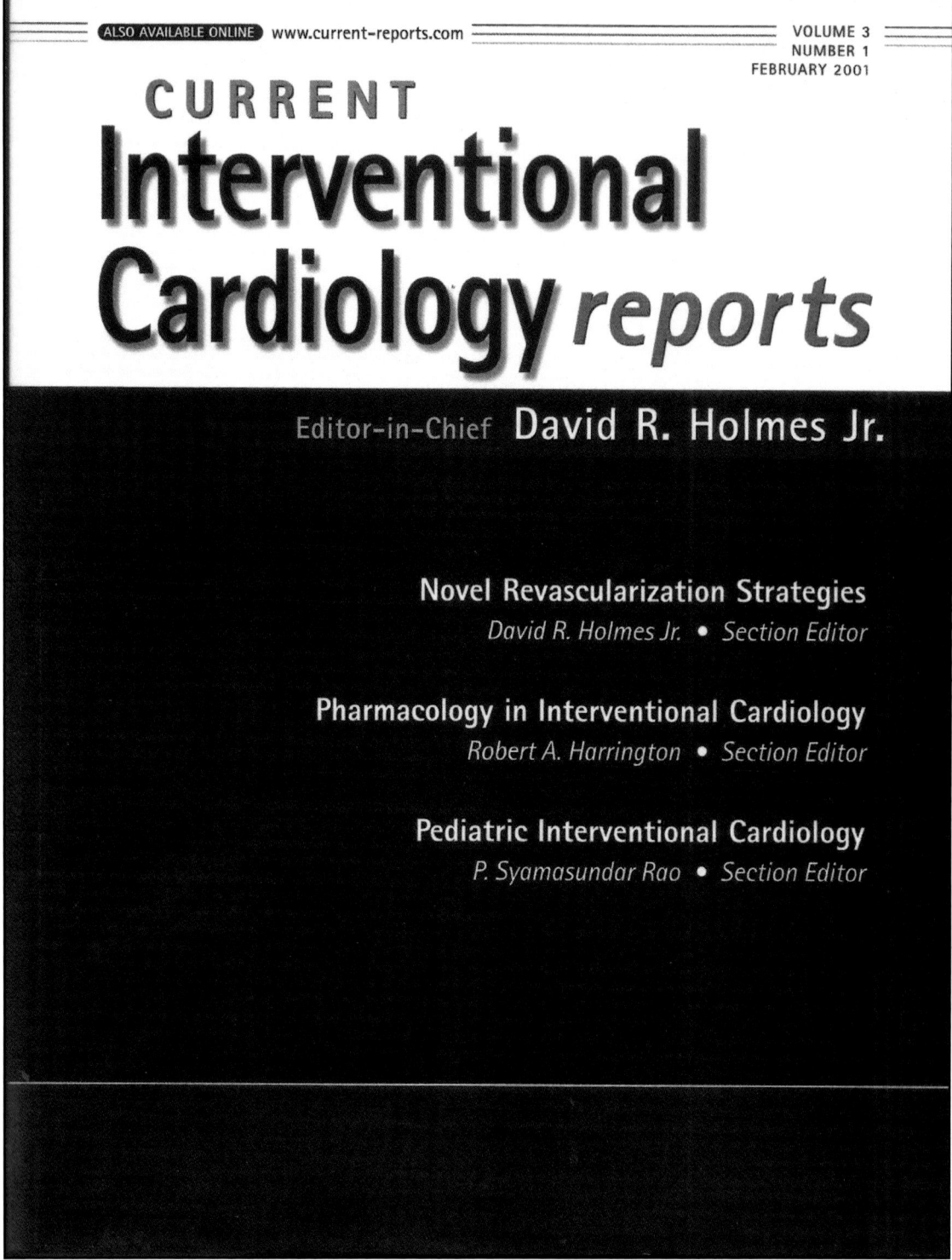

Figure 14. Photograph of the cover page of *The Current Interventional Cardiology Reports* (Vol. 3, No. 1, 2001) in which a special section on "Pediatric Interventional Cardiology" that I organized and edited was published.

AD HOC EDITORIALS

These editorials[2,4-8,13,50,55,56,58,60,63] were written on a given subject that is considered to be of importance at that particular time. The editorials discussed the role of balloons, blades, plugs and umbrellas in the management of heart disease in infants and children,[2] how big a balloon and how many balloons should be used for pulmonary valvuloplasty,[4] indications for balloon pulmonary valvuloplasty,[5] which types of aortic coarctations should be balloon-dilated,[6] the methods and results of balloon angioplasty/valvuloplasty in CHD,[7,55] the issue of whether the use of the term "tricuspid atresia" is appropriate,[8] whether balloon angioplasty should be used instead of surgery for treatment of native aortic coarctation,[13] when and how atrial septal defects should be closed in adults,[50] methods and results of percutaneous occlusion of cardiac septal defects in children,[56] role of stents in the management of heart disease in children,[58] future directions in the management of aortic coarctation in young patients,[60] and prevention of sudden death in athletes.[63] The interested reader may review these papers at their discretion.[2,4-8,13,50,55,56,58,60,63]

EDITORIALS ON CONCURRENTLY PUBLISHED PAPERS

In general, these editorials[10-12,14,15,17-23,25-29,31-34,36-41,43-48,51-54,57,59,61,64] were requested by the Editor-in-Chiefs of the respective journals to be published concurrently with the original papers written by other investigators. The commentary generally included a historical perspective of the topic under question, review of the findings of the study along with a critique, and a perspective of the subject. These editorials discussed the following subjects:

1. Static balloon dilation of restrictive atrial septal defects (ASDs).[10,12]

2. Aortic rupture following balloon angioplasty of aortic coarctation.[11]

3. Balloon valvuloplasty in the neonate with critical pulmonary stenosis.[14]

4. Methods to use for transcatheter occlusion of patent ductus arteriosus.[15,17,22,32,45]

5. Role of stents in the treatment of aortic coarctation.[18]

6. History of pediatric therapeutic catheterization.[19]

7. Balloon pulmonary valvuloplasty.[20,36,43]

8. Transcatheter treatment of coarctation of the aorta (Balloon angioplasty of native coarctation of the aorta).[21,29]

9. Transcatheter closure of ASDs.[23,25,26,37,48]

10. Balloon angioplasty of fixed sub-aortic stenosis.[27]

11. Balloon aortic valvuloplasty.[28,64]

12. Coil occlusion of patent ductus arteriosus.[31]

13. Absorbable pulmonary artery band in tricuspid atresia.[33]

14. Concurrent balloon dilatation of stenosed aortopulmonary Gore-Tex shunts and branch pulmonary arteries.[34]

15. Balloon angioplasty in re-coarctation involving transverse aortic arch: Should protective balloon in the carotid artery be used?[38]

16. Percutaneous occlusion of complex atrial septal defects.[39,59]

17. Transcatheter management of platypnea-orthodeoxia syndrome.[40]

18. Cardiac function in juvenile rheumatoid arthritis.[41]

19. Cardiac function after percutaneous closure of patent foramen ovale (PFO).[44]

20. Protein-losing enteropathy following the Fontan operation.[46]

21. Perimembraneous ventricular septal defect closure with the Amplatzer device.[47]

22. Stents in the management of aortic coarctation in young children.[51]

23. Transcatheter interventions in critically ill neonates and infants with aortic coarctation.[52]

24. Left ventricular function after percutaneous occlusion of ASDs.[53]

25. Quest for the Ideal ASD/PFO closure device.[54]

26. Atrial electromechanical delay measured by tissue Doppler imaging in patients with secundum ASDs.[57]

27. Is intracardiac echocardiography essential for monitoring stent deployment across aortic coarctation?[61]

28. In the interest of conserving space, the above topics will not be detailed here, but the interested reader can refer to these publications.[10-12,14,15,17-23,25-29,31-34,36-41,43-48,51-54,57,59,61,64]

LETTERS TO THE EDITOR

I have contributed many letters to the editor.[65-102] The purpose of these letters varied from letter to letter and were constructed to present original data not suitable for a full paper, to point out omitting/ignoring previously published works of other investigators, misquoting prior publications, performing wrong type of statistical analysis, errors of interpretation of the data presented and/or a combination thereof. The interested reader may review these publications,[65-102] as they see fit.

REFERENCES

1. Rao PS, "Foreword to pediatric cardiology seminar," *Paediatrician 1978*; 7:1-2.

2. Rao PS, "Balloons, blades, plugs and umbrellas in the treatment of heart disease in infants and children (Editorial)," *Ann Saudi Med 1987*; 7:85-7.

3. Rao PS, "Preface to the pediatric cardiology issue," *Indian J. Pediatr 1988*; 55:7-9.

4. Rao PS, "How big a balloon and how many balloons for pulmonary valvuloplasty (Editorial)," *Am Heart J 1988*; 116:577-80.

5. Rao PS, "Indications for balloon pulmonary valvuloplasty (Editorial)," *Amer Heart J 1988*; 116:1661-2.

6. Rao PS, "Which aortic coarctations should we balloon-dilate? (Editorial)," *Amer Heart J 1989*; 117:787-9.

7. Rao PS, "Balloon angioplasty/valvuloplasty in congenital heart disease (Editorial)," *J Invasive Cardiol 1990*; 2:129-36.

8. Rao PS, "Is the term "tricuspid atresia" appropriate? (Editorial)," *Am J Cardiol 1990*; 66:1251-4.

9. Rao PS, "Pediatric cardiology symposium (Editorial)," *Indian J Pediat 1991*; 58:439-440.

10. Rao PS, "Static balloon dilation of restrictive atrial septal defects (Editorial)," *J Saudi Heart Assoc 1992*; 4:55-8.

11. Rao PS, "Aortic rupture following balloon angioplasty of aortic coarctation (Editorial)," *Am Heart J 1993*; 125:1205-6.

12. Rao PS, "Static balloon dilation of atrial septum (Editorial)," *Am Heart J 1993*; 125:1826-7.

13. Rao PS, "Should balloon angioplasty be used instead of surgery for native aortic coarctation? (Editorial)," *Br Heart J 1995*; 74:578-9.

14. Rao PS, "Balloon valvuloplasty in the neonate with critical pulmonary stenosis (Editorial)," *J Am Coll Cardiol 1996*; 27:479-80.

15. Rao PS, "Which method to use for transcatheter occlusion of patent ductus arteriosus? (Editorial)," *Cathet Cardiovasc Diag 1996*; 39:49-51.

16. Rao PS, "Catheter-based therapy in children with heart defects (Editorial)," *J Invasive Cardiol 1996*; 8:A4-6.

17. Rao PS, "Transcatheter occlusion of patent ductus arteriosus: Which method to use and which ductus to close? (Editorial)," *Am Heart J 1996*; 132:905-9.

18. Rao PS, "Stents in the treatment of aortic coarctation (Editorial)," *J Am Coll Cardiol 1997*; 30:1853-5.

19. Rao PS, "Commentary on Mullins CE. History of pediatric interventional catheterization: Pediatric therapeutic catheterization," *Pediat Cardiol 1998*; 19:8.

20. Rao PS, "Commentary on Rome JJ. Balloon pulmonary valvuloplasty," *Pediat Cardiol 1998*; 19:25.

21. Rao PS, "Commentary on Ovaert C, et al, "Transcatheter treatment of coarctation of the aorta: A review," *Pediat Cardiol 1998*; 19:45.

22. Rao PS, "Commentary on Shim D, Beekman RH, III. Transcatheter management of patent ductus arteriosus," Pediat Cardiol 1998; 19:72.

23. Rao PS, "Commentary on Latson LA. Per-catheter ASD closure," *Pediat Cardiol 1998*; 19:94.

24. Rao PS, "Symposium on pediatric cardiology (Editorial)," *Indian J Pediat 1998*; 65:11-12.

25. Rao PS, "Transcatheter closure of atrial septal defect: Are we there yet? (Editorial)," *J Am Coll Cardiol 1998*; 31:1117-9.

26. Rao PS, "Closure devices for atrial septal defect: Which one to choose? (Editorial)," *Indian Heart J 1998*; 50:379-83.

27. Rao PS, "Balloon angioplasty of fixed subaortic stenosis (Editorial)," *J Invasive Cardiol 1999*; 11:197-9.

28. Chopra PS, Rao PS, "Balloon aortic valvuloplasty in children (Editorial)," J Invasive Cardiol 1999; 11:277-9.

29. Rao PS, "Balloon angioplasty of native coarctation of the aorta (Editorial)," *J Invasive Cardiol 2000*; 12:407-9.

30. Rao PS, "Interventional pediatric cardiology: Introduction (Editorial)," *J Invasive Cardiol 2001*; 13:29-30.

31. Rao PS, "Coil occlusion of patent ductus arteriosus (Editorial)," *J Invasive Cardiol 2001*; 13:36-8.

32. Rao PS, "Transcatheter closure of moderate-to-large patent ductus arteriosus (Editorial)," *J Invasive Cardiol 2001*; 13: 303-306.

33. Rao PS, "Absorbable pulmonary artery band in tricuspid atresia (Editorial)," *Ann Thorac Surg 2001*; 71:361-2.

34. Rao PS, "Concurrent balloon dilatation of stenosed aortopulmonary Gore-Tex shunts and branch pulmonary arteries (Editorial)," *J Am Coll Cardiol 2001*; 37:948-950.

35. Saxena A and Rao PS, "The practice of pediatric cardiology – Symposium on pediatric cardiology (Editorial)," *Indian J Pediat 2002*; 69:313-4.

36. Rao PS, "Balloon pulmonary valvuloplasty (Editorial)," *J Saudi Heart Assoc 2003*; 15:1-4.

37. Rao PS, "Catheter closure of atrial septal defects (Editorial)," *J Invasive Cardiol 2003*; 15:398-400.

38. Rao PS, "Balloon angioplasty in recoarctation involving transverse aortic arch: Should protective balloon in the carotid artery be used? (Editorial)," *Cath Cardiovasc Intervent 2003*; 60:534-5.

39. Nagm AM and Rao PS, "Percutaneous occlusion of complex atrial septal defects (Editorial)," *J Invasive Cardiol 2004*; 16:123-5.

40. Rao PS, "Transcatheter management of platypnea-orthodeoxia syndrome (Editorial)," *J Invasive Cardiol 2004*; 16:583-4.

41. Gupta M and Rao PS, "Cardiac function in juvenile rheumatoid arthritis (Editorial)," *J Postgrad Med 2004*; 50:266-7.

42. Rao PS, "Introduction of pediatric cardiology symposium – I: Pediatric Cardiology (Editorial)," *Indian J Pediatr 2005*; 72:493.

43. Rao PS, "Balloon pulmonary valvuloplasty in children (Editorial)," *J Invasive Cardiol 2005*; 17:323-325.

44. Rao PS and Lorch S, "Cardiac function after percutaneous closure of patent foramen ovale (Editorial)," *J Invasive Cardiol 2007*; 19:255-6.

45. Rao PS, "Percutaneous closure of patent ductus arteriosus: State of the art (Editorial)," *J Invasive Cardiol 2007*; 19:299-302.

46. Rao PS, "Protein-losing enteropathy following the Fontan operation (Editorial)," *J Invasive Cardiol 2007*; 19:447-8.

47. Rao PS, "Perimembraneous ventricular septal defect closure with the Amplatzer device (Editorial)," *J Invasive Cardiol 2008*; 20:217-8.

48. Rao PS, "Continued development of devices for transcatheter closure of atrial septal defects (Editorial)," *J Invasive Cardiol 2008*; 20:284-5.

49. Rao PS, "Focus: Structural heart disease in adults (Editorial)," *J Invasive Cardiol 2008*; 20:A6-A11.

50. Rao PS, "Focus: Atrial septal defects, Structural heart disease in adults (Editorial)," *J Invasive Cardiol 2009*; 21:A6-A10.

51. Rao PS, "Stents in the management of aortic coarctation in young children (Editorial)," *J Am Coll Cardiol 2009*; 2:884-6.

52. Rao PS, "Transcatheter interventions in critically ill neonates and infants with aortic coarctation (Editorial)," *Annals of Pediat Cardiol 2009*; 2:116-9.

53. Rao PS and Lorch S, "Left ventricular function after percutaneous occlusion of atrial septal defects (Editorial)," *Echocardiography 2010*; 27:351-3.

54. Balaguru D and Rao PS, "Quest for the Ideal ASD/PFO Closure Device Continues (Editorial)," *J Invasive Cardiol 2010*; 22:188-9.

55. Rao PS, "Balloon valvuloplasty and angioplasty in pediatric practice," *Pediatr Therapeut 2011*, Vol. 1, Issue 3. DOI: 10.4172/2161-0665.1000e103

56. Rao PS, "Percutaneous occlusion of cardiac defects in children," *Pediatr Therapeut 2012*, Volume 2, Issue 3. DOI: 10.4172/2161-0665.1000e107

57. Biliciler-Denktas G and Rao PS, "Atrial electromechanical delay measured by tissue Doppler imaging in patients with secundum atrial septal defects (Editorial)," *Echocardiography 2013*; 30:619-20. DOI: 10.1111/echo.12251

58. Rao PS, "Stents in the management of heart disease in children (Editorial)," *Pediat Therapeut 2013*, 3(2):e120. Available at DOI: 10.4172/2161-0665.1000e120.

59. Rao PS, "Transcatheter closure of complex atrial septal defects (Editorial)," *Echocardiography 2014*; 31:1173-6.

60. Rao PS, "Future directions in the management of aortic coarctation in young patients," *Pediat Therapeut 2014*; 4: e125. Available at DOI:10.4172/2161-0665.1000e125.

61. Rao PS, "Is intracardiac echocardiography essential for monitoring stent deployment across aortic coarctation? (Editorial)," *Echocardiography 2015*; 32:731-3. Available at DOI: 10.1111/echo.12905, Epub 2015, February 13, PMID: 25684662.

62. Rao PS, "What does the pediatrician needs to know about heart defects in children? (Editorial)," *Indian J Pediatr. 2015*, September 14 [Epub ahead of print], No abstract available, PMID: 26365157.

63. Rao PS, "Prevention of sudden death in athletes," *Pediat Therapeut 2015*, August 20; 5:e129. Available at DOI: 10.4172/2161-0665.1000e129

64. Rao PS, "Balloon aortic valvuloplasty (Editorial)," *Indian Heart Journal 2016*; 68:592-5.

65. Rao PS, "Left ventricular obstruction in double outlet right ventricle (Letter)," *Amer Heart J 1972*; 83:389-90.

66. Rao PS, "Imperforate Ebstein's anomaly of the tricuspid valve (Letter)," *Brit Heart J 1976*; 38:1108.

67. Rao PS, "Complications of pulmonary vein angiography (Letter)," *Brit Heart J 1980*; 43:124.

68. Rao PS, Moore HV and Strong WB, "Surgery for mitral atresia and interatrial obstruction without pulmonic stenosis (Letter)," *Circulation 1980*; 62:201-2.

69. Rao PS, "Physiologically advantageous ventricular septal defects (Letter)," *Pediatr Cardiol 1983*; 4:59-62.

70. Rao PS and Whisennand HW, "Chylopericardium (Letter)," *Ann Thorac Surg 1983*; 36:494.

71. Rao PS, "Chylopericardium following Blalock-Taussig anastomosis (Letter)," *J Thorac Cardiovasc Surg 1984*; 87:642.

72. Rao PS, "Anomalous connection of the right superior vena cava to the left atrium (Letter)," *J Amer Coll Cardiol 1984*; 4:650-1.

73. Rao PS, "Comparison of single and double balloon valvuloplasty in children with aortic stenosis (Letter)," *J Am Coll Cardiol 1989*; 13:1216-7.

74. Rao PS, "Balloon rupture during valvuloplasty (letter)," *Am Heart J 1990*; 119:1441.

75. Rao PS, "Balloon angioplasty of native coarctations (Letter)," *Am J Cardiol 1990*; 66:1401.

76. Rao PS and Thapar MK, "Balloon pulmonary valvuloplasty (Reply to Letter)," *Am Heart J 1991*; 121:1839-40.

77. Rao PS, "Tricuspid atresia with common arterial trunk (Letter)," *Internat J Cardiol 1991*; 30:367-8.

78. Rao PS, "Pseudoaneurysm following balloon angioplasty (Letter)," *Cathet Cardiovasc Diag 1991*; 23:150-3.

79. Rao PS, "Balloon angioplasty of native aortic coarctation (Letter)," *Internat J Cardiol 1991*; 31:363-7.

80. Rao PS, "Subaortic obstruction after pulmonary artery banding in patients with tricuspid atresia and double-inlet left ventricle and ventriculoarterial discordance (Letter)," *J Am Coll Cardiol 1991*; 18:1885-6.

81. Rao PS, "Fatal aortic rupture following balloon angioplasty of aortic recoarctation (Letter)," *Br Heart J 1991*; 66:406-7.

82. Rao PS, "Spontaneous closure of ventricular septal defects (Letter)," *Pediat Cardiol 1992*; 13:190-1.

83. Rao PS, "Balloon dilatation of supravalvar pulmonary stenosis after arterial switch procedure for complete transposition (Letter)," *Br Heart J 1992*; 67:204-5.

84. Rao PS, "Balloon angioplasty of native aortic coarctation (Letter)," *J Am Coll Cardiol 1992*; 20:749-52.

85. Rao PS and Chopra PS, "Balloon angioplasty of aortic coarctation (Letter)," *Ann Thorac Surg 1992*; 54:599-602.

86. Rao PS, "Balloon angioplasty of aortic recoarctation (Letter)," *Am J. Cardiol 1993*; 71:256.

87. Rao PS, "Neurologic complications following balloon angioplasty (Letter)," *Pediat Cardiol 1993*; 14:63-4.

88. Rao PS, "Technique of balloon pulmonary valvuloplasty in the neonate (Letter)," *J Am Coll Cardiol 1994*; 23:1735.

89. Rao PS and Chopra PS, "Reply - The jury is still out regarding balloon therapy for native aortic coarctation (Letter)," *J Am Coll Cardiol 1994*; 24:1589-90.

90. Rao PS, "Afterload reduction for dilated cardiomyopathy (Letter)," *Pediat Cardiol 1995*; 16:51.

91. Rao PS, "Intussception of catheter sheath (Letter)," *Pediat Cardiol 1995*; 16:207.

92. Rao PS and Sideris EB, "Transcatheter occlusion of cardiac defects (Letter)," *Br Heart J 1995*; 73:585-6.

93. Rao PS, "Static balloon dilatation of the atrial septum (Letter)," *Pediat Cardiol 1996*; 17:349-50.

94. Rao PS, "Reply - Should balloon angioplasty be used instead of surgery for native aortic coarctation (Letter)," *Heart 1997*; 77:86-8.

95. Rao PS, "Balloon pulmonary valvuloplasty (Letter)," *Cathet Cardiovasc Diag 1997*; 40:427-8.

96. Rao PS and Jureidini SB, "Predictors of outcome of balloon angioplasty of native aortic coarctation (Letter)," *Circulation 1997*; 96:1057-9.

97. Rao PS and Sideris E.B, "Transcatheter closure of atrial septal defects (Letter)," *Heart 1999*; 82:644.

98. Rao PS, "Late pulmonary insufficiency after balloon dilatation of the pulmonary valve (Letter)," *Cathet Cardiovasc Intervent 2000*; 49:118-9.

99. Rao PS and Sideris EB, "Infant buttoned device (Letter)," *Cathet Cardiovasc Intervent 2000*; 50:125-6.

100. Rao PS, "Catheter-based device closure of Fontan fenestration (Letter)," *Cathet Cardiovasc Intervent 2001*; 52:407.

101. Rao PS, "Anterograde Transumbilical Venous Balloon Aortic Valvuloplasty (Letter)," *Cath Cardiovasc Intervent 2002*; 56:439.

102. Rao PS, "Anterograde balloon aortic valvuloplasty in the neonate via the umbilical vein (Letter)," *Cath Cardiovasc Intervent 2003*; 59:291-2.

103. Rao PS, "When and how should atrial septal defects be closed in adults?" *J Invasive Cardiol 2009*; 21:76-82.

CHAPTER 9

REVIEWS

INTRODUCTION

I published a number of reviews[1-132] over the years. Some of these reviews were commissioned by Chief Editors of the respective journals and others were initiated by me because of the importance of that particular subject at that particular time. Brief summaries of these reviews will be presented; however, if a given subject was dealt with in the prior chapters or in the book titled "Pediatric Cardiology: How It Has Evolved Over the last 50 Years," the reader will be referred to the respective chapter.

PHYSIOLOGICAL BASIS OF DIURETIC DRUGS

This review was prepared while I was in pediatric training, prior to starting fellowship in pediatric cardiology, as an assignment for the senior resident seminar. The selection of this particular subject was predicated on ensuing pediatric cardiology fellowship. The reason for selecting *The Journal of Indian Medical Association*[1] for publication was because of my plan to return to India following my training. The manuscript began with defining the components of the nephron followed by a detailed description of kidney function. Then, the review focused on the mechanism of action of each of the diuretic classes (as available in early 1970s), including osmotic diuretics (mannitol), acid forming salts (ammonium chloride), proximal tubular inhibitors (organic mercurials, thiazides, ethacrynic acid, furosemide, xanthines, and carbonic anhydrase inhibitors), and distal tubular inhibitors (aldosterone antagonists and aldosterone blocking agents). While the focus of the paper was on the mechanism of action, discussion of indications for use, dosages, onset of and duration of diuresis, and side effects of the diuretics was also included.[1]

PREVENTIVE ASPECTS OF HEART DISEASE IN INFANTS AND CHILDREN

Preventive aspects of heart disease in infants and children were reviewed in multiple publications,[2,8,9,12] resulting in culmination of a booklet in *The Current Problems in Pediatrics* in 1977.[13] In these reviews prevention of congenital heart disease (CHD), rheumatic fever, bacterial endocarditis, atherosclerosis, cardiac non-disease and miscellaneous were addressed.[2,8,9,12,13]

Congenital Heart Disease

Known causes of CHD as of that time were maternal rubella, ingestion of thalidomide during pregnancy, chromosomal anomalies and somatic syndrome complexes. Appropriate preventive measures are immunization with live-attenuated rubella vaccine and avoidance of unnecessary medications during pregnancy. Analysis of chromosomes and genetic counseling in families with an infant with Down's Syndrome may be helpful. Prenatal diagnosis of hereditary defects associated with CHD seems to be a promising area of prevention. The outlined etiologic factors account for less than five percent of CHD. Multi-factorial inheritance (genetic-environmental interaction) may be responsible for the majority of the CHD. Appropriate genetic counseling and quoting the risk of recurrence may be helpful to the parents. A greater understanding of the etiology and pathogenesis of CHD may produce more effective strategies for prevention. These reviews were nearly four decades old and the author has hoped for substantial advancement by this time. While significant understanding of gene mutations and extensive research on gene mapping has taken place, very few clinically applicable methods to prevent classic CHD are currently in vogue.

Acute Rheumatic Fever

Primary Prevention. Acute rheumatic fever (ARF) is causally related to group A ß-hemolytic streptococcal throat infection. Prevention of first attacks of ARF (primary prevention) by prompt identification and adequate treatment of streptococcal pharyngitis was recommended.

Secondary Prevention. Prevention of recurrences of ARF in patients who had prior ARF is described as the secondary prevention. This is best done with monthly intramuscular injections of long-acting Benzathine penicillin. Oral penicillin may be effective, but is associated with higher rates of recurrence than with intramuscular injections and this is probably related to noncompliance when oral regimen was pursued. Patients with penicillin allergy may receive oral sulfadiazine.

While the ARF is practically non-existent in the developed countries at the present time, it continues to be significant in developing countries.

Bacterial Endocarditis

Oro-dental or other surgical procedures produce transitory bacteremia and these bacteria may lodge on the diseased or deformed heart valves or endocardium and cause endocarditis. Antibiotics are recommended for preventing endocarditis in any patient with a congenital or acquired heart defect one to two hours prior to, and for two days following any potentially bacteremia-producing procedure. Types of antibiotics used are tailored to the bacteremia producing procedure. Recently, however, some of these recommendations were modified by the American Heart Association.

Atherosclerosis

The etiology of atherosclerosis was not clearly established. In longitudinal epidemiologic studies, the concept of "risk factors" was developed, which indicates any personal characteristic(s) that is associated with a higher than average incidence of atherosclerosis. The major risk factors identified were hyperlipidemia, hypertension, and smoking. The minor risk factors were sedentary living habits, obesity, hyperglycemia, family history of premature (≤ 50 years of age) atherosclerotic event, and psycho-social tension. Risk factor modification for the adult population to reduce the incidence of atherosclerosis appears to be generally accepted. Despite lack of concrete evidence for effectiveness of risk factor modification in the pediatric age group, many groups of workers recommend such a modification. These include a low fat and low-cholesterol diet for all children (beyond infancy), screening for hyperlipidemia and prompt treatment if detected, routine blood pressure recording in the pediatrician's office, lowering of dietary salt intake, discouraging cigarette smoking, prevention (or early treatment) of obesity, encouraging moderate exercise, and monitoring carbohydrate tolerance of the progeny of diabetic patients. Identification of children at risk by a family history of premature onset of an atherosclerotic event may be more practical because of a higher yield. These and the progeny of persons with hypertension, diabetes mellitus and hyperlipidemia should be screened for hyperlipidemia, hypertension (and treated appropriately if present) and counseled as to proper nutrition, exercise, and avoidance of smoking. Health education of children and the population at large with regard to the current knowledge of risk factors of coronary heart disease and possible methods of prevention is necessary if programs for prevention of atherosclerosis are to be effective. Even though these reviews were more than four decades old, these recommendations are still valid.

Cardiac Non-disease

When dealing with children with functional (innocent) heart murmurs and mild organic heart disease, the pediatrician and the pediatric cardiologist should provide appropriate counseling to ensure that Cardiac Non-disease is not produced.

Miscellaneous

Finally, the miscellaneous group includes prevention of adverse psychological effects of heart disease and prevention of irreversible damage to cardiovascular structures and complications in patients with congenital or acquired heart disease by timely and appropriate psychological, medical and/or surgical intervention.

EARLY IDENTIFICATION OF THE NEONATE WITH SERIOUS HEART DISEASE

Prompt identification of neonates with significant CHD, their transport to a medical center equipped to diagnose and treat such infants and immediate diagnosis, and medical/trans-catheter/surgical management, as appropriate (Figure 1) is highly important if we are to accrue the benefits of advances in the recent diagnostic and therapeutic techniques. These concepts were reviewed from time to time to educate primary care physicians[3,7,22,89,90] and was reviewed in different journals.

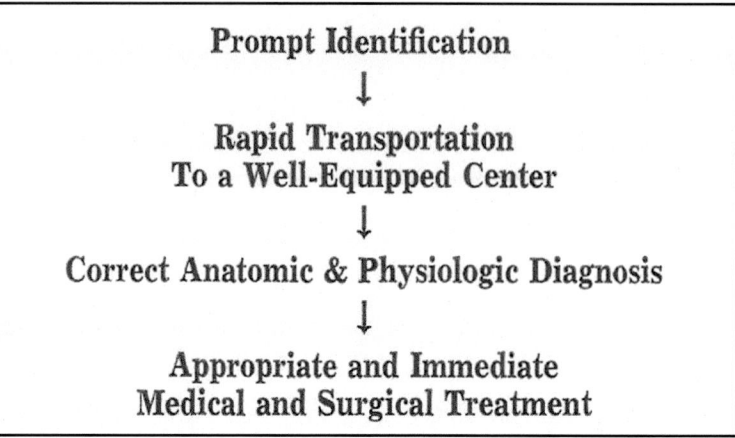

Figure 1. Steps essential in the management of heart disease in neonates.
Reproduced from Rao PS and Strong WB, *J Med Assoc of Georgia 1974*;
63:430-3.

These reviews emphasized that early detection of newborn infants with serious heart disease is the first important step in their subsequent accurate diagnosis and prompt treatment. The presentations focused on the early identification of functionally important cardiac abnormality by careful attention to color, respiratory pattern, activity and other physical findings by the physician caring for the newborn infants. Functional abnormality of the cardiovascular system is recognized by the presence of cyanosis, signs of congestive heart failure, respiratory distress (tachypnea, hyperpnea, retractions) and/or lethargy and lack of spontaneous movement. Chest x-ray and blood gas determination are also helpful tools in this regard. The role of auscultation and electrocardiogram is de-emphasized as far as their usefulness is concerned in the identification of the neonate with heart disease by the primary physician.

Once an infant with CHD is identified, immediate transfer to a regional pediatric cardiology center equipped to care for neonatal CHD babies should arranged. While the transport facilities were not well developed in the beginning, they gradually improved over time. During the process of identification and transfer, prevention of hypothermia, monitoring for and prompt treatment of hypoglycemia and hypocalcemia and monitoring acid-base status and treating it if abnormal (metabolic acidosis – $NaHCO_3$; respiratory acidosis – suction, intubation, assisted ventilation) should be undertaken. Once the infant arrives at the tertiary care center, correct anatomic and physiologic diagnosis followed by appropriate and immediate medical and/or surgical treatment should be instituted.[3,7,22,89,90] These principles, as outlined in my reviews in the past, remain valid today; although, a new tool, pulse oximetry screening for detecting CHDs in the newborn, as reviewed elsewhere,[133] seems to be effective in detecting otherwise unidentified cases.

DIGITALIS TOXICITY IN INFANTS AND CHILDREN

Two major types of digitalis intoxication are recognized in the pediatric patients: First is accidental glycoside ingestion, and the second is therapeutic use of digoxin in children with heart disease. Two illustrative cases were presented in this review, representing the above two types. Evaluation of the patient includes clinical signs and symptoms, serum electrolytes, electrocardiogram (ECG) and serum digoxin levels. Early recognition and treatment of digitalis toxicity is essential. The clinical usefulness of serum digoxin levels in the management of children with suspected digitalis toxicity was discussed as were the methods of management.[4] With remarkable decrease in the use of digoxin in the management of congestive heart failure (CHF) at the present time, digoxin toxicity is not frequently seen in pediatric cardiology practice today.

INFECTIVE ENDOCARDITIS

I was involved in reviews of infective endocarditis (IE) of all age groups[5] at UCLA Medical Center, Los Angeles, California, and infective endocarditis in the pediatric patients[14,15] at the Medical College of Georgia Hospitals, Augusta, Georgia.

The first review involved fifty consecutive patients with sub-acute bacterial endocarditis (SBE) seen between 1965 and 1970. Data were summarized concerning the clinical picture, changes in etiology and antibiotic sensitivities and therapy, laboratory diagnosis, and complications in one figure and thirteen tables. The study has documented the changing nature of SBE over the years. The study also examined recurrent SBE and a new phenomenon, endocarditis occurring in otherwise normal hearts.[5] In this review, the literature was examined with emphasis on newer modifications in the diagnosis and therapy. These center around the variations in clinical picture, infected site in patients with heart disease and those with normal hearts, endocarditis associated with cardiac operations, and particularly, the increasing incidence of infection on grafts used in cardiovascular repair. The indications and hazards of emergency operation for infected graft material were also examined. The continuing emergence of new strains of bacteria and fungi was discussed in terms of altered patient immunity, increased use of antibiotics and more radical surgical and medical procedures. Finally, a short section was presented on current concepts and recommendations concerning prevention and prophylaxis for endocarditis. Infective endocarditis continues to be a changing disease in which the former classical picture is seldom seen. Clinical suspicion and early diagnosis remain the most important factors in determining success of either the medical or the surgical treatment.

The second of the reviews[14,15] also involved fifty patients with SBE, but was confined to children seen at the Medical College of Georgia Hospitals, Augusta, Georgia. Data were summarized in one figure and eight tables. The peak incidence of IE was between eleven and fifteen years. Both sexes were equally affected. Patients with congenital or acquired heart disease tend to have hemodynamic trauma to the endocardium and vascular endothelium. These sites form the nidus for circulating bacteria of either spontaneous origin or the result of oro-dental, genitourinary or other surgery or procedures and produce vegetations characteristic of infective endocarditis. The location of the vegetation is dependent upon the predisposing cardiac lesion. Embolic phenomenon is another cardinal feature of endocarditis and may occur in any organ system. Although, a large variety of microbes have been known to cause endocarditis, streptococci and staphylococci remain the most frequent offenders. Clinical diagnosis of infective endocarditis is difficult because of the insidious onset and varied clinical features. A high degree of suspicion is essential for early diagnosis. Any patient with known heart disease and unexplained fever should be a suspect for endocarditis. Splenomegaly, petechiae and embolic phenomena support this diagnosis. New or changing murmurs, splinter hemorrhages, Osler's nodes, Janeway's lesions and Roth's spots may be present. Elevated sedimentation rate, microscopic hematuria, leukocytosis with a shift-to-the-left, and anemia may further support the diagnosis. Congenital or acquired heart disease and fever are all that will be present in many cases. Only isolation of the causative agent from the blood can confirm the diagnosis. General principles of management include selection of antibiotics based on the antibiotic sensitivities of the causative organism, use of bactericidal rather than bacteriostatic drugs, usage of a combination of two or more antibiotics to enhance the synergic bactericidal activity, and their administration by intravenous route for prolonged periods (six weeks). Monitoring the serum bactericidal activity to confirm the biological effectiveness of the antibiotics used and adjusting the level from 1:8 to 1:16 was recommended. Specific drug therapy for each type of endocarditis was discussed. Supportive measures and indications for surgical intervention were also discussed. A summary of preventive aspects of infective endocarditis that were in vogue at that time was also presented.[14,15]

PRESSURE AND ENERGY IN CARDIOVASCULAR CHAMBERS

Issues related to pressure and energy in cardiovascular chambers,[6] both in terms of "Pressure Gradient in the Absence of Obstruction/Stenosis" and "Lack of Pressure Gradient in the Presence of Multiple Obstructions," were discussed in the chapter on "Cardiac Catheterization and Cineangiography" in the book titled "Pediatric Cardiology: How It Has Evolved Over the last 50 Years" and will not be repeated here.

CARDIAC CATHETERIZATION IN INFANCY AND CHILDHOOD

Cardiac catheterization in infancy and childhood[10] was also reviewed in the chapter on "Cardiac Catheterization and Cineangiography" in the book titled "Pediatric Cardiology: How It Has Evolved Over the last 50 Years" and will not be repeated here.

POLYSPLENIA SYNDROME

In Polysplenia Syndrome, there are two or more splenic masses of equal size, each of which is smaller than the normal spleen, but the total amount of splenic tissue is equal to a normal-sized spleen. The review describes the extra-cardiac anomalies and cardiac defects seen with Polysplenia Syndrome, comparing/contrasting with those of Asplenia Syndrome.[11] This is followed by a detailed presentation of clinical diagnosis of Polysplenia Syndrome.[11]

PRESENT STATUS OF SURGERY IN CONGENITAL HEART DISEASE

Present status of surgery in CHD was initially reviewed in 1981,[16] and the subject was revisited in 1991.[43] In the first paper,[16] a brief review of the historical aspects of surgery for CHD was first presented. Palliative procedures were designed to improve physiologic abnormalities, such as systemic artery (or venous) to pulmonary artery shunts of various types to augment pulmonary blood flow, banding of the pulmonary artery to decrease the pulmonary blood flow and balloon, blade, or surgical atrial septostomy to improve intra-cardiac mixing have been carried out with success. The role of prostaglandin E₁ (PGE₁) for ductal dilation in patients with severe right ventricular out-flow tract obstruction, including our initial experience (Figure 2) was described. The recommendations for dosage of PGE₁ infusion (0.05 to 0.1 mcg/kg/min) and the ductal dependent lesions in which PGE₁ is useful were tabulated (Table I). In babies with pulmonary oligemia, Blalock-Taussig shunt or its latest modifications was recommended in contradistinction other types of shunts.[16]

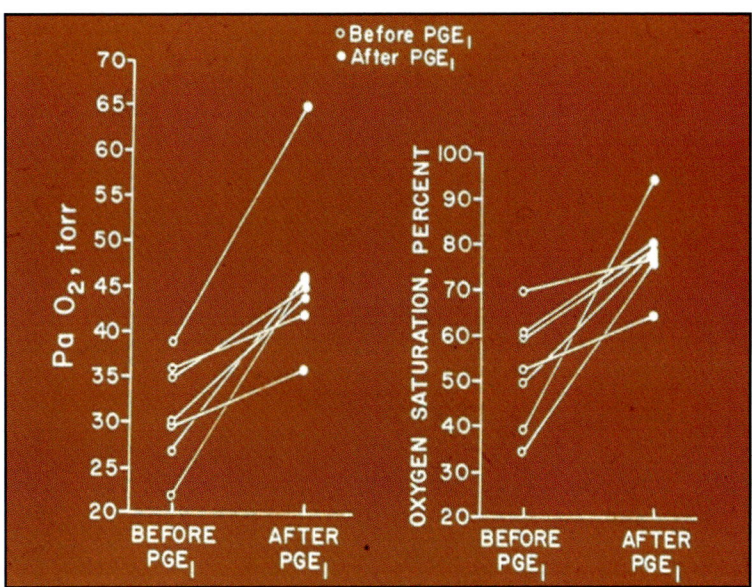

Figure 2. . The effect of prostaglandin E₁ (PGE₁) infusion on the systemic arterial tension (PaO₂) (left panel) and oxygen saturation (right panel) in seven infants with cyanotic congenital heart disease and ductal dependent pulmonary blood flow. Note significant increase in PaO₂ and O₂ saturation in each case. Open circles represent values before PGE₁ and closed circles, after PGE₁ administration. Reproduced from Rao PS, Indian J Pediatr 1981; 49:349-63.

Table I. Lesions with Ductal Dependent Pulmonary Blood Flow

Pulmonary atresia with intact ventricular septum
Pulmonary atresia with ventricular septal defect
Severe tetralogy of Fallot
Complex CHD with pulmonary atresia or severe stenosis
Tricuspid atresia
Critical pulmonary stenosis
Ebstein's anomaly of tricuspid valve
Hypoplastic right ventricle

CHD, Cyanotic Heart Disease. Reproduced from Rao PS, *Indian J Pediatr 1981*; 49:349-63.

With regard to corrective surgery, it was stated that most of the CHD can be corrected by open heart surgical techniques; the defects that can be operated without prior palliative surgery (Table II) and those that require prior palliation (Table III) were listed. The surgical mortality rates for common acyanotic and cyanotic CHD, as observed at the Medical College of Georgia in Augusta and from the literature were tabulated in tables IV and V, respectively of the original publication,[16] for the interested reader. It was noted that the post-operative mortality has declined over the years and the mortality rate for the simple defects was less than 5 percent and for complex defects it is slightly higher, around 10 percent, as of the time of the review.[16]

Table II. Lesions Which Can be Primarily Repaired Without Prior Palliative Procedures

1. Acyanotic lesions
a. *Left to right to shunt*
Atrial septal defect
Ventricular septal defect
Patent ductus arteriosus
Endocardial cushion defect
Partial anomalous pulmonary venous connection
b. *Obstructive lesions*
Aortic stenosis
Coarctation of the aorta
Interrupted aortic arch
Pulmonic stenosis
2. Cyanotic lesions
Tetralogy of Fallot
Total anomalous pulmonary venous connection
Single atrium
Truncus arteriosus
Double outlet right ventricle

Reproduced from Rao PS, *Indian J Pediatr. 1981*; 49:349-63.

Table III. Lesions Requiring Prior Palliation

Transposition of the great arteries
Pulmonary atresia
Tricuspid atresia
Single ventricle
Double outlet right ventricle

Reproduced from Rao PS, *Indian J Pediatr 1981*; 49:349-63.

Then, recent surgical advances, as of the time of that review were discussed and include early total surgical correction for tetralogy of Fallot, Mustard and Jatene operations for the transposition of the great arteries, Fontan operation and its newer modifications for tricuspid atresia, intra-ventricular septation or modified Fontan for single ventricle, new operations for hypoplastic left heart syndrome and newer prosthetic valves, particularly left ventricular apex to descending aorta conduit. In the final part of the paper, potential for non-surgical, catheter closure atrial septal defect (ASD) and patent ductus arteriosus (PDA) was reviewed.[16]

In the second review published in 1991,[43] a decade after the first review, largely updates the initial review. The historical aspects, palliative management, and corrective surgery for most defects are similar to those described in the first review. Advances in surgical management of cyanotic CHD, namely, early primary correction of tetralogy of Fallot (TOF), arterial switch procedure for transposition of the great arteries (TGA), Fontan operation for tricuspid atresia and single ventricle, Norwood procedure and cardiac transplantation for hypoplastic left heart syndrome (HLHS) were reviewed. Advances in prosthetic valves and improved techniques for myocardial preservation were also examined.[43]

DEXTROCARDIA: SYSTEMATIC APPROACH TO DIFFERENTIAL DIAGNOSIS

In this paper, a systematic approach is provided to the clinician with an appropriate formulation for evaluating patients with dextrocardia.[17] Initially definitions of various terms used, namely, dextrocardia, levocardia, mesocardia, situs solitus, situs inversus, situs inversus totalis, isolated dextrocardia and isolated levocardia were presented. It was stated that the diagnostic approach is similar in dextrocardia, levocardia, and mesocardia. A reasonable diagnosis may be arrived by answering five questions:

1. Why is the heart on the right side of the chest? (Is it intrinsic dextrocardia or dextroposition of the heart?)

2. What is the visceroatrial situs?

3. Where are the ventricles located in relation to each other?

4. What is the visceroatrial-to-ventricular relationship?

5. What is the conotruncal relationship?

In the majority of cases, physical examination, chest x-ray, ECG, echocardiogram, and cardiac catheterization with selective cineangiography may be required for complete diagnosis. However, a reasonable and almost complete diagnosis may be made by noninvasive means. Multiple figures showing examples of most of the scenarios were presented in this review. Once these five questions are answered, the presence of other defects such as ventricular septal defect (VSD), pulmonary stenosis (PS) and other defects may be determined by conventional means.

Following the discussion of visceroatrial situs, features of asplenia and polysplenia syndrome were also reviewed. In more recent book chapters,[134-136] the concepts were re-emphasized and new illustration supplied. Also, some modifications of the questions have been introduced, which are given as follows:

1. Is it intrinsic dextrocardia or dextroposition of the heart?

2. What is the visceroatrial situs?

3. Ventricular relationship: Are there two ventricles or one?;
   If two, where are the ventricles located in relation to each other

4. What is the status of atrioventricular (AV) connections

5. How are the great arteries related to each other and with ventricles?

6. What is the conotruncal relationship?[134-136]

ECHOCARDIOGRAPHIC EVALUATION OF LEFT VENTRICULAR FUNCTION

Echocardiographic evaluation of the left ventricular function[18,20] was reviewed in the chapter on "Echocardiography" in the book titled "Pediatric Cardiology: How It Has Evolved Over the last 50 Years" and will not be repeated here.

VASODILATOR THERAPY FOR CARDIAC FAILURE IN PEDIATRIC PRACTICE

The major determinants of ventricular function are preload or ventricular end-diastolic volume, contractile state of the myocardium (which is the innate force of the myocardial contraction and is independent of the load on the ventricle), afterload, or intra-ventricular systolic tension during ventricular ejection, and heart rate. As of early 1980s, particularly in the pediatric cardiac practice, conventional treatment regimens of congestive heart failure (CHF) have included manipulation of preload by diuretics/salt restriction, contractile state of the myocardium with digitalis and other inotropic agents and heart rate by anti-arrhythmic drugs to decrease the heart rate and chronotropic agents to increase the heart rate.[19] Manipulation of afterload to treat CHF has not been used as of that time, although, I alluded to this concept in chapter in Conn's Current Therapy[137] as an experimental therapy in infants and children.

In this paper,[19] the afterload was defined and the initial efforts in using this concept to treat CHF in children were reviewed. The role of sodium nitroprusside, nitroglycerine, prazosin and hydralazine as vasodilator and afterload-reducing agent was reviewed.[19] I later studied and concluded that hydralazine, as vasodilator and afterload-reducing agent, is a valuable addition in the management of primary myocardial disease (PMD) in infants and children,[138] as reviewed in detail in the chapter on "Echocardiography" in the book titled "Pediatric Cardiology: How It Has Evolved Over the last 50 Years." Subsequently, I switched to angiotensin-converting enzyme (ACE) inhibitors such as captopril instead of vasodilators such as hydralazine as afterload reducing agents to treat dilated cardiomyopathy.[139] Currently, afterload reduction with ACE inhibitors has become almost first-line therapy in managing CHF in children.

PATHOPHYSIOLOGIC CONSEQUENCES OF CYANOTIC HEART DISEASE

Patho-physiological consequences (Table IV) of CHD were reviewed in 1983.[21] Cyanotic CHDs usually have multiple defects of the heart that result in right-to-left shunt causing arterial oxygen de-saturation. Obstruction to pulmonary blood flow as seen in tetralogy of Fallot, complete admixture of pulmonary and systemic venous returns as in total anomalous pulmonary venous return and double-inlet left ventricle, and parallel rather than in-series circulation such as transposition of the great arteries (TGA) are the common causes of right-to-left shunts and cyanosis. The magnitude of arterial de-saturation is dependent upon the severity of the right ventricular outflow tract obstruction or the degree of intra-cardiac mixing.

Table IV. Pathophysiologic Consequences of Cyanotic Congenital Heart Disease

Arterial oxygen desaturation
Cyanosis
Clubbing
Erythrocytosis
Relative anemia
Polycythemia
Hypercyanotic spells
Squatting
Cerebrovascular accidents
Brain abscess
Coagulation problems
Hyperuricemia
Gout

Reproduced from Rao PS, *Indian J Pediat 1983*; 50:479-87.

Compensatory mechanisms ensue in cyanotic CHD; some of these are beneficial to the patients, but when over-compensation occurs, complications tend to dominate the clinical scenario. Cyanosis is a clinical sign of arterial de-saturation. Chronic cyanosis results in clubbing. The chronic arterial hypoxemia increases red blood cell production by stimulating erythropoietin from the kidneys (Figure 3). If this is excessive, polycythemia will result. If iron sources are inadequate, relative anemia results. Monitoring hemoglobin levels during follow-up of cyanotic CHD is important. Severe polycythemia may require erythrophoresis instead of simple blood-letting; the volume of blood to be exchanged is calculated as shown in Figure 4.[21] In patients with relative anemia, oral iron supplements may become necessary.[21]

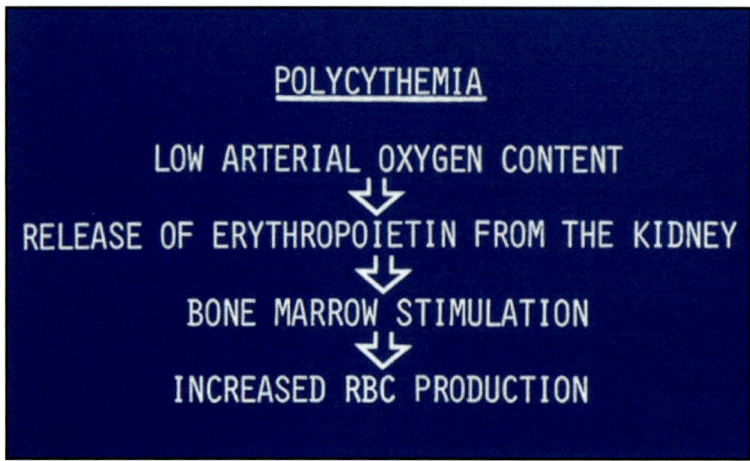

Figure 3. The mechanism of polycythemia in cyanotic congenial heart disease.
Modified from Rao PS, *Indian J Pediat 1983*; 50:479-87.

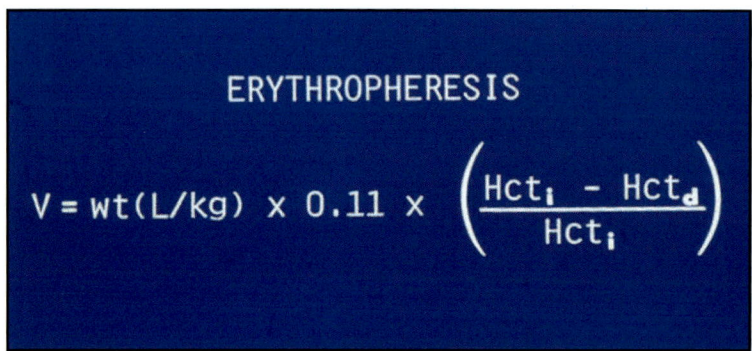

Figure 4. Calculation of the volume of blood to be exchanged is shown.
Modified from Rao PS, *Indian J Pediat 1983*; 50:479-87.

Hypercyanotic spells may develop in patients with tetralogy of Fallot and other cyanotic CHD with right ventricular outflow obstruction with a large inter-ventricular communication; the mechanism, clinical features and management were discussed for the interested reader.[21] Squatting is seen in children; this may be considered the equivalent of spell syndrome of infancy.[21] The right to left shunts also predispose to cerebrovascular accidents, strokes and brain abscess. Long-standing hypoxemia and polycythemia result in coagulation abnormalities, hyper-uricemia, gout, and uric acid nephropathy. Each of these were discussed in this review.[21] These complications may be prevented by maintaining an optimal level of hemoglobin, avoiding dehydration, and by performing timely palliative or corrective surgery.[21] With the advent of early correction of cyanotic CHD, these complications are seen less often at the present time.

TRANSCATHETER MANAGEMENT OF PEDIATRIC HEART DISEASE

Transcatheter management of pediatric heart disease was reviewed in a number of papers[23,27,28,30] in the early phases of development of these procedures. In these reviews, it was stated that transcatheter therapy is now available for many cardiovascular disorders in infants and children. This had come about because both material and technology are available for developing innovative catheters and because pediatric patients with heart disease are being managed more aggressively.

Rashkind's balloon atrial septostomy has been widely used over the last two-and-a-half to three decades to enlarge interatrial communications. In older infants and children in whom the lower margin of the patent foramen ovale is thick and muscular and cannot be torn by the balloon, transcatheter blade (or knife) atrial septostomy can be performed successfully.

Several devices have been designed to close the patent ductus arteriosus and atrial septal defect via catheters. Variable success has been reported with these devices. Further, refinement of these devices and additional clinical trials are necessary prior to their general use.

Balloon dilatation of stenotic lesions has been successful over the last few years. In general, valvular stenotic lesions appear to be amenable to relief by balloon dilatation, while central arterial (aorta and pulmonary artery) stenotic lesions exhibit a variable result and venous (pulmonary or systemic) stenotic lesions respond least favorably.

There has been a limited, but successful, experience in selective embolization of abnormal blood vessels in the pediatric patient; this procedure has been used for a variety of problems.

Removal of inadvertently embolized polyethylene catheters and other materials in the cardiovascular system is possible with several catheter techniques. Prevention by meticulous attention to inserting and securing the intravenous catheters, use of radio-opaque catheters to locate easily in the event of inadvertent embolization, and prompt removal once embolized (because of high incidence of serious complication) is recommended.

Transcatheter His bundle ablation for controlling junctional automatic ectopic tachycardias unresponsive to conventional measures and potential applicability of such a technique to ablate the Kent bundle were also discussed in brief.

Finally, the recent use of transcatheter laser techniques to produce an atrial septal defect and to relieve stenotic lesions in postmortem hearts and in experimental animals was reviewed; this technique appears to have potential clinical applicability.[23,27,28,30]

COMPREHENSIVE MANAGEMENT OF PULMONARY ATRESIA WITH INTACT VENTRICULAR SEPTUM

Comprehensive management of pulmonary atresia with intact ventricular septum[24] was presented as a lecture at the International Symposium on Heart Disease in Neonates and Children, held at Riyadh Armed Forces Hospital, Riyadh, Saudi Arabia, in November 1984 and was subsequently published in the booklet of the proceedings of this symposium.[140] At the behest of several international experts, this material was submitted to and published in Annals of Thoracic Surgery.[24] The prognosis for patients with pulmonary atresia with intact ventricular septum is poor with or without conventional surgical intervention. Therefore, a comprehensive program of medical and surgical treatment is necessary to improve long-term outlook for these infants. Such a program consists of management of the neonate at initial presentation with prompt administration of prostaglandins and institution of a combination of surgical procedures (isolated pulmonary valvotomy, valvotomy plus modified Blalock-Taussig shunt, Blalock-Taussig shunt plus balloon atrial septostomy, or Blalock-Taussig shunt alone) depending on the results of morphological analysis of the right ventricle; this treatment regimen is designed to relieve hypoxemia, encourage right ventricular growth, and provide adequate egress of blood from the right atrium.

Another important element of management is to perform follow-up hemodynamic and angiographic studies when the patient is between six and twelve months old to ensure that the objectives of the comprehensive program are being met.

Finally, a definitive repair should be offered. This can be done by using (staged surgical repair using right ventricle) or bypassing (staged surgical correction by right ventricular bypass - Fontan) the right ventricle, depending on whether the right ventricle can support the pulmonary circuit.[24]

In summary, a comprehensive program of medical and surgical treatment incorporating the principles discussed in this review is mandatory if the objectives are to increase the number of long-term survivors and to improve their quality of life.[24] These concepts and results were updated in subsequent reviews.[77,141]

PEDIATRIC CARDIOLOGY UPDATE: RECENT THERAPEUTIC ADVANCES

In this paper, recent advances in therapy of cardiac disease in infants and children as of mid-1980s was reviewed.[25] These advances were arbitrarily divided into five categories:

1. Treatment of CHF,

2. Therapy of tachyarrhythmias,

3. Pharmacological manipulation of the ductus arteriosus,

4. Transcatheter management of pediatric heart disease, and

5. Advances in surgical treatment of CHD.

In this review, the first three topics were discussed.

Treatment of CHF

The major determinants of cardiac function are the preload, contractile state of the heart, afterload, and heart rate. Conventional treatment of cardiac failure has depended upon manipulation of the preload (diuretics and salt restriction) and contractile state of the myocardium (digitalis) without dealing with the afterload. The principles of afterload reduction and their use in the treatment of severe CHF in children were discussed. New inotropic agents, namely, dobutamine, amrinone and milrinone were also briefly discussed.

Advances in Therapy of Tachy-arrhythmias

The advances at the time of this review include high-dose propranolol, verapamil, phenytoin, amiodarone, and patient-activated and automatic overdrive pacemakers for supraventricular tachycardia. Other advances are surgical or cryothermic ablation of accessory conduction pathways, AV node, or automatic focus to prevent recurrences of ventricular or supraventricular tachycardia.

Pharmacological Manipulation of the Ductus Arteriosus

Because ductal patency is influenced by prostaglandins, particularly in the early life, infusion of prostaglandin E_1 and E_2 to dilate the ductus in situations where it is hemodynamically advantageous (Table V and Figure 2), and administration of indomethacin, a prostaglandin synthesis inhibitor, in conditions where the ductus should be obliterated such as for premature infants (Figure 5 and 6), are useful.

Table V. Ductus-Dependent Cardiac Defects

A. Ductus-dependent pulmonary blood flow
1. Pulmonary atresia with intact ventricular septum
2. Pulmonary atresia with ventricular septal defect
3. Severe tetralogy of Fallot
4. Complex cyanotic heart disease with pulmonary atresia or severe stenosis
5. Tricuspid atresia
6. Critical pulmonary stenosis
7. Ebstein's anomaly of tricuspid valve
8. Hypoplastic right ventricle
B. Ductus-dependent systemic blood flow
1. Interruption of the aortic arch
2. Severe coarctation of the aorta
3. Hypoplastic left-heart syndrome

Reproduced from Rao PS, *Saudi Med J 1986*; 7:306-20.

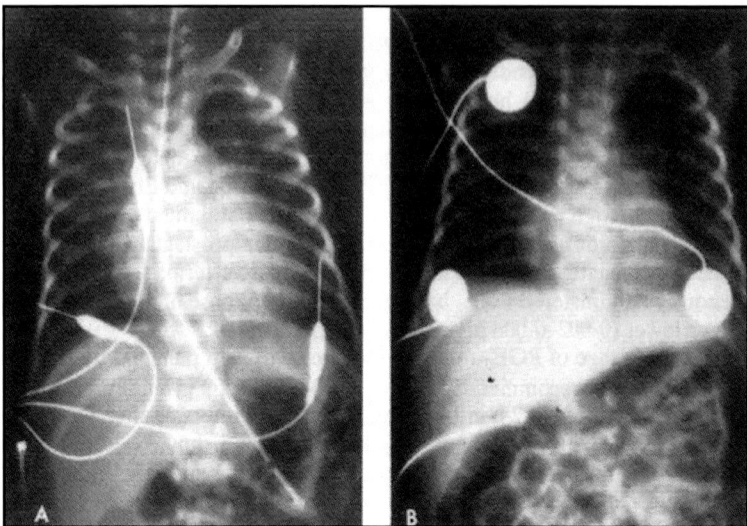

Figure 5. Chest roentgenograms of a 5-day-old premature infant with a large patent ductus arteriosus. Note cardiomegaly and increased pulmonary blood flow prior to indomethacin (A). The cardiac size has decreased markedly after indomethacin (B). This was accompanied by marked improvement in the infant's clinical status. Reproduced from Rao PS, *Saudi Med J 1986*; 7:306-20.

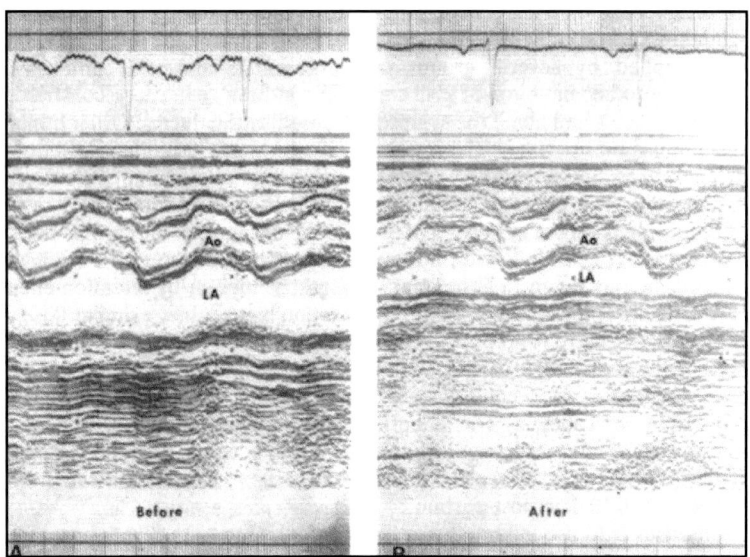

Figure 6. Echocardiograms of the same infant shown in figure 5; these were recorded at the same time of obtaining chest X-rays. Note the enlarged left atrium (LA) and increased LA/Aortic (Ao) ratio prior to indomethacin (A), both of which have decreased after indomethacin (B). Reproduced from Rao PS, *Saudi Med J 1986*; 7:306-20.

Algorhythm for orderly management of premature infant with hemodynamically significant PDA is shown in Table VI.[25]

Table VI. Management of Premature Infant With PDA

A. A. Premature infant with hyaline membrane disease

↓

B. Requirement of greater FI0$_2$ and increased ventilatory support
Appearance of a murmur
Hyperdynamic precordium and bounding pulses
Cardiomegaly on chest X-ray
Increased LA size and LA/Ao ratio with normal or increased LV shortening fraction
on an echocardiogram

↓

C. 24-48 h of fluid restriction, diuretics and possibly digoxin

↓

D. No improvement or worsening of signs listed in B
Increasing size LA and LV
Decreasing LV shortening fraction

↓

E. Indomethacin administration

Reproduced from Rao PS, *Saudi Med J 1986*; 7:306-20.

MITRAL VALVE PROLAPSE SYNDROME

A review of mitral valve prolapse was prepared at the request of the editor of *The Indian Journal of Pediatrics*.[26] The term "mitral valve prolapse" was used to describe a constellation of auscultatory findings, namely, non-ejection systolic click and late systolic murmur with or without electrocardiographic changes. More recently, characteristic echocardiographic findings were also described. Although, mitral valve prolapse is associated with a number of conditions, it is most commonly seen as an isolated finding. The etiology of isolated mitral valve prolapse is unknown. The incidence in the pediatric population appears to be in the order of 1·4 percent, much lower than 6·3 percent reported in adult populations; however, the characteristic preponderance in females is maintained in children. Mitral valve prolapse is usually detected on routine examination with only few children presenting symptoms related to the cardiovascular system. Typical auscultatory features of non-ejection systolic click followed by late systolic murmur are present in 60 percent of patients. Characteristic features are seen on M-mode and two-dimensional echocardiograms (see Figures 1 and 2 of Reference 26). The clinical course is benign during childhood and adolescence. The long-term natural history of mitral valve prolapse in pediatric population is not clearly established.[26] An extended review of this subject was presented in a book chapter in 1994.[142]

DOPPLER ECHOCARDIOGRAPHY IN NON-INVASIVE DIAGNOSIS OF HEART DISEASE IN INFANTS AND CHILDREN[29]

This subject[29] was reviewed in the chapter on "Echocardiography" in the book titled "Pediatric Cardiology: How It Has Evolved Over the last 50 Years" and will not be repeated here.

BALLOON VALVULOPLASTY AND ANGIOPLASTY IN INFANTS AND CHILDREN

A number of reviews of balloon valvuloplasty and angioplasty in infants and children[31,33,35,38] were written culminating in presenting an extensive review of the subject in booklet form.[143] Similar reviews were also published elsewhere.[67,80,144,145] In these reviews, historical aspects, indications, technique, immediate and follow-up results, complications, mechanism of balloon dilatation, and causes of restenosis for each of the cardiac lesion were discussed, although the extent of the detail provided varied from one publication to the other.[31,33,35,38,143-145]

The technique of balloon dilatation of stenotic lesions of the heart and great vessels in infants and children has been available since 1982. This technique has been used extensively in isolated valvar pulmonic stenosis with excellent immediate and reasonably good intermediate-term follow-up results. Refinements in the technique may further decrease the restenosis rate. Balloon pulmonary valvuloplasty is now the procedure of choice in the treatment of moderate to severe valvar pulmonic stenosis. Although, good immediate and intermediate-term follow-up results of balloon angioplasty of aortic coarctation have been reported, recommendation for use of this technique as the treatment of choice has been clouded by reports of development of aneurysms at the site of coarctation dilatation. I believed (at that time) that balloon coarctation angioplasty is the treatment of choice in neonates and small infants, while general use of this technique in both native and post-operative coarctation in older children should await longer follow-up results in a larger number of children. Balloon dilatation of aortic valve stenosis and branch pulmonary artery stenosis produced reasonable immediate results, but long-term results are needed prior to making definitive recommendations. However, this technique is attractive for neonates with critical aortic obstruction. I recommended balloon valvuloplasty of pulmonary stenosis in association with other congenital heart defects, though reported by only a few groups of investigators, as an effective alternative to surgical aorta-to-pulmonary anastomosis because of the good immediate and follow-up results. Despite good results with many other lesions, there was not enough experience with children with each of these defects to make a definitive recommendation.

The indications for balloon dilatation of stenotic lesions of the heart and great vessels are essentially the same as those for surgical therapy. The technique of balloon angioplasty/valvuloplasty should now be added to the therapeutic armamentarium available to the pediatric cardiologist for the management of infants and children with heart disease. Thus far, only one to two year follow-up results are available. Five to ten year follow-up results to document long-term effectiveness of balloon dilatation for all stenotic lesions are needed. Miniaturization of currently bulky dilating catheter systems and improving rapidity of inflation and deflation of balloons are necessary for increasing the safety and effectiveness of this technique in infants and children. Meticulous attention to the details of the technique and additional refinement of the procedure will further reduce the complication rate. For vascular lesions with poor results with balloon angioplasty (peripheral pulmonary artery or pulmonary vein stenosis), intravascular stents (which are currently being tested in animal models and humans) may prove valuable to keep the stenotic lesions open. Transcatheter laser technique to relieve stenotic lesions and visualization of these lesions, while relieving the obstruction by a dual fiber optic catheter, have been used in postmortem stenotic lesions and animal models. Further development and refinement of these techniques in animal models, followed by clinical trials, is necessary prior to their application in infants and children with obstructive lesions of the heart and great vessels. The transcatheter techniques offer promise as excellent alternatives to open or closed heart surgery in the treatment of several CHDs.[31,33,35,38,143-145]

BALLOON PULMONARY VALVULOPLASTY: A REVIEW

I prepared an extensive review of balloon pulmonary valvuloplasty in 1988[32] and presented indications, multiple aspects of the technique (balloon diameter, length, number of balloons to be used, balloon inflation pressure, and duration of balloon inflation), follow-up results, mechanism of valvuloplasty, role in patients with dysplastic pulmonary valves, applicability at different ages, applicability to patients with restenosis following prior surgery, electrocardiographic and echocardiographic evaluation of follow-up results, comparison with surgical results, applicability to complex CHD with pulmonary stenosis, and porcine heterograft stenosis.

Balloon pulmonary valvuloplasty has been used successfully over the last few years for the relief of moderate to severe valvar pulmonic stenosis in neonates, infants, children, and adults. Both immediate and intermediate term follow-up results have been well documented by cardiac catheterization studies. Electrocardiographic and Echo-Doppler evaluation at follow-up is reflective of the results and may avoid the need for re-catheterization. The results of balloon valvuloplasty are either comparable to or better than those reported with surgical valvuloplasty. The causes of restenosis have been identified, and appropriate modifications in the technique, particularly the recommended use of a balloon/annulus ratio of 1.2 to 1.4, should give better results than previously documented. Complications of the procedure have been minimal. Further refinement of the catheters and technique may reduce the complication rate even further. The indications for balloon valvuloplasty have not been clearly defined, but should probably be similar to those used for surgical valvotomy; only patients with moderate to severe valvar pulmonic stenosis are candidates for balloon valvuloplasty. Previous surgery and pulmonary valve dysplasia are not contraindications for balloon valvuloplasty. The procedure is also applicable to pulmonary stenosis associated with other complex cardiac defects and stenosis of bioprosthetic valves in pulmonary position. Miniaturization of balloon/catheter systems to further reduce the complication rate and documentation of favorable result at five to ten year follow-up are necessary. Additional updates in the form of reviews and book chapters were provided[58,68,88,146-152] over the years for the interested reader.

BALLOON ANGIOPLASTY OF AORTIC COARCTATION: A REVIEW

An extensive review of balloon angioplasty of aortic coarctation was prepared in 1989[34] and I presented historical aspects, indications, immediate and intermediate-term results in both native and post-surgical recoarctation, applicability to adult patients, mechanism of angioplasty, complications, causes of restenosis, remodeling of aorta following angioplasty, Echo-Doppler and magnetic resonance imaging (MRI) evaluation of follow-up results, and comparison with surgery.

Since the initial report of balloon coarctation angioplasty in 1982, several workers used this technique in native coarctation and post-operative recoarctation. Immediate and intermediate-term follow-up results are generally good with a small probability for recoarctation and aneurismal formation at the site of coarctation. The causes of recoarctation were identified and include age less than one year, isthmus hypoplasia, and a small coarcted aortic segment. Despite good immediate and follow-up results, recommendations for use of balloon angioplasty as a treatment procedure of choice are clouded by the reports of development of aneurysms at the site of coarctation. I felt that balloon coarctation angioplasty is the treatment of choice in neonates and small infants, while general use of this technique in both native and post-operative coarctations in older children should await follow-up results in larger numbers of children. Miniaturization of currently bulky catheter systems and improving rapidity of inflation/deflation of balloons are necessary for increasing the safety and effectiveness of this technique in infants and children. Meticulous attention to the details of the technique and further refinements of the procedure are likely to reduce the complication rate further. As the year's pass-by, I updated the material and provided additional information in multiple reviews and book chapters.[41,51,63,73,80,82,86,117,153-160]

CAUSES OF RESTENOSIS FOLLOWING BALLOON ANGIOPLASTY/VALVULOPLASTY: A REVIEW

The causes of restenosis following balloon angioplasty/valvuloplasty were reviewed in 1989 and published in 1990.[36] The purpose of this review was to examine the causes of the recurrence of pulmonary stenosis, aortic coarctation and aortic stenosis following balloon dilation. Both the published and unpublished data acquired by us was used for analysis.

Pulmonary Stenosis

During a fifty-five-month period ending May 1988, sixty-two children aged seven days to twenty years, underwent balloon valvuloplasty of valvar pulmonary stenosis. On the basis of the results of six to thirty-four month follow-up catheterization data in forty children, they were divided into: Group I with good results (pulmonary valve gradient of 30 mmHg or less), thirty-three patients; Group II with poor results (gradient greater than 30 mmHg), seven patients. Fourteen different variables were examined by multivariate logistic regression analysis to identify factors associated with restenosis. The risk factors were as follows: (1) Residual pulmonary valve gradient in excess of 30 mm Hg immediately following balloon valvuloplasty, and (2) Balloon to pulmonary valve annulus ratio of 1.2 or less. Dysplastic pulmonary valves did not seem to play a role in recurrence and this may have been due to the use of large balloons in patients with dysplastic valves. These data suggest that balloon/annulus ratio of 1.2 or less is the cause for pulmonary valve restenosis at intermediate-term follow-up and such recurrence can be expected if immediate post-valvuloplasty pulmonary valve gradient is in excess of 30 mmHg.

Aortic Coarctation

During a thirty-five-month period ending December 1987, thirty children, aged fourteen days to thirteen years, underwent balloon angioplasty of unoperated aortic coarctations. On the basis of results of six to thirty month follow-up catheterization data in twenty children, they were divided into: Group A with good results (gradient ≤ 20 mmHg and no recoarctation on angiograms), thirteen patients; Group B with fair and poor results (gradient > 20 mmHg with or without recoarctation on angiography), seven patients. Thirty different variables were examined by multivariate logistic regression analysis and four factors were identified as risk factors for the development of recoarctation, which are as follows: 1. Age less than twelve months, 2. Aortic isthmus less than half the size of ascending aorta, 3. Coarcted aortic segment smaller than 3.5 mm prior to dilatation, and 4. Coarcted aortic segment less than 6 mm after angioplasty. The identification of the risk factors may help in the selection of patients for balloon angioplasty. Avoiding or minimizing the number of risk factors may help reducing the probability of re-coarctation following the balloon angioplasty.

Valvar Aortic Stenosis

Seventeen infants and children with valvar aortic stenosis underwent percutaneous balloon aortic valvuloplasty over a forty-month period ending December 1988. On the basis of the follow-up results in seventeen children, they were divided into two groups: Group I with good results (gradients ≤ 49 mmHg), thirteen patients; and Group II with poor results (gradients > 50 mmHg), four patients. All four patients in Group II required repeat balloon valvuloplasty or surgical valvotomy; none from Group I required these procedures. Seventeen biographic, anatomic, physiologic and technical variables were examined by a multivariate logistic regression analysis to identify factors associated with restenosis, and these risk factors were as follows: 1. Age ≤ 3 years; and 2. Immediate post-valvuloplasty aortic valvar gradient ≥ 30 mmHg. Recognition of the risk factors may help identify the potential candidates for recurrence. Attempts to reduce the immediate post-balloon valvuloplasty gradients to less than 30 mmHg may prevent recurrences at intermediate term follow-up.

Summary and Conclusions

In this review, we examined the causes of recurrence at intermediate-term follow-up after balloon dilatation of stenotic pulmonary and aortic valves and aortic coarctation. For each lesion, a set of risk factors that predispose to recurrence were identified. For valvar pulmonary stenosis, a balloon/annulus ratio less than 1.2 and an immediate post-valvuloplasty pulmonary valvar gradient in excess of 30 mmHg were identified as the risk factors. Age less than one year, hypoplastic aortic isthmus, absolute size of coarcted segment < 3.5 mm and immediate post-angioplasty coarcted segment < 6.0 mm have been seen with recoarctation following balloon angioplasty. In valvar aortic stenosis, the identified factors were age ≤ 3 years and immediate post-valvuloplasty aortic valvar gradient ≥ 30 mmHg. Identification of risk factors may help in the selection of patients for the balloon dilatation procedures. Also, identification of the risk factors may help reduce the chances for recurrence in that a more appropriate-sized balloon may be chosen or the end-point of immediate result, i.e. residual gradient, may be selected in a manner conducive to reduction of the chances for recurrence.[36] Some of these data were published previously[161,162] and those that were not published in peer-reviewed journals were later published in peer-reviewed journals.[163,164]

BALLOON AORTIC VALVULOPLASTY: A REVIEW

A review of balloon aortic valvuloplasty was prepared in 1989[37] and I presented historical aspects, indications, immediate and intermediate-term results, applicability at different ages, applicability to patients with restenosis following prior surgery, applicability to sub-valvar stenosis, mechanism of valvuloplasty, complications, influence of technical factors, causes of restenosis, echocardiographic evaluation of follow-up results, and comparison with surgical results.

The procedure of balloon aortic valvuloplasty has been used in infants, children, and adults since its first description in 1983. Immediate results reported by several workers and intermediate term results by a few workers appear encouraging. Complications are minimal; although, potential for arterial complications and aortic insufficiency should be recognized. Significant restenosis rates at intermediate-term follow-up have been reported and could be minimized by reducing the risk factors associated with recurrence. Echo-Doppler studies are useful in follow-up evaluation of balloon valvuloplasty. The results seem to compare favorably with those following surgical valvotomy. The indications are essentially the same as those used for surgery; a gradient in excess of 70 mmHg irrespective of symptoms or a gradient greater than or equal to 50 mmHg with symptoms or ST-T wave changes. Previous surgical valvotomy is not a contraindication for balloon valvuloplasty. The technique is applicable to subaortic membranous stenosis as well. Thus far, only one to two year follow-up results are available. Five to ten year follow-up results to document long-term effectiveness of balloon aortic valvuloplasty are needed. Miniaturization of currently bulky dilating catheter systems and improving rapidity of inflation/deflation of balloons are necessary to increase safety and effectiveness of these techniques in infants and children. Meticulous attention to the details of the technique and further refinement of the procedure may further increase effectiveness and reduce the complication rate.[37] These data were updated time to time in journal articles and book chapters[59,115,165-173] for the interested reader.

PERINATAL CIRCULATORY PHYSIOLOGY

Perinatal circulatory physiology and influence of post-natal changes on clinical manifestations and management of neonatal heart disease was reviewed in 1991.[39] While postnatal circulation utilizes the lungs for gas exchange, fetal circulation uses the placenta for gas exchange. Low placental vascular resistance, high pulmonary vascular resistance (PVR), and fetal circulatory pathways namely, umbilical vessels, ductus venosus, foramen ovale, and ductus arteriosus facilitate gas exchange in the placenta and promote distribution of oxygenated blood to the vital organs of the fetus, such as the brain and the heart. Mechanical factors, prostaglandins, and low PO_2 in the lungs maintain fetal circulation.

Most heart defects, even when they are severe, do not unduly affect the fetus because of the non-restrictive foramen ovale and dutcus arteriosus. However, cardiac development may be affected by abnormalities of flows, obstructive lesions, and possibly high pulmonary artery O_2 saturations.

Circulatory changes following birth are detachment of the placenta, maturation of the pulmonary circulation, and closure of the fetal circulatory pathways. Each of these were described in detail.

Circulatory changes following birth noticeably influence the clinical presentation and clinical course of the neonate with CHDs. Spontaneous closure of the ductus arteriosus unfavorably influences the following: 1. Inter-circulatory mixing in TGA, 2. Pulmonary blood flow in a variety of cardiac defects that have severe pulmonary stenosis or atresia (Table V A), and, 3. Systemic perfusion in hypoplastic left heart syndrome (HLHS) and obstructive lesions of the aortic arch (Table V B). Intravenous infusion of PGE_1 is successful in maintaining the patency of the ductus arteriosus. Since the dependable effectiveness of PGE_1 may last for only a few days to a few weeks, more permanent solutions should be sought, and these include corrective surgery, surgical aortopulmonary shunts, and ductal stents, depending on the clinical scenario.

Restriction or closure of the foramen ovale negatively affects the following: 1. Inter-circulatory mixing in TGA, 2. Left-to-right shunting in obstructive lesions of the left heart, and 3. Right-to-left shunting in obstructive lesions of the right heart and total anomalous pulmonary venous connection (TAPVC). Restrictive foramen ovale may be dealt with by various types of transcatheter interventional or surgical septectomy techniques, depending on the clinical situation.

The PVR plays a vital role in neonates with large inter-circulatory communications, HLHS, and other defects, and appropriate adjustments in the management plan should be made to address issues related to PVR.[39] Additional updates were provided in the ensuing reviews and book chapters.[98,99,104,105,174-176]

EVALUATION OF CARDIAC MURMURS IN CHILDREN

A detailed review of evaluation of cardiac murmurs in children was provided in 1991[40] and included discussion of prevalence at different ages, my approach to auscultation, classification of the murmurs (systoic [Figure 7], diastolic [Figure 8], and continuous [Figure 9]), causes of these murmurs (Tables VII, VIII, IX, X, XI and XII), and differential diagnosis (Tables 3 and 4 of Reference 40).

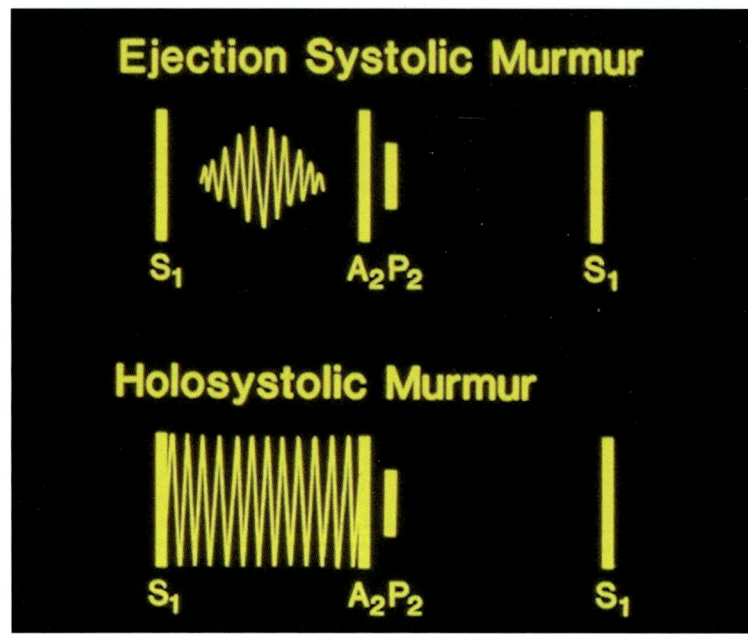

Figure 7. Auscultatory diagrams of systolic murmurs. Ejection systolic murmur (top) begins shortly after the first heart sound (Sl) and ends shortly before the second heart sound (A2, aortic component; P2, pulmonary component), whereas a holosystolic murmur (bottom) begins with and obscures the Sl and may last throughout the systole (as in the diagram) or may stop short of A2. Modified from Rao PS, *Indian J Pediat 1991*; 58:471-89.

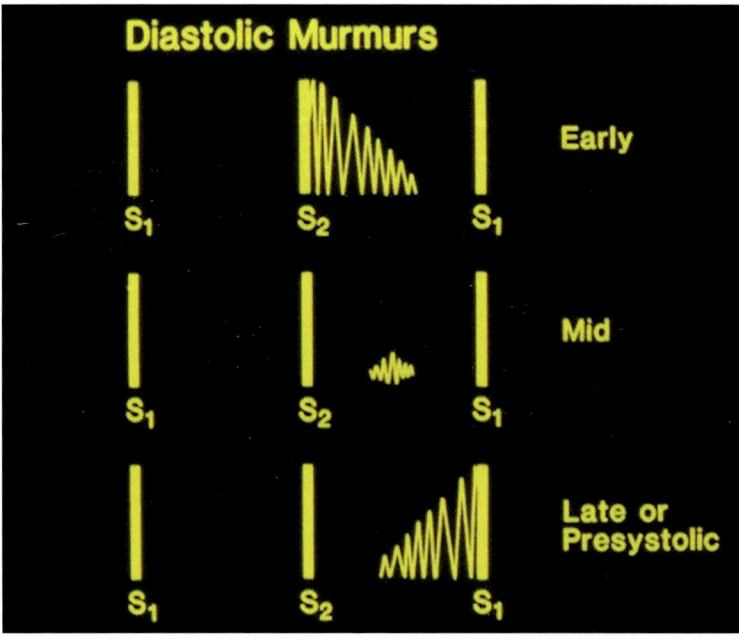

Figure 8. Diagrammatic representation of diastolic murmurs; early, mid and late (or pre-systolic) diastolic murmurs are shown. Modified from Rao PS, *Indian J Pediat 1991*; 58:471-89.

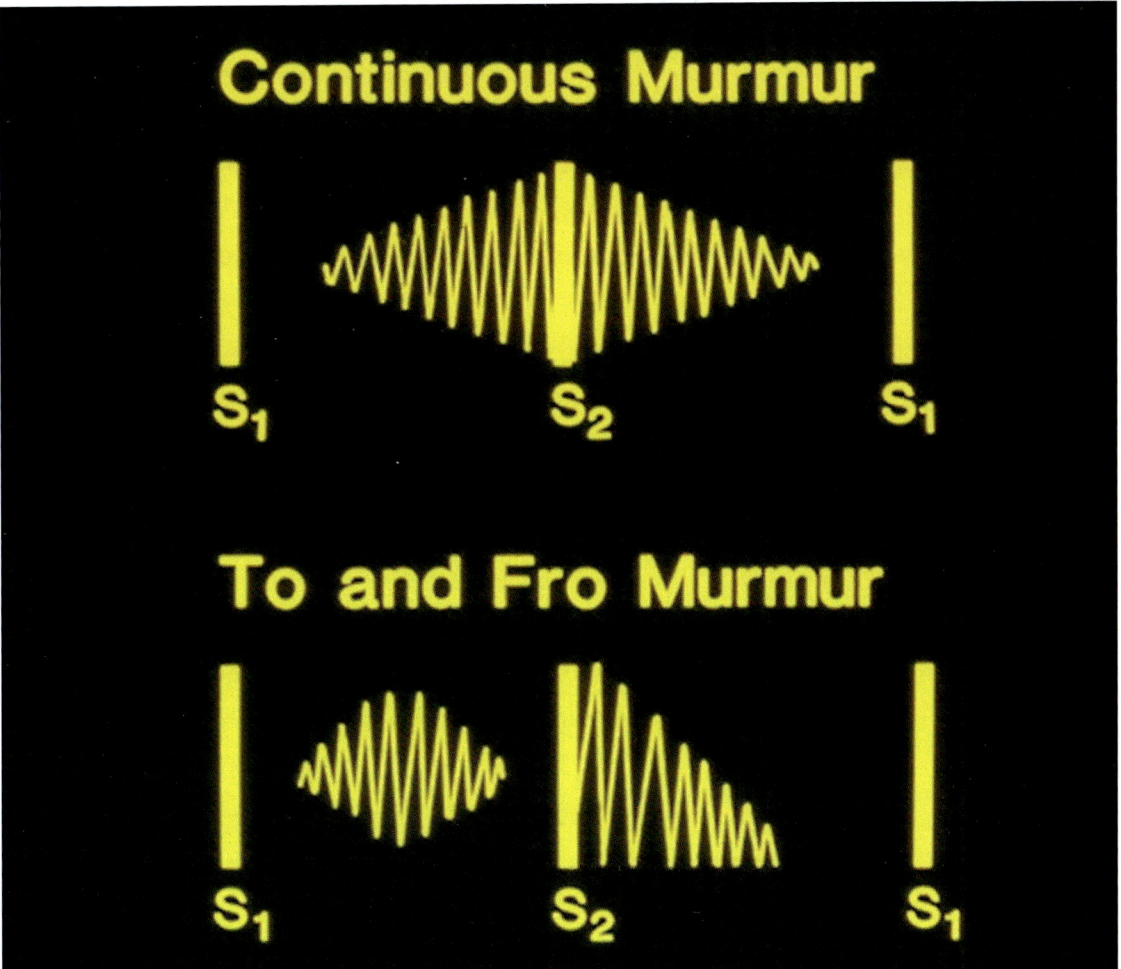

Figure 9. The continuous murmur (top) begins in systole, crescendos up to the second heart sound (S2) and decrescendos to a varying distance into the diastole. In contradistinction to this murmur, the to-and-fro murmur (bottom) consists of an ejection systolic murmur with a separate early diastolic decrescendo murmur; note that there is a definite gap between the end of the ejection murmur and S2. Modified from Rao PS, *Indian J Pediat 1991*; 58:471-89.

Table VII. Causes of Ejection Systolic Murmurs

Common Causes
Aortic stenosis
Coarctation of the aorta
Pulmonic stenosis
Atrial septal defect
Functional or innocent murmur
Less Common Causes
Mitral prolapse syndrome
Acyanotic tetralogy of Fallot
Patent ductus arteriosus

Reproduced from Rao PS, *Indian J Pediat 1991*; 58:471-89.

Table VIII. Causes of Holosystolic Murmurs

Ventricular septal defect
Mitral insufficiency
Tricuspid insufficiency

Reproduced from Rao PS, *Indian J Pediat 1991*; 58:471-89.

Table IX. Causes of Early Diastolic Murmurs

Aortic insufficiency
Pulmonary insufficiency
Pulmonary hypertension (Graham-Steel murmur)

Reproduced from Rao PS, *Indian J Pediat 1991*; 58:471-89.

Table X. Causes of Mid-Diastolic Murmurs

1. Large flow across the mitral valve
a. Ventricular septal defect
b. Patent ductus arteriosus
c. Mitral insufficiency
2. Rheumatic mitral valvulitis (Carey Coombs murmur)
3. Aortic insufficiency (Austin Flint murmur)
4. 4. Mitral stenosis
5. Large flow across the tricuspid valve   Atrial septal defect
a. Anomalous pulmonary venous connection (partial or total)
b. Tricuspid insufficiency
6. Tricuspid stenosis

Reproduced from Rao PS, *Indian J Pediat 1991*; 58:471-89.

Table XI. Causes of Presystolic Murmurs

Mitral stenosis, rheumatic and congenital
Tricuspid stenosis, congenital and rheumatic
Left (or right) atrial myxoma

Reproduced from Rao PS, *Indian J Pediat 1991*; 58:471-89.

Table XII. Causes of Continuous Murmurs

Common Causes
Patent ductus arteriosus
Venous hum
Surgical aortopulmonary shunts
Less Common Causes
Aortopulmonary window
Persistent truncus arteriosus
Hemitruncus
Embryonic Collateral vessels in pulmonary atresia with ventricular septal defect
Coronary arteriovenous fistula
Ruptured sinus of Valsalva aneurysm
Pulmonary arteriovenous fistula
Peripheral pulmonary artery stenosis
Coarctation of the aorta
Obstructed venous return

Reproduced from Rao PS, *Indian J Pediat 1991*; 58:471-89.

It was concluded that cardiac murmur is a common finding and the murmurs are the most common reason for detection of cardiac disease in children. The murmurs were divided into systolic, diastolic and continuous types. Careful evaluation of the murmur and other associated findings will often result in making a reasonably correct diagnosis. Occasionally, the use of non-invasive and invasive studies may become necessary for accurate diagnosis. However, these studies may often be required for quantification and is conducted prior to transcatheter or surgical intervention.[40]

TRANSCATHETER OCCLUSION OF CARDIAC SEPTAL DEFECTS

A number of reviews on transcatheter occlusion of cardiac septal defects (ASDs, VSDs and PDAs) and abnormal vascular connections[42,47,49,50,54,62,64-66,70-72,74,75,81,87,91,106,109,114,116,127,129] were published in the past and these subjects were discussed in detail in the chapters on "Atrial Septal Defect," "Patent Ductus Arteriosus," "Ventricular Septal Defect," and "Miscellaneous Transcatheter Occlusions," in the book titled "Pediatric Cardiology: How It Has Evolved Over the last 50 Years" and will not be repeated.

CORRECTIVE SURGERY FOR TRICUSPID ATRESIA: WHICH MODIFICATIONS OF FONTAN-KREUTZER PROCEDURE SHOULD BE USED? A REVIEW[44]

Which modifications of Fontan-Kreutzer procedure should be used for correction of tricuspid atresia was reviewed in the section on "Insights into Surgical Approaches" of the chapter on "Tricuspid Atresia" in the book titled "Pediatric Cardiology: How It Has Evolved Over the last 50 Years" and will not be repeated here.

TRANSCATHETER MANAGEMENT OF CYANOTIC CONGENITAL HEART DEFECTS (CHD): A REVIEW

Transcatheter management of cyanotic CHD was reviewed in 1992.[45] Since this subject was discussed in the section on "Pulmonary Stenosis Associated with Other Heart Defects" in the chapter on "Pulmonary Stenosis" in the book titled "Pediatric Cardiology: How It Has Evolved Over the last 50 Years," it will only be briefly reviewed here. In this review, the role of transcatheter methods in the management of cyanotic CHDs was discussed. In patients with inter-ventricular right-to-left shunting secondary to pulmonary outflow tract obstruction (most commonly tetralogy of Fallot), balloon dilatation may be an effective palliative procedure in a substantial proportion of patients, obviating the need for a palliative shunt; detailed discussion may be found in the chapter on "Pulmonary Stenosis" as mentioned above. Infundibular myectomy with atherectomy catheter in tetralogy of Fallot patients may become a useful adjunct in the management of these infants, although there is an extremely limited experience with this technique.[45]

Cyanotic children with interatrial right-to-left shunt secondary to severe valvar pulmonary stenosis respond to balloon pulmonary valvuloplasty in a manner similar to that seen with isolated pulmonary valve stenosis. In these patients, balloon valvuloplasty is the treatment of choice and may be corrective in most cases.[177]

In patients with a narrowed Blalock-Taussig shunt, balloon angioplasty may improve pulmonary oligemia and systemic arterial hypoxemia and may obviate the need for a second systemic-to-pulmonary artery shunt. Balloon angioplasty is recommended if the patient's cardiac defect is not amenable to surgical correction at a low risk, either because of the size of the patient or because of the complexity of the cyanotic heart defect.

In patients with pulmonary valve atresia, initial opening of the atretic pulmonary valve by either laser or surgery with subsequent balloon dilatation is potentially beneficial in reducing the total number of surgical procedures that these children are likely to require. However, further clinical trials are needed prior to their general use.[45]

Based on my personal experience and this review, it appears that transcatheter methods have a definitive role in the management of certain types of cyanotic CHDs. They help avoid or postpone the need for palliative and corrective surgery. Selection criteria for use of transcatheter methods require further refinement. Both immediate and follow-up results on a larger number of patients are necessary to define the safety and effectiveness of these procedures more accurately.[45]

TRANSCATHETER TREATMENT OF PULMONARY OUTFLOW TRACT OBSTRUCTION: A REVIEW

The role of transcatheter methods in the management of pulmonary outflow tract obstruction were discussed in this review,[46] although there is some overlap with the prior review.[45] Balloon pulmonary valvuloplasty for relief of isolated pulmonary valve stenosis has been successfully used by many investigators and is the procedure of choice for the management of these lesions. Supravalvar pulmonary stenosis, if discrete, can be relieved by balloon dilatation. Cyanotic children with interatrial right-to-left shunts secondary to severe valvar pulmonary stenosis respond in a manner similar to that observed with isolated pulmonary valve stenosis. In these patients, balloon valvuloplasty is the treatment of choice and may be corrective in most patients. In patients with interventricular right-to-left shunting, secondary to pulmonary outflow tract obstruction and in patients with narrowed BT shunts, balloon dilatation may be an effective palliative procedure in a substantial proportion of patients obviating the need for an initial or second palliative shunt. Balloon dilatation is recommended if the patient's size or cardiac anatomy make them unsuitable for safe total surgical correction. In patients with pulmonary atresia, either initial opening of the atretic pulmonary valve by laser or by surgery with subsequent balloon dilatation are potentially beneficial in reducing the total number of surgical procedures that these children are likely to require. However, further clinical trials are needed before their general use.[46]

ECHOCARDIOGRAPHIC EVALUATION OF LEFT HEART OUTFLOW OBSTRUCTIONS

In collaboration with Dr. Gautam Singh of St. Louis University, the strengths and pitfalls of two-dimensional and Doppler echocardiography in evaluation of left heart outflow obstructions,[48] and echocardiographic evaluation of coarctation of the aorta in adults[56] were reviewed. Similarly, ultrasound as an adjunct to cardiac intervention in the pediatric patient[55] was also reviewed. The interested reader may review the respective publications.[48,55,56]

SHOULD BALLOON ANGIOPLASTY BE USED AS A TREATMENT OF CHOICE FOR NATIVE AORTIC COARCTATIONS[51]

This subject was addressed in the chapter on "Coarctation of the Aorta" in the book titled "Pediatric Cardiology: How It Has Evolved Over the last 50 Years" and will not be further dealt with here.

ROLE OF STENTS IN THE MANAGEMENT OF CHDS[52,76,113]

The role of stents in the management of congenital heart defects was reviewed in detail in the section on "Reviews and Book Chapters" of the chapter on "Stents" in the book titled "Pediatric Cardiology: How It Has Evolved Over the last 50 Years" and will not be repeated here.

CRITICAL PULMONARY STENOSIS IN THE NEONATE: ROLE OF TRANSCATHETER MANAGEMENT[53]

The role of transcatheter management of critical pulmonary stenosis in the neonate was discussed in the section on "Critical Pulmonary Stenosis in the Neonate" of the chapter on "Pulmonary Stenosis" and in the chapter on "Neonatal Interventions" in the book titled "Pediatric Cardiology: How It Has Evolved Over the last 50 Years" and will not be reviewed again.

INTERVENTIONAL PEDIATRIC CARDIOLOGY: STATE OF THE ART AND FUTURE DIRECTIONS

An extensive review of the state of art of interventional pediatric cardiology as of late 1990s was provided.[57] Although the interventional pediatric cardiology began in the early 1950s, it was not until the mid-1980s that a full spectrum of transcatheter interventions in children could be undertaken including balloon atrial septostomy, which has been in usage since 1966. Enormous developments have occurred even from the mid-1980s to date. In this review, current state-of-the-art for each broad area of therapeutic catheterization was presented. A large variety of lesions could be opened-up or closed as the case may be, and the results of these interventions were either similar to or better than those reported for the alternative surgical therapy. Indeed, therapeutic catheterization techniques have replaced the conventional surgery for many lesions and are threatening to do so for others. However, long-term follow-up results are scanty and are needed. Further miniaturization of catheters/sheaths used in interventional pediatric cardiology and development of new technology for the lesions, which are not amenable to currently available transcatheter methods are awaited. The future seems to be bright for interventional pediatric cardiology.

It was concluded that since the initial description of Rashkind balloon septostomy in the mid-1960s and more recently the modification of coronary artery balloon technology to treat congenital valvar and vascular lesions, enormous advances have occurred in the interventional technology for the pediatric patients. Further miniaturization of the catheter systems, refinement of the techniques and evaluation of long-term results are likely to take place in the next decade, thus making the procedures safer, more effective and more appropriate than they are now.

CHEST PAIN IN CHILDREN

Chest pain in children was reviewed in 1998.[60] Chronic chest pain is a complaint that frequently prompts referral to pediatric cardiology clinics although very few pediatric patients with this symptom will be found to have cardiac disease. This review discussed the common non-cardiac and cardiac causes of chest pain (Table XIII). Each of the causative factors were briefly described followed by clinical evaluation by history and physical examination and management. Guidelines on the office management of this group of patients as well as the indications for referring patients for evaluation and treatment by the sub-specialist was also presented.

Table XIII. Chest Pain in Children

Idiopathic
Musculoskeletal
Muscle sprain
Costochondritis
Trauma
Slipping rib syndrome
Psychogenic
Respiratory
Pneumonia
Pneumothorax
Asthma
Chronic cough
Gastrointestinal
Esophagitis
Foreign body
Cardiac
Arrhythmias
Coronary artery lesions
Congenital heart disease
Severe aortic stenosis or pulmonic stenosis
Hypertrophic cardiomyopathy
Pericarditis
Myocarditis
Rupture of sinus of Valsalva
Mitral valve prolapse
Kawasaki disease
Pulmonary vascular obstructive disease
Miscellaneous
Sickle cell disease
Shingles
Thoracic tumor

Reproduced from Balfour IC, Rao PS, *Indian J Pediat 1998*; 65:21-26.

Many patients with chest pain will not have a readily identifiable cause for their pain. Fortunately, the pain is self limiting; although, it may persist for months. Once a cardiac cause has been excluded, the patient and family should be reassured to allay their fears. Some patients may respond to trial of a two-week course of an anti-inflammatory agent if the pain is of musculoskeletal origin. It is sometimes helpful to have the patient and/or parents keep a diary recording the time of the day when the pain occurs, its relationship to activity, meals, etc., and aggravating and relieving factors. If the pain persists on follow-up and is severe or causes significant impairment of the patient's lifestyle, then referral to a sub-specialist is appropriate. Further evaluation of the patient would depend on the suspected etiology of the pain. Patients with possible exercise induced bronchospasm should be evaluated by exercise testing and pre and post exercise lung function studies. If the etiology is thought to be gastro-intestinal, then a barium series or gastroduodenoscopy may be indicated. Chest pain is a common complaint in children, particularly adolescents. Fortunately, the pain is rarely caused by cardiac disease. For most patients, the only evaluation necessary is a detailed history and physical examination.[60]

CONGENITAL CORONARY ARTERY ANOMALIES

A review of congenital coronary artery abnormalities was presented in 1998[61] describing normal coronary artery anatomy, imaging by Echo-Doppler studies, classification of coronary artery anomalies (Table XIV), detailed description of each these anomalies and their management.

Table XIV. Classification of Congenital Coronary Artery (CA) Anomalies

A. Anomalous origin of CA (origin from other than the aorta)
B. Aberrant CA (origin from the aorta, but from the contra-lateral aortic sinus of Valsalva with variation in the epicardial course).
C. Bridging (when the epicardial CA dips within the myocardial layers)
D. Ostial stenosis or atresia (these conditions may be isolated or may occur in association with other congenital heart defects).
E. Coronary arteriovenous fistula

Reproduced from Jureidini SB, Marino CJ, Rao PS, *Indian J Pediat 1998*; 65:217-29.

Congenital coronary artery abnormalities are rare and account for 0.1 to 2 percent of CHD. They may pose significant risk of mortality or morbidity to the patient. The pediatrician and the pediatric cardiologist should be aware of their subtle presentations and diagnostic steps to be undertaken to pinpoint the diagnosis. Exercise-induced symptoms such as chest pressure, chest pain, arrhythmia, collapse or aborted cardiac arrest should be considered with utmost care, and a suspicion of coronary artery anomaly should be raised. Echocardiography is a reliable non-invasive technique in diagnosing most of these conditions. The echocardiographer should become familiar with the normal coronary artery anatomy and the pattern of normal coronary artery flow by color flow mapping and spectral Doppler so that any abnormality can be diagnosed in time. Prevention of serious complications from these abnormalities can be achieved by making the appropriate diagnosis and performing timely surgical intervention as indicated.[61]

LONG-TERM FOLLOW-UP RESULTS AFTER BALLOON DILATATION OF PULMONIC STENOSIS, AORTIC STENOSIS AND COARCTATION OF THE AORTA: A REVIEW.

Whereas acute and intermediate-term follow-up results after balloon valvuloplasty/angioplasty in children have been well documented, there is little long-term follow-up data. Therefore, I reviewed our experience on long-term follow-up results along with that of others.[63]

Long-term follow-up results of balloon pulmonary valvuloplasty suggest low residual gradients and high re-intervention-free rates of 85 percent at ten years, but with a high prevalence of pulmonary insufficiency. The previous view that balloon valvuloplasty is the treatment modality of choice is supported by these data, but a recommendation to obtain longer-term (ten to twenty years) follow-up data to evaluate the significance of pulmonary insufficiency has emerged.

Following balloon aortic valvuloplasty, the late follow-up data suggest mild residual gradient; significant prevalence of restenosis, requiring reintervention; generally lower re-intervention-free rates when compared with pulmonary valve data; and, most importantly, progression of aortic insufficiency at late follow-up. Further investigation of causes of late aortic insufficiency may be necessary to ensure validity of the current thesis that transcatheter balloon dilatation is the choice option of therapy for valvar aortic stenosis in children.

Balloon angioplasty of native aortic coarctation produces low residual gradients and normal blood pressure in the majority of patients at late follow-up, although recoarctation, requiring repeat intervention, and aneurysms in a small percentage of patients, some requiring surgery and femoral artery compromise, were observed at intermediate-term follow-up. There is a reasonable consensus that balloon angioplasty of native coarctation is a viable option in children, but controversy continues to exist with regard to its utility in neonates and infants.

Late follow-up results of balloon dilatation of postsurgical aortic recoarctation also indicate low residual gradients and normotensive patterns in the majority of patients. But, recoarctations and aneurysms in some patients along with a requirement for surgery to relieve aortic arch or isthmic narrowing do exist. Balloon angioplasty is the preferred treatment option in the management of postsurgical aortic coarctation. Stenting, when more experience is gained, may serve as a useful adjunct with potential for replacement of surgery.[63]

In summary, data indicate low residual gradients and low to moderate re-intervention rates in all stenotic lesions and normal blood pressure in the majority of patients with coarctation at late follow-up. Development of semilunar valve insufficiency in patients with valvar stenoses, aneurismal formation in those with aortic coarctation, and femoral artery compromise for lesions requiring trans-femoral arterial dilatation are of concern and may need continued study. Overall, balloon dilatation is a useful technique in the management of stenotic lesion of the heart in children.[63]

For additional review of the above four defects, the reader is referred to the chapters on "Pulmonary Stenosis," "Aortic Stenosis," and "Coarctation of the Aorta" in the book entitled "Pediatric Cardiology: How It Has Evolved Over the last 50 Years."

CURRENT STATUS OF BALLOON ANGIOPLASTY FOR NEONATAL AND INFANT AORTIC COARCTATION

Balloon angioplasty of native aortic coarctation in children is now generally accepted as the initial management option, but its use in the neonate and young infant remains controversial. In order to objectively assess this matter, a review of previously published reports and an analysis of my own experience in recent years was undertaken.[73] Balloon angioplasty has been shown to be effective in immediate relief of obstruction. During intermediate-term follow-up, recurrence of obstruction was encountered in a significant number of patients, but such recurrence has been successfully treated either by repeat balloon angioplasty or by surgery. The procedure is not associated with mortality, although there are occasional exceptions recorded in the literature. Arterial complications occur when femoral artery is used for balloon angioplasty. Aneurysms are uncommon following balloon angioplasty in neonates and young infants. These data indicated that complication rates are in an acceptable range and the procedure is considered safe. Comparison with surgical therapy revealed similar mortality rates and similar degree of relief of obstruction, but slightly lower morbidity and complication rates with balloon than with surgical therapy. Data from our recent experience suggests effective palliation, defined as no need for surgical intervention for four weeks or longer, in 96 percent patients. But, recurrence was observed during short-term follow-up in 45 percent patients. The recurrence, however, has successfully been treated with repeat balloon angioplasty or surgical therapy. Trans-umbilical artery and trans-venous anterograde approaches were devoid of femoral artery complications, while such complications are seen in infants undergoing the procedure via the femoral artery. Recent introduction of balloon catheters that can be introduced through three-French sheaths may decrease arterial complications. Biodegradable stents, when they become available, may prevent or reduce recoarctation. Based on the available data, it may be concluded that balloon angioplasty is an acceptable alternative to surgical treatment in the initial management of native aortic coarctation in the neonate and young infant. Availability of smaller-sized balloon catheters and potential for biodegradable stents may further improve on the current limitations of balloon therapy.[73] For additional details, the reader is referred to the chapter on "Coarctation of the Aorta" in the book titled "Pediatric Cardiology: How It Has Evolved Over the last 50 Years."

WHAT IS NEW IN PEDIATRIC CARDIOLOGY? AND RECENT ADVANCES IN PEDIATRIC CARDIOLOGY

Recent advances in pediatric cardiology were reviewed in two separate papers[78,79] by me and my associates in a symposium on "Advances in Pediatrics." In the first of the two papers,[78] what may be called medical advances (Table XV) were reviewed. Enormous advances in the diagnosis and management of heart disease in pediatric patient have taken place during the last four decades. In this review, we concentrated on the developments within the last five to ten years of the review date.

Table XV. Medical Advances in Pediatric Cardiology

1. Non-invasive evaluation
a. Echocardiography
b. Cardiac Magnetic Resonance imaging
2. Molecular and genetic aspects of congenital heart disease
3. Management of congestive heart failure
a. Medical Management
b. Mechanical Support for the Failing Ventricle
4. Pulmonary Hypertension
5. Acquired Heart Disease
a. Kawasaki disease
b. Acute Rheumatic fever
c. Anthracycline cardiotoxicity
6. Hypertrophic Cardiomyopathy

Reproduced from Gupta ML, Lantin-Hermosa MR, Rao PS, *Indian J Pediat 2003*; 70:41-9.

The ultrasound technology for the evaluation of the heart has come a long way from the early A-mode and M-mode capabilities to Doppler (pulsed, continuous wave and color), two-dimentional and three-dimentional capabilities as well as tissue Doppler. Specialized echocardiograhic techniques have been developed and include transesophageal echocardiography (TEE), intracardiac echocardiography (ICE), stress echocardiography, intravascular ultrasound (IVUS) and fetal echocardiography. Each of these techniques have their value in the evaluation of a particular subset of individuals. MRI has become useful in evaluating CHD issues not adequately addressed by echocardiographic techniques and is slowly becoming the primary mode of investigation in some institutions. Recent advances in molecular genetics and defining the familial patterns have led to finding that certain genetic and molecular factors are linked to CHD and arrhythmia, thus providing opportunity for improved genetic counseling and future gene therapy. Medical treatment of CHF targets not only the augmentation of ventricular contractility (positive inotropy), but also addresses the neurohumoral derangement associated with it. Advances in understanding of pulmonary hypertension, non-invasive diagnosis and the newly described pulmonary vasodilators was reviewed. Similarly advances in understanding of and treatment of Kawasaki disease, acute rheumatic fever and anthracyclin cardio toxicity was discussed. Finally, advances in medical, surgical and transcatheter therapy for hypertrophic cardiomyopathy were addressed.

In the second paper,[79] electrophysiological, transcatheter and surgical advances (Table XVI) were the focus of the review. Greater understanding of the arrhythmias, development of non-pharmacological treatment, namely catheter ablation and internal cardioverter-defibrillator (ICD) and miniaturization pacemakers and ICDs have occurred in the last decade so that the methods could be applied to smaller and more complex patient population. Surgery has been the traditional treatment option for palliation and correction of congenital and acquired heart defects in infants and children. During the last one to one-and-a-half decades, a remarkable number of transcatheter methods were developed and refined. These developments during the last decade were reviewed and include long-term results of balloon dilatation procedures, transcatheter closure of ASDs, PDAs, and VSDs, percutaneous valve replacement, intravascular stents to manage vascular obstructive lesions that cannot be satisfactorily balloon-dilated, catheter completion of Fontan procedure, myocardial reduction in hypertrophic cardiomyopathy, and other miscellaneous procedures. Recent advances in the transcatheter modes of therapy have added a new dimension to the management of neonates, infants and children with heart disease. They should now be added to the armamentarium available to the Pediatrician and Pediatric Cardiologist in the management of cardiac problems in the pediatric patient. Surgical methods and concepts have been greatly refined such that surgery can be undertaken even in the sickest and most complex patient. The majority of CHDs can be corrected by open heart surgery; some require prior palliation and others can be operated without prior palliation. Recent advances in surgery for each of the defects (Table XVI, 3) were reviewed.[79]

Table XVI. Electrophysiologic, Transcatheter and Surgical Advances

1. Pediatric Arrhythmia & Electrophysiology
a. Bradycardia
b. Tachyarrhythmia
c. Advances in genetics
2. Transcatheter Therapy
a. Long-term results of balloon angioplasty
b. Device closure of cardiac septal defects
c. Transcatheter valve replacement
d. Stents
e. Catheter completion of Fontan
f. Myocardial reduction in hypertrophic cardiomyopathy
g. Miscellaneous
3. Surgery
a. Tetralogy of Fallot
b. Transposition of the Great Arteries
c. Tricuspid Atresia and Other Single Ventricle Lesions
d. Pulmonary Atresia with Intact Ventricular Septum
e. Hypoplastic Left Heart Syndrome   L Truncus Arteriosus
f. Severe Aortic Valve Disease
g. Cardiac Transplantation

Reproduced from Rao PS, et al, *Indian J Pediat 2003;70:557-64.*

DIAGNOSIS AND MANAGEMENT OF ACYANOTIC HEART DISEASE

Diagnosis and management of acyanotic CHD was reviewed in two separate papers[83,84] in a symposium on "Pediatric Cardiology." In the first of the two papers,[83] obstructive lesions were addressed, while the second paper[84] dealt with left-to-right shunt lesions. In both these papers, a brief description of the anatomy, clinical features (symptoms and physical findings), ECG, Echo-Doppler findings, catheterization and angiographic features, and management of most commonly encountered acyanotic obstructive[83] and left to right shunt[84] lesions were discussed. Mild lesions, especially in children are usually asymptomatic while neonates and infants with severe lesions may present with symptoms. Ejection systolic murmurs in patients with pulmonary and aortic stenosis and decreased femoral pulses and blood pressure difference (> 20 mmHg) between arms and leg in patients with aortic coarctation are usually seen. Clinical diagnosis is not difficult and the diagnosis can be confirmed and quantified by non-invasive echocardiographic studies. Whereas surgical intervention was used in the past, balloon dilatation appears to be effective in the treatment of these obstructive lesions.

Most commonly encountered acyanotic, left-to-right shunt lesions were discussed in the second paper.[84] Patients with small defects, especially in childhood, are usually asymptomatic, while moderate to large defects in infancy may present with symptoms. Hyperdynamic precordium, widely split and fixed second heart sound, ejection systolic murmur at the left upper sternal border and a mid-diastolic flow rumble at the left lower sternal border are present in ASDs. Holosystolic murmur at the left lower border is characteristic for a VSD, whereas a continuous murmur at the left upper sternal border is distinctive for PDA. Clinical diagnosis is not usually difficult and the diagnosis can be confirmed and quantified by non-invasive echocardiographic studies. Whereas surgical intervention was used in the past, transcatheter methods are increasingly used for closure of ASDs and PDA. Small VSDs may not need to be closed, whereas medium and large defects may require surgical closure. Transcatheter closure of both muscular and membranous ventricular septal defects is feasible by transcatheter methodology, but these techniques were experimental at the time of that writing.[84]

CURRENT PERSPECTIVES ON KAWASAKI DISEASE

Current perspectives on Kawasaki disease (KD) was also presented in a symposium on "Pediatric Cardiology."[85] The etiology of KD remains unknown despite several years of dedicated research in this direction. Recently, corona virus infection and genetic polymorphisms have been implicated. Since first description of the disease there have been few changes in the diagnostic criteria (Table XVII), except for newer recommendations of fever of at least four instead of five days duration. Recently, Laboratory (Table XVIII) and Echocardiography (Table XIX) Criteria were added to aid in the diagnosis of incomplete KD where all the historical diagnostic criteria are not present; this is now called the "incomplete form of KD" as opposed to "atypical form of KD." The word "atypical" is reserved for unusual presentations of KD such as those with hemophagocytic syndrome or nerve palsy. The treatment of KD includes infusion of high dose immunoglobulin. Patients non-responsive to immunoglobulin therapy are labeled as having "immunoglobulin resistant KD." The treatment of immunoglobulin resistant KD can be challenging and new therapies have tried with some success. Late outcomes after four decades of treating these patients have recently been published. There has been some concern about increased risk for premature atherosclerosis in patients with childhood KD who had coronary artery abnormalities.[85]

Table XVII. Diagnostic Clinical Criteria for Kawasaki Disease

Clinical Criteria
1. Fever of at least five days duration.
2. Polymorphous exanthema
3. Bilateral bulbar conjunctiva injection
4. Oral cavity and lip changes.
5. Changes in the extremities with swelling of palms and soles (membranous desquamation in the convalescent stage)
6. Cervical lymphadenopathy of greater than 1.5 cm

Reproduced from Gupta-Malhotra M, Rao PS, *Indian J Pediatr 2005*; 72:621-29.

Table XVIII. Laboratory Criteria for Diagnosis of Incomplete Kawasaki Disease

Supplemental Laboratory Criteria
1. Serum albumin of > 3g/dL
2. Anemia for age
3. Elevation of alanine aminotransferase
4. Elevated platelets after seven days of > 45,000/mm^3
5. Elevated white blood cell count of > 15,000/mm^3
6. Urine with > 10 white blood cells/high-power field

Reproduced from Gupta-Malhotra M, Rao PS, *Indian J Pediatr 2005*; 72:621-29.

Table XIX. Echocardiography Criteria for Diagnosis of Incomplete Kawasaki Disease

Supplemental Echocardiographic Criteria
1. Perivascular brightness
2. Z-scores of left anterior descending or right coronary artery between 2 and 2.5
3. Lack of vessel tapering
4. Decreased left ventricular function
5. Mitral regurgitation
6. Pericardial effusion

Reproduced from Gupta-Malhotra M, Rao PS, *Indian J Pediatr 2005*; 72:621-29.

AN APPROACH TO THE DIAGNOSIS OF CYANOTIC NEONATE FOR THE PRIMARY CARE PROVIDER

Cyanosis is a chief sign of CHD in the newborn. At the outset, it was emphasized that:

1. Complex physiologic and anatomic alterations take place during and immediately after birth, 2. Severe cyanotic CHD can exist without a cardiac murmur, 3. A loud murmur does not automatically suggest that the reason for the distress in the baby is related to a heart defect, 4. When a murmur is detected, it is not necessarily characteristic for a specified CHD, and 5. Lack of cardiomegaly on a chest roentgenogram does not eliminate severe CHD.[89] Recent recommendations for pulse oximetry screening of the neonates also help identify infants with CHDs.[133] The causes of cyanosis (Table XX) may be categorized into respiratory (Table XXI), cardiac (Table XXII), and central nervous system (Table XXIII) disorders, persistent pulmonary hypertension and a miscellaneous group of abnormalities (Table XXIV).

Table XX. Causes of Cyanosis

• Respiratory disorders
• Cyanotic heart defects
• Persistent fetal circulation
• Central nervous system disorders
• Miscellaneous

Reproduced from Rao PS. Neonatology Today 2007; 2(6):1-7.

Table XXI. Respiratory disorders Causing Cyanosis

A. Pulmonary parenchymal diseases
• Hyaline membrane disease
• Aspiration Syndrome
• Pneumonia
• Rare disorders like pulmonary hemorrhage or Wilson-Mikety Syndrome
Diseases causing mechanical interference with lung function
• Diaphragmatic hernia
• Pneumothorax and pneumomediastinum
• Tracheo-esophageal fistula
• Lobar emphysema

Reproduced from Rao PS, *Neonatology Today 2007*; 2(6):1-7.

Table XXII. Heart Defects Causing Cyanosis

A. Decreased pulmonary vascular markings
• Tetralogy of Fallot
• Pulmonary atresia (stenosis) with intact ventricular septum
• Tricuspid atresia
• Complex pulmonary stenosis
B. Increased pulmonary vascular markings
• Transposition of the great arteries
• Hypoplastic left heart syndrome
• Coarctation of the aorta syndrome
• Multiple left-to-right shunts
Severe pulmonary venous congestion
• Total anomalous pulmonary venous connection (infradiaphragmatic type)
• Hypoplastic left heart syndrome (with intact atrial septum)
• Severe coarctation of the aorta

Reproduced from Rao PS, *Neonatology Today 2007*; 2(6):1-7.

Table XXIII. Central Nervous System Disorders Causing Cyanosis

• Intracranial hemorrhage
• Intracerebral malformations
• Severe intracranial infections
• Primary seizure disorders

Reproduced from Rao PS, *Neonatology Today 2007*; 2(6):1-7.

Table XXIV. Miscellaneous Disorders Causing Cyanosis

• Polycythemia
• Hypoglycemia
• Methemoglobinemia
• Shock and sepsis
• Maternal drugs

Reproduced from Rao PS, *Neonatology Today 2007*; 2(6):1-7.

A preponderance of babies may be diagnosed by their well-documented clinical and laboratory features. In some neonates, a straight-forward diagnosis is not achievable and in such babies, examination of PO_2 response to 100 percent O_2 and continuous positive airway pressure (CPAP) may help differentiate cardiac from non-cardiac cyanosis. After making a diagnosis of a cardiac baby, cautious analysis of pulmonary vascular marking on a chest roentgenogram may assist classification into sub-groups. Further scrutiny of ECG and other clinical data may facilitate coming up with a realistically correct diagnosis. Echo-Doppler studies can undoubtedly help in reaching a precise diagnosis and is the next step. The exercise presented above is an approach that should be undertaken when echocardiogram is not readily accessible; this may also be utilized prior to the arrival of an echocardiographer.[89]

PRINCIPLES OF MANAGEMENT OF THE NEONATE WITH CONGENITAL HEART DISEASE

Advances in the neonatal care, non-invasive diagnosis, appreciation of pathophysiology of CHD, anesthesia, medical and surgical treatment make it possible to either correct or successfully palliate most CHD manifesting in the neonatal period. Prompt identification, rapid transport to a tertiary care center equipped to manage complex CHD, urgent and precise diagnosis and quick and suitable treatment are essential. The neonatologist or primary care physician providing care for the cyanotic/distressed neonate is in a position to organize the multifaceted care with the pediatric cardiologist, anesthesiologist, pediatric cardiovascular surgeon, and other consultants.[90]

General treatment measures during the course of recognition, transfer to and care at the tertiary care facility was reviewed in the section on "Early Identification of the Neonate with Serious Heart Disease" above. Treatment of cyanosis and CHF was then addressed.[90] Following institution of the supportive care, the type management is dependent on the hemodynamic abnormality produced by the CHD itself along with the associated cardiac anomalies and was discussed under the following categories: Decreased pulmonary flow, increased pulmonary flow, poor mixing, and intra-cardiac obstruction. Infusion of PGE_1 and modified Blalock-Taussig shunt for the baby with decreased pulmonary blood flow (Table VA), anti-congestive measures and banding of the pulmonary artery for neonates with markedly increased pulmonary blood flow (Table XXV), relief of inter-atrial obstruction (Table XXVI), either by catheter-based or surgical means, as required should be provided. Also, relief or bypass of inter-ventricular obstruction (Table XXVII) may become necessary.

Table XXV. Complex Neonatal Heart Defects* Requiring Pulmonary Artery Banding

1. Swiss-cheese type of ventricular septal defects
2. Double inlet left ventricle (Single ventricle)
3. Double outlet right ventricle
4. Tricuspid atresia with a large ventricular septal defect

* Without associate pulmonary stenosis. Reproduced from Rao PS, *Neonatology Today 2007*; 2(8):1-10.

Table XXVI. Interatrial Obstruction

1. Pulmonary atresia
2. Tricuspid atresia
3. Mitral atresia
4. Hypoplastic left heart syndrome
5. Total anomalous pulmonary venous connection

Reproduced from Rao PS, *Neonatology Today 2007*; 2(8):1-10.

Table XXVII. Inter-ventricular Obstruction

1. Tricuspid atresia
2. Double inlet left ventricle
3. Double outlet right (or left) ventricle

Reproduced from Rao PS, *Neonatology Today 2007*; 2(8):1-10.

With regard to specific heart defects, transcatheter and/or surgical correction, as deemed appropriate should be undertaken; management of a number of these defects were reviewed and include, critical pulmonary stenosis, critical aortic stenosis, coarctation of the aorta, infra-diaphragmatic TAPVC, TGA, tetralogy of Fallot (TOF), interrupted aortic arch, VSD, PDA, patent foramen ovale (PFO), HLHS, double inlet left ventricle and other single ventricle lesions, tricuspid atresia, pulmonary atresia with intact ventricular septum, truncus arteriosus, Ebstein's anomaly of the tricuspid valve, and syndrome of absent pulmonary valve.[90]

ROLE OF INTERVENTIONAL CARDIOLOGY IN NEONATES[92-97]

This subject was reviewed in the chapter on "Neonatal Catheter Interventions" in the book titled "Pediatric Cardiology: How It Has Evolved Over the last 50 Years" and will not be discussed here.

CARDIAC EMERGENCIES IN PEDIATRIC PRACTICE

A review of pediatric cardiac emergencies was prepared when I was a PALS instructor in the early 1990s at the University of Wisconsin and subsequently the review was published in *Physician's Digest*,[100] *Neonatology Today*,[101] *Emergency Medicine*,[123] and most recently as a textbook chapter in the author's book on *Perinatal Cardiology*.[178] Two of these reviews[100,123] address cardiac emergencies in the entire pediatric population, while the others two[101,178] focus on the neonate.

Life-threatening emergencies involving the cardiovascular system in children are many and sometimes complex and their successful management depends upon prompt and accurate diagnosis so that appropriate therapeutic measures can be instituted. More commonly encountered emergencies are listed in Table XXVIII. Management of cardio-respiratory arrest and shock are essentially similar to that in the adult and therefore was not dealt with in these reviews. Detailed description of hypercyanotic spells, arrhythmias, cyanosis in the newborn, CHF, cerebro-vascular accidents and brain abscess and their management was addressed in these reviews.

Table XXVIII. List of Cardiac Emergencies in Pediatric Practice

1. Cardiopulmonary arrest
2. Shock
3. Hypercyanotic spells
4. Arrhythmias
5. Cyanosis in the newborn
6. Congestive heart failure
7. Cerebrovascular accidents
8. Brain Abscess

Reproduced from Rao PS, *Physician's Digest 200 (June-July)*; 17(2):30-36.

In the more recent reviews,[101,178] a new topic, cardiac emergencies in the babies with a functional single ventricle was added. In these infants, the systemic and pulmonary circulations function in-parallel, rather than in-series circuits of normal circulation. Too much pulmonary blood flow produces systemic hypo-perfusion and markedly reduced pulmonary blood flow produces severe hypoxemia and therefore, a delicate balance of the blood flows between the two circulations should be maintained. Conditions such as dehydration, acidosis, or fever upset the balance between the two circulations and cause a patient to become critically ill. Obstructed aorto-pulmonary shunts also adversely affect these patients. Significant inter-stage mortality is attributed to these events. Awareness of these issues with palliated single ventricle physiology patients and aggressive evaluation and management of even minor illnesses is emphasized to maximize successful outcomes.

Conditions such as pericardial effusion with or without cardiac tamponade and congenital complete heart block are also important cardiac emergencies, but were not addressed in these reviews.[100,101,123.178]

DIAGNOSIS AND MANAGEMENT OF CYANOTIC CONGENITAL HEART DISEASE

Diagnosis and management of cyanotic CHD was reviewed in the *Indian Journal of Pediatrics* in another Symposium on Cardiology in 2009. In the first the two papers,[102] the most commonly encountered cyanotic heart defects in children, namely, TOF, TGA, and tricuspid atresia were reviewed. In the second paper,[103] less commonly encountered cyanotic cardiac lesions, namely, TAPVC, truncus arteriosus, HLHS, pulmonary atresia with intact ventricular septum, double outlet right ventricle, univentricular hearts (double inlet left ventricle), pulmonary atresia associated other complex cardiac defects, interrupted aortic arch, and syndrome of absent pulmonary valve were reviewed. Pathology, pathophysiology, clinical features, non-invasive and invasive laboratory studies and management of each of defects were discussed.[102,103] The clinical and non-invasive laboratory features are sufficiently characteristic for making the diagnosis and invasive cardiac catheterization and angiographic studies are not routinely required, but may be needed either to define features not clearly defined by non-invasive studies or as a part of catheter-based intervention. Following the diagnosis, some of these patients require immediate treatment for stabilization and all require subsequent corrective and/or palliative surgical therapy. Surgical correction or effective palliation can be undertaken with relatively low risk. However, residual defects, some requiring repeat catheter or surgical intervention, are present in a significant percentage of patients and therefore, continued follow-up after surgery is mandatory.[102,103]

WHEN AND HOW SHOULD ATRIAL SEPTAL DEFECTS BE CLOSED IN ADULTS[106]

This subject was reviewed in the chapter on "Atrial Septal Defects" in the book titled "Pediatric Cardiology: How It Has Evolved Over the last 50 Years" and will not be reviewed here.

TRANSPOSITION OF THE GREAT ARTERIES IN THE NEONATE[107,179]

Transposition of the great arteries is a CHD in which the aorta arises from the right ventricle, while the pulmonary artery comes off of the left ventricle. It is the most common cyanotic CHD in the neonate. In this condition, the systemic and pulmonary circulations are parallel instead of the normal circulation, which is in series. This anomaly is classified into TGA with intact ventricular septum, TGA with VSD, and TGA with VSD and PS. The intact ventricular septum patients present in the very early neonatal period, while the other two may present with symptoms slightly latter. Cyanosis is the major symptom in intact septum patients, while hearing failure is the presenting symptom in VSD patients. TGA with VSD and PS have a variable presentation. Murmurs are notably absent in intact septum babies, while loud holosystolic or ejection systolic murmurs dominate in the other two groups. While the chest x-ray and ECG are helpful in the diagnosis, echocardiographic studies are confirmatory in the diagnosis and quantification of the associated defects. PGE_1 infusion to open the ductus and/or balloon atrial septostomy to enlarge the PFO may sometimes be required for palliation. Corrective surgery by arterial switch (Jatene) procedure is necessary in TGA patients with intact septum and those with VSD, whereas Rastelli procedure may be required for patients with VSD and PS.[107,179]

TETRALOGY OF FALLOT (TOF) IN THE NEONATE[108]

TOF is the most common cyanotic CHD beyond one year of age and constitutes 10 percent of all CHDs. In the neonate however, it is less common than transposition of the great arteries. TOF is a constellation of four abnormalities: 1. VSD, 2. PS, 3. Right ventricular hypertrophy, and 4. Dextroposition of the aorta. Because the VSD is large, the systolic pressures in both ventricles are equal and for practical purposes both ventricles act as one functional chamber. The quantity of blood flow into the systemic and pulmonary circuits depends upon their respective resistances. The level of systemic vascular resistance and the resistance offered by the right ventricular outflow tract stenosis determine the flows. The more severe the PS, the less is the pulmonary flow. There are several variants of TOF with differences in presentation in the neonatal period; neonatal TOF may be classified as: Type I, Classic TOF; Type II, TOF with pulmonary atresia; Type III, TOF with MAPCAs; Type IV, TOF with absent pulmonary valve syndrome.

The majority of classic TOF patients are either acyanotic or minimally cyanotic in the neonatal period and do not require surgical intervention as a neonate. The initial management of TOF with pulmonary atresia (ductal dependent) is by prompt infusion of PGE_1 to keep the ductus open. Once the baby is stabilized, a permanent way to provide pulmonary blood flow should be made. In those patients whose cardiac defect could not be corrected in the neonatal period, a modified Blalock-Taussig (BT) shunt using an interposition Gore-Tex graft between the right or left subclavian arteries and the ipsilateral pulmonary artery is current surgical procedure of choice. Ductal stenting is an attractive non-surgical option, but because of limited experience and generally long and tortuous ducti, ductal stent is not currently the first-line therapeutic choice. In rare babies with membranous valvar pulmonary atresia, perforation of the atretic valve along with balloon dilatation, similar to that advocated for pulmonary atresia with intact ventricular septum, may be attempted. The initial management of patients with TOF and MAPCAs depends on the extent of pulmonary blood flow. The majority of patients will maintain acceptable arterial oxygen saturations in the range of 80 percent to 90 percent and may not require intervention in the neonatal period. Patients with decreased pulmonary flow and hypoxemia may need PGE$_1$ and BT shunt. Patients with increased pulmonary flow may need anti-congestive treatment. The definitive management of TOF with MAPCAs includes combined staged approach with surgery and interventional catheterization to establish antegrade pulmonary blood flow from the right ventricle, rehabilitate the pulmonary arteries, and closure of the VSD. Symptomatic neonates with TOF and syndrome of absent pulmonary valve require ventilatory support to stabilize the patient followed by total surgical correction under cardiopulmonary bypass, including closure of the VSD, relief of PS by a transannular pericardial patch as necessary and partial resection and plastic repair of aneurysmally dilated pulmonary arteries.[108]

HYPOPLASTIC LEFT HEART SYNDROME (HLHS) IN THE NEONATE[110]

Hypoplastic left heart syndrome is a constellation of left heart anomalies including diminutive left ventricle with under development of mitral and aortic valves and a small and hypoplastic aorta. A PFO and a PDA are usually present and are required for survival. Coarctation of the aorta may also be present. Pulmonary venous blood crosses the atrial septum and mixes with systemic venous blood in the right atrium and from there transmitted into the right ventricle and the pulmonary artery. The pulmonary and the systemic circulations are connected in parallel by the ductus arteriosus and the blood exiting in the right ventricle is distributed into the lungs via the branch pulmonary arteries and into the body via the ductus arteriosus. HLHS comprises 1.2 percent to 1.5 percent of all CHDs and is uniformly lethal unless it is promptly identified, treated with PGE$_1$ and surgically palliated. They are clinically identified either by prenatal ultrasound or present with symptoms after birth as the ductus begins to close. The time of presentation depends on the degree of atrial level obstruction, ductal patency and the level of pulmonary vascular resistance. The diagnosis can usually be made with Echo-Doppler studies. The initial management of HLHS is by prompt infusion of PGE$_1$ to keep the ductus open. Balancing the pulmonary and systemic circulation to maintain adequate systemic perfusion and ensuring adequacy of patent foramen ovale for easy egress of left atrial blood while waiting for surgery are the next tasks. Surgical management is either by multi-stage surgical procedures, consisting of Norwood procedure (Stage I) in the neonatal period, hemi-Fontan or bidirectional Glenn procedure (Stage II) at about six months of age, and Fontan conversion (Stage III) one year later or orthotopic heart transplantation. Currently, the actuarial survival rate of infants treated with these surgical approaches is 70 perent at five years and is similar to that of infants with other complex forms of congenital heart disease in whom a two-ventricle repair is not possible.[110]

TRICUSPID ATRESIA (TA) IN THE NEONATE [111]

TA is the third most common cyanotic CHD. Significant differences in the associated defects and consequent physiology result in varied clinical presentations. The diagnosis is fairly simple and can frequently be made by clinical features and simple studies such as chest X-ray and ECG, which can be confirmed by Echo-Doppler studies. Aggressive treatment to normalize the pulmonary blood flow and to correct associated defects such as coarctation of the aorta should be carried out at the time of initial presentation. Careful follow-up and management in an attempt to preserve (or normalize) cardiac structures and function (for example, pulmonary artery pressure and anatomy, and left ventricular function) should be pursued. Lastly, undertaking staged, modified Fontan-Kreutzer operation (total cavo-pulmonary connection with an extra-cardiac conduit and fenestration) before any deterioration of the left ventricular function should noticeably improve the prognosis for TA patients. [111] Further details may be found in the chapter on "Tricuspid Atresia" in the book titled "Pediatric Cardiology: How It Has Evolved Over the last 50 Years."

CONSENSUS ON TIMING OF INTERVENTION FOR COMMON CONGENITAL HEART DISEASES: ACYANOTIC HEART DEFECTS [112]

This was an invited paper and the review started by stating that CHD is a common congenital anomaly occurring in 0.6% and 0.8% of live births and that 50 percent of these defects may be managed by observation, simple medications, and follow-up without any major therapeutic intervention, while the remaining 50 percent require surgical or transcatheter intervention to address these anomalies in an attempt to prevent mortality, decrease morbidity, and avoid permanent damage to the heart or pulmonary vasculature. The review addresses how and when to treat the most common CHD; the Part I discusses acyanotic heart defects112 and discussion of cyanotic CHD was included in a subsequent paper. The acyanotic defects may be subdivided into obstructive and left-to-right shunt lesions; methods of management of six most common acyanotic CHD were described. By and large, the indications and timing of intervention are decided by the severity of the lesion. Balloon pulmonary valvuloplasty is the treatment of choice for valvar pulmonary stenosis and the indication for intervention is peak-to-peak systolic pressure gradient > 50 mmHg across the pulmonary valve. For aortic valve stenosis, balloon aortic valvuloplasty appears to be the first therapeutic procedure of choice; the indications for balloon dilatation of aortic valve are peak-to-peak systolic pressure gradient across the aortic valve in excess of 70 mmHg irrespective of the symptoms or a gradient ≥ 50 mmHg with either symptoms or electrocardiographic ST-T wave changes indicative of myocardial perfusion abnormality. The indications for intervention in coarctation of the aorta are significant hypertension and/or congestive heart failure along with a pressure gradient in excess of 20 mmHg across the coarctation; the type of intervention varies with age at presentation and the anatomy of coarctation: Surgical intervention for neonates and young infants, balloon angioplasty for discrete native coarctation in children, and stents in adolescents and adults. Long segment coarctations or those associated with hypoplasia of the isthmus or transverse aortic arch require surgical treatment in younger children and stents in adolescents and adults. For post-surgical aortic recoarctation, balloon angioplasty in young children and stents in adolescents and adults are the treatment options.

Transcatheter closure methods are currently preferred for ostium secundum atrial septal defects (ASDs); the indications for occlusion are right ventricular volume overload by echocardiogram. Ostium primum, sinus venosus and coronary sinus ASDs require surgical closure. For all ASDs, elective closure around the age of four to five years is recommended or as and when detected beyond that age. For the more common perimembranous VSDs of large size, surgical closure should be performed prior to six to twelve months of age. Muscular VSDs may be closed with devices. Patent ductus arteriosus (PDA) may be closed with Amplatzer Duct Occluder if they are moderate to large and Gianturco coils if they are small. Surgical and video-thoracoscopic closure are the other available options at some centers. In the presence of pulmonary hypertension appropriate testing to determine suitability for closure should be undertaken.

The treatment of acyanotic CHD with currently available medical, transcatheter and surgical methods is feasible, safe and effective and should be performed at an appropriate age in order to prevent damage to cardiovascular structures.[112]

CONSENSUS ON TIMING OF INTERVENTION FOR COMMON CONGENITAL HEART DISEASES: PART II - CYANOTIC HEART DEFECTS[120]

This review was intended to discuss how and when to treat the most common cyanotic CHD;[120] the discussion of acyanotic heart defects was presented in the first paper.[112] By and large, the indications and timing of intervention are decided by the severity of the lesion. While some patients with acyanotic CHD may not require surgical or transcatheter intervention because of spontaneous resolution of the defect or mildness of the defect, the majority of cyanotic CHD patients will require intervention, mostly surgical.

Total surgical correction is the treatment of choice for TOF patients; although, some patients may require initial palliation with a modified Blalock-Taussig shunt. For TGA, arterial switch (Jatene) procedure is the treatment of choice; although, Rastelli procedure is required for patients who have associated VSD and PS. Some of these babies may require PGE_1 infusion and/or balloon atrial septostomy prior to corrective surgery. In tricuspid atresia patients, most babies require palliation at presentation either with a modified Blalock-Taussig shunt or pulmonary artery banding followed later by staged Fontan (bidirectional Glenn followed later by extracardiac conduit Fontan procedure usually with a fenestration). Truncus arteriosus babies are treated by closure of VSD along with right ventricle to pulmonary artery conduit; palliative banding of the pulmonary artery is no longer recommended. Total anomalous pulmonary venous connection babies require anastomosis of the common pulmonary vein with the left atrium at presentation. Other defects discussed include HLHS, pulmonary atresia with intact ventricular septum, double outlet right ventricle, double inlet left ventricle, interrupted aortic arch, and Ebstein's anomaly of the tricuspid valve. These defects are also addressed, mostly by staged correction or complete repair depending upon the anatomy/physiology. Treatment of cyanotic CHD with currently available medical, transcatheter and surgical methods is feasible, safe and effective and should be performed at an appropriate age in order to prevent damage to cardiovascular structures.

HISTORICAL ASPECTS OF TRANSCATHETER TREATMENT OF HEART DISEASE IN CHILDREN[114]

In this review, the historical aspects of transcatheter treatment heart disease in children was addressed.[114] The very first transcatheter intervention to treat congenital cardiac defects was reported by Rubio-Alvarez et al in 1953, when they performed pulmonary valvotomy using a modified ureteral catheter. A decade later Dotter, Rashkind, Porstmann and their associates described progressive dilatation of peripheral arterial stenotic lesions, balloon atrial septostomy and transcatheter occlusion of patent ductus arteriosus, respectively. The purpose of this review was to present these and other historical developments of catheter-based interventions in the treatment of heart disease in children.

Historical aspects of the following: 1. Balloon angioplasty/valvuloplasty of valvar pulmonary stenosis, valvar aortic stenosis, fixed subaortic stenosis, native aortic coarctation, postsurgical aortic recoarctation, branch pulmonary artery stenosis, mitral stenosis, cyanotic heart defects with pulmonary oligemia, stenotic bioprosthetic valves, congenital tricuspid and mitral stenosis, truncal valve stenosis, subvalvar pulmonary stenosis, supravalvar pulmonary stenosis (congenital membranous or postoperative), stenosis of the aorta (Leriche syndrome, atherosclerotic and Takayasu's arteritis), baffle obstruction following Mustard or Senning procedure (both systemic and pulmonary venous obstructions), superior and inferior vena caval obstructions, pulmonary vein stenosis, pulmonary venoocclusive disease, vertical vein stenosis in total anomalous pulmonary venous connection, pulmonary venous obstruction following repair of total anomalous pulmonary venous obstruction, specially designed pulmonary artery bands, cor triatriatum, cor triatriatum dexter, and coronary artery stenotic lesions that develop after Kawasaki disease; 2. Stents to enlarge stenotic lesions of branch pulmonary arteries, systemic veins, systemic and pulmonary venous pathways after Mustard procedure, aorta, right ventricular outflow conduits, pulmonary veins and native right ventricular outflow tract or to keep the ductus arteriosus open in patients with pulmonary atresia and hypoplastic left heart syndrome and maintaining patency of stenosed aorto-pulmonary collaterals; 3. balloon/blade atrial septostomy, balloon angioplasty of the atrial septum, transseptal puncture and atrial septal stents were presented.[114] For a more detailed review of the historical aspects of transcatheter treatment heart disease in children, the reader is referred to a more recent publication.[180]

TOTAL ANOMALOUS PULMONARY VENOUS CONNECTION (TAPVC) IN THE NEONATE[118]

In TAPVC, all pulmonary veins drain into systemic veins, most commonly they drain into a common pulmonary vein, which is then connected to the left innominate vein, superior vena cava, coronary sinus, portal vein or other rare sites. TAPVC is the fifth most common cyanotic CHD and occurs in 0.6 to 1.2 per 10,000 live births. Irrespective of the type, all pulmonary venous blood eventually gets back into right atrium, mixes with systemic venous return and gets redistributed to the systemic (via patent foramen ovale) and pulmonary (via tricuspid valve) circulations. The TAPVC is classified based on the anatomic location to which the connecting veins drain, namely, supra-diaphragmatic (supra-cardiac and cardiac) or infra-diaphragmatic and physiologic, based on obstruction to the pulmonary venous return, namely, obstructive or non-obstructive. The supra-diaphragmatic forms are generally non-obstructive and the infra-diaphragmatic forms are almost always obstructive. Connection to the left innominate vein is the most common type of TAPVC. Infra-diaphragmatic type is most common form in the neonate.

The obstructive types present within the first few hours to days of life with signs of severe pulmonary venous congestion and manifest severe tachypnea, tachycardia and cyanosis. Examination reveals rales in the lung fields and a loud pulmonary component of the second heart sound. The non-obstructive TAPVC patients, on the other hand usually present with signs of CHF later in the first month of life. On examination, they have very mild or no visible cyanosis and may have clinical signs of heart failure. Other findings on examination are similar to those seen in patients with secundum atrial septal defect. Clinical and chest x-ray findings are suggestive of the diagnosis and can be confirmed by echocardiographic studies.

In the obstructive type, initial stabilization by intubation and ventilation with high airway pressure should be undertaken. This is followed by emergent surgical correction by anastomosis of the common pulmonary vein with the left atrium. In the non-obstructive type, control of congestive heart failure and stabilization of the patient, followed by elective or semi-elective surgery is recommended. Follow-up to detect development of pulmonary venous obstruction is recommended.[118]

WHAT AN ADULT CARDIOLOGIST SHOULD KNOW ABOUT CYANOTIC CONGENITAL HEART DISEASE?[119]

This subject will be reviewed in the chapter on "Adult Congenital Heart Disease" and will not be discussed here.

TRUNCUS ARTERIOSUS IN THE NEONATE[121]

Truncus arteriosus is an uncommon cyanotic heart defect with a prevalence of less than 1 percent of all CHDs and is characterized by a single blood vessel (truncus) originating from the heart, which in turn gives rise to the aorta, pulmonary arteries and coronary arteries and is usually associated with a large VSD in the conal ventricular septum. This anomaly is generally classified (Collette and Edwards) based on the origin and distribution pulmonary arteries form the truncus, namely, Types I, II, III and IV. These babies are usually asymptomatic at birth and may be detected because of a cardiac murmur or cyanosis. As the PVR decreases, the pulmonary blood flow increases and the babies may show signs of congestive heart failure. Clinical findings include mild cyanosis, a single second heart sound, an ejection systolic click and an ejection systolic murmur at the left upper sternal border. If there is associated severe truncal valve regurgitation, interrupted aortic arch or anomalous and rapid fall in PVR, the presentation is earlier and the symptomatology is severe. ECG is either normal or shows biventricular hypertrophy. Chest X-ray shows cardiomegaly and increased pulmonary vascular markings and associated right aortic arch is virtually diagnostic of truncus. Echocardiographic studies are useful in confirming the diagnosis and in the definition of pulmonary artery anatomy and of the associated defects. Medical management depends on the status of pulmonary blood flow, presence of associated truncal valve insufficiency and interrupted aortic arch, and these should be addressed with anti-congestive measures, afterload reducing agents and intravenous administration of PGE_1 to open the ductus, respectively. Total surgical correction around the age of two weeks is recommended. The results are generally good; although, the need for re-intervention later in life is frequent.[121]

CHILDHOOD HYPERTENSION: A REVIEW[122]

This is a review of hypertension in children.[122] Following introduction, a detailed discussion of definition, prevalence, diagnosis, role of ambulatory BP monitoring, etiology, causes of primary and secondary hypertension, methods of evaluation, and treatment of childhood hypertension was presented.[122] Prevalence of hypertension in children has increased significantly in recent times, in part related to the epidemic of childhood obesity. Identification and treatment of hypertension in childhood is likely to favorably impact on cardiovascular disease in adulthood. Identification of hypertensive children continues to be problematic because of incomplete blood pressure screening during routine pediatric clinical visits.

The blood pressure norms are based on age, gender and height specific values in contradistinction to adults where a single value suffices. Childhood hypertension is either primary or secondary and is categorized as pre-hypertension (between 90th to 95th percentile), Stage 1 (95th to 99th percentile plus 5 mmHg) and Stage 2 (≥ 99th percentile plus 5 mmHg) hypertension. Ambulatory blood pressure monitoring is useful in confirming the diagnosis and in helping diagnose white coat and masked hypertension. Once diagnosed as definitive hypertension, the causes of secondary hypertension (Table XXIX) should be determined and appropriately treated. In children with primary hypertension, a combination of lifestyle changes (diet and exercise) and drug therapy (Table 2 of Reference 122) should be instituted depending upon the stage of the hypertension. Continued follow-up to ensure compliance with treatment regimen and to monitor blood pressure control is mandatory.[122]

Table XXIX. Causes of Secondary Hypertension in Children

Renovascular hypertension

    Renal artery or vein stenosis or thrombosis

    Fibromuscular dysplasia

    Arteritis (Takayasu's, Kawasaki, Moyamoya)

    Renal vessel compression – Tumor, post-trauma, or surgery

Renal Parenchymal Diseases

    Congenital renal malformations

    Glomerulonephritis

    Systemic vasculitis (SLE, HSP)

    Acute or chronic renal failure

Cardiovascular

    Coarctation of the aorta

    Mid aortic hypoplasia

    Syndromes associated with increased risk for aortic hypoplasia (William, Turner's)

Endocrine

    Catecholamine excess (Pheochromocytoma, Neuroblastoma)

    Corticosteroid excess (Iatrogenic, Cushing's disease, CAH)

    Hyperthyroidism

    Hypercalcemia (malignancy, hyperparathyroidism)

Medications

    Steroids

    Cyclosporine, tacrolimus

    ADHD Medications

    Oral contraceptives

    Erythropoietin

    Illicit Drugs

Miscellaneous:

    Neurologic (Elevated ICP, seizures, Guillan Barre', Dysautonomia)

    Post-ECMO

    Chronic Lung Disease

    Obstructive Sleep Apnea

ADHD, Attention deficit hyperactivity disorder; CAH, Congenital adrenal hyperplasia; ECMO, Extra-corporeal membrane oxygenation; HSP, Henoch-Schonlein purpura; ICP, Intra cranial pressure; SLE, Systemic lupus erythematosis.
Reproduced from Banker A, Gupta-Malhotra M, Rao PS, *J Hypertens 2013*; 2:128. Available at DOI:10.4172/2167-1095.1000128.

In summary, increasing prevalence of elevated BP and obesity in children and adolescents is likely to adversely impact on the hypertensive cardiovascular disease in adulthood. Secondary hypertension should be treated as and when the cause is identified. With regard to primary hypertension, prompt identification, exclusion of secondary hypertension, non-pharmacological (diet and exercise) intervention followed by drug therapy, as necessary are essential to address pediatric hypertension. Continued follow-up is mandatory in most patients.[122]

EBSTEIN'S ANOMALY OF THE TRICUSPID VALVE IN THE NEONATE[124]

Ebstein's anomaly is a rare congenital heart disease and is characterized by downward displacement of the septal and posterior leaflets of the tricuspid valve, leading to varying degrees of tricuspid regurgitation and right atrial enlargement. Clinical manifestations vary depending upon the severity of the lesion. Chest x-ray shows severe cardiac enlargement, mostly due to right atrial enlargement, which is commensurate with the severity of tricuspid regurgitation. ECG shows tall and peaked P waves indicating right atrial enlargement, and right bundle branch block. Features of WPW syndrome with short PR interval and delta wave may be present in some patients. Echocardiogram demonstrates tricuspid valve displacement and is useful in confirming the diagnosis. The degree of tricuspid regurgitation and right atrial size can also be assessed. Celemajer index (ratio of area of right atrium [RA] + atrialized portion of right ventricle [RV] to the combined area of RV, left ventricle [LV] and left atrium [LA]) is useful in grading the severity of Ebstein's and in predicting the prognosis.

Mild forms may be asymptomatic and may not need any treatment. Moderate forms may be managed with relative ease. Severe forms of the disease are a challenge to manage. In the presence of severe cyanosis in the neonate, initial treatment to augment pulmonary blood flow using PGE_1 infusion (0.05 – 0.1 mcg/kg/min) is done until PVR decreases. Use of inhaled nitric oxide (NO) in the first few days of life to reduce PVR may be helpful in severe cases associated with high PVR. A few neonates may require surgical systemic-pulmonary shunt to maintain adequate pulmonary blood flow and thus, maintain adequate systemic oxygen saturation. Anti-arrhythmic medications may be necessary for treatment of atrial flutter or supraventricular tachycardia (SVT), when such are present. Every attempt should be made to avoid surgery in neonatal period. In extremely severe cases, Starnes procedure may be required; Starnes procedure is a RV-exclusion procedure consisting of patch-closure of tricuspid valve and Blalock-Taussig shunt to provide pulmonary blood flow. Multiple approaches for repair of tricuspid valve in Ebstein's anomaly were referenced in this review and all such procedures are reserved for older children and adolescents. Prognosis depends on severity of the lesion, age at presentation and type of surgical repair. Surgical outcomes have improved over time but, early presentation as fetus and newborn is associated with poor prognosis.[124]

FONTAN OPERATION: INDICATIONS, SHORT AND LONG TERM OUTCOMES[125]

Since the initial description of the Fontan operation in early 1970s, it had undergone a number of modifications and currently staged, total cavo-pulmonary connection with fenestration has become the most commonly used method of diverting the vena caval blood flow into the lungs. The functioning ventricle, whether it is left or right, is allowed to supply systemic circulation. In Stage I, at presentation in the neonatal period or early infancy, appropriate palliation (modified BT shunt for patients with pulmonary oligemia, pulmonary artery banding in babies with pulmonary plethora and Norwood operation for patients with HLHS) or observation depending upon the patho-physiology of the defect complex is undertaken. In Stage II, bidirectional Glenn by diverting the superior vena caval (SVC) flow into both lungs is performed at about the age of six months. In Stage IIIA, the inferior vena caval (IVC) blood flow is diverted into the lungs, usually by an extra-cardiac conduit along with a fenestration, usually between the ages of two and four years. In Stage IIIB, the fenestration is occluded by transcatheter methodology six to twelve months after Stage IIIA. Because of substantial inter-stage morbidity and mortality, careful follow-up of these babies with prompt and aggressive management of inter-current illnesses and symptoms of hypoxemia is mandatory.

The indications for selecting Fontan route are cardiac defects with only one functioning ventricle. The mor-bidity and mortality associated with early types of Fontan has substantially decreased since the introduction of staged, total cavo-pulmonary connection with fenestration. However, many complications such as, arrhythmias, obstructed Fontan pathways, cyanosis and paradoxical emboli, thrombus formation, development of collateral ves-sels and protein losing enteropathy may develop during long-term follow-up of Fontan patients and these should be promptly diagnosed and addressed.[125]

THE JOURNEY OF AN INDIAN PEDIATRIC CARDIOLOGIST[126]

The life journey of an Indian pediatric cardiologist, who bestowed considerable attention to the development of new knowledge and train/teach physicians around the world while providing care of patients with heart disease over a forty-five-year period, was reviewed. This appraisal focuses particular attention on the scientific contribu-tions to the literature. These include spontaneous closure of physiologically advantageous VSDs, various issues related to a congenital heart defect namely, tricuspid atresia and transcatheter and interventional pediatric cardiac procedures.[126]

RECENT ADVANCES IN MANAGING SEPTAL DEFECTS: ATRIAL SEPTAL DEFECTS

This was another invited review[127] in which we discussed the management of ASD, paying particular atten-tion to the most recent developments. It was stated that there are four types of ASDs, namely, ostium secun-dum, ostium primum, sinus venosus, and coronary sinus defects. The fifth type, patent foramen ovale, which is present in 25 percent to 30 percent of normal individuals, may be considered a normal variant, although it may be the seat of paradoxical embolism, particularly in adults and was not addressed in this review.

The indication for closure of the ASDs, by and large, is the presence of right ventricular volume overload. In asymp-tomatic patients, the closure is usually performed at four to five years of age. While there was some earlier contro-versy regarding ASD closure in adult patients, currently it is recommended that ASDs in adults be closed at the ti me of presentation.

Each of the four defects was briefly described followed by presentation of management, whether by surgical or per-cutaneous approach, as the case may be. Of the four types of ASDs, only the ostium secundum defect is amenable to percutaneous occlusion. For ostium secundum defects, transcatheter closure has been shown to be as effective as surgical closure, but with the added benefits of decreased hospital stay, avoidance of a sternotomy, lower cost, and more rapid recovery. There are several FDA-approved devices in use today for percutaneous closure, including the Amplatzer® Septal Occluder (ASO), Amplatzer® Cribriform device, and Gore HELEX® device. The ASO is most commonly used for ostium secundum ASDs, the Gore HELEX® is useful for small to medium defects, and the cribriform device is utilized for fenestrated ASDs. The remaining types of ASDs usually require surgical correction. All of the available treatment modes are safe and effective and prevent the development of further cardiac complications.[127]

RECENT ADVANCES IN MANAGING SEPTAL DEFECTS: VENTRICULAR SEPTAL DEFECTS AND ATRIOVENTRICULAR SEPTAL DEFECTS.[129]

This is second of the reviews discusses the management of VSDs and atrioventricular septal defects (AVSDs). There are several types of VSDs: Perimembranous, supracristal, atrioventricular septal, and muscular. The indications for closure are moderate to large VSDs with enlarged left atrium and left ventricle or elevated pulmonary artery pressure (or both) and a pulmonary-to-systemic flow ratio greater than 2:1. Surgical closure is recommended for large perimembranous VSDs, supracristal VSDs, and VSDs with aortic valve prolapse. Large muscular VSDs may be closed by percutaneous techniques. A large number of devices have been used in the past for VSD occlusion, but currently Amplatzer Muscular VSD Occluder is the only device approved by the US Food and Drug Administration for clinical use. A hybrid approach may be used for large muscular VSDs in small babies. Timely intervention to prevent pulmonary vascular obstructive disease (PVOD) is germane in the management of these babies.

There are several types of AVSDs: Partial, transitional, intermediate, and complete.

Complete AVSDs are also classified as balanced and unbalanced. All intermediate and complete balanced AVSDs require surgical correction, and early repair is needed to prevent the onset of PVOD. Surgical correction with closure of atrial septal defect and VSD, along with repair and reconstruction of atrioventricular valves, is recommended. Palliative pulmonary artery banding may be considered in babies weighing less than 5 kg and those with significant co-morbidities. The management of unbalanced AVSDs is more complex, and staged single-ventricle palliation is the common management strategy. However, recent data suggest that achieving two-ventricle repair may be a better option in patients with suitable anatomy, particularly in patients in whom outcomes of single-ventricle palliation are less than optimal.

The majority of treatment modes in the management of VSDs and AVSDs are safe and effective and prevent the development of PVOD and cardiac dysfunction.[129]

ROLE OF ECHOCARDIOGRAPHY IN THE EVALUATION OF PRETERM INFANTS WITH PATENT DUCTUS ARTERIOSUS[128,130]

The ductus arteriosus is a muscular structure that connects the main pulmonary artery with the descending thoracic aorta. In the fetal circulation, the ductus diverts less oxygenated blood from the pulmonary artery into the descending aorta, umbilical arteries and placenta for oxygenation. The ductus closes spontaneously shortly after birth, but persistence patency beyond seventy-two hours after birth is defined as a PDA. The ductal patency is more frequent in the preterm than in the term babies; the lower the gestational age, the higher the incidence. The PDA causes left to right shunt, mainly proportional to the minimal ductal diameter. Such a shunt may cause pulmonary and cardiac compromise. While clinical features, chest roentgenogram and serum BNP levels may help identifying a PDA, hemodynamically significant PDAs may be best detected and quantified by Echo-Doppler studies. The Echo-Doppler protocol includes performing two-dimensional (2D), M-mode, and Doppler examination in parasternal long and short axis, apical four-chamber and two-chamber, subcostal and suprasternal notch views. Pulsed, continuous wave and color Doppler in multiple views are recorded with particular attention to define the size of the PDA and its hemodynamic effects. Recording maximal Doppler flow velocity magnitudes across the ductus is also undertaken. Doppler recordings that are useful in estimation of pulmonary arterial pressures should also be made. Finally, recording the patterns of descending aortic diastolic flow should also be undertaken in order to demonstrate normal anterograde diastolic flow, absent diastolic flow or retrograde diastolic flow, as the case may be.

The LA, LA:Ao ratio (< 1.4:1) and LV are likely to be normal in size in small PDAs, and the LV function is normal. The LA and LV are dilated and LA:Ao ratio is increased (>1.6:1) in large PDAs. In the beginning, the LV function is normal or hyperdynamic and with time, LV function may deteriorate resulting in increased LV end-diastolic and LA pressures with consequent deterioration of the respiratory status. In moderate PDAs, the values in are in middle with moderate dilatation of LA (LA:Ao ratio of 1.4 to 1.6) and LV. In most, the LV function is preserved.

The minimal ductal diameter is small with high Doppler velocity across it in small PDAs whereas the minimal ductal diameter is large with low Doppler velocity across the ductus in large PDAs. These values are in the middle in moderate sized PDAs. In small PDAs, the PA pressures are usually normal, while they are likely to be high in large PDAs. While the above assertions are largely correct, the PA pressures also depend upon the degree of pulmonary parenchymal disease. In addition, in very low birth weight infants, the PA pressure may not be elevated parallel to the pulmonary parenchymal disease because of under-developed pulmonary vasculature in the premature.

Finally, normal anterograde descending aortic diastolic flow is seen in small PDAs, whereas the descending aortic diastolic flow is either retrograde or no normal anterograde descending aortic diastolic flow is seen in large PDAs.

In summary, the size of the LA, LA:Ao ratio, the diameter of the LV, estimated pulmonary artery pressures, minimal ductal diameter, Doppler flow velocity across the PDA and descending aortic Doppler flow pattern help us to identify the size of the PDA. When a medium to large PDA is present along with respiratory compromise, a hemodynamically significant PDAs may be diagnosed.[128,130]

MANAGEMENT OF CONGENITAL HEART DISEASE: STATE OF THE ART

These were another set of invited reviews in which I discussed state of the art of the management of CHD.[131,132] In the first of these reviews addressing acyanotic CHD, it was stated: Since the description of surgery for patent ductus arteriosus in late 1930s, an enumerable number of advances have taken place in the management of CHDs. In the first review,[131] the current status of treatment of seven most common acyanotic CHDs was reviewed. Discussion included indications for and timing of intervention and methods of intervention. The indications are by and large determined by severity of the lesion. Pressure gradients in obstructive lesions and magnitude of shunt in left to right shunt lesions are used to assess the severity of the lesion. The timing of intervention is different for each lesion and largely dependent upon when the criteria for indications for intervention were met. Appropriate medical management is necessary in most patients. Transcatheter methods are preferable in some defects, while surgery is a better option in some other defects. The currently available medical, transcatheter and surgical methods to treat acyanotic CHD are feasible, safe and effective.[131]

In the second of the reviews,[132] management of the most common cyanotic CHDs was discussed. While the need for intervention in acyanotic CHD is by and large determined by the severity of the lesion, most cyanotic CHDs require intervention, mostly by surgery. Different types of tetralogy of Fallot require different types of total surgical corrective procedures, and some may require initial palliation, mainly by modified Blalock-Taussig shunts. Babies with transposition of the great arteries with intact ventricular septum as well as those with VSD need arterial switch (Jatene) procedure, while those with both VSD and PS should be addressed by Rastelli procedure. These procedures may need to be preceded by prostaglandin infusion and/or balloon atrial septostomy in some babies. Infants with tricuspid atresia require initial palliation either with a modified Blalock-Taussig shunt or banding of the pulmonary artery and subsequent staged Fontan (bidirectional Glenn and fenestrated Fontan with extra-cardiac conduit). Neonates with total anomalous pulmonary venous connection are managed by anastomosis of the common pulmonary vein with the left atrium either electively in non-obstructed types or as an emergency procedure in the obstructed types. Babies with truncus arteriosus are treated by surgical closure of VSD along with right ventricle to pulmonary artery conduit. The other defects, namely, hypoplastic left heart syndrome, pulmonary atresia with intact ventricular septum, double outlet right ventricle, double inlet left ventricle, and univentricular hearts largely require multistage surgical correction. The currently existing medical, transcatheter and surgical techniques to manage cyanotic CHD are safe and effective and can be performed at a relatively low risk.[132]

REFERENCES

1. Rao PS, "Physiological basis of diuretic drugs," *J Indian Med Ass 1971*; 56:100-7.

2. Rao PS, "Preventive aspects of congenital heart disease," *Paediatrician 1973*; 2:224-38.

3. Vincent WR and Rao PS, "Early identification of the neonate with suspected serious heart disease," *Paediatrician 1973*; 2:239-250.

4. Lee MH and Rao PS, "Digitalis toxicity in infants and children," *Paediatrician 1973*; 2:306-16.

5. Linde LM and Rao PS, "A modern view of infective endocarditis," *Cardiovasc Clinics 1973*; Vol. 5, No. 2:15-34.

6. Linde LM and Rao PS, "Pressure and energy in cardiovascular chambers," *Chest 1974*; 66:176-8.

7. Rao PS and Strong WB, "Early identification of the neonate with heart disease," *J Med Assoc Georgia 1974*; 63:430-3.

8. Strong WB, Rao PS, Steinbauch M, "Primary prevention of atherosclerosis: A challenge to the physician caring for children," *Southern Med J 1975*; 68:319-27.

9. Rao PS, "Prevention of pediatric heart disease," *Paediatrician 1975*; 4:320-42.

10. Rigby JJ and Rao PS, "Cardiac catheterization in infancy and childhood," *Paediatrician 1975*; 4:343-55.

11. Rao PS and Leonard T, "Polysplenia syndrome," *Cardiology Digest 1976*; 11(3):14-22, (March).

12. Rao PS, "Preventive aspects of heart disease in infants and children," *South Med J 1977*; 70:728-40.

13. Rao PS, "Prevention of Heart Disease in Infants and Children," Current Problems in Pediatrics, Vol. 7, May 1977, pp. 1-48, *Yearbook Medical Publisher, Inc.*, Chicago, USA.

14. Thapar MK, Rao PS, Linde LM, Feldman D, "Infective endocarditis: I. Incidence, etiology, pathology and clinical features," *Paediatrician 1978*; 7:65-84.

15. Rao PS, Thapar MK, Linde LM, Feldman D, "Infective endocarditis: II. Diagnosis and treatment," *Paediatrician 1978*; 7:85-99.

16. Rao PS, "Present status of surgery in congenital heart disease," *Indian J Pediatr 1981*; 49:349-63.

17. Rao PS, "Dextrocardia: Systematic approach to differential diagnosis," *Amer Heart J 1981*; 102:389-403.

18. Rao PS, Kulangara RJ, "Echocardiographic evaluation of global left ventricular performance in infants and children," *Indian Pediat 1982*; 19:21-32.

19. Rao PS, "Vasodilator therapy for cardiac failure in pediatric practice," *Indian J Pediat 1982*; 49:843-8.

20. Rao PS, "Non-invasive evaluation of left ventricular function in infants and children," *Saudi Med J 1983*; 4:195-209.

21. Rao PS, "Pathophysiologic consequences of cyanotic heart disease," *Indian J Pediat 1983*; 50:479-87.

22. Rao PS, "Management of the neonate with suspected serious heart disease," *King Faisal Specialist Hospital Med J 1984*; 4:209-16.

23. Rao PS, "Surgery without thoracotomy: Transcatheter management of pediatric heart disease," *Indian J Pediatr 1984*, 51:703-714.

24. Rao PS, "Comprehensive management of pulmonary atresia with intact ventricular septum," *Ann Thorac Surg 1985*; 40:409-13.

25. Rao PS, "Pediatric cardiology update: Recent therapeutic advances," *Saudi Med J 1986*; 7:306-20.

26. Rao PS, "Mitral valve prolapse síndrome," *Indian J Pediat 1987*; 54:140-4.

27. Rao PS, "Transcatheter management of heart disease in infants and children," *Pediat Rev Comm 1987*; 1:1-18.

28. Rao PS, "Transcatheter therapy of cardiac defects in infants and children," *Indian J Pediatr 1988*; 44:137-140.

29. Rao PS, "Doppler echocardiography in non-invasive diagnosis of heart disease in infants and children," *Indian J Pediatr 1988*; 55:80-95.

30. Rao PS, "Transcatheter treatment of heart disease in infancy and childhood," *Wisconsin Med J 1988*; 87:28-30.

31. Rao PS, "Balloon dilatation in infants and children with cardiac defects," *Cath Cardiovasc Diag 1989*; 18:136-49.

32. Rao PS, "Balloon pulmonary valvuloplasty: A review," *Clin Cardiol 1989*; 12:55-74.

33. Rao PS, "Medical Progress: Balloon valvuloplasty and angioplasty in infants and children," *J Pediat 1989*; 114:907-14.

34. Rao PS, "Balloon angioplasty of aortic coarctation: A review," *Clin Cardiol 1989*; 12:618-28.

35. Rao PS, "Balloon valvuloplasty and angioplasty for congenital and acquired heart defects in children," *Bull Saudi Heart Assoc 1990*; 2:10-22.

36. Rao PS, "Causes of restenosis following balloon angioplasty/valvuloplasty: A review," *Pediatr Rev Comm 1990*; 4:157-72.

37. Rao PS, "Balloon aortic valvuloplasty: A review," *Clinical Cardiol 1990*; 13:458-66.

38. Rao PS, "Balloon valvuloplasty in neonates and children," *Saudi Heart Bulletin 1990*; 1:55-70.

39. Rao PS, "Perinatal circulatory physiology," *Indian J Pediat 1991*; 58:441-51.

40. Rao PS, "Evaluation of cardiac murmurs in children," *Indian J Pediat 1991*; 58:471-89.

41. Rao PS and Chopra PS, "Role of balloon angioplasty in the treatment of aortic coarctation," *Ann Thorac Surg 1991*; 52:621-31.

42. Rao PS, "Transcatheter occlusion of cardiac septal defects," *Indian J Pediat 1991*; 58:605-21.

43. Chopra PS and Rao PS, "Surgical management of congenital heart disease: Current trends," *Indian J Pediat 1991*; 58:623-40.

44. Chopra PS and Rao PS, "Corrective surgery for tricuspid atresia: Which modifications of Fontan-Kreutzer procedure should be used? A review," *Am Heart J 1992*; 123:758-67.

45. Rao PS, "Transcatheter management of cyanotic congenital heart defects: A review," *Clin Cardiol 1992*; 15:483-96.

46. Rao PS, "Transcatheter treatment of pulmonary outflow tract obstruction: A review," *Progress Cardiovasc Dis 1992*; 35:119-158.

47. Rao PS, "Transcatheter occlusion of atrial septal defects and patent ductus arteriosus: Now a reality in India," *Indian J Pediat 1993*; 60:615-23.

48. Singh GK, Marino CJ, Rao PS, "Left Heart outflow obstruction, aortic stenosis and coarctation of the aorta: An Echocardiographic assessment," *Pediat Ultrasound Today 1996*; 1:61-76.

49. Rao PS, Sideris EB, "Transcatheter occlusion of patent ductus arteriosus: State of the art," *J Invasive Cardiol 1996*; 8:278-88.

50. Sideris EB, Rao PS, "Transcatheter closure of atrial septal defects: Role of buttoned devices." *J Invasive Cardiol 1996*; 8:289-96.

51. Rao PS, "Should balloon angioplasty be used as a treatment of choice for native aortic coarctations?" *J Invasive Cardiol 1996*; 8:301-13.

52. Chandar JS, Wolfe SB, Rao PS, "Role of stents in the management of congenital heart defects," *J Invasive Cardiol 1996*; 8:314-25.

53. Jureidini SB, Rao PS, "Critical pulmonary stenosis in the neonate: Role of transcatheter management," *J Invasive Cardiol 1996*; 8:326-31.

54. Siblini G, Rao PS, "Coil embolization in the management of cardiac problems in children," *J Invasive Cardiol 1996*; 8:332-40.

55. Singh GK, Marino C, Rao PS, "Ultrasound as an adjunct to cardiac intervention in the pediatric patient," *J Invasive Cardiol 1996*; 8:341-9.

56. Singh GK, Marino CJ, Rao PS, "Echocardiographic evaluation of coarctation of the aorta in adults," *Cardiac Ultrasound Today 1997*; 3:111-24.

57. Rao PS, "Interventional pediatric cardiology: State of the art and future directions," *Pediat Cardiol 1998*; 19:107-24.

58. Rao PS, "Balloon pulmonary valvuloplasty," *J Intervent Cardiol 1998*; 11:303-18.

59. Rao PS, "Balloon aortic valvuloplasty," *J Intervent Cardiol 1998*; 11:319-29.

60. Balfour IC, Rao PS, "Chest pain in children," *Indian J Pediat 1998*; 65:21-26.

61. Jureidini SB, Marino CJ, Rao PS, "Congenital coronary artery anomalies," *Indian J Pediat 1998*; 65:217-29.

62. Rao PS, Sideris EB, "Buttoned device closure of the atrial septal defect," *J Intervent Cardiol 1998*; 11:467-84.

63. Rao PS, "Long-term follow-up results after balloon dilatation of pulmonic stenosis, aortic stenosis and coarctation of the aorta: A review," *Progr Cardiovasc Dis 1999*; 42:59-74.

64. Chopra PS and Rao PS, "History of the development of atrial septal occlusion devices," *Current Intervent Cardiol Reports 2000*; 2:63-9.

65. Zamora R, Rao PS, Sideris EB, "Buttoned device for atrial septal defect occlusion," *Current Intervent Cardiol Reports 2000*; 2:167-76.

66. Rao PS, "Summary and comparison of atrial septal defect closure devices," *Current Intervent Cardiol Reports 2000*; 2:367-76.

67. Rao PS, "Nonsurgical management of pulmonary and aortic stenosis in children with transluminal balloon dilatation techniques," *Gulf Med Coll Ajaman Health J 2000*; 2:18-24.

68. Balfour IC, Rao PS, "Pulmonary stenosis," *Current Treatment Options Cardiovasc Med 2000*; 2:489-98.

69. Rao PS, "Tricuspid atresia," *Current Treatment Options Cardiovasc Med 2000*; 2:507-20.

70. Sideris EB, Rao PS, "Buttoned Device Occlusion of Patent Ductus Arteriosus," *Current Intervent Cardiol Reports*, 3:71-79, 2001.

71. Rao PS, "Summary and comparison of patent ductus arteriosus closure devices," *Current Intervent Cardiol Reports 2001*; 3:268-74.

72. Sideris EB, Haddad J, Rao PS, "The Role of the 'Sideris' devices in the occlusion of ventricular septal defects," *Current Intervent Cardiol Reports 2001*; 3:349-53.

73. Rao PS, "Current status of balloon angioplasty for neonatal and infant aortic coarctation," *Progress Pediat Cardiol 2001*; 14:35-44.

74. Rao PS, Sideris EB, "Centering-on-demand buttoned device: Its role in transcatheter occlusion of atrial septal defects," *J Intervent Cardiol 2001*; 14:81-9.

75. Sideris EB, Rao PS, Zamora R, "The Sideris' buttoned device for transcatheter closure of patent ductus arteriosus," *J Intervent Cardiol 2001*; 14:239-46.

76. Rao PS, "Stents in the management of congenital heart disease in the pediatric and adult patients," *Indian Heart J 2001*; 53:714-30.

77. Rao PS, "Pulmonary atresia with intact ventricular septum," *Current Treatment Options in Cardiovasc Med 2002*; 4:321-36.

78. Gupta ML, Lantin-Hermosa MR, Rao PS, "What is new in pediatric cardiology?" *Indian J Pediat 2003*; 70:41-9.

79. Rao PS, Gupta ML, Balaji S, "Recent advances in pediatric cardiology - electrophysiology, transcatheter and surgical advances," *Indian J Pediat 2003*; 70:557-64.

80. Rao PS, "Current status of cardiac interventions for pediatric congenital heart disease – Part I: Balloon valvuloplasty/angioplasty," *Pediatric Cardiology Newsletter 2004*; 6 (No.1 January-June):1-4.

81. Rao PS, "Current status of cardiac interventions for pediatric congenital heart disease – Part II: Percutaneous closure of cardiac septal defects," *Pediatric Cardiology Newsletter 2004*; 6 (No. 2, July-December):1-5.

82. Rao PS, "Balloon angioplasty for native aortic coarctation in neonates and infants," *Cardiology Today 2005*; 9:94-99.

83. Rao PS, "Diagnosis and management of acyanotic heart disease: Part I - obstructive lesions," *Indian J Pediatr 2005*; 72:496-502.

84. Rao PS, "Diagnosis and management of acyanotic heart disease: Part II - left-to-right shunt lesions," *Indian J Pediatr 2005*; 72:503-12.

85. Gupta-Malhotra M, Rao PS, "Current perspectives on Kawasaki disease," *Indian J Pediatr 2005*; 72:621-29.

86. Rao PS, "Coarctation of the Aorta," *Current Cardiol Reports 2005*; 7:425-34.

87. Rao PS, "Expanding application of devices in congenital heart disease management," *Cardiol Today 2006*; 10:249-66.

88. Rao PS, "Percutaneous balloon pulmonary valvuloplasty: State of the art," *Cath Cardiovasc Intervent 2007*; 69:747-63.

89. Rao PS, "The growing problem of the newborn: An Approach to the diagnosis of cyanotic neonate for the primary care provider," *Neonatology Today 2007*; 2(6):1-7.

90. Rao PS, "Principles of management of the neonate with congenital heart disease," *Neonatology Today 2007*; 2(8):1-10.

91. Rao PS, Techniques for closure of large atrial septal defects. Cath Cardiovasc Intervent 2007; 70: 329-30.

92. Rao PS, "Role of interventional cardiology in neonates: Part I. Non-surgical atrial septostomy," *Neonatology Today 2007*; 2(9):9-14.

93. Rao PS, "Role of interventional cardiology in neonates: Part II - Balloon angioplasty/valvuloplasty," *Neonatology Today 2007*; 2(10):1-12.

94. Rao PS, "Role of interventional cardiology in the treatment of neonates: Part III," *Neonatology Today 2007*; 2(11):1-10.

95. Rao PS, "Role of interventional cardiology in neonates: Part I. Non-surgical atrial septostomy," *Congenital Cardiol Today 2007*; 5(12):1-12.

96. Rao PS, "Role of interventional cardiology in neonates: Part II - Balloon angioplasty/valvuloplasty," *Congenital Cardiol Today 2008*; 6(1):1-14.

97. Rao PS, "Role of interventional cardiology in the treatment of neonates: Part III," *Congenital Cardiol Today 2008*; 6(2):1-10.

98. Rao PS, "Perinatal circulatory physiology: It's influence on clinical manifestations of neonatal heart disease – Part I," *Neonatology Today 2008*; 3(2):6-12.

99. Rao PS, "Perinatal circulatory physiology: It's influence on clinical manifestations of neonatal heart disease – Part II," *Neonatology Today 2008*; 3(3):1-10.

100. Rao PS, "Cardiac emergencies in pediatric practice," *Physician's Digest 200 (June-July)*; 17(2):30-36.

101. Rao PS, "Neonatal cardiac emergencies: Management strategies," *Neonatology Today 2008*; 3(12):1-5.

102. Rao PS, "Diagnosis and management of cyanotic congenital heart disease: Part I," *Indian J Pediat 2009*; 76:57-70.

103. Rao PS, "Diagnosis and management of cyanotic congenital heart disease: Part II," *Indian J Pediat 2009*; 76:297-308.

104. Rao PS, "Perinatal circulatory physiology: It's influence on clinical manifestations of neonatal heart disease – Part I," *Congenital Cardiol Today 2009*; 7(4):1-9.

105. Rao PS, "Perinatal circulatory physiology: It's influence on clinical manifestations of neonatal heart disease – Part II," *Congenital Cardiol Today 2009*; 7(5):1-11.

106. Rao PS, "When and how should atrial septal defects be closed in adults," *J Invasive Cardiol 2009*; 21:76-82.

107. Rao PS, "Transposition of the great arteries in the neonate," *Neonatology Today 2010*; 5(8):1-8.

108. Alapati S, Rao PS, "Tetralogy of Fallot in the neonate," *Neonatology Today 2011*; 6(5): 1-10.

109. Rao PS, "Percutaneous closure of patent ductus arteriosus — Current status," *J Invasive Cardiol 2011*; 23(12):517-20.

110. Alapati S, Rao PS, "Hypoplastic left heart syndrome in the neonate," *Neonatology Today 2011*; 6(12):1-9.

111. Rao PS, Alapati S, "Tricuspid atresia in the neonate," *Neonatology Today 2012*; 7(5):1-12.

112. Rao PS, "Consensus on timing of intervention for common congenital heart diseases: Part I - Acyanotic heart defects," *Indian J Pediatr. 2013*; 80 (1):72-8 [Epub ahead of print; June 30, 2012], PMID: 22752706, [PubMed - as supplied by publisher].

113. Sahu R and Rao PS, "Transcatheter stent therapy in children: An update." *Pediatr Therapeut 2012*; S5:001. DOI: 10.4172/2161-0665.S5-001.

114. Rao PS, "Historical aspects of transcatheter treatment of heart disease in children," *Pediatr Therapeut 2012*; S5:002. DOI:10.4172/2161-0665.S5-002

115. Agu NC, Rao PS, "Balloon aortic valvuloplasty," *Pediatr Therapeut 2012*; S5:004. Available at DOI: 10.4172/2161-0665.S5-004.

116. Yarrabolu TR, Rao PS, "Transcatheter closure of patent ductus arteriosus," *Pediatr Therapeut 2012*; S5:005. Available at DOI: 10.4172/2161-0665.S5-005

117. Doshi AR, Rao PS, "Coarctation of aorta - Management options and decision making," *Pediatr Therapeut 2012*; S5:006. Available at DOI: 10.4172/2161-0665.S5-006

118. Whitfield CK, Rao PS, "Total anomalous pulmonary venous connection in the neonate," *Neonatology Today 2013*; 8(2):1-7.

119. Rao PS, "What an adult cardiologist should know about cyanotic congenital heart disease?" J Cardiovasc Dis Diag 2013; 1:104. Available at DOI:10.4172/jcdd.1000104.

120. Rao PS, "Consensus on timing of intervention for common congenital heart diseases: Part II - Cyanotic heart defects" *Indian J Pediatr Volume 2013*; 80(8):663-74. Available at DOI: 10.1007/s12098-013-1039-2

121. Rao PS, Balaguru D, "Truncus arteriosus in the neonate," *Neonatology Today 2013*; 8(9):1-6.

122. Banker A, Gupta-Malhotra M, Rao PS, "Childhood hypertension: A review," *J Hypertens 2013*; 2:128. Available at DOI:10.4172/2167-1095.1000128.

123. Yates MC, Rao PS, "Pediatric cardiac emergencies," *Emergency Med 2013*; 3:164. Avilable at doi:10.4172/2165-7548.1000164.

124. Balaguru D, Rao PS, "Ebstein's anomaly of the tricuspid valve in the neonate," *Neonatology Today 2015*; 10(2):1-6.

125. Rao PS, "Fontan operation: Indications, short and long term outcomes," *Indian J Pediatr. 2015 June 20*, [Epub ahead of print] PMID: 26088549.

126. Rao PS, "The journey of an Indian pediatric cardiologist: Dr. K.C. Chaudhuri Lifetime Achievement Award/Oration at AIIMS," *Indian J Pediat 2017*, New Delhi, September 2017; Available at DOI 10.1007/s12098-017-2452-8.

127. Rao PS, Harris AD, "Recent advances in managing septal defects: Atrial septal defects," *F1000 Faculty Rev:2042,* 2017; 6:2042, PMID: 29250321. Available at DOI: 10.12688/ f1000research.11844.1.

128. Rao PS, "Role of echocardiography in the evaluation of preterm infants with patent ductus arteriosus," *Neonatology Today 2018*; 14(1):1-10.

129. Rao PS, Harris AD, "Recent advances in managing septal defects: Ventricular septal defects and atrio-ventricular septal defects," *F1000 Res. 2018 Apr 26; 7. pii: F1000 Faculty Rev-498.* Available at DOI: 10.12688/f1000research.14102.1, eCollection 2018, Review, PMID: 29770201.

130. Rao PS, "Role of echocardiography in the evaluation of preterm infants with patent ductus arteriosus," *Congenital Cardiology Today 2018*; 16(4):1-10.

131. Rao PS, "Management of congenital heart disease: State of the art—Part I—Acyanotic heart defects, *Children (Basel) 2019*; 6, 42. Available at DOI:10.3390/children6030042, PMID: 30857252.

132. Rao PS, "Management of congenital heart disease: State of the art—Part II—Cyanotic heart defects," *Children (Basel) 2019*; 6, 54. Available at DOI:10.3390/children604005. PMID: 30987364

133. Vidyasagar D, "Pulse oximetry screening for detecting congenital heart defects in the newborn," In. Rao PS, Vidyasagar D. (eds.), Perinatal Cardiology: A Multidisciplinary Approach – Chapter 9, Minneapolis, MN, *Cardiotext Publishing 2015*.

134. Rao PS, "Cardiac malpositions including heterotaxy syndromes," In. Rao PS, Vidyasagar D. (eds.), Perinatal Cardiology: A Multidisciplinary Approach – Chapter 36, Minneapolis, MN, *Cardiotext Publishing 2015*.

135. Rao PS, "Cardiac malposition," In: Gupta P, Menon PSN, Ramji S, Lodha R (eds.), *PG Textbook of Pediatrics*, Jaypee Brothers Medical Publishers (P) Ltd., New Delhi, India, 2015, pp.1807-1816.

136. Rao PS, "Cardiac malposition," In: Gupta P, Menon PSN, Ramji S, Lodha R (eds.), *PG Textbook of Pediatrics*, 2nd edn., Jaypee Brothers Medical Publishers (P) Ltd., New Delhi, India, 2018.

137. Rao PS, Strong WB, "Congenital heart disease," In: Current Therapy 1981, Conn HF (ed.), *W.B. Saunders 1981*, Philadelphia, PA, pp. 185-209.

138. Rao PS, Andaya WG, "Chronic afterload reduction in infants and children with primary myocardial disease," *J Pediat 1986*; 108:530-4.

139. Rao PS, "Afterload reduction for dilated cardiomyopathy (Letter)," *Pediat Cardiol 1995*; 16:51.

140. Rao PS, "Current management of pulmonary stenosis and atresia with intact ventricular septum," In: Heart Disease in Neonates and Children, Al Fagih, MR (ed.), *The Medicine Group 1985*, Oxford, England, pp. 109-120.

141. Balaguru D, Rao PS, "Pulmonary atresia with intact ventricular septum," In. Rao PS, Vidyasagar D (eds.), Perinatal Cardiology: A Multidisciplinary Approach – Chapter 34, Minneapolis, MN, *Cardiotext Publishing 2015*.

142. Kambam J, Rao PS, "Mitral valve prolapse syndrome (Barlow's syndrome)," In: Cardiac Anesthesia for Infants and Children, Kambam J (ed.), *Mosby-Year Book 1994*, St. Louis, MO, pp. 354-360.

143. Rao PS, "Balloon angioplasty and valvuloplasty in infants, children and adolescents," Current Problems in Cardiology, *YearBook Medical Publishers, Inc. 1989*, Chicago; 14(8): 417-500.

144. Rao PS, "Balloon valvuloplasty and angioplasty of stenotic lesions of the heart and great vessels in children," In: Advances in Pediatrics, Barness LA; DeVivo DC, Morrow G, III, Oski F, Rudolph AM (eds.), *Year Book Medical Publishers, Inc. 1990*, Chicago, IL, Vol. 37, pp. 33-76.

145. Rao PS, "Percutaneous balloon valvuloplasty/angioplasty in congenital heart disease," In: Percutaneous Valvuloplasty and Related Techniques, Bashore TM and Davidson CT (eds.), Williams & Wilkins, Baltimore, MD, 1990, pp. 251-277.

146. Rao PS, "Percutaneous balloon pulmonary valvuloplasty," In: Percutaneous Balloon Valvuloplasty, Cheng T (ed.), *Igaku-Shion Med Publishers 1992*, New York, pp. 365-420.

147. Rao PS, "Balloon pulmonary valvuloplasty for isolated pulmonic stenosis," In. Rao PS, Transcatheter Therapy in Pediatric Cardiology – Chapter 6, *Wiley-Liss, Inc. 1993*, New York, pp. 59-104.

148. Rao PS, "Pulmonary valve in children," In: Handbook of Cardiovascular Interventions, Bertrand M, Serruys P, Sigwart U (eds.), *Churchill Livingstone 1996*, London, pp. 273-310.

149. Rao PS, "Pulmonary valve disease. In: Valvular Heart Disease," 3rd edn., Alpert JS, Dalen JE, Rahimtoola S (eds.), *Lippincott Raven 2000*, Philadelphia, PA, pp. 339-376.

150. Rao PS, "Pulmonary valve stenosis," In: Percutaneous Interventions in Congenital Heart Disease, Sievert H, Qureshi SA, Wilson N, Hijazi Z (eds.), *Informa Health Care 2007*, Oxford, UK, pp. 185-195.

151. Rao PS, "Pulmonary valve disease: Pulmonary valve stenosis," In: Sievert H, Qureshi SA, Wilson N, Hijazi Z (eds.), Interventions in Structural, Valvular and Congenital Heart Disease – Chapter 31, *CRC Press 2014*, pp. 297-308. Print ISBN: 978-1-4822-1563-2; eBook ISBN: 978-1-4822-1564-9.

152. Rao PS, "Balloon valvuloplasty for pulmonary stenosis," In. Vijayalakshmi IB (ed.), Cardiac Catheterization and Imaging (From Pediatrics to Geriatrics), *Jaypee Publications 2015*, New Delhi, India, pp. 149-174.

153. Rao PS, "Balloon angioplasty of native aortic coarctation," In. Rao PS, Transcatheter Therapy in Pediatric Cardiology, *Wiley-Liss, Inc. 1993*, New York, pp. 153-196.

154. Rao PS, "Balloon angioplasty of aortic recoarctation following previous surgery," In. Rao PS, Transcatheter Therapy in Pediatric Cardiology – Chapter 11, *Wiley-Liss, Inc. 1993*, New York, pp. 197-212.

155. Rao PS, "Coarctation of the aorta," In: Secondary Forms of Hypertension, Ram CVS (ed.), Seminars in Nephrology, Kurtzman NA (ed.), *W.B. Saunders 1995*, Philadelphia, PA, 15(2):81-105.

156. Rao PS, "Aortic coarctation," In: Handbook of Cardiovascular Interventions, Bertrand M, Serreys P, Sigwart U (eds.), *Churchill Livingston 1996*, London, pp. 757-781.

157. Rao PS, "Coarctation of aorta," In: Lang F (ed.), *Encyclopedia of Molecular Mechanisms of Disease Springer-Verlag 2009*, Berlin, Heidelberg, New York, Tokyo. ISBN: 978-3-540-67136-7 (Print) 978-3-540-29676-8 (Online).

158. Doshi AR, Rao PS, "Coarctation of aorta-Management options and decision making," *Pediatr Therapeut 2012*; S5:006. Available at DOI: 10.4172/2161-0665.S5-006.

159. Rao PS, "Coarctation of the aorta," In. Rao PS, Vidyasagar D (eds.), Perinatal Cardiology: A Multidisciplinary Approach – Chapter 38, Minneapolis, MN, *Cardiotext Publishing 2015*.

160. Rao PS, "Percutaneous management of aortic coarctation," In. Vijayalakshmi IB (ed.), Cardiac Catheterization and Imaging (From Pediatrics to Geriatrics), *Jaypee Publications 2015*, New Delhi, India, pp. 433-471.

161. Rao PS, Thapar MK, Kutayli F, "Causes of restenosis following balloon valvuloplasty for valvar pulmonic stenosis," *Am J Cardiol 1988*; 62:979-82.

162. Rao PS, Thapar MK, Kutayli F, Carey P, "Causes of recoarctation following balloon angioplasty of unoperated aortic coarctations," *J Amer Coll Cardiol 1989*; 13:109-15.

163. Rao PS, Thapar MK, Wilson AD, Levy JM, Chopra PS, "Intermediate-term follow-up results of balloon aortic valvuloplasty in infants and children with special reference to causes of restenosis," *Am J Cardiol 1989*; 64:1356-60.

164. Rao PS, Koscik R, "Validation of risk factors in predicting recoarctation following initially successful balloon angioplasty for native aortic coarctation," *Am Heart J 1995*; 130:116-21.

165. Galal O, Rao PS, Al-Fadley F, Wilson AD, "Follow-up results of balloon aortic valvuloplasty in children with special reference to causes of late aortic insufficiency," *Am Heart J 1997*; 113:418-27.

166. Rao PS, "Balloon aortic valvuloplasty," *J Intervent Cardiol 1998I*; 11:319-29.

167. Chopra PS, Rao PS, "Balloon aortic valvuloplasty in children (Editorial)," *J Invasive Cardiol 1999*; 11:277-279.

168. Agu NC, Rao PS, "Balloon aortic valvuloplasty," *Pediatr Therapeut 2012*; S5:004. Available at DOI: 10.4172/2161-0665.S5-004.

169. Rao PS, "Balloon aortic valvuloplasty (Editorial)," *Indian Heart Journal 2016*; 68(5):592–595.

170. Rao PS, "Balloon valvuloplasty for aortic stenosis," In. Rao PS, Transcatheter Therapy in Pediatric Cardiology, *Wiley-Liss, Inc. 1993*, New York, pp.105-27.

171. Singh GK, Rao PS, "Left heart outflow obstructions," In: Cardiology, Crawford MH, DiMarco JP (eds.), *Mosby International 2001*, London, pp. 7-11.1 to 7-11.9.

172. Singh GK, Rao PS, "Left heart outflow obstructions," In: Cardiology, 2nd edn., Crawford MH, DiMarco JP, Paulus WJ (eds.), *Mosby International 2004*, Edinburgh, pp. 1317-26.

173. Singh GK, Rao PS, "Left heart outflow obstructions" In: Cardiology, 3rd edn., Crawford MH., DiMarco JP, Paulus WJ. (eds.), *Mosby Elsevier 2010*, ISBN 978-0-7234-3485-6, Edinburgh, UK, pp. 1507-1518.

174. Rao PS, "Fetal and neonatal circulation," In: Cardiac Anesthesia for Infants and Children – Chapter 2, Kambam J (ed.), *Mosby-Year Book 1994*, St. Louis, MO, pp. 10-19.

175. Rao PS, "Perinatal circulatory physiology," In. Rao PS, Vidyasagar D. (eds.), Perinatal Cardiology: A Multidisciplinary Approach – Chapter 1, *Cardiotext Publishing* 2015, Minneapolis, MN.

176. Rao PS, "Role of Perinatal circulatory physiology on clinical manifestations and management of neonatal heart disease," In. Rao PS, Vidyasagar D. (eds.), Perinatal Cardiology: A Multidisciplinary Approach – Chapter 2, *Cardiotext Publishing 2015*, Minneapolis, MN.

177. Rao PS, Wilson AD, Thapar MK, Brais M, "Balloon pulmonary valvuloplasty in the management of cyanotic congenital heart defects," *Cathet Cardiovasc Diag 1992*; 25:16-24.

178. Rao PS, "Neonatal cardiac emergencies: Management strategies," In. Rao PS, Vidyasagar D (eds.), Perinatal Cardiology: A Multidisciplinary Approach – Chapter 8, *Cardiotext Publishing 2015*, Minneapolis, MN.

179. Rao PS, "Transposition of the great arteries in the neonate," *Congenital Cardiology Today 2010*; 8(8):1-10.

180. Rao PS, "History of transcatheter interventions in pediatric cardiology," In. Vijayalakshmi IB (ed.), Cardiac Catheterization and Imaging (From Pediatrics to Geriatrics), *Jaypee Publications 2015*, New Delhi, India, pp. 3-20.

CHAPTER 10

MONOGRAPHS, BOOKS, BOOK CHAPTERS, AND OTHER PUBLICATIONS

INTRODUCTION

This chapter reviews monographs and books I wrote/edited (Figures 1 and 2). The published monographs and books are listed in Table I and each of these will be summarized in this chapter. In addition, I had the privilege of editing several seminars/symposia for a number of journals. I have also contributed chapters to several books, multiple papers in journals as well as electronic communications, which will be briefed at the end of this chapter.

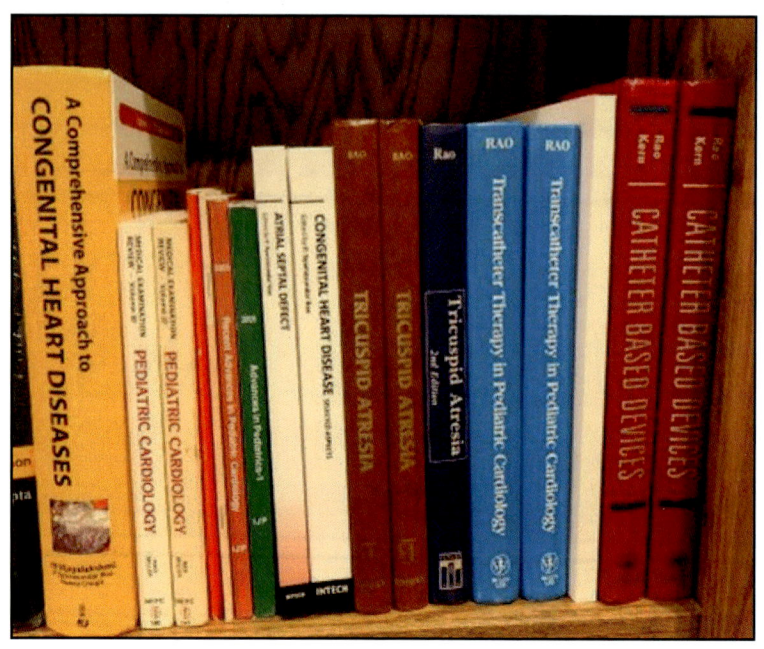

Figure 1. Photograph of books that I wrote or edited.

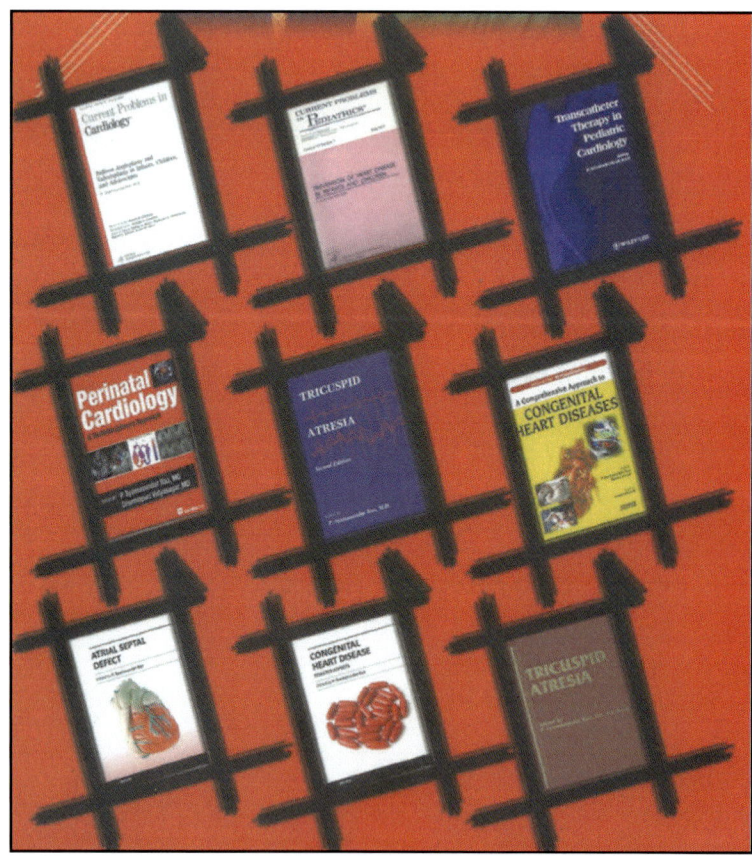

Figure 2. Some of my books framed by an artist.

Table I. Monographs and Books Published by Me

1. Rao PS, "Prevention of Heart Disease in Infants and Children," Current Problems in Pediatrics, Vol. 7, *Yearbook Medical Publisher, Inc.,* May 1977, Chicago, USA.

2. Rao PS and Miller MD, "Medical Examination Review," Pediatric Cardiology, *Medical Examination Publishing Co., Inc., 1980,* New York, USA.

3. Rao PS, "Tricuspid Atresia," *Futura Publishing Co. 1982*, Kisco, Mount New York.

4. Rao PS, "Balloon Angioplasty and Valvuloplasty in Infants, Children and Adolescents," Current Problems in Cardiology, *YearBook Medical Publishers, Inc., 1989*, Chicago, 14(8): 417-500.

5. Rao PS, "Tricuspid Atresia," 2nd edn., *Futura Publishing Co. 1992*, Mt. Kisco, NY.

6. Rao PS, "Transcatheter Therapy in Pediatric Cardiology," *Wiley-Liss, Inc., 1993*, New York.

7. Rao PS, Kern MJ. (eds.), "Catheter Based Devices for Treatment of Noncoronary Cardiovascular Disease in Adults and Children," *Lippincott, Williams & Wilkins 2003*, Philadelphia, PA.

8. Rao PS, Saxena A (eds.), "Recent Advances in Pediatric Cardiology," *Indian Journal of Pediatrics 2005*, New Delhi, India.

9. Rao PS (ed.), "Perinatal Cardiology for the Neonatologist," *MHHCS Press*, April 2011, Houston, TX.

10. Rao PS (ed.), "Congenital Heart Disease - Selected Aspects," ISBN 978-953-307-472-6; InTech, Rijeka, Croatia, January 2012.

11. Rao PS (Editor). Atrial Septal Defect, ISBN 978-953-51-0531-2; InTech, Rijeka, Croatia, April 2012.

12. Vijayalakshmi IB, Rao PS, Chugh R (eds.), "A Comprehensive Approach to Management of Congenital Heart Diseases," *Jaypee Publications 2013*, New Delhi, India.

13. Rao PS, Vidyasagar D (eds.), Perinatal Cardiology: A Multidisciplinary Approach, *Cardiotext Publishing*, Minneapolis, MN.

14. Vijayalakshmi IB, Rao PS, Chugh R (eds.), "A Comprehensive Approach to Management of Congenital Heart Diseases," 2nd edn., Jaypee Publications 2019, New Delhi, India.

PREVENTION OF HEART DISEASE IN INFANTS AND CHILDREN

This was the first monograph that I wrote and it was published in 1977 (Figure 3). This review is a culmination of multiple publications,[1-4] resulting in publication of a booklet in Current Problems in Pediatrics.[5] This subject was discussed in the Chapter on "Reviews" and will not be repeated here.

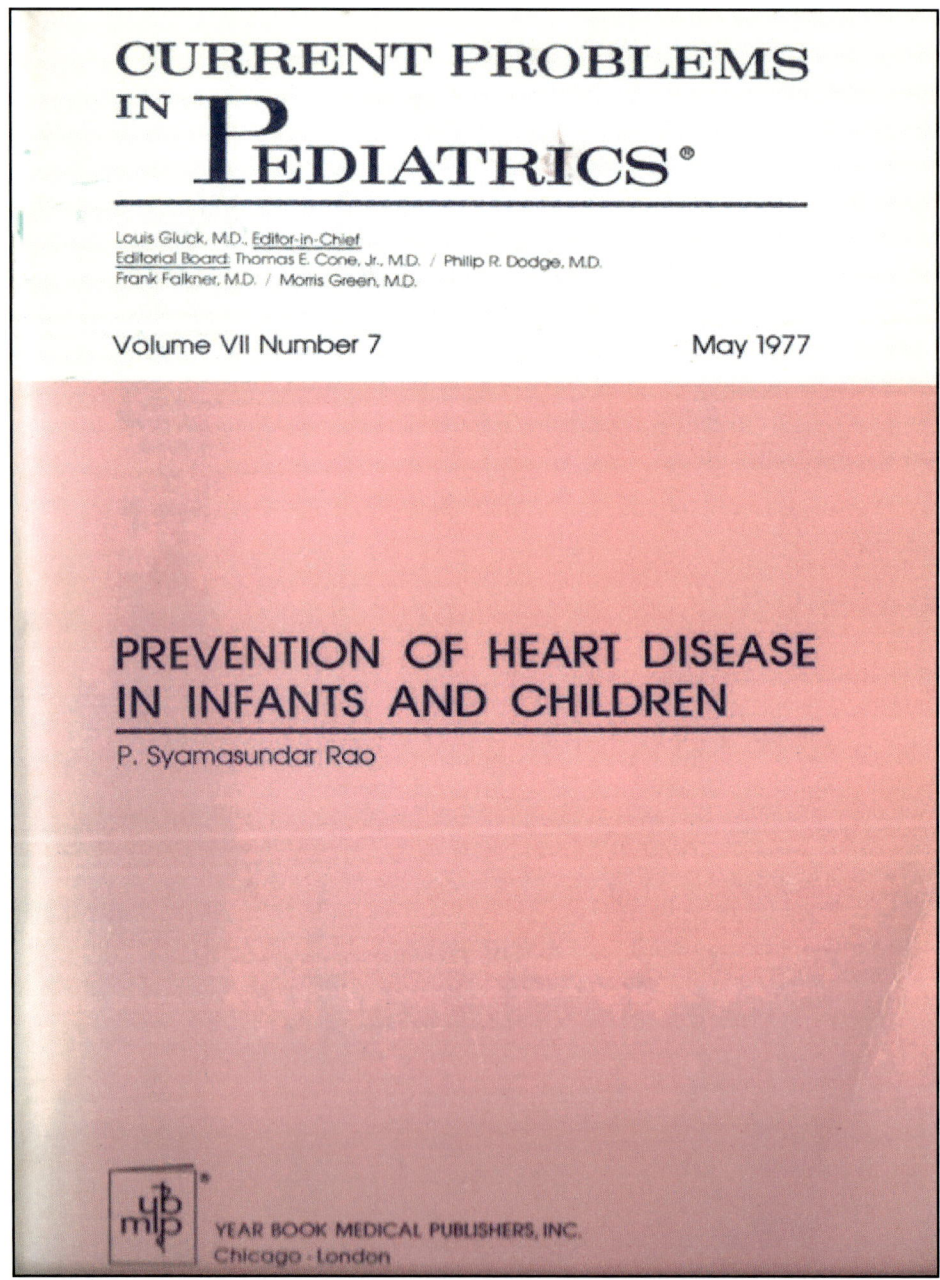

Figure 3. Photograph of monograph titled "Prevention of Heart Disease in Infants and Children" in *Current Problems in Pediatrics* published in 1977.

MEDICAL EXAMINATION REVIEW - PEDIATRIC CARDIOLOGY

A multiple choice questions book with referenced answers was prepared with the help of Max Miller, EdD, an educational specialist and published by the Medical Examination Publishing Company, Inc., in 1980 (Figure 4).[6] In the preface to the book, it was stated that over the past three decades the diagnostic techniques and therapeutic measures (both medical and surgical) for congenital heart defects (CHDs) have advanced to such a degree that virtually every CHD can be "corrected" and the few that cannot be corrected can be effectively palliated. During the same time span significant advances have also occurred in the etiologic and preventive aspects of rheumatic fever and other types of cardiac diseases affecting infants and children. Because of these advances there is a greater need for the house-officer, general practitioner, family practitioner, pediatrician and internist to be familiar with cardiac problems in infants and children so that they can identify and provide appropriate (at least initial) care to these infants and children. The advances mentioned above have also resulted in survival of larger numbers of these patients for longer periods and, therefore, we will have increasing numbers of adolescents and young adults who will require cardiac care, especially from the internist and adult cardiologist.

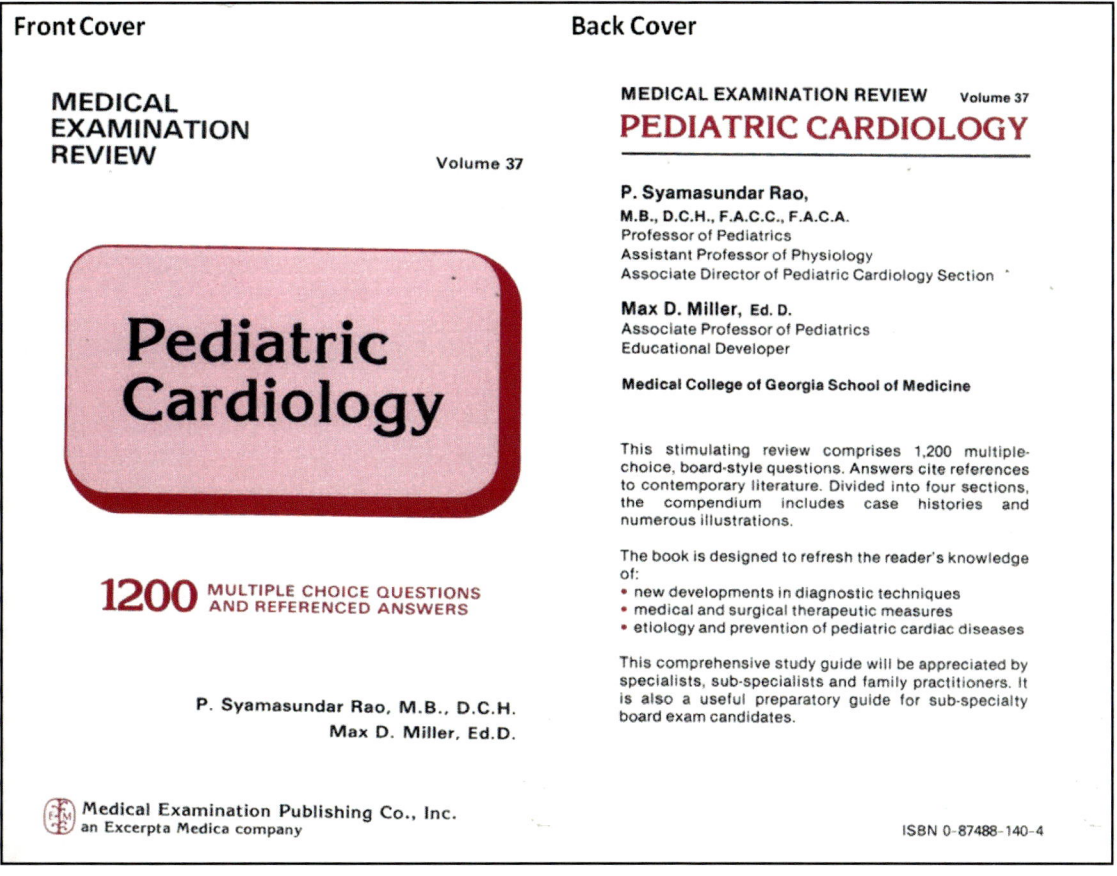

Figure 4. Photograph of the book titled "Medical Examination Review, Pediatric Cardiology" published by the *Medical Examination Publishing Co., Inc.,* in 1980. Both front and back covers are shown.

Although there is some overlap, the first half of this book was aimed for the generalist, and the second half towards the physician more interested in cardiac problems in the young, whether he/she be a pediatric cardiologist or an adult cardiologist. A total of 1,200 multiple choice questions were presented and forty-four references were provided. For each question, the source of correct answer was provided so that the reader may able to verify the answer and pursue further investigation of the subject of their interest. Although, an attempt was made to cover the entire spectrum of problems, editorial bias and limited space may have resulted in inadvertent omission of some subjects. Also, because of the overlap, minor repetition was unavoidable. In those cases where the questions presented appear too simple or too easy, it should be understood that our aim in these questions was only to make sure that the reader's knowledge in these areas is reinforced. Conversely, some questions may appear complicated or highly sophisticated for the generalist and perhaps these were aimed at the pediatric cardiologist. We hoped that most readers, whether they be generalists or specialists, will be able to acquire new knowledge or at least confirm what they know is correct. However, we did not recommend that this book be a substitute to regular textbook reading, organized courses of study or preceptorships.

We expressed our appreciation to our associates Drs. William B. Strong and Wesley Covitz for allowing the use of some of their clinical material, and to Mrs. Beth Parrish and Miss Jean Matthai for their excellent secretarial assistance in preparing the manuscript.

A book review published in the *European Heart Journal* is shown in figure 5.

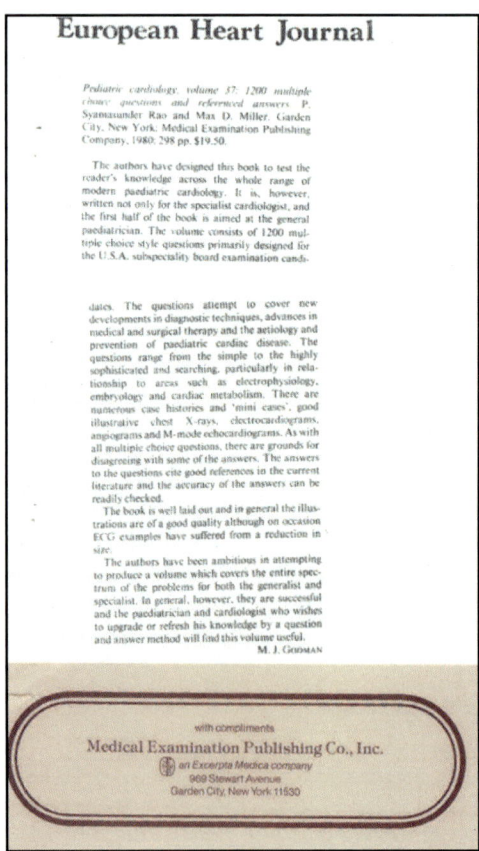

Figure 5. Book review of "Medical Examination Review - Pediatric Cardiology"
published in the *European Heart Journal*.

TRICUSPID ATRESIA

The first book on tricuspid atresia was published in 1982; this was partly written and finalized during my sabbatical from my professorial position at the Medical college of Georgia (Figure 6).[7]

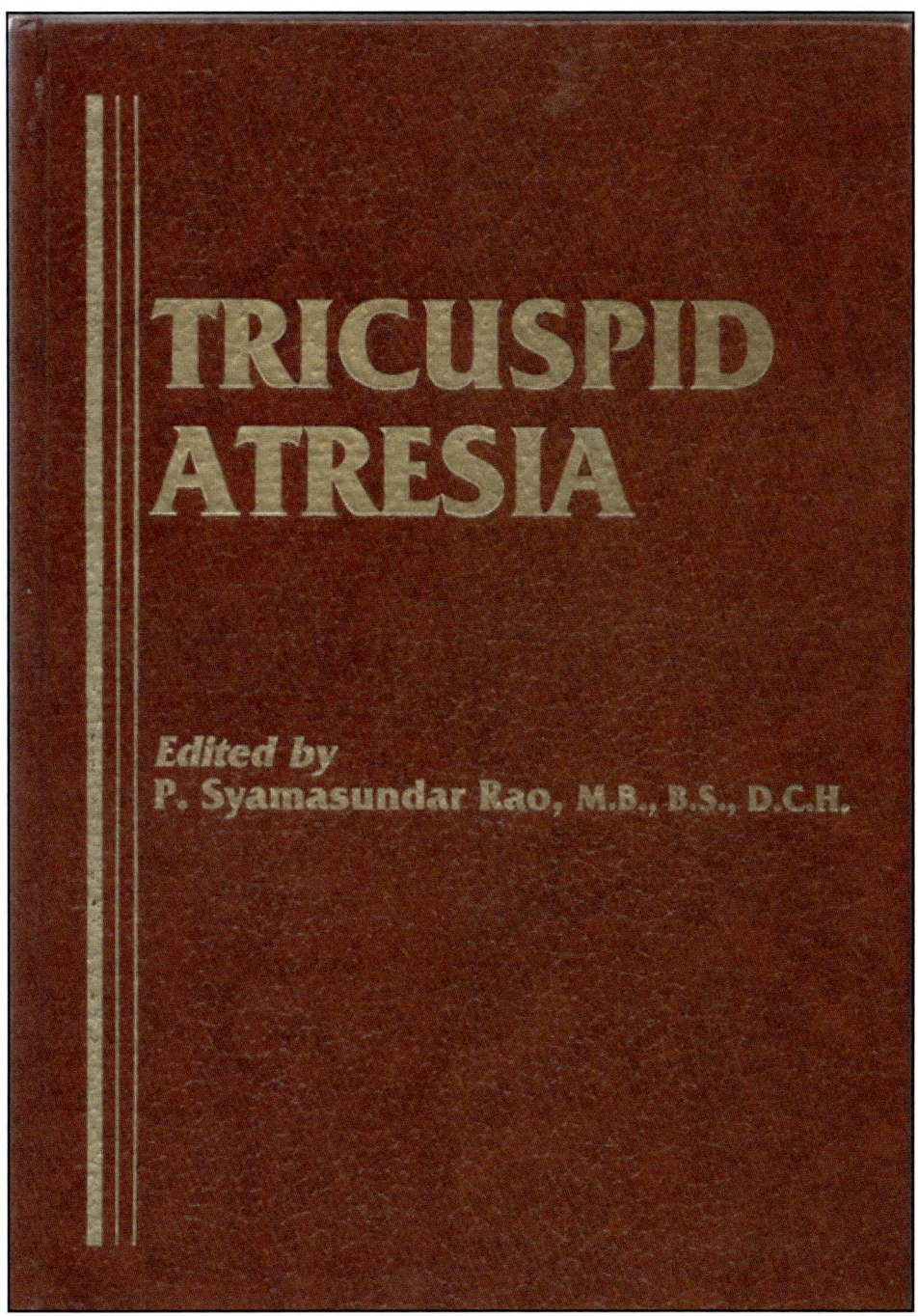

Figure 6. Photograph of the book titled "Tricuspid Atresia" published by *Futura Publishing Co.*, in 1982.

Eleven of the twenty-one chapters were contributed by myself and my associates. In the final chapter on "Conclusions and Future Directions," I stated the following: Over the past three and a half decades, significant advances in cardiovascular physiology, diagnostic techniques, and medical and surgical therapeutic measures have occurred such that almost every CHD can be "corrected," and the few that cannot be corrected can be effectively palliated. In 1971, Fontan and Kreutzer independently described physiologic correction of tricuspid atresia; this has markedly improved the prognosis of a very large percentage of patients with tricuspid atresia. This recent advance in surgery has stimulated further interest in this lesion.

The population prevalence of tricuspid atresia is 1 in 10,000. There does not appear to be any sex preponderance for this defect. No geographic differences in prevalence were observed, nor was there any evidence for racial predilection. The prevalence rate of tricuspid atresia among CHDs has decreased; this apparent decrease appears to be related to identification of a greater number of other types of CHDs.

All anatomic types of tricuspid atresia (based on valve morphology), including the most common muscular variety, are physiologically very similar. Only the Ebstein's type of tricuspid atresia is different from the rest with regard to "corrective" surgical approach; the Ebstein's type will require excision of the atretic tricuspid valve with prosthetic valve replacement, whereas the other anatomic types will have to have a Fontan type of operation.

The electrocardiographic (ECG) feature of abnormally superior QRS vector with counterclockwise loop was not completely explained by the conduction system abnormalities found at postmortem examination. The preliminary epicardial mapping studies performed at our institution appear to explain the abnormally superior vector.

Different classifications have previously been proposed by several investigators; our classification, which includes the concepts expounded by Kuhne, Edwards, and Burchell and Keith and their associates, appears to unify the basic themes. Hopefully, this classification will be useful for all and will be used by most workers in the field.

Originally described roentgenographic and ECG findings continue to be helpful, in their own way, in the diagnosis and follow-up of patients with tricuspid atresia. Echocardiography and nuclear angiography have added a new dimension in the diagnosis and management of these patients. Particularly useful is our ability to obtain repeated non-invasive measurement of left ventricular (LV) function. The availability and use of balloon-tipped catheters has immensely helped in obtaining the needed physiologic information, i.e., pulmonary artery pressure and resistance. Occurrence of frequent left-to-right shunting is now documented and appears to be the result of instantaneous pressure differences between the atria.

Spontaneous diminution of the size of the ventricular septal defect (VSD) occurs quite frequently, which causes pulmonary oligemia in Type I patients and subaortic obstruction in Type II patients.

Many types of palliative surgical procedures are currently available. Most of the operations used to augment pulmonary blood flow are either unpredictable initially or produce long-term complications precluding latter successful physiologic correction. We recommended Blalock-Taussig (BT) shunt for initial palliation in preference to the classic Glenn procedure; this is based on the knowledge that if the VSD closes after the Glenn operation, the left pulmonary artery (PA) is without blood flow. Furthermore, recent use of microsurgical techniques, subclavian arterioplasty and the use of Gore-Tex graft to extend the length of the subclavian artery made it applicable to all age groups, including the newborn. Prostaglandin E_1 (PGE_1) is of great value in temporarily palliating neonates whose pulmonary or systemic blood flow is ductal dependent. The recently described operation to relieve obstruction at the VSD level (also pulmonary infundibular and valvar level) by Annechino appears to be the most physiologic and logical solution to the problem; perhaps this will become the palliative procedure of choice in Type I patients. The procedures described by Fontan and Kreutzer for physiologic correction of tricuspid atresia have undergone many modifications and refinements, and the morbidity and mortality appear to be improving. There are some long-term follow-up studies following the Fontan type operation, but studies on much larger numbers of patients with longer follow-up period are needed.

The preliminary studies on epicardial mapping have, to a great extent, appeared to have explained the specific QRS abnormality seen in most cases of tricuspid atresia. Further studies in larger numbers of patients and mapping of tricuspid atresia patients with inferiorly oriented QRS vectors are needed to fully understand the ECG abnormality. More accurate measurement of LV functional parameters and their correlation with operative success and long-term survival are also needed. There appear to be "cardiomyopathic" changes of the left ventricle (LV) in some patients with tricuspid atresia. Whether these are causally related to a specific anatomic or physiologic abnormality should be determined. Techniques for evaluation of LV functional reserve with ability to identify minor deviations of this reserve capacity should be further developed. Perhaps, at the first sign of such an abnormality, we should perform corrective surgery. Understanding of the hemodynamics of right atrium to PA connection with subsequent emptying left atrium may immensely help us in the post-operative management. Ability to support right atrial function (by balloon pumping, etc.) in the post-operative period may help salvage some Fontan patients that are now not being benefited. Long-term follow-up studies of the several modifications of the Fontan procedure are needed to assess which of these is most likely to offer best long-term results. Further studies on the frequency and effect of calcification of porcine valves and development of peel in the conduit in patients that have undergone Fontan type of procedure may help resolve whether valved or non-valved conduit or pericardial material are better choices. Similarly, evaluation of the advantages and disadvantages of right atrium to right ventricular (RV) anastomosis versus right atrium to PA anastomosis should be made.

Until these problems are resolved, palliative procedures should be performed with an aim to restore and preserve the anatomy and physiology as close to normal as possible such that a complete correction can be performed safely and the infant and the child are allowed to grow up to be a normal adult.

BALLOON ANGIOPLASTY AND VALVULOPLASTY IN INFANTS, CHILDREN, AND ADOLESCENTS

I began using transcatheter techniques to relieve obstructive lesions of the heart in early 1980s with resultant publication of multiple papers in 1985, 1986, 1987, and 1988.[8-26] These studies along with those of other workers in the field were put together as a monograph in 1989 (Figure 7).[27]

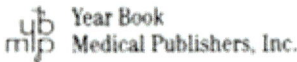

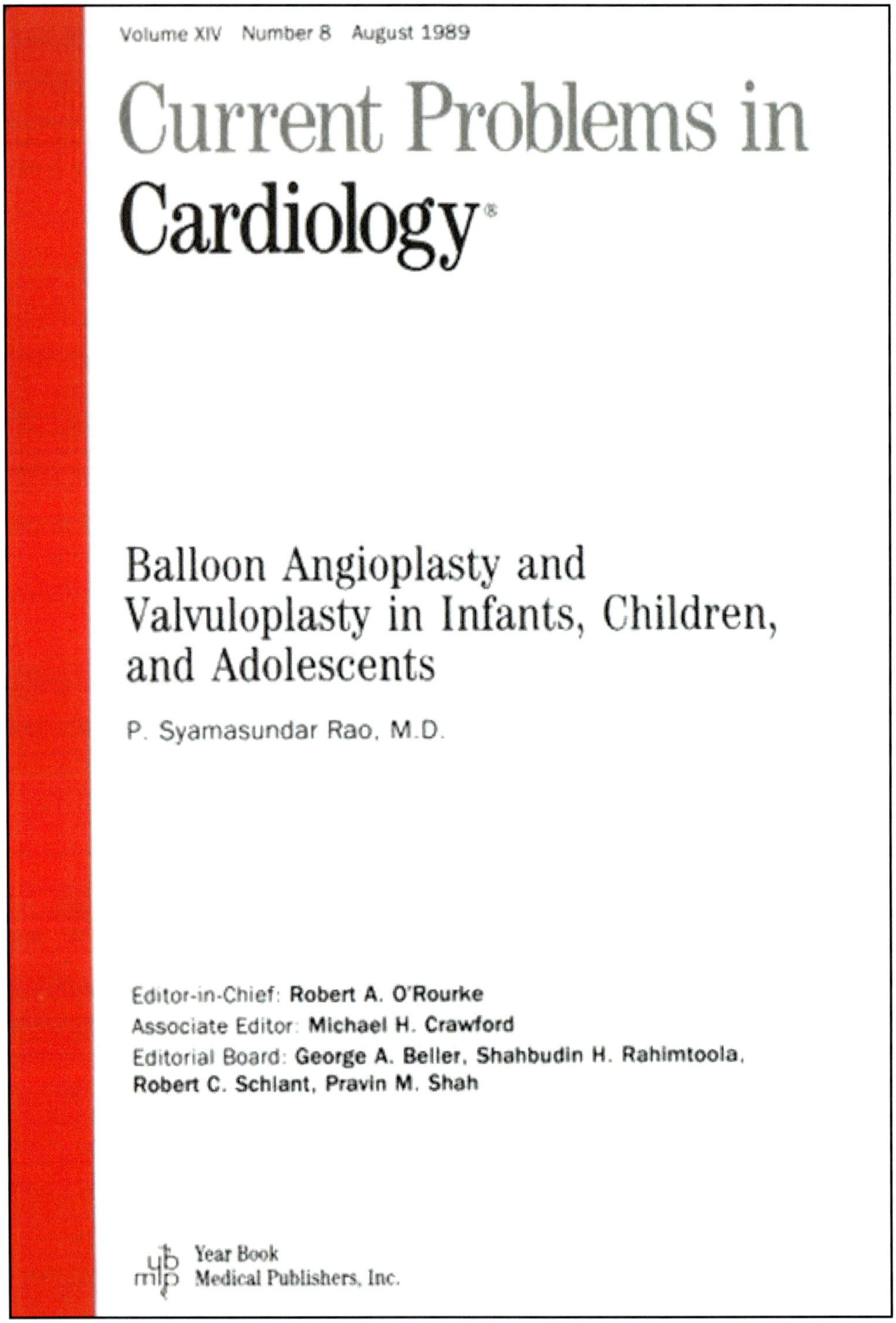
Volume XIV Number 8 August 1989

Current Problems in Cardiology®

Balloon Angioplasty and Valvuloplasty in Infants, Children, and Adolescents

P. Syamasundar Rao, M.D.

Editor-in-Chief: **Robert A. O'Rourke**
Associate Editor: **Michael H. Crawford**
Editorial Board: **George A. Beller, Shahbudin H. Rahimtoola, Robert C. Schlant, Pravin M. Shah**

Year Book Medical Publishers, Inc.

Figure 7. Photograph of monograph titled "Balloon Angioplasty and Valvuloplasty in Infants, Children and Adolescents" in *Current Problems in Cardiology* published in 1989.

The monograph may be summarized as follows: The technique of balloon dilatation of stenotic lesions of the heart and great vessels in infants and children has been available since 1982. This technique has been used extensively in isolated valvar pulmonary stenosis (PS) with excellent immediate and reasonably good intermediate-term follow-up results. Refinements in the technique may further decrease the restenosis rate. Balloon pulmonary valvuloplasty is now the procedure of choice in the treatment of moderate to severe valvar PS. Although good immediate and intermediate-term follow-up results of balloon angioplasty of aortic coarctation have been reported, recommendation for use of this technique as the treatment of choice has been clouded by reports of development of aneurysms at the site of coarctation dilatation. At that time, I believed that balloon coarctation angioplasty is the treatment of choice in neonates and small infants, while general use of this technique in both native and postoperative coarctation in older children should await longer follow-up results in a larger number of children. Balloon dilatation of aortic valve stenosis and branch PA stenosis produced reasonable immediate results, but long-term results are needed prior to making definitive recommendations. However, this technique is attractive for neonates with critical aortic valve obstruction. We recommended balloon valvuloplasty of PS in association with other CHDs, though reported by only a few groups of investigators, as an effective alternative to surgical aorta-to-pulmonary anastomosis because of the good immediate and follow-up results. Despite good results with many miscellaneous obstructive lesions, there is not enough experience with children with each of these defects to make a definitive recommendation.

The indications for balloon dilatation of stenotic lesions of the heart and great vessels are essentially the same as those used for surgical therapy. The technique of balloon angioplasty/valvuloplasty should now be added to the therapeutic armamentarium available to the pediatric cardiologist for the management of infants and children with heart disease. Thus far, only one to two year follow-up results are available. Five to ten year follow-up results to document long-term effectiveness of balloon dilatation for all stenotic lesions are needed. Miniaturization of currently bulky dilating catheter systems and improving rapidity of inflation and deflation of balloons are necessary for increasing the safety and effectiveness of this technique in infants and children. Meticulous attention to the details of technique and further refinement of the procedure will further reduce the complication rate. For vascular lesions with poor results with balloon angioplasty (peripheral PA or pulmonary vein stenosis), intravascular stents (which are currently being tested in animal models and humans) may prove valuable to keep the stenotic lesions open. Transcatheter laser technique to relieve stenotic lesions and visualization of these lesions while relieving the obstruction by dual fiber-optic catheters have been used in postmortem stenotic lesions and animal models. Further development and refinement of these techniques in animal models, followed by clinical trials, are necessary prior to their application in infants and children with obstructive lesions of the heart and great vessels. The transcatheter techniques offer promise as excellent alternatives to open or closed heart surgery in the treatment of several CHDs.[27]

TRICUSPID ATRESIA, 2ND EDITION

Ten years following the publication of the first tricuspid atresia book, I decided to update the book in view of significant advances in the management of tricuspid atresia (Figure 8).[28]

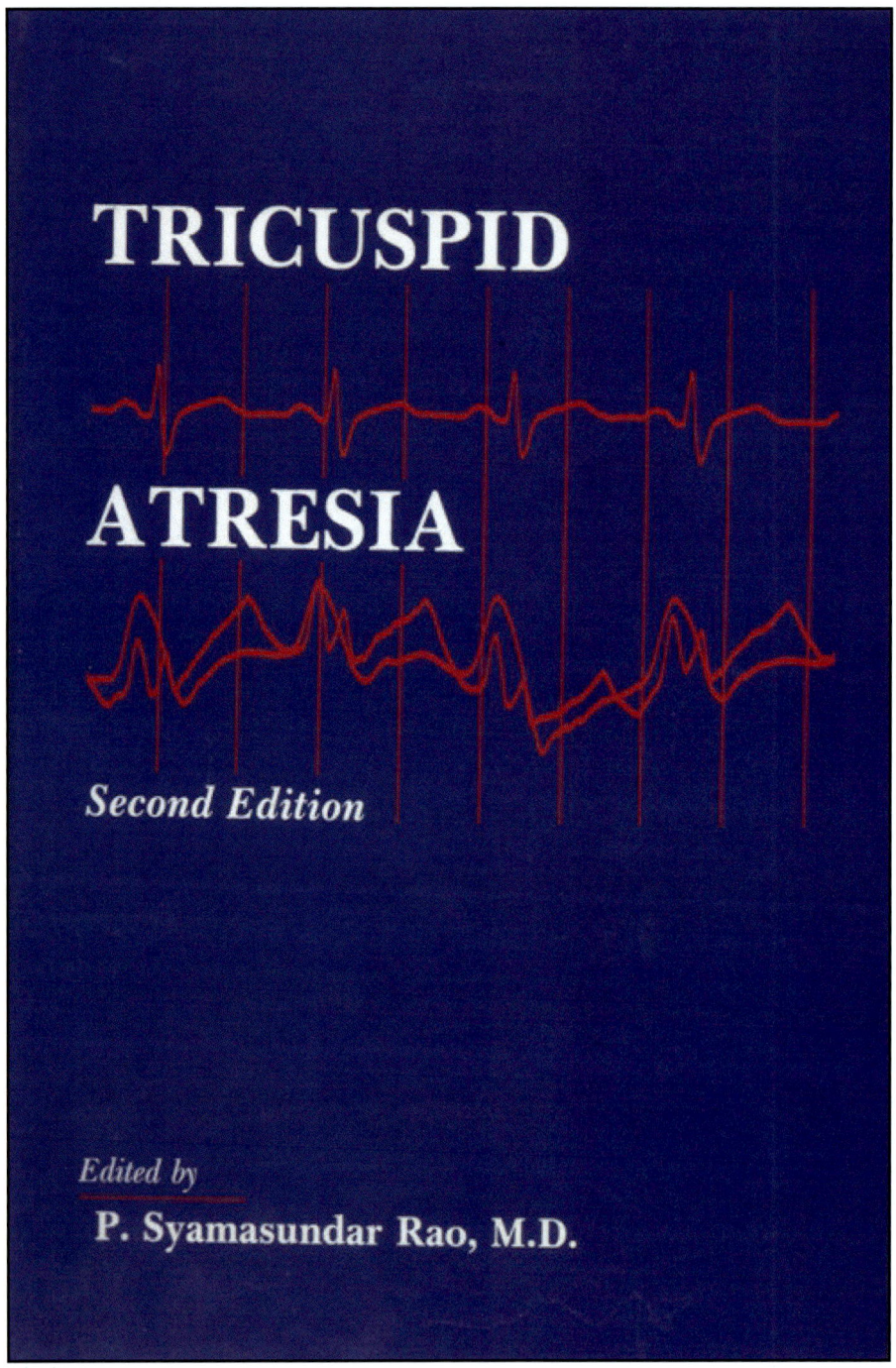

Figure 8. Photograph of book titled "Tricuspid Atresia, Second Edition" published by *Futura Publishing Co.*, in 1992.

Thirteen of the twenty-five chapters were contributed by me and my associates. In the final chapter on "Conclusions and Future Directions," I stated the following: Over the last four and a half decades a large number of advances have taken place in the understanding of the pathophysiology, non-invasive and invasive diagnosis, and medical and surgical therapy of CHDs. Consequently, almost all CHDs can be "corrected" and a few that cannot be corrected can either be palliated or considered for heart transplantation. In 1971, Fontan and Kreutzer independently described physiologic correction of tricuspid atresia which is now widely used all over the world. There has been a dramatic improvement in the prognosis of a large percentage of patients with tricuspid atresia. This prompted me to organize, edit, and publish a book (the first edition) on this cardiac defect.[7] Since the publication of the book in 1982, further advances in the understanding of this lesion have occurred and therefore, this second edition was prepared to gather together all that is known about this lesion.

There has been debate as to whether the term, tricuspid atresia, should be used to describe this well known clinical entity and whether this is a part of single ventricle complex, univentricular heart or univentricular atrioventricular connection and so on and so forth. I strongly felt that tricuspid atresia is a distinct entity and presented available evidence to support this view in the first edition of the book. The anatomical data provided by Wenink and colleagues from Leiden and echocardiographic data have for sure convinced me and others (Editorial: *American Journal of Cardiology*, 66: 1251, 1990) that tricuspid atresia is indeed an appropriate and correct term to describe the clinical and pathologic entity under discussion.

The nineteenth century historical aspects so elegantly described by the late William J. Rashkind were reproduced from the first edition,[7] and rightly so. Based on this excellent review, the first documented case of tricuspid atresia was that of Kreysig in 1817, although the 1812 report by the editors of *London Medical Review* appears to fit the description of tricuspid atresia, but they did not use the specific term for us to be sure of the diagnosis. In addition, Rashkind's review suggested that long descriptive names were used to describe this disease entity in the nineteenth century and the phrase "tricuspid atresia" is a twentieth century term.

I have added data from several papers to the previous analysis of demographic features of tricuspid atresia and this did not change the prevalence figures. The population prevalence of tricuspid atresia continues to be 1 in 10,000 live births; the autopsy and clinical prevalence rates remain at 2.9 percent and 1.4 percent of CHDs, respectively. There is not a gender preponderance for the more common variety of tricuspid atresia with normally related great arteries, while male preponderance may be present in patients with associated transposition of the great arteries (TGA). There is no evidence for differences in geographic or racial predilection for this lesion. There is a decrease in tricuspid atresia prevalence rate among CHDs; this appears to be related to a greater number of other types of CHDs identified rather than due to a decrease in the number of tricuspid atresia cases seen.

Although, there have not been any significant advances in the understanding of normal development of tricuspid valve, a theme has evolved with regard to the morphogenesis of tricuspid atresia; tricuspid valve stenosis, tricuspid atresia with well-developed, but fused valve leaflets and muscular (the so-called absent connection or classical) tricuspid atresia represent a spectrum of morphologic abnormality (See Chapters 1 and 4) caused by a similar embryologic insult. The eventual type of tricuspid atresia would be dependent upon the time of onset of embryologic abnormality. Further research into embryologic mechanism of development of tricuspid atresia and causes of such embryologic aberration should be pursued.

Six anatomic types of tricuspid atresia based on valve morphology have been described and these are clinically and hemodynamically indistinguishable from each other. Some of these types can be differentiated from each other by echocardiographic and/or angiographic findings and such distinction may be clinically useful in that some types (for example, valvular, Ebstein's and perhaps atrioventricular canal types) may be amenable for biventricular correction in contradistinction to univentricular Fontan-Kreutzer repair.

Clinical features are largely dependent upon the associated defects and orderly assortment of these defects is of great value in the clinical management. In an attempt to resolve this issue, different classifications have been proposed by several investigators including our group. The classification I proposed a decade ago, included the concepts expounded by Kuhne, Edwards and Burchell, and Keith et al. The major grouping is based on the positional anomalies of great arteries: Type I, normally related great arteries; Type II, d-TGA; Type III, mal-positions of the great arteries other than d-transposition; Type IV, truncus arteriosus. Each type and subtypes of Type III (l-TGA, double outlet right ventricle, double outlet left ventricle, d-malposition of the great arteries, and I-malposition of the great arteries) were subdivided: Subgroup a. pulmonary atresia, Subgroup b. PS or pulmonary hypoplasia, and Subgroup c, normal PAs. The status of the atrial and ventricular septae (whether defects are present or not) and other associated defects are then enumerated for each case. This classification appears to unify the basic themes and maintains uniformity, yet is comprehensive and takes into account all variations of great artery anatomy. Some workers have adopted our classification, many have referenced it, but it has not been used as widely as I anticipated. I was hopeful that this unified classification will be used by most, if not by all workers in the field.

Tricuspid atresia is not a single defect, but is a defect complex. A systematic approach to the diagnosis is needed and attention should be paid to intra-cardiac organization, including segmental analysis, great artery relationship, septal defects, outflow tract obstruction and other associated defects including persistent left superior vena cava, aortic coarctation and juxtaposition of the atrial appendages.

Tricuspid atresia is the third most common cyanotic CHD. There are significant variations in the associated cardiac defects and physiology resulting in different clinical presentations. More than half of the patients present with symptoms on the first day of life and 80 percent would have had symptoms by the end of first month of their life. The diagnosis is relatively simple and can often be made on clinical features and simple laboratory studies such as chest roentgenogram and ECG; although, echocardiography, cardiac catheterization and selective cineangiography may be necessary to define anatomic and physiologic detail.

The clinical course of patients with tricuspid atresia is characterized by significant mortality in the first year of life from hypoxemia, congestive heart failure (CHF) or palliative surgery or a combination thereof. Following this initial mortality, a stable plateau is achieved with a second bout of mortality beyond fifteen years of age. The later appears to be declining with the institution of corrective surgery and the prospect for long-term survival into young adulthood and beyond appears to be encouraging.

The ECG feature of abnormally superior vector with counterclockwise loop (the so-called left axis deviation) is not completely explained by the conduction system abnormalities found at postmortem studies. Epicardial mapping and intramural activation studies performed by our group appear to explain the abnormally superior vector: Right-to-left phase asynchrony of the ventricular activation due to right-to-left ventricular disproportion and late, and unopposed, activation of the superior (anterolateral) basal portions of the LV secondary to asymmetric distribution of the LV mass favoring the superior wall. I hoped that similar epicardial mapping studies on a larger number of patients, both with superiorly and inferiorly oriented QRS vectors, by ours or by other groups will be conducted to further delineate causes of abnormally superior vector in tricuspid atresia. Our group broke up, with each member at different institutions, and no further studies were performed by our group. To my knowledge, no other investigator performed similar studies; although, studies of the electrocardiographic body surface potential maps by Liebman et al have to some extent confirmed our observations.

Originally described roentgenographic and ECG features continue to be helpful, in their own way, in the diagnosis and follow-up of patients with tricuspid atresia. Greater use of two-dimensional (2D) echocardiographic studies than in the past and the application of various modes of Doppler studies (pulsed, continuous wave and color) has helped in the assessment of anatomic and physiologic parameters of tricuspid atresia. Radionuclide imaging techniques have been helpful in specific situations. Thus, non-invasive testing is of value in the diagnosis and management of children with tricuspid atresia. As a diagnostic tool, it is most useful in the differentiation of complex lesions. As a management tool, it is useful in assessing the need for, success of, and complications of palliative and/or corrective surgery.

Exercise testing in conjunction with echocardiographic and radionuclide imaging is useful in the evaluation of tricuspid atresia patients with regard to heart rate, blood pressure, working capacity, oxygen consumption, and cardiac index response to exercise. LV function reserve, and improvement following palliative and corrective surgery can also be assessed. However, there have been only a limited number of studies in a limited number of patients. Studying the same patients, both before and after Fontan, may allow analysis of effects of various pre-operative and intraoperative variables on the long-term result, which in turn may allow optimal patient selection and timing of surgical intervention.

With the availability of non-invasive studies just reviewed, invasive studies are not being performed for diagnostic purposes as often as in the past. Cardiac catheterization and selective cineangiography have been very useful in the evaluation of tricuspid atresia patients, particularly prior to considering corrective surgery. Preoperative evaluation should not only confirm the diagnosis and define the associated defects, but also specifically evaluate each of the hemodynamic and angiographic criteria outlined by Choussat and others. Particular attention should be directed towards PA pressure, resistance, and anatomy, LV function, and assessment of sub-aortic obstruction at VSD level in Type II patients. The availability of flow directed balloon-tipped catheters and other devices and axial cineangiographic views have immensely helped in obtaining the needed physiologic and anatomic information. Physiologic left-to-right shunt at atrial level in a significant proportion of tricuspid atresia patients is of interest and appears to be related to instantaneous pressure differences between the atria. Follow-up hemodynamic and angiographic studies after Fontan operation are sparse but reveal minimal residua. Long-term follow-up hemodynamic and angiographic studies in a larger and representative group of patients are necessary for a better understanding of long-term outlook following the Fontan-Kreutzer procedure.

LV function has been studied by echocardiographic, radionuclide, and cineangiographic methods. The LV volume overloading appears to be due to the dual circulation work and the extent of overloading appears to be proportional to pulmonary blood flow. LV ejection fraction was observed to be decreased and is related to age, pulmonary-to-systemic flow ratio and hypoxemia. Conventional measures of LV function did not seem to have a consistent relationship with poor outcome following surgery, although some studies suggest that inappropriate LV muscle hypertrophy predisposes to poor outcome following surgery. Most measures of LV function that have been investigated are load-dependent and may, to some extent, explain discrepancy among studies and the inability to predict surgical outcome. Load-insensitive measures of LV function need to be studied in a large number of patients and results of such studies may provide clues to the role of LV function in this anomaly.

Spontaneous closure of the VSD occurs quite frequently in tricuspid atresia; both functional and anatomic closures have been documented. Such a closure causes pulmonary oligemia in Type I patients and sub-aortic obstruction in Type II patients. The incidence of VSD closure in tricuspid atresia is similar to that observed with isolated defects. There are surgical implications to spontaneous VSD closure, and these should be considered when palliative or corrective surgery is planned.

The majority of tricuspid atresia patients present with symptoms in the neonatal period and infancy and are not candidates for corrective surgery at initial presentation. Palliative procedures to normalize pulmonary blood are usually needed at the time of presentation or at a variable time period thereafter. PGE_1 is of great value in temporarily palliating neonates, whose pulmonary or systemic flow is ductal dependent. Pulmonary oligemia can be treated with several surgical shunt procedures. I was generally opposed to Potts/Waterston type of procedures because of their adverse long-term effects, precluding later successful physiologic correction. BT shunt is the procedure of choice for initial palliation; this is in preference to classic Glenn procedure because spontaneous closure of VSD following Glenn leaves the left pulmonary circuit without blood flow. If additional palliation is needed prior to the time of the Fontan-Kreutzer procedure, another BT shunt, Glenn procedure, or enlargement of the restrictive VSD with right ventricular outflow tract reconstruction (Annechino's procedure) should be considered.

Pulmonary plethora should be treated by PA banding in order to control CHF and to prevent pulmonary vascular obstructive disease. In Type I patients, banding is rarely necessary. In Type II patients, potential for sub-aortic obstruction at the VSD level exists. If a restrictive VSD is present, bypassing the sub-aortic obstruction by Stancel procedure should be considered instead of PA banding.

Interatrial obstruction is relatively rare in tricuspid atresia and when present, can be treated by balloon or blade atrial septostomy. Surgical septectomy is rarely necessary. As mentioned above, interventricular obstruction by restrictive VSD can occur and its management during palliate management has already been alluded to. At the time of physiologic correction, restrictive nature of the VSD should be carefully scrutinized in Type II patients and if present, the obstruction should be relieved either by resection of the outlet septum or bypassed by a Stancel type of procedure.

Experimental observations beginning in the 1940s have laid foundation for the physiologic rationale for the Fontan-Kreutzer operation. Experimental data also suggest that a four chamber, four valve heart can be achieved in tricuspid atresia provided the hypoplastic right ventricle is at least 25 percent to 30 percent of normal value. Based on other experimental data from animal studies, inferences with regard to post-operative care can be drawn as follows: a) Low left atrial pressure should be aimed for by maintaining sinus rhythm, and supporting LV function by inotropes and afterload reducing agents; b) low pulmonary vascular resistance should be sought by mild respiratory alkalosis and low blood viscosity (hematocrit 30-35 percent); c) maintain adequate right atrial pressure by colloid infusion to achieve adequate cardiac output; d) mechanical ventilation may be well tolerated by post-Fontan patients, but the positive end-expiratory pressure should not exceed 6 torr.

Fontan and Kreutzer have independently developed physiologic correction of tricuspid atresia in human subjects. This surgical procedure is most commonly referred to as Fontan operation, while others call it the Fontan-Kreutzer procedure. Brevity and perhaps priority of publication favor the former. However, because of use of "Kreutzer's" principle (See Chapter 19) in "Fontan" circulation and because the concepts and human applications have been developed independently by these two groups of investigators, I prefer to use the latter term, Fontan-Kreutzer. Since the development of these initial operations, a large number of modifications have been devised. At that time, it was not clear which of the four commonly used corrective operations are best for the patient on long-term basis. Limited data suggest that direct right atrial to PA anastomosis is preferable unless a respectable sized right ventricle is present, when a right atrial to RV valved conduit (preferably homograft) anastomosis may be the procedure of choice. But it is clear that some form of Fontan-Kreutzer is the preferred definitive treatment option for tricuspid atresia patients. It improves oxygen saturation, decreases LV volume work and ablates right-to-left shunt, thus eliminating the potential for paradoxical embolism. Operative mortality is low (5 percent or less) for patients with ideal criteria, while a higher mortality is expected if one or more criteria are exceeded. The vast majority of late survivors are in good condition. Systemic venous congestion, "protein-losing enteropathy," arrhythmia (see below), and need for re-operation, particularly in the sub-group with valved or non-valved Dacron conduits continue to plague the follow-up results. Continued collection of follow-up data and refinement of selection criteria are necessary. However, it is clear that Fontan-Kreutzer procedure improves patient survival and quality of life.

Post-operative arrhythmias following Fontan-Kreutzer repair, both immediate and late have been noted. In some studies, 40 percent to 50 percent of the patients were noted to have arrhythmia; the majority of the risk factors for development arrhythmia are residual hemodynamic abnormalities. Supraventricular tachycardia and atrial flutter are the most frequent rhythm abnormalities with occasional patients exhibiting sick sinus node syndrome, atrial and junctional ectopic beats and atrioventricular block. Ventricular arrhythmia and sudden death have also been reported. Limited number of patients underwent detailed electrophysiologic studies following Fontan-Kreutzer. Electrophysiologic abnormalities were detected in at least two-thirds of the patients studied; although, the study patients were not necessarily representative of the total group that underwent corrective surgery. Significant electrophysiologic abnormalities include sinus node dysfunction (increased corrected sinus node recovery time and prolonged sinoatrial conduction time), delayed intra-atrial conduction, prolonged atrial refractory period, and inducible supraventricular tachycardia. The abnormalities appear to be related to extensive atrial surgery and chronically elevated right atrial pressure. Monitoring for arrhythmia during follow-up is recommended. Further studies to identify patients at risk for development of serious arrhythmia are needed.

While most patients with tricuspid atresia present with symptoms during infancy and childhood and are seen and cared for by the pediatrician and pediatric cardiologist, many of them will grow into adolescence and adulthood because of advances in palliative and "corrective" surgical therapy and will need medical care by the internist and adult cardiologist. Therefore, services of' physicians skilled in diagnosis and treatment of patients with congenital cardiac disease in the adult patient are necessary. Liaison between adult and pediatric cardiologists may help promote optimal care for these patients graduating into adulthood. Accurate diagnosis based on clinical, non-invasive and invasive studies are necessary in most of these patients. They should be evaluated to decide on the need for appropriate palliative and corrective surgical therapy with the objective of improving symptoms and preventing damage to cardiovascular structures. For those that had undergone a previous Fontan-Kreutzer procedure, periodic evaluation to detect long-term residual complications of the surgery such as systemic venous congestion, arrhythmia and LV dysfunction and treat such abnormalities as indicated.

It is important to recognize issues of sexuality, contraception, and pregnancy as they relate to cyanotic CHDs in general and tricuspid atresia in particular. Inclusion of a program of sexual education, contraceptive counseling and family planning within the overall medical care of adolescents and young adults with CHDs is essential. Early sexual education and contraceptive counseling will help in preventing unwanted pregnancies and grave complications of contraindicated types of contraception. If pregnancy has occurred, early diagnosis is essential for the management and prevention of complications. A planned team approach including the assistance of pediatrician or internist, obstetrician and cardiologist, and a specialized center with capabilities of management of high-risk pregnancy is mandatory. Pregnancy outcome in the unoperated tricuspid atresia patient is dismal. Although, positive outcome after Fontan-Kreutzer has been documented and is probably related to minimal residual complications and preserved LV function. Further data are needed for making a definitive recommendation for Fontan-Kreutzer patients as a group.

Although a reasonable understanding of the normal development of the atrio-ventricular (AV) valves exist, the mechanisms of embryogenesis of tricuspid atresia are hypothetical and largely speculative. Further research to investigate mechanism involved in the morphogenesis of tricuspid atresia and causes of such altered development is needed.

Preliminary studies on epicardial mapping and intramural activation performed at our institution, to a great extent, explained the QRS abnormality seen in most cases of tricuspid atresia. Further studies in a larger number of patients with abnormally superior vector ("left axis deviation") and mapping on tricuspid atresia patients with inferiorly oriented QRS vectors are needed to fully understand the ECG abnormalities in this defect complex.

Evaluation of LV function has largely been accomplished with load-dependent measures, although load-independent measures have been utilized recently. Correlation of such load-independent measures of LV function with the outcome of surgery and long-term survival are in order. Also, simpler methods to measure LV contractility, which are load-independent should be developed. Techniques of evaluation of LV function reserve by exercise testing or other means, though available, have been utilized in only a limited number of patients. Identification of deviations of the functional reserve capacity from normal and correlating with surgical outcome may be necessary. There appears to be "cardiomyopathic" changes in some patients with tricuspid atresia. Whether these are causally related to a specific anatomic or physiologic abnormality should be investigated.

Development of sub-aortic stenosis in Type II patients is well documented, but the palliative and corrective surgery for such obstruction has been less than ideal. Innovative approaches to this problem should be sought.

Excellent selection criteria for suitability for Fontan-Kreutzer have been developed. Innovative surgeons have exceeded a number of these criteria and still maintained good results. Further refinement of these criteria, examining indices such as that proposed by Mair and development of new ones are essential to continue further improvement of surgical outcome and long-term prognosis.

A greater understanding of the hemodynamics of Fontan-Kreutzer operation may help in the post-operative care of these patients. Ability to support right atrial function such as balloon pumping, etc., in the post-operative period may help salvage some Fontan-Kreutzer patients that are not being benefited.

There are several types of Fontan-Kreutzer operations that are currently being performed; atrio-pulmonary or atrio-ventricular anastomosis with direct connection or valved or non-valved conduit interposition. There is limited data with regard to early and late mortality, need for re-operation, long-term functional capacity, post-operative residual complications and arrhythmia for each of the surgical options. Such information is of value in deciding on the most appropriate type of Fontan-Kreutzer to be used in a given patient. Such information may help resolve whether direct anastomosis, valved (heterografts or homografts), non-valved conduit or pericardial material are better choices. Thus, long-term invasive and non-invasive studies following Fontan-Kreutzer procedure are needed. Other problems following these operations, namely long-term systemic venous congestion, arrhythmia, poor LV function, protein losing enteropathy should also be investigated and risk factors predisposing to such complications should be determined.

A greater understanding of the issues of sexuality, contraception and pregnancy by the cardiologist taking care of patients with tricuspid atresia or any cyanotic heart defect and incorporation of educational and counseling aspects pertaining to these issues within the overall medical care of adolescents and adults are necessary. Data on the pregnancy in the patient following Fontan-Kreutzer are sparse and therefore, all such pregnancies and their outcome should be carefully documented.

Until these problems are resolved and answers to questions raised are cleared, palliative procedures should be performed with the aim to preserve and restore the anatomy and physiology as close to normal as possible such that a complete correction can be performed safely and the infant and child allowed to grow up to be a healthy adult.[28]

TRANSCATHETER THERAPY IN PEDIATRIC CARDIOLOGY

While I have contributed a number of reviews[27,29-42] detailing transcatheter methods of management of heart disease in children, it was felt that a more comprehensive treatment of this subject in a book format was in order and this book is the product of such a thought.[43] The purpose of this book was to unify and review the decade of advances in interventional pediatric cardiology and to present the state-of-the-art of this exciting new discipline (Figure 9).[43] Although, a substantial portion of the volume deals with balloon angioplasty/valvuloplasty, the book includes chapters dealing with balloon and blade atrial septostomy, transcatheter closure of cardiac septal defects, selective embolization of abnormal blood vessels, transcatheter removal of foreign bodies, transcatheter ablation of conduction bundles, and other transcatheter measures. While a number of chapters have been written by me and my associates, I took the liberty to tap the resources and expertise of other workers in the field. A section on international experience was also included. Although the presentations focus on the pediatric age group, the same principles, by and large, can be applied to adult patients with congenital or acquired stenotic lesions. Attempts to avoid repetition have been made, but some degree of duplication was unavoidable to preserve the continuity of discussion.

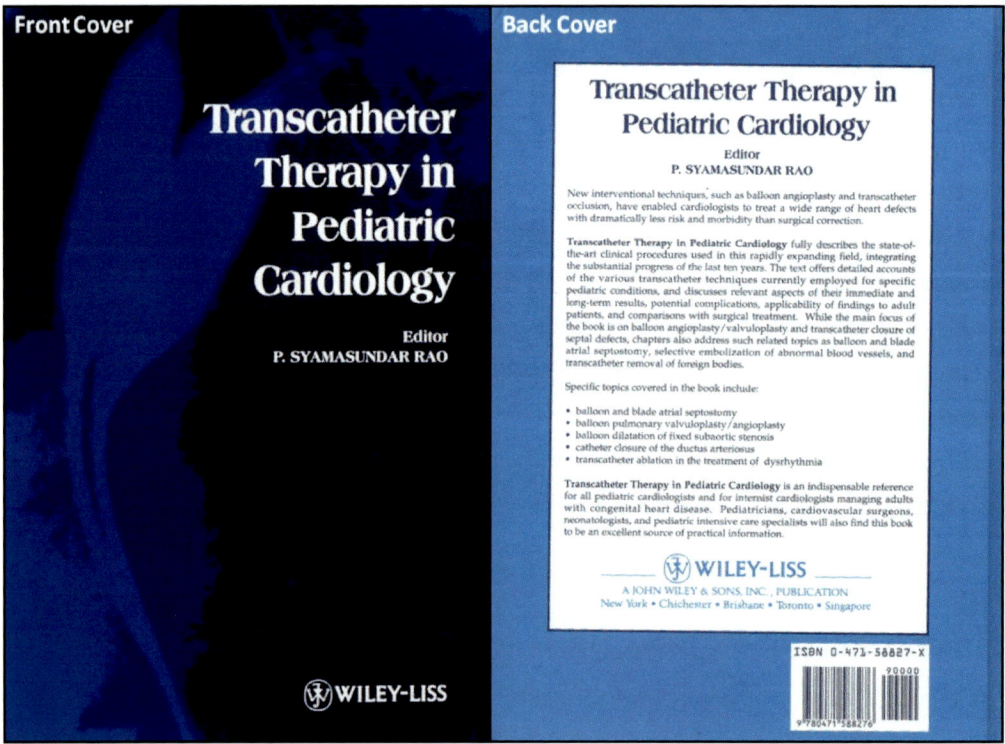

Figure 9. Photograph of book titled "Transcatheter Therapy in Pediatric Cardiology" published by *Wiley-Liss, Inc.,* in 1993. Both front and back covers are shown.

It is hoped that this book will provide useful information to the pediatric cardiologists and to the internist cardiologists caring for adults with CHD in their day-to-day management of patients with CHDs. It should serve as a reference work to many physicians in pediatrics, cardiovascular surgery, neonatology, and pediatric intensive care. The volume should also serve as a source material for other health care professionals, including nurses, social workers, catheterization laboratory technologists, and echocardiography technologists. It is hoped that this book will answer many questions in interventional pediatric cardiology, stimulate further interest in transcatheter therapy, and promote research to resolve unsettled issues in this new and exciting field.

The conventional treatment option for congenital or acquired lesions of the heart is surgical correction. Since the early 1950s, concurrent with the development of surgical techniques, investigators have attempted to replace the more invasive surgical techniques with less invasive transcatheter treatment modes. In 1953 and 1954, Rubio-Alvarez and his colleagues described a technique by which pulmonary and tricuspid valve stenoses could be relieved via a catheter; they used a ureteral catheter with a wire. A decade later, Dotter and Judkins introduced a gradual dilatation technique to open up stenotic atherosclerotic lesions of the peripheral arteries. In the next decade, Gruntzig and his coworkers extended these principles and developed a double-lumen catheter with a non-elastic balloon and used it to dilate stenotic lesions of the iliac, popliteal, femoral, renal, and coronary arteries. Shortly thereafter, in 1982, Kan and her associates extended these dilatation techniques to children with pulmonary valve stenosis. This appears to have produced a rapid increase in the use of balloon dilatation techniques in the pediatric patients. Concurrent with the development of these techniques, other investigators attempted either to open or to close cardiac septal defects. In 1966, Rashkind and Miller described a dynamic balloon dilatation technique to enlarge the patent foramen ovale (PFO). This life-saving technique was extensively used in neonates with TGA. For patients in whom this balloon septostomy technique is not adequate, Park et al. developed a blade septostomy technique. This is useful in older infants and children and in patients with thick interatrial septae. Porstmann (1967), King (1976), Rashkind (1979, 1983), and their associates, on the other hand, developed devices that could be deployed via catheters and occlude atrial and ventricular defects and patent ductus arteriosus (PDA). These initial historic attempts have been followed by clinical trials and refinement of techniques by many investigators around the world.

Rashkind's balloon atrial septostomy has been used extensively in the palliation of the neonate with TGA and intact ventricular septum. The improved mixing at the atrial level allowed the transposition patients to grow up to an age and size at which a venous switch procedure (Mustard or Senning) could safely be performed. Since the advent and extensive use of the arterial switch procedure (Jatene) in the early neonatal period, balloon septostomy has not been used as extensively as in the past. But, this procedure is still useful in temporizing a sick, hypoxemic, and acidotic neonate. It is also used for palliation if the arterial switch procedure cannot be performed on an urgent basis. The septostomy technique is also useful in the management of other conditions such as tricuspid or mitral atresia, hypoplastic right or left heart syndrome, and total anomalous pulmonary venous connection (TAPVC), all with interatrial obstruction. Balloon atrial septostomy is the initial procedure of choice in all situations in which an adequate interatrial communication is deemed necessary.

While the balloon atrial septostomy is generally successful, it does fail to create an adequate interatrial opening in some patients. By and large, this appears to be related to a thick interatrial septum, especially in older infants and children. To circumvent this problem, Park developed a blade septostomy catheter that can be utilized to cut (literally) the interatrial septum, which is then followed up by balloon atrial septostomy to enlarge the atrial defect further. The majority of time the procedure is carried out through an open, but restrictive, atrial defect. However, the procedure can also be performed in patients with an intact atrial septum following transseptal puncture. Park's initial clinical trials, collaborative studies, and experience reported by multiple other workers around the world have demonstrated that the method is feasible, effective, and safe. Attention to details of the technique and biplane fluoroscopy are essential to the safety and success of the procedure.

The technique of balloon angioplasty/valvuloplasty used in relieving obstructive lesions is reasonably well standardized. The indications for employing these procedures are similar to those used for surgical intervention. Obtaining informed consent from the parents and/or patient is essential. An intravenous line and type and cross-match for blood are generally required. Surgical stand-by is generally not recommended. We perform the procedure with sedation of the patient with a mixture of meperidine, promethazine, and chlorpromazine (supplemented with intermittent doses of midazolam), while a limited number of interventional pediatric cardiologists use ketamine or general anesthesia. The procedure involves positioning a balloon dilatation catheter across the site of obstruction and inflating it. Sequential balloon inflation with 3, 4, and 5 atm of pressure of five second duration, five minutes apart is recommended. Higher inflation pressures may be used if the balloon catheter manufacturer states that higher pressures are tolerated by the balloon. Appropriate choice of balloon size remains critical to achieving good results and preventing complications. Further miniaturization of balloon/catheter systems and meticulous attention to the details of the technique are necessary for successful relief of obstruction and reduction of complication rates. Limited applications of newer transcatheter technologies, such as double-blade valvotomy, laser, and atherectomy catheter device, have been reported in the treatment of children with heart disease.

While the interventional cardiologist does not need to become a physicist, some understanding of the catheter and balloon material, dilating forces of the balloon, and implications of use of different sizes, types, and numbers of balloons is necessary to optimize the effects of balloon dilatation procedures. The effects of complete, but transient obstruction to blood flow during balloon inflation are minimal and are well tolerated by most patients. Minimizing adverse effects of such obstruction, while maximizing the benefits of radial forces of balloon dilatation, is the key to the success of the balloon dilatation procedures. The response of the stenotic site depends not only on the radial forces of balloon dilatation but also on the morphology and pathologic process of the lesion being dilated. Commissural splitting is the most frequently observed response following balloon valvuloplasty. However, valve tears and dehiscence of valve leaflets have also been reported. These latter effects are likely to be problematic when aortic or mitral valves are the sites of damage. Such adverse effects may be secondary to uni-commissural valves or related to the technique of valvuloplasty. Disruption of intimal and medial layers of the aortic wall appears to be the mechanism of action of controlled injury by balloon dilation of aortic coarctation.

Pulmonary valve stenosis is one of the first congenital stenotic lesions to be balloon dilated and is one of the first for which balloon valvuloplasty is generally accepted as a therapeutic procedure of choice. There is some difference of opinion as to the indications for balloon therapy. I believe that indications for balloon intervention should be similar to those for surgery. A moderate degree of pulmonary valve obstruction with a gradient ≥ 50 mmHg and a normal cardiac index are what I would require for considering balloon intervention. Previous surgery, mild pulmonary valve dysplasia, and Noonan syndrome are not contraindications for balloon valvuloplasty. Excellent relief of obstruction of valve stenosis by pulmonary balloon valvuloplasty has been documented in neonates, infants, children, and adults. Immediate and intermediate-term results are available, but there are limited long-term follow-up data. ECG and Echo-Doppler evaluations at follow-up are reflective of the results; re-catheterization may not be necessary to evaluate results. The results of balloon valvuloplasty are either comparable with or better than those reported with surgical valvotomy. Complications of the procedure are minimal. The causes of restenosis have been identified, and appropriate modification of the technique, particularly use of a balloon/annulus ratio of 1.2 to 1.4, may produce better results than previously documented. Infundibular reaction may be present in older patients and in patients with severe obstruction and can most often be treated with adequate valvuloplasty and ß-blocking drugs, with rare need for surgery. Further miniaturization of the balloon/catheter systems, further refinements of the procedure, and meticulous attention to details of the technique may further increase the success rate and decrease the complication rate. Documentation of favorable results for five to ten years following balloon dilatation is necessary. Balloon pulmonary valvuloplasty is an excellent alternative to open or closed heart surgery in most, if not all, patients with PS.

Balloon valvuloplasty was initially utilized for aortic stenosis (AS) by Lababidi, but has not been used as frequently as balloon pulmonary valvuloplsty. Several workers have utilized it for relief of aortic valve obstruction in neonates, infants, children, and adults. Immediate and intermediate-term results have produced reduction of aortic valve gradients by 60 percent of prevalvuloplasty values. Previous surgical valvotomy does not adversely affect the result. Complications are minimal, although the potential for complications, such as arterial occlusion, especially in young children, and aortic insufficiency should be recognized. Significant restenosis rates at intermediate-term follow-up have been reported and could be minimized by reducing risk factors associated with recurrence. Echo-Doppler studies are helpful in follow-up evaluation of balloon dilatation of aortic valve. The balloon therapy compares favorably with surgical valvotomy. The indications for balloon valvuloplasty are essentially the same as those used for surgical intervention, namely, peak-to-peak gradients ≥ 70 mmHg, irrespective of symptoms, and gradients ≥ 50 mmHg with associated symptoms and/or ST - T wave abnormalities suggestive of myocardial ischemia. The procedure is particularly useful in neonates and young infants in view of the high mortality rate associated with surgery in these sick infants. Thus far, only short-term follow-up results are available. Five to ten year follow-up results to document longer term effectiveness of balloon aortic valvuloplasty are needed. Some reduction in the size of the balloon catheter systems has taken place. Further decrease in the size of the catheter and greater rapidity of inflation/deflation of balloons are necessary for increasing the safety and effectiveness of the balloon dilatation procedures, particularly in younger children.

Inoue introduced balloon mitral valvotomy to relieve mitral valve obstruction in 1984, shortly after the introduction of balloon valvuloplasty to treat congenital valvar obstructions. The majority of the reported experience is in adult patients with rheumatic mitral stenosis. In general, the indications for balloon intervention are symptoms in patients with moderate to severe stenosis (mitral valve area ≤ 1.5 cm^2) without evidence for left atrial thrombus or moderate to severe mitral regurgitation. Balloon dilatation with conventional single and double balloons and with Inoue balloons has been reported. The balloons are most commonly inserted antegrade by transseptal technique. Decrease in pressure gradient across the mitral valve, increase in mitral valve area, and improvement in symptoms have been documented after balloon mitral valvuloplasty. Complication rate is low and includes minimal mortality (< 2 percent), cardiac tamponade (1 percent to 3 percent), thrombo-embolism (0 percent to 4 percent), and severe mitral insufficiency requiring surgery (1 percent to 4 percent). Residual atrial septal defects (ASDs) with left-to-right shunting have been noted, but these are small, with negligible hemodynamic consequence. Short-term follow-up results are encouraging; long-term results are not available. Based on the available data, percutaneous balloon mitral valvuloplasty appears to be a valid alternative to surgical commissurotomy in the relief of stenotic mitral valve. Balloon valvuloplasty has also been applied to rheumatic tricuspid valve stenosis. The reported experience is small but favorable. An increase in cardiac output and improvement in symptoms were noted in most cases. Complications are minimal. Percutaneous tricuspid valvuloplasty appears to be a reasonable alternative to surgery for the relief of tricuspid valve stenosis unless there is associated severe tricuspid regurgitation.

Suarez de Lezo et al. in 1986 applied balloon dilatation techniques to relieve discrete sub-aortic stenosis. Several other workers have since used this technique with success. Because of the potential for development of aortic insufficiency, indication for intervention is set at a slightly lower level of obstruction (peak-to-peak gradients ≥ 40 mmHg) than for valvar stenosis. The immediate results appear excellent, as are the intermediate-term follow-up results when the sub-aortic membrane is discrete and thin (Type I). When the sub-aortic obstruction is a fibro-muscular (Type II) or tunnel (Type III) type, both the immediate and follow-up results are poor. With the discrete, thin sub-aortic membrane, balloons larger than the aortic valve annulus may be safely used, provided there is no associated valvar AS. The mechanism of action is tearing of the sub-aortic membrane. It was concluded that balloon angioplasty may be a preferable initial procedure in the treatment of membranous sub-aortic obstruction.

Because of the initially reported poor result and concern for the development of aneurysms, there is considerable controversy with regard to the use of balloon angioplasty for treatment of native aortic coarctation. This initial concern seems to be abating, and at present, more medical centers are performing this procedure than in the past. Immediate and intermediate-term follow-up results of balloon angioplasty are generally good, with a small chance for recoarctation and aneurismal formation at the site of coarctation. Echo-Doppler and nuclear magnetic resonance imaging (MRI) techniques are useful adjuncts to cardiac catheterization and selective cineangiography in the evaluation of follow-up results. The causes of recoarctation have been identified and include age of less than one year, hypoplasia of the aortic isthmus, and a very small coarcted segment prior to and immediately after balloon angioplasty. The aorta appears to remodel itself to approach a near-normal aortic shape following successful balloon dilatation. Complications of the procedure are modest in degree, although arterial complications in the neonate and young infant may be significant. A substantial miniaturization of balloon catheter systems has taken place. Further miniaturization may be necessary to decrease the arterial complications. Meticulous attention to the technique, including appropriate balloon choices and avoidance of manipulation of the tips of catheters and guide wires in the region of freshly dilated coarctation, are likely to reduce the complication rate further. Despite some of these problems, I opined that balloon angioplasty is an effective and safe alternative to surgical intervention for native coarctation, particularly in the neonate and young infant. Periodic assessment of this recommendation is in order as more data are accumulated. Five to ten year follow-up data, assessment of the causes and the natural history of aneurysms occurring after balloon angioplasty, and actuarial evaluation of surgical versus balloon angioplasty are needed to achieve this objective.

Balloon dilatation of aortic recoarctation following previous surgery is next only to valvar PS with regard to the acceptability by cardiologists as a therapeutic alternative to surgery. Immediate results seem excellent with an acceptable complication rate. The results and risks appear comparable with those seen with repeat surgical intervention. Follow-up results are available in only a limited number of patients, with recurrence and aneurismal formation rates of 2.5 percent and 9 percent, respectively. The high recurrence rates appear to be related to the use of small balloons in the early experience of some of the investigators. These and arterial complication rates are likely to diminish because of progressive improvement of the balloon catheter technology and a greater understanding by cardiologists of the angioplasty technique. Most cardiologists agree that balloon angioplasty is the treatment of choice for management of aortic recoarctations. A peak-to-peak systolic pressure gradient across the operative site in excess of 20 mmHg with angiographic demonstration of discrete narrowing is an indication for balloon dilatation. Use of heparin, appropriate choice of balloon diameter, and avoidance of manipulation of the tips of guide wire and catheter in the vicinity of freshly dilated recoarctation are important technical features of balloon angioplasty. Periodic evaluation for evidence of re-narrowing and for development of aneurysms is necessary; these may be performed by clinical, Echo-Doppler, MRI, and angiographic studies. The mechanism of effectiveness of angioplasty appears to be intimal and medial disruption produced by controlled injury through radial forces of balloon inflation. Further miniaturization of balloon/catheter systems, a better understanding of the technique of balloon angioplasty, longer duration of follow-up in a larger number of patients than is currently available, and cause and natural history of aneurysm formation following angioplasty are important in further advancing balloon angioplasty as a successful therapeutic option for the management of post-operative aortic recoarctation.

Peripheral PA stenosis is one of the few lesions in which balloon dilatation has not produced excellent results. This is related to the elastic nature of branch PA stenotic lesions in the congenital obstructions and fibrosis around the PA in the postsurgical obstructions. It is generally more difficult to position a balloon dilatation catheter across branch PA stenotic lesions than across other lesions. With the availability of extra-stiff guide wires and low-profile balloon angioplasty catheters, this technical difficulty has decreased. Even with adequate technique, balloon angioplasty success can be expected in approximately 50 percent of the patients. However, the follow-up studies are few, and therefore long-term results are unknown. Recently, balloon-expandable stents have been used with success in relieving branch PA stenoses. Although there is limited experience with stents, they are likely to be useful in patients in whom balloon angioplasty is not successful.

Transcatheter treatment methodology appears useful in the management of several types of cyanotic CHDs. The role of Rashkind's balloon atrial septostomy and Park's blade atrial septostomy in promoting interatrial mixing and relieving atrial obstruction has already been alluded to. Cyanotic children with interatrial right-to-left shunting secondary to severe valvar PS respond to balloon pulmonary valvuloplasty in a manner similar to that observed with isolated pulmonary valve stenosis. In these patients, balloon valvuloplasty is the treatment of choice and may be corrective in the majority of patients. In a substantial proportion of patients with inter-ventricular right-to-left shunting secondary to pulmonary outflow tract obstruction, balloon pulmonary valvuloplasty may be an effective palliative procedure, obviating the need for palliative shunt. Balloon dilatation of narrowed classic or modified BT shunts is also feasible and augments pulmonary blood flow and improves systemic arterial oxygen saturation. I recommend either balloon valvuloplasty of the stenotic pulmonary valve or narrowed Blalock-Taussig shunt if the patient's size or cardiac anatomy make a cyanotic heart defect unsuitable for safe total surgical correction. In patients with pulmonary atresia, opening of the atretic pulmonary valve by either laser or initial surgery and follow-up with balloon dilatation are potentially beneficial in reducing the total number of surgical procedures that these children are likely to require. The preliminary data seem to indicate potential for these methods; further clinical trials are required prior to adopting them for general use.

Calcific degeneration and obstruction of bio-prosthetic valves have been documented; this appears to occur more frequently and more rapidly in younger children than in older children and adults. Conventional treatment of choice is repeat valve replacement. Recently, balloon valvuloplasty techniques have been utilized to relieve the obstruction of the biological valves in an attempt to avoid or postpone surgery for repeat valve replacement. All varieties of heterografts and homografts can be balloon dilated. The largest experience is with bio-prosthetic valve conduits in the pulmonary position. Although the results are not uniformly successful, repeat valve replacement was avoided or at least postponed for several years in some patients. The indication for intervention is a peak-to-peak systolic pressure gradient ≥ 50 mmHg across the pulmonary bio-prosthetic valve. A balloon size equal to the size of the bio-prosthesis should be used. Relief of valvar obstruction may unmask additional obstructive lesions at the proximal or distal anastamosis. These should be sought out and, if feasible, balloon dilated concurrently. The high incidence of balloon rupture associated with pulmonary heterograft dilatation is of concern; appropriate precautions should be taken to prevent or reduce balloon ruptures. Follow-up results are few and are needed. There are also reports of balloon dilatation of stenotic heterografts in the tricuspid position. Acute improvement in valve stenosis was observed in most, but nearly one-half of them required additional intervention within months after balloon valvuloplasty. Because of limited experience with this lesion, definitive recommendations with regard to the role of balloon dilatation of tricuspid heterograft stenosis cannot be made. Balloon dilatation of mitral and aortic heterograft valve stenosis has also been performed. The results are unpredictable. This and the potential for dislodgement of calcific debris and fractured valve cusps and the consequent systemic embolization warrant a limited role of balloon valvuloplasty procedures in the management of left heart bio-prosthetic valve obstruction. However, the development of embolic-protecting devices may resolve the latter issue. Mechanisms of relief of obstruction following balloon dilatation have been studied and include commissural splitting and valve leaflet fracture. Because of limited experience with balloon dilatation of prosthetic biologic valve stenoses, it is imperative that careful documentation of both immediate and follow-up results is made. Additional clinical trials are necessary prior to the adoption of the balloon valvuloplasty technique as a procedure of choice in the management of bio-prosthetic valve stenosis.

As discussed above, balloon angioplasty/valvuloplasty techniques have been applied with reasonable success in relieving several congenital and acquired stenotic lesions of the heart and great vessels. There are other lesions that are either uncommon or for which balloon dilatation has not frequently been utilized. These lesions, namely, congenital tricuspid and mitral valve stenosis, truncal valve stenosis, stenotic ductus arteriosus, restrictive PFO, subvalvar PS, supravalvar PS (congenital or postoperative), stenosis of the aorta (Takayasu's arteritis), baffle obstructions following a Mustard or Senning procedure (both systemic venous and pulmonary venous), superior and inferior vena caval obstructive lesions, pulmonary vein stenosis, pulmonary veno-occlusive disease, pulmonary venous obstruction following repair of TAPVC, cor triatriatum dexter, and coronary artery stenotic lesions post-Kawasaki disease, can also be balloon dilated. The indications are generally those used for surgical intervention. The reported experience with each of the above lesions is limited. In most, there is effective relief of obstruction after balloon dilatation. Follow-up results are scanty. Further clinical trials are necessary to advocate the use of balloon dilatation technique as a preferred alternative to surgical intervention. There have also been attempts to devise pulmonary bands that could initially be placed surgically to produce effective relief of pulmonary over circulation and later opened up (dilated) by balloon angioplasty if the offending lesion (e.g., VSD) resolves spontaneously.

While the balloon dilatation techniques have rapidly been adopted in effecting enlargement of stenotic lesions of the heart, transcatheter methods of closure of septal defects have not gained quick acceptance. This is related in part to the cumbersome nature of the techniques and in part to leaving a foreign body in the heart. Since King's initial description of paired umbrellas to close the ASDs, a variety of devices have been developed and tested in animal models and in clinical trials. Until recently, Clamshell Septal Umbrella and "buttoned" devices were the only two ASD closing devices approved by the FDA for investigational use. Approximately 400 Clamshell devices have been implanted in a multicenter trial. At the time of this writing, the FDA suspended clinical trials with this device because of breakage of wire hinges at follow-up. Therefore, the buttoned device is the only ASD closure prosthesis currently under approval for clinical trials. To date, approximately hundred buttoned devices have been implanted, with success in 90 percent of the patients. With further clinical trials and further refinement of the device, it is likely to be clinically useful in the treatment of ASDs. There are also multiple types of PDA closing devices; many were tried in animal models, and a few of these have been applied to human subjects. Porstmann's Ivalon plug and Rashkind's double-disc device are available for use. In the United States, Rashkind's device is available for investigational use; it is likely to be released soon by the FDA for general use. A "buttoned" device, similar to that used for ASD closure, has also been utilized for closure of PDA as a custom-made device; approval by the FDA for clinical trials of this device is awaited. Closure of the VSDs, though more cumbersome than ASD and PDA closure, can be accomplished by use of several of the above-described devices. Much larger clinical experience than is currently available is needed for adopting the method for general use.

In summary, attempts to replace surgical treatment of cardiac septal defects with transcatheter methods began more than twenty-five years ago. Several types of devices and device delivery systems have been developed and refined to some degree. Safety and efficacy have been reasonably good, but most of the available devices and delivery systems are bulky and cumbersome. Some miniaturization of the devices has taken place, and some are more suitable for clinical use today than in the past. Further clinical trials to examine the safety and effectiveness and further miniaturization of the devices are required prior to routine application of these techniques in the treatment of certain cardiac septal defects.

Transcatheter embolization techniques were initially developed for treatment of neurovascular conditions. These have since been extended to a variety of vascular abnormalities seen in pediatric patients. Multiple types of embolic materials have been utilized; however, Gianturco coils and detachable balloons were the most commonly used devices. Systemic collateral vessels to the lungs in patients with tetralogy of Fallot (TOF) with pulmonary atresia, pulmonary arteriovenous malformations, BT shunt that is no longer needed, systemic arteriovenous fistulae, vein of Galen malformation, coronary arteriovenous fistula, and systemic vessels supplying the sequestered lung in Scimitar Syndrome are but some of the lesions that have been successfully treated by transcatheter embolization techniques. There is a limited number of reports on a limited number of patients, but the acute results are generally good. Complications are rare, but include embolization to an undesirable site, transient infarction, and infection. There are extremely few reports on long-term effects. These embolization techniques do have advantage over surgery, but no systematic study comparing the two modes has been made. However, based on the available data, the embolization techniques are considered as the initial choice for treatment of these conditions.

Since the initial introduction by Myers in 1945 of indwelling intravascular catheters, polyethylene catheters have become a source of inadvertent embolization. The incidence of embolization has increased with the widespread use of these catheters in critically ill patients for the purpose of monitoring and fluid administration. Recognition of this problem resulted in the modification of the catheter systems, with improvement. But new sources of emboli have emerged with widespread use of cardiac catheterization and, more recently, with interventional procedures. Retained intra-vascular/intra-cardiac foreign bodies cause serious complications, including death. The consensus at this time is that all foreign bodies should be retrieved. Initially, a surgical approach was necessary to extract the foreign bodies. Since the first description by Thomas and colleagues in the mid 1960s of percutaneous, nonsurgical removal of the foreign body, several other types of retrieval sets have been described. Guide-wire loop snare (or a modification of it), helical baskets, and endoscopic forceps are the most commonly utilized retrieval devices. More recently Nittinol goose-neck snares have been introduced for foreign body retrieval. Approximately 90 percent of the foreign bodies can be retrieved through transcatheter methods. Complications associated with foreign body retrieval are minimal. The prevention of embolization through meticulous attention to the details of the technique of placing, securing, and removal of intravenous lines is important. Use of radio-opaque catheters is a must so that they can be easily visualized and removed through transcatheter techniques in the event of inadvertent embolization. Initially, the retrieval devices were bulky, but their sizes have been reduced for safe usage in the pediatric patient.

Refractory dysrhythmias are now amenable through transcatheter treatment. Multiple forms of energy, including direct current, laser, microwave, cryothermia, and radiofrequency, have been used in catheter ablation. Currently, radiofrequency ablation appears to be the most commonly utilized. Ablation techniques have been used in the treatment of both automatic focus and re-entry tachycardias in childhood. Accurate diagnosis through careful mapping studies is needed prior to transcatheter ablation. Although there is limited experience with these techniques, the experience is encouraging and compares favorably to that with surgical ablation.

In the last section of this book, several international experts describe their experiences with balloon dilatation of stenotic lesions of the heart. The results are generally similar to those reported by the USA workers. These international experiences enrich the discussions presented in the preceding chapters.

In this book, I have included most, if not all, transcatheter techniques available for treatment of congenital and acquired cardiac anomalies seen in infancy and childhood. Many of these techniques are equally applicable to adult patients. There has not been an extensive experience with the transcatheter techniques, mostly because of the relatively recent availability of the techniques to the practicing cardiologist. There is also a need for better understanding by the practicing cardiologist of the balloon technology, with particular reference to the types and sizes of balloon catheters, the balloon sizes available, and the choice of balloon size that is most appropriate in a given case. Acute results have been generally good. There is a limited number of reports, on a limited number of patients, describing intermediate-term follow-up results. There are practically none describing long-term results. The long-term results are needed to assess the efficacy of the techniques.

For the most part, the catheter systems are bulky and have a high potential for vascular injury. Recently, a significant miniaturization of the catheter systems has taken place, and, I believe, with further research and development, additional reduction in the size of the catheters, balloons, and devices is feasible. This would increase the safety and effectiveness of the transcatheter treatment modes.

Many of the catheter modes of treatment are replacing "standard" surgical procedures. However, there has not been a careful, prospective comparison between surgical and transcatheter therapeutic modalities. It is doubtful if such a comparative study is feasible at this stage of technology development.

While it may not be feasible to have a double-blind, controlled comparison of surgical versus transcatheter therapy, it is certainly possible to collect data prospectively to evaluate the immediate and follow-up results. Because the number of patients treated at each institution is small, registries have been established in the United States and Europe. While such registries increase the numbers, vagaries of variations in the technique and difficulties in data acquisition have been stumbling blocks to the rapid acquisition of results. Further miniaturization of catheter systems and careful, long-term (at least five and ten year) follow-up studies are feasible and should be attempted.

For lesions that are not currently amenable to presently available transcatheter methods, other methods should be sought. Some attempts in this direction are being made, and include stents and laser application. Such efforts should continue.[43]

A book review published in *Doody's Annual Health Science Book Review* is shown in figure 10.

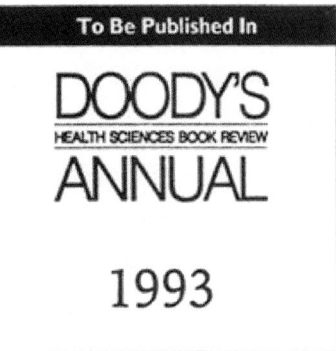

Rao / Transcatheter Therapy in Pediatric Cardiology

Author: Rao, P. Syamasundar, MD (Univ of Wisconsin Medical School)

Bibliographic Data: John Wiley & Sons, Inc, 1993, 1st ed. Imprint: Wiley-Liss. ISBN: 0-471-58827-X, LCCN: 92-48794, NLM: WS 290 T772, LC: RJ426.C64T73, Monograph, 23 chpt, 509 pp, 570 indx, 1821 ref, 56 tbl, 219 fig, 31 cntrb, 7" x 10", Hard Cover, $99.95.

Doody's Notes: Primary Audience: Pediatric Cardiologists. Secondary Audience: Cardiologists. There are 215 one-color figures and 4 four-color figures consisting predominantly of line drawings and radiographs, with some halftones. Nearly all of the contributors are pediatric cardiologists from depts of pediatrics at medical centers in North America (Johns Hopkins, the Univ of Wisconsin, Univ of Texas-Houston, the Univ of South Carolina), the Middle East, Spain, Hong Kong and India.

Reviewer's Expert Opinion: Description: This book provides a comprehensive review of most interventional cardiac procedures for congenital and acquired diseases in pediatric patients. Purpose: This book clearly outlines the indications, methods, and available clinical data for most interventional cardiac catheterization procedures. This book is a useful complement to a small number of texts already available in this area. The author has done a very good job in meeting the intended objectives. Audience: This book will be useful to pediatric cardiologists, pediatric cardiac surgeons, and trainees in these disciplines. Certain chapters will be valuable references for practicing pediatricians if they wish to evaluate the safety and efficiency of angioplasty. Features: The methods section of each chapter is clearly outlined and will be most useful to the trainee or inexperienced operator. The quality of the angiograms and valvuloplasty procedures is excellent. The references are complete and up-to-date. The author's comments for nearly every chapter are overdone. The index and table of contents are quite complete. Assessment: This book provides a useful resource for pediatric cardiologists who are practicing in the new discipline of interventional catheterization. It is recommended for fellows-in-training because of the clear illustrative angiography provided, current references, and multiauthored approach to a large number of procedures. Rating: 96

Reviewer: Vincent R. Zales, MD (Children's Memorial Hospital)

Figure 10. Book review of "Transcatheter Therapy in Pediatric Cardiology" published in *Doody's Annual Health Science Book Review.*

CATHETER BASED DEVICES FOR TREATMENT OF NON-CORONARY CARDIOVASCULAR DISEASE IN ADULTS AND CHILDREN

Since the publication of the book on "Transcatheter Therapy in Pediatric Cardiology,"[43] a large proliferation of device technology has occurred, especially in the last decade of the twentieth century. I collaborated with Dr. Morton Kern, an adult interventional cardiologist at the St. Louis University School of Medicine to organize and edit this book (Figure 11).[44]

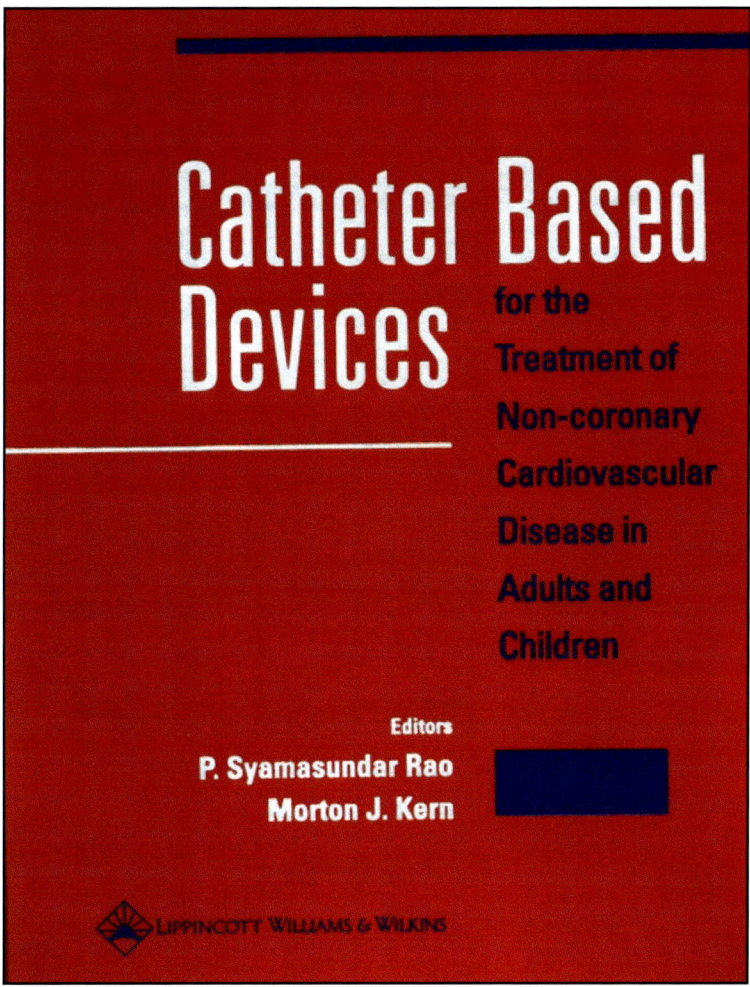

Figure 11. Photograph of the book titled "Catheter Based Devices for Treatment of Noncoronary Cardiovascular Disease in Adults and Children" published by *Lippincott, Williams & Wilkins* in 2003.

The purpose of this book was to bring together all the available transcatheter implantable device technology and present the state-of-the-art of this new discipline. Since there are many other books and monographs dealing with coronary artery interventions, this book was designed only to address treatment of non-coronary cardiovascular disease in both children and adults. We have gathered experts from around the world to contribute to this book; in the majority of chapters, we have been able to get either the inventor of the device/method or a major investigator of a particular device or method to write the chapters. The device description, indications for implantation and results of each device were discussed, along with alternative management strategies, if any. The devices that are generally considered a "pediatric" device will include a section dealing with device application in adult subjects.

The book is divided into six sections. The first section discusses transcatheter occlusion of ASDs. The second section deals with closure of PDA by transcatheter route. The next section describes transcatheter closure of both congenital and post-myocardial infarction VSDs and paravalvular leaks. The role of intravascular stents in the management of congenital and acquired stenotic vascular obstructive lesions in both children and adults was reviewed in section four. The fifth section deals with a number of diverse topics, including vascular embolization, device management of arrhythmias, vena caval filters to prevent pulmonary embolism, vascular closure devices, transcatheter implantation of prosthetic valves, and other miscellaneous devices. Role of echocardiography was discussed in this and other sections.

The conventional treatment of choice for acquired and congenial cardiac defects is surgical correction. Since the early 1950s, concurrent with the development of open-heart surgical techniques, several investigators attempted to develop transcatheter methodologies to replace invasive surgical procedures. A number of transcatheter methods, including pulmonary and tricuspid valvotomy by Rubio-Alverez and his colleagues, gradational dilatation of atherosclerotic lesions of peripheral arteries by Dotter and Judkins, balloon atrial septostomy by Rashkind, occlusion of PDA by Porstmann, device occlusion of ASDs by King, and coil occlusion of blood vessels by Gianturco, have been described. However, it was not until Gruntzig's clinical use of a double-lumen catheter with non-elastic balloon (percutaneous trans-luminal angioplasty) that interventional technology was applied widely to treat cardiac disease in both adult and pediatric patients. The decade of 1980s witnessed development, proliferation, and refinements of balloon angioplasty techniques, and the 1990s saw the mushrooming of transcatheter device implantation technology. In this book, we attempted to bring together the descriptions of all the available transcatheter implantable devices. This book did not include coronary artery device applications because many other monographs and books dealt with that subject.

Following pioneering efforts of King, Rashkind, and their colleagues in the mid-1970s, a number of transcatheter ASD occluding devices have been described. These include the Clamshell septal occluder, buttoned device, monodisk device, modified Rashkind PDA device, ASDOS (ASD occluding system), Angel Wing Das device, Amplatzer Septal Occluder, CardioSEAL device, Starflex device, Helex device, and PFO-Star. Most of the devices have undergone experimentation in animal models to test their feasibility, safety, and efficacy. This experience was followed by clinical trials in human subjects with approval of local Institutional Review Boards (IRBs) and the Food and Drug Administration (FDA) with investigational device exemption (IDE) in the United States or CD Mark in Europe. Some of the devices have been discontinued either because of investigators' assessment of lack of safety or efficacy or because of instructions from the regulatory authorities. Other devices were modified or redesigned.

Following my description of historical developments of ASD occluding devices, Dr. Rome described the Clamshell device and its utility in occluding the ASDs. I then discussed the buttoned device, its modifications, and results. The role of ASDOS in closing ASDs was reviewed by Dr. Babic and his colleagues. Drs. Das, Harrison, and O'Laughlin provide insight into the design, application, and modifications of the Angel Wing Das device, now the Guardian Angel device. The method of implantation and results of the Amplatzer Septal Occluder were reviewed by Drs.

Hamdan, Cao, and Hijazi. Drs. Bennhagen, McLaughlin, and Benson described the CardioSEAL and Starflex devices and their role in closure of the ASDs. This is followed by the description of the Helex device by Drs. Latson, Wilson, and Zahn. Dr. Sideris brought wireless devices to our attention. Drs. Ewert and Berger reviewed their experience in closing ASDs without fluoroscopy. I provided a summary of ASD closure devices.

At the time of this writing, the FDA approved none of the devices for general clinical use. At the present time, several devices are under FDA approved clinical trials with IDE. These include the Amplatzer Septal Occluder, centering-on-demand buttoned device, CardioSEAL, STARflex, and Helex devices (By the time of review of the proof of the chapter, FDA approved Amplatzer Septal Occluder for closure of ostium secundum ASDs).

There are a few studies comparing a limited number of devices, used consecutively as the new devices become available. There were no prospective, randomized clinical trials using all the available devices to provide a comparison of their feasibility, safety, and effectiveness. It also appears unlikely that such a clinical trial is feasible at this juncture.

There are claims of superiority of one device over the others. But a careful comparison of the previously conducted studies in Chapter 11 suggested that the feasibility, safety, and effectiveness of most of the devices are similar. There are minor differences in the size of the delivery sheath, ease of implantation, cost, and availability.

At the time of this writing, the FDA approved none of the devices for general clinical use, with the exception of Amplatzer. Approval of other devices is anticipated in the near future. The availability of several devices may help facilitate randomized clinical studies that may provide data to evaluate which is the better (best) device. However, it is more likely that such trials may not be feasible. Also, it is possible that a particular device may be useful for a "given" type of defect, whereas another device may be suitable for another type of defect.

In addition to occluding ostium secundum ASD, the devices have been utilized to occlude PFO/ASD presumed to be the site of paradoxical embolism, PFO/ASDs causing right-to-left shunt following surgical or transcatheter intervention, Fontan fenestrations, PFO/ASDs responsible for platypnea-orthodeoxia syndrome, and PFOs causing neurologic decompression illness in divers. Drs. Schrader, Fossbender, and Strasser describe the role of PFO-Starr in closing the PFOs presumed to be the site of paradoxical embolism causing cerebrovascular accidents (CVAs) and transient ischemic attacks (TIAs) in young people. Drs. Windecker and Meier discuss the issues related to prevention of recurrence of CVAs and TIAs presumably secondary to paradoxical embolism through the atrial septum with particular attention to device closure. I presented a discussion of closure of PFO/ASDs with right-to-left shunt. Dr. Bitar and I described transcatheter treatment of platypnea-orthodeoxia syndrome. In the final chapter of this section, Dr. Banarjee and his associates discuss the role of three-dimensional echocardiographic reconstruction in transcatheter closure of atrial defects.

Thus, device closure of not only ostium secundum ASD, but also atrial defects responsible for actual and presumed right-to-left shunt is feasible, safe, and effective. However, with the current technology it is not feasible to address sinus venosus and ostium primum ASDs.

Since the initial description of transcatheter closure of PDAs by Porstmann and associates, a number of devices have been described to achieve transcatheter occlusion. A number of devices have been designed and tested in animal models but did not reach the stage of human application, and these have been reviewed in Chapter 25. In addition, a number of devices have undergone clinical trials, including Porstmann's Ivalon foam plug, Rashkind's hooked single umbrella, the Rashkind PDA occluding system, Botallo-Occluder, buttoned device, Clamshell ASD occluder, Gianturco coils, detachable coils, Duct-Occlud pfm, polyvinyl alcohol foam plug mounted on titanium pin, infant PDA buttoned device, Gianturco-Grifka vascular occlusion device, Amplatzer Duct Occluder, folding plug buttoned device, and wireless PDA devices. Of these, Porstmann's Ivalon foam plug, both Rashkind's hooked single-umbrella and double-umbrella devices, Botallo-occluder, Clamshell ASD device, regular buttoned device, infant buttoned device, and polyvinyl foam plug were discontinued or modified after initial clinical trials.

I detailed historical developments in transcatheter PDA occlusion. Dr. Qureshi describes the Rashkind device and its role in closure of PDA prior to its discontinuation. I also reviewed various modifications of the buttoned device and the result of closure of PDAs. Drs. Schneider and Moore reviewed Gianturco coil occlusion of PDA. Drs. Sreeram and Yap provided insight into the usage of detachable coils in occluding PDAs. Drs. Le, Neuss, and Freudenthal described the Duct-Occlud device and its modification and their utility in ductal closure. The role of the Gianturco-Grifka vascular occlusion device in occluding tubular PDA was discussed by Dr. Grifka. Drs. Sandhu and King described the Amplatzer Duct Occluder and its role in PDA closure. Finally, I provided a summary of PDA closure devices and presented an approach to the choice of closure methods in occluding PDAs based on its size and shape.

Gianturco coils were initially used on an off-label application and they subsequently became available for general clinical use. Detachable coils and the Gianturco-Grifka vascular occlusion device are currently available for general clinical use. Several PDA-occluding devices are undergoing FDA-approved clinical trials with IDE and include the Duct-occlud, the folding-plug buttoned device, and the Amplatzer Duct Occluder.

Very small and small PDAs can be occluded safely and effectively with either free or detachable Gianturco coils. Some investigators prefer detachable coils because of greater control during delivery and to "prevent" embolization. Careful review of the data, however, suggests that the prevalence of coil dislodgment/embolization is not significantly different from that of free coils, and therefore the advantage cited does not seem to exist. I personally prefer free 0.038-inch Gianturco coils for very small to small PDAs, 0.052-inch coils (delivered with a biopsy forceps via 4F long sheath) for small to moderate PDAs, and devices for moderate-to-large PDAs. As and when data become available on the devices in clinical trials, an appropriate selection of devices for closure of moderate-to-large PDAs will be feasible.

Continued use of and gaining experience with the use of coils for closure of small PDAs and approval of some of the devices for moderate to large PDAs in the near future are anticipated.

Since the report of Rashkind and Cuoso in the mid-1970s of transcatheter closure of experimentally created VSDs with single-umbrella and double-umbrella devices, a number of devices have been used by other workers. The Rashkind PDA occluder, Clamshell Septal Occluder, buttoned device, Amplatzer muscular VSD occluder, CardioSEAL, STARflex devices, and Nit-occlud have been utilized to close the VSD.

Dr. Goh discussed the role that the Rashkind and Clamshell devices played in occluding VSDs before their discontinuation. Dr. Sideris described the use of the buttoned device in closure of muscular and perimembranous VSDs. Drs. Waight, Cao, and Hijazi reviewed the utility of the Amplatzer muscular VSD occluder in transcatheter occlusion of muscular VSDs. Drs. Marshall and Perry provided data on the usefulness of the CardioSEAL and STARflex devices in closing VSDs. Dr. Le and his colleagues described a new VSD occluding device, Nit-occlud, and presented data on its experimental use and preliminary clinical trials. Dr. Landzberg presented an approach to occlude post-myocardial infarction VSDs. He also provided information on device closure of paravalvular leaks.

None of the devices are available for general clinical use. CardioSEAL is available for use under humanitarian device exemption (HDE). Nit-occlud is in clinical trials in Europe. Other devices, namely, buttoned device, Amplatzer muscular VSD occluder, and STARflex are in FDA approved clinical trials with IDE in the United States.

Isolated defects and defects associated with other complex heart disease have been addressed. In the latter situation, catheter closure served as an adjunct to surgery. Congenital and post-myocardial infarction VSDs have been tackled. The experience with VSD closure is not as extensive as that with ASD and PDA closures, presumably related to complexity of the procedure and lack of anatomic suitability of most VSDs for device closure.

Since the advent of the balloon dilatation in 1977 to mechanically alter the shape of coronary artery conduits, the field of interventional cardiology has consistently and steadfastly moved forward, developing new means to address both acquired and congenital heart disease and eliminate the morbidity and mortality of surgery. Approximately seven years following introduction of the balloon catheter, Palmaz produced a tubular steel-etched stent system that, when expanded with a balloon catheter, formed a metallic scaffold to be permanently implanted, opening the diseased arterial system.

Continued efforts from this landmark achievement have made the stent a mainstay of everyday interventional adult and pediatric cardiology. As the technology of coronary stents evolved, so did the clinical applications. A wide variety of peripheral and central arterial deformities and diseases involving the pulmonary artery, aortic coarctation, PDA, pulmonary and systemic venous obstruction, as well as bidirectional cavopulmonary shunts, and stenosed synthetic conduits are now treated by stenting. Moreover, the success of placing large-diameter stents either covered or uncovered, facilitated non-surgical treatment of many congenital cardiac conditions, requiring either reconstruction of narrowed conduits or closure of abnormal connections. In both adults and children this technologic advance has become commonplace.

In addition to management of arterial disease, a number of miscellaneous techniques of catheter-based non-coronary interventions are applied to arrhythmia management, pulmonary embolism prevention with vena caval filters, vascular closure for arterial punctures, and implantation of prosthetic valves through percutaneous approaches. Coupled to device placement is the increased use of refined and enhanced imaging of these clinical dilemmas with trans-esophageal echocardiography (TEE). Both the device and imaging advances propelled the field toward more minimally invasive methods to manage complex heart disease.

As the data on stents have been acquired, it is appropriate to concentrate on the outcomes of stents for the various manifestations of extra-cardiac and peripheral vascular abnormalities. Late Dr. Hausdorf described important mechanical and biophysical aspects of stenting as they may be applied to pulmonary arteries, coarctations, ductal connections, and venous obstructions. Drs. Coulson, Everett, and Owada presented information on the recent technical developments, including all the available stents and balloons, particularly for use in congenital and post-surgical cardiovascular anomalies.

For clinical management, Drs. McMahon and Nihill described management of pulmonary artery stenosis and its sub-branches using stenting. Drs. Jayakumar and Hellenbrand provided further insight into the management of coarctation using large stents in children. Dr. Ruiz elucidated new stenting techniques to assess and treat PDA in most of the complex CHDs encountered in the pediatric cardiac catheterization laboratory. Unique to this field is the information regarding the treatment of systemic and pulmonary venous obstruction using self-expanding and balloon-expandable stents, presented by Dr. Ing. Further insight was provided with a specific device, the NuMed CP stent, for CHDs, as described by Dr. Cheatham. I discussed the role of new stents in the treatment of vascular obstructive lesions in children.

Of great interest to the adult interventional cardiologist will be the information on the management of peripheral arterial stenosis. Drs. Vale, Bashir, and Rosenfield describe the wide use of stents in these patients. The application of stents to the carotid artery, now an everyday practice, was reviewed by Dr. Iyer and his associates. Infra-renal aortic aneurysms, once the exclusive province of the vascular surgeon, may now be managed by interventional cardiologists and radiologists using covered stents, as described by Drs. White, Lennox, and May. In years to come, these methods will be highly influenced by new materials and coatings applied to stents. Drs. Tsuji and Tamai described prospects for the future using biodegradable stents.

In the miscellaneous section contributing to our understanding of catheter-based devices for treatment of non-coronary cardiovascular disease, several premier interventionalists place in perspective the current status of devices for arrhythmia management, embolization of unwanted blood vessels, and application of vena caval filters for the prevention of pulmonary embolus.

Dr. Sandborn reported his wide experience with vascular closure devices, reviewing the different mechanisms of femoral arterial closure with the immediate and long-term outcomes for these tools. Needless to say, most adult vascular closure devices would not suffice for children, but have potential for use. These closure devices have been a great boon to the adult cardiologist concerned with complications of vascular access, especially retroperitoneal hematoma after intense anticoagulation during percutaneous coronary intervention (PCI).

Probably the most important new area in the next decade will be that of prosthetic valve implantation through a transcatheter approach. Drs. Pavcnik, Boudjemline, and Bonnhoeffer described the percutaneous methods of implanting prosthetic valves in both the aortic and pulmonary positions. I briefly reviewed several unique applications of device technology not included in the prior chapters, namely, percutaneous completion of Fontan, use of covered stents to treat aortic coarctation, device closure of aortopulmonary windows, devices to keep that atrial septal defect open, transcatheter management of pulmonary oligemia, and percutaneous closure of left atrial appendage to prevent strokes in patients with atrial fibrillation.

While it is clear that stents have risen as the mainstay of treatment of narrowed conduits in any location within the body, new devices continue to emerge. These devices well described herein are designed to solve problems that formerly could be addressed only by surgery. These devices will be the future of the field. It is important for all interventionalists in this area to observe, follow, and critique the changes in materials, methods, and results for implantation of new occluding devices and stents and valvular substitutes, in a fashion similar to that of surgery, the quality of procedures.

This volume on catheter-based non-coronary device interventions may lead to new ideas and the next developments in non-coronary catheter-based devices. Understanding the current data provides the basis from which improved care can be delivered to both adults and children needing these approaches.[44]

RECENT ADVANCES IN PEDIATRIC CARDIOLOGY

At the request of the Chief Editor of the *Indian Journal of Pediatrics*, Dr. Anita Saxena of All India Institute of Medical Sciences (AIMS), New Delhi and I organized and edited a Symposium in Pediatric Cardiology.[45] These papers along with other papers were put together into a monograph by the *Indian Journal of Pediatrics* (Figure12) and titled "Recent Advances in Pediatric Cardiology."[46]

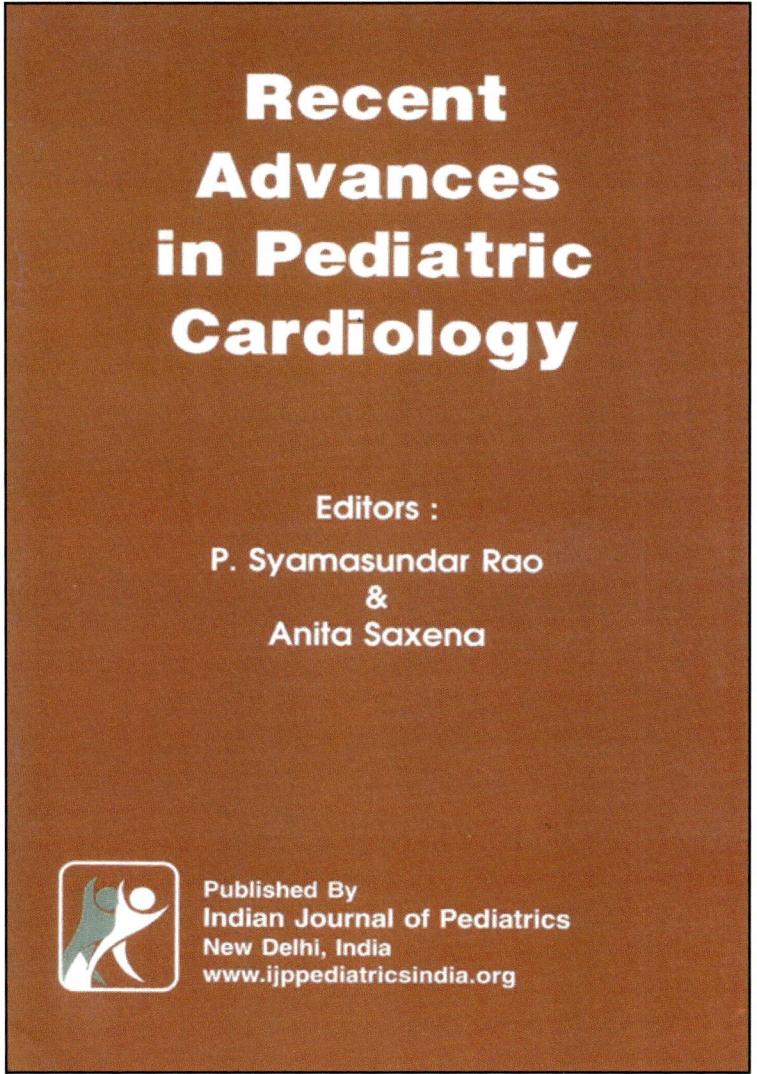

Figure 12. Photograph of monograph titled "Recent Advances in Pediatric Cardiology" published by the *Indian Journal of Pediatrics* in 2005.

I expressed distinct pleasure and honor to serve as the Guest Editor and organize the Pediatric Cardiology symposia of the *Indian Journal of Pediatrics (IJP)* since the mid-1980s. Initially, the focus was to educate the practicing pediatricians regarding the general issues of congenital and acquired heart disease, scientific basis of the management approaches, and updating recent advances. Worldwide, the sub-specialty of pediatric cardiology has witnessed tremendous growth and expansion. Recent advances include better understanding of genetics and environmental etiology, availability of highly sensitive non-invasive diagnostic tools, progress in transcatheter interventional procedures and ability to perform complicated surgical procedures in neonates and infants. For delivering excellent pediatric cardiac care, however, close interaction and collaboration of the pediatric cardiologists with neonatologists, pediatricians, general/family practitioners (who care for children), anesthesiologists and cardiac surgeons is mandatory. Keeping this in mind, the *IJP* publishes symposia on various aspects of pediatric cardiology from time to time; an example is the recent pediatric cardiology symposium published in June and July 2005 issues of the Journal. And, updating its features on Pediatric Cardiology, the Journal wished to release its book, "Recent Advances in Pediatric Cardiology," at the time of Pediatric Congress to be held in New Delhi in January 2006. For this purpose, the Journal invited Dr. Saxena and me to organize this book.[46] We accepted the responsibility they accorded us and thanked the Editors of the *IJP* for this distinct honor and privilege. This book simply brings together many of the recently published articles in the pediatric cardiology symposia, with some additional papers to complement the already published materials.

In the first two papers, I discussed the clinical features of the most common types of acyanotic heart defects, both obstructive and left-to-right shunt lesions, followed by commonly used laboratory studies, which confirm the diagnosis and quantify the severity of the problem; the latter will help on deciding the need for catheter or surgical intervention. Transcatheter therapy may be successfully applied to most obstructive lesions and a large number of left-to-right shunt lesions. The few who are not candidates for transcatheter intervention may require surgical intervention. As the technology gets better, more and more of these defects will become amenable to transcatheter treatment.

In the next paper, Dr. Usha Krishnan from the New York Medical College, Valhalla, New York, NY, discussed management options for patients with the so-called single ventricle which, by the way, constitutes a variety of complex CHDs, including tricuspid atresia, double inlet left ventricle, HLHS, unbalanced AV canal, heterotaxy syndromes and many other defects in which one of the ventricles is too small to support the pulmonary or systemic circulation, respectively. The management, as the author rightly pointed out, is by a multistage Fontan approach, necessarily required because of the fact that the pulmonary artery pressures are high and sometimes their size are not suited for single stage correction at presentation. Untreated, the prognosis of patients with functionally single ventricle is poor. Recent advances in medical and surgical therapy, particularly the application of the "Fontan" principle, have markedly improved the long-term outlook of these children. Palliative procedures to normalize the pulmonary blood flow (BT or similar aorta-pulmonary shunt for patients with pulmonary oligemia, and PA banding for patients with pulmonary plethora), and to relieve inter-atrial and/or inter-ventricular obstruction should be undertaken promptly. Norwood procedure is required for patients with HLHS. Staged total cavo-pulmonary connection (modified Fontan) to bypass the right atrium and right ventricle by bi-directional Glenn procedure initially followed by extra-cardiac conduit diversion of inferior vena caval flow into the pulmonary arteries appears to be the current procedure of choice in the surgical management of single ventricle lesions. Total cavo-pulmonary diversion appears to be superior to conventional Fontan-Kreutzer operations, but long-term follow-up results are currently not available and are needed to confirm this impression. There is an attempt to undertake some of these Fontan steps with transcatheter means; this technique is evolving.

Then, Dr. Reena Lantin from the University of Texas/Houston Medical School, Houston, Texas, TX, presented a lucid discussion outlining what a primary care physician should do to take care of his/her patients with cardiac defects. She discussed the role of primary care physician in taking care of milder forms of heart defects that do not require transcatheter or surgical intervention as well as those that need rapid intervention. Particularly useful are her recommendations regarding anticipated problems of patients who had undergone cardiac surgery and the emphasis she placed on the team approach in collaborative management of the patients along with pediatric cardiologists and cardiac surgeons.

Dr. Savitri Shrivastava of Escorts Heart Institute and Research Center, New Delhi, discussed the optimal timing of intervention in blue babies. This is a relevant issue for neonatologists or pediatricians who are the first health care providers for a blue baby. In this article, Dr. Shrivastava described various types of CHDs and their clinical recognition. Cyanotic CHDs were grouped into five headings depending on the underlying hemodynamic disturbance. She then discussed various surgical and non-surgical interventional procedures currently available for the treatment of these babies. She rightly pointed out that "blue babies are doomed" is a myth and is no more true in today's era of technological achievements. Dr. Shrivastava concluded by emphasizing that most of cyanotic CHDs are amenable to definitive treatment if timely intervention is performed. The pediatrician needs to have a high index of suspicion and an aggressive approach when confronted with a blue baby.

Dr. Reeni Soni of University of Manitoba, Winnipeg, Canada, and Dr. Saxena discussed the current status of fetal echocardiography. Fetal echocardiography, initially introduced in the 1980s has come a long way over the years. It is not only a tool for diagnosing a structural heart defect in fetus, but also an immense help in diagnosing and guiding management of fetal arrhythmias. A negative scan also has great importance, as it is very reassuring for a family with a previous child affected with CHD. The current status of fetal echocardiography also enables navigation in cardiac interventions, such as fetal aortic valve balloon dilatation to prevent LV hypoplasia. It surely will be of great help if and when fetal cardiac surgery becomes a reality.

Dr. Michal Kantoch of the University of Alberta, Edmonton, Alberta, Canada, discussed another important topic, the diagnosis and management approach to supraventricular tachycardia (SVT) in children. The underlying mechanism for SVT varies according to the age of the child and so does the management. Tachyarrhythmia is a common problem at all ages, encountered by the pediatricians in the emergency room. The treating physician must be familiar with the initial mode of treatment for interrupting the tachycardia. Dr. Kantoch discussed the role of vagal maneuvers, adenosine and other drugs for acute management. He then goes on to discuss the chronic management with oral drugs. For older children who continue to have episodes of tachyarrhythmia, radiofrequency ablation procedure is useful and was also detailed.

The next article is on current perspectives on Kawasaki disease, jointly written by Dr. Monesha Gupta-Malhotra of University of Texas/Houston Medical School, Houston, TX and me. The topic is of increasing importance to pediatricians in India, as the previously held belief that the Kawasaki disease does not occur in India is not true anymore. Again, one needs to keep a high index of suspicion since there is no single confirmatory test for definitive diagnosis. Fulfillment of five out of the six clinical criteria is necessary for making a diagnosis of a typical Kawasaki disease. The authors also discussed the so-called "incomplete form" of Kawasaki disease seen in as many as 10 percent of cases. The role of echocardiogram has been discussed which further helps in diagnosing this condition. The treatment with intravenous immunoglobulin is well known, but failure to respond to immunoglobulin is seen in 10 percent of cases, necessitating pulsed steroid therapy. This article also provided a review of short and long term follow up of Kawasaki disease, an important information for pediatricians counseling the families with affected children.

The article by Dr. Saxena focused on the current status of CHD in India. By all estimates, the burden of CHD in India is enormous, and the infrastructure and resources are grossly inadequate. There are only fourteen centers with established cardiac care programs for neonates and infants in whole of India as against an ideal number of 200. Less than 2 percent of all infants born with CHD are privileged enough to get specialized cardiac care in one of these centers. The most important remedial measure is to increase awareness regarding recognition of CHD amongst the primary health care providers, i.e., the pediatricians. Furthermore, we desperately need a mechanism by which this very expensive care is financed and/or subsidized. A national registry or a database for defining the demography of CHD, results of cardiac surgery and results of non-surgical cardiac interventions will also be useful. All this is necessary for a holistic view of issues related to CHD in India, leading to its optimal management.

Dr. Sumeet Sharma of the University of Texas/Houston Medical School and I discussed the methods of closure of PDA with special emphasis on transcatheter occlusion. The discussion, by design, excludes the PDA of the premature infant. Various devices that were designed and tested for transcatheter occlusion were listed, and the devices that are currently in use were described and their implantation procedures detailed. A discussion of selection of method of closure based on the shape and size of the ductus is included. Closure of silent PDAs is not recommended. Very small to small PDAs can be successfully closed with the free or detachable Gianturco coils. Small to moderate PDAs may need multiple coils or larger wire diameter (0.52-in) coils. Options for closure of moderate-to-large PDAs are devices, video-thoracoscopic interruption and conventional surgical closure. Amplatzer Duct Occluder was approved by the FDA and is useful in closing moderate to large PDAs. A few other devices are undergoing FDA approved clinical trials. Availability of the method or device and expertise at a given institution at a given time are likely to determine the method selected.

Dr. Anjan Batra of University of Indiana/Riley Children's Hospital, Indianapolis, IN, discussed pacemaker therapy in children. There is a growing population of children and young adults with conduction abnormalities, and pacing is an integral part of their management, which may significantly reduce their morbidity and mortality. The current pacemakers are more sophisticated and complex and are being used for indications other than heart block, such as termination of tachycardia and improvement of heart failure. Dr. Batra states that it is important to understand the newer pacing modalities and individualized therapy. Small size and complex anatomy pose many limitations and technical challenges related to the placement of a pacemaker. He concluded that technical innovations are helping us overcome some of these challenges.

In the last two articles of this book, Drs. Gupta, Lantin, Balaji (Oregon Health and Sciences University, Portland, OR), and I reviewed the recent advances in pediatric cardiology. These papers are updated versions of the advances published in *IJP* in 2003. These are arbitrarily divided into medical, electrophysiological, transcatheter and surgical advances. There is certainly overlap between these and other papers in the book, but this was unavoidable in the interest of preserving continuity of the discussions.

These discussions in the "Recent Advances in Pediatric Cardiology," we hope will not only be useful for the practicing pediatric cardiologists, but also useful in giving a fund of information to the practicing pediatricians and enhance their existing knowledge, which in turn may help them provide better care for their (and our) patients.[46]

PERINATAL CARDIOLOGY FOR THE NEONATOLOGIST

This monograph was prepared to provide state-of-the-art knowledge about the diagnosis and management of the neonate with CHD to the trainees in pediatrics, pediatric cardiology and neonatology, and neonatologists and was printed by Memorial Hermann Printing Services (Figure 13);[47] the papers included reviews published in *Neonatology Today* and *Congenital Cardiology Today* by me and my associates with additional papers from the other faculty at the University of Texas Medical School/Children's Memorial Hermann Hospital and meant to be distributed locally. The contents of this monograph will be reviewed along with the review of the book, "Perinatal Cardiology: A Multidisciplinary Approach."[48]

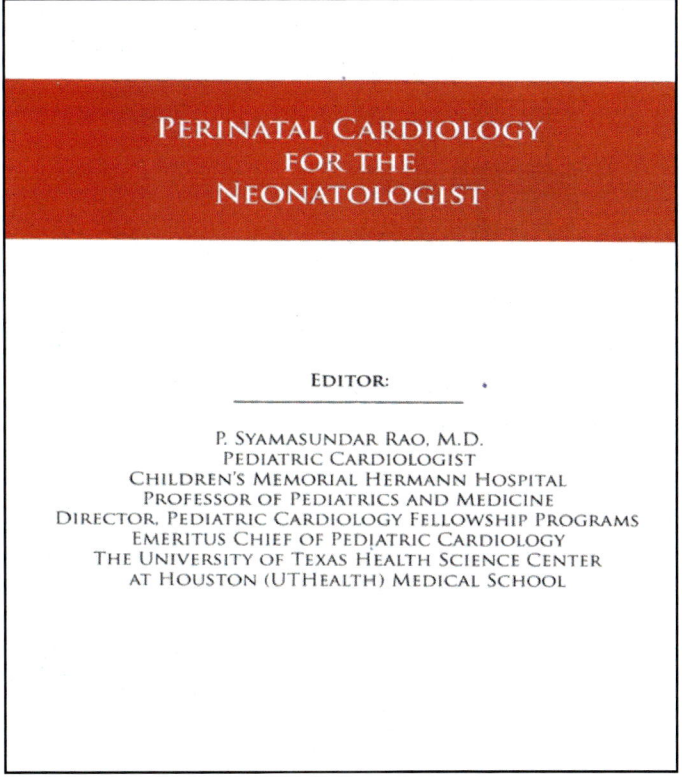

Figure 13. Photograph of monograph titled "Perinatal Cardiology for the Neonatologist" published by the *MHHCS Press* in 2011.

CONGENITAL HEART DISEASE - SELECTED ASPECTS

This book was edited by the author at the request of InTech (Figure 14)[49] and consists of multiple papers from clinicians and investigators around the world.

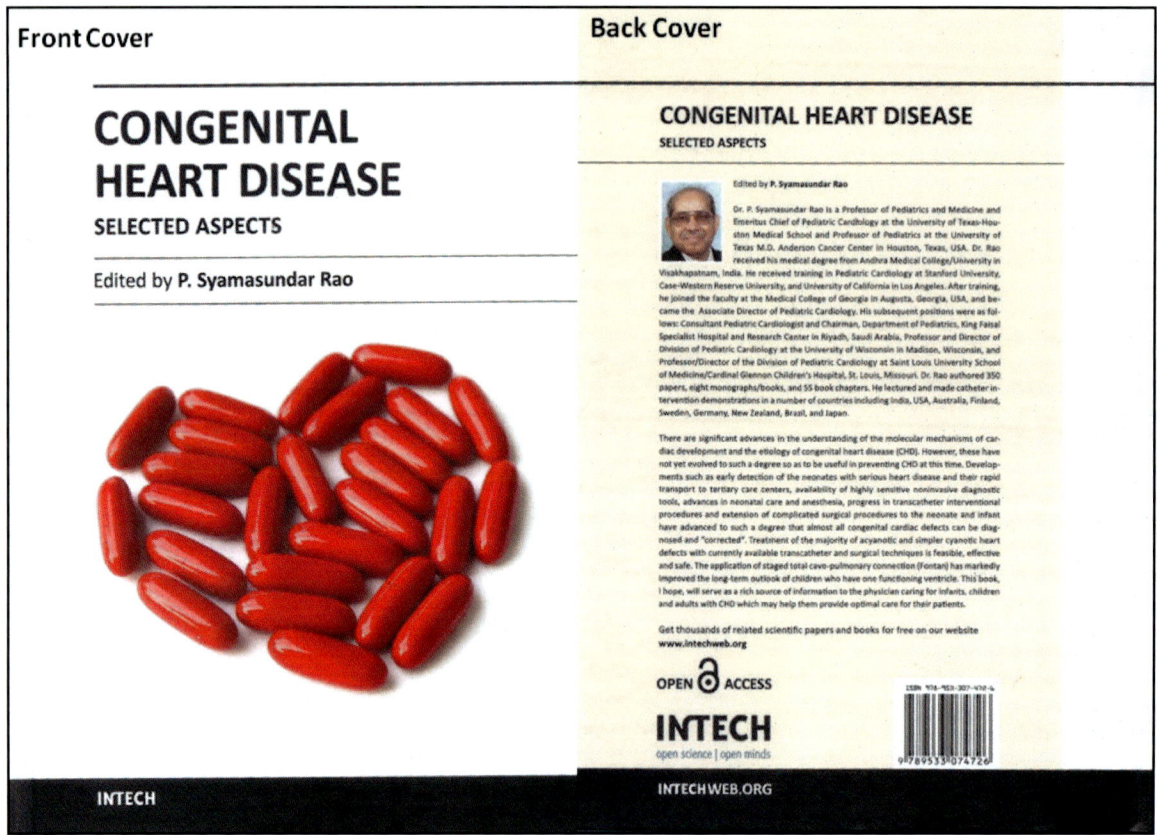

Figure 14. Photograph of book titled "Congenital Heart Disease - Selected Aspects" published by *InTech* in 2012. Both front and back covers are shown.

CHD may be defined as an anatomic malformation of the heart or great vessels, which occurs during intrauterine development, irrespective of the age at presentation. VSD and coarctation of the aorta are typical examples of CHDs. The reported incidence of CHDs varies between 0.6 percent and 0.8 percent of live births. This would result in birth of 30 to 35,000 infants with CHD each year in the United States alone. CHDs are more common than well-known congenital anomalies such as congenital pyloric stenosis, cleft lip, Down syndrome and congenital dislocation of the hip. Nearly 50 percent of these babies can be managed with simple medications, observation and follow-up without any major therapeutic intervention. However, the remaining 50 percent, in the past, required surgical intervention, some under cardiopulmonary bypass. Since the advent of transcatheter techniques, 50 percent of these babies (i.e., 25 percent of the total) can be managed with less invasive, percutaneous, transcatheter techniques.

Developments such as early detection of the neonates with serious heart disease and their rapid transport to tertiary care centers, availability of highly sensitive non-invasive diagnostic tools, advances in neonatal care and anesthesia, progress in transcatheter interventional procedures and extension of complicated surgical procedures to the neonate and infant have advanced to such a degree that almost all CHDs can be diagnosed and "corrected." The defects that could not be corrected could be effectively palliated. For achieving excellence in cardiac care, however, close interaction and collaboration of the pediatric cardiologists with neonatologists, pediatricians, general/family practitioners (who care for children with CHD), internists (who care for adults with CHD), anesthesiologists and cardiac surgeons is mandatory. Education of physicians caring for children and adults with CHD continues to be important in achieving optimal care for the patients with heart disease.

Because of vastness of the subject, all issues related to CHDs cannot be discussed in their entirety and therefore, only selected aspects were included in this book. The book is divided into several sections, which include an overview of CHDs, prevalence and etiology, some individual heart defects, management of some of the CHDs, international issues, and miscellaneous topics. While there are significant advances in the understanding molecular mechanisms of cardiac development and of the etiology of CHD, these have not progressed to such a degree so as to be clinically useful in preventing CHD at this time. Consequently, several chapters were devoted to this subject.

In the first section on overview of CHDs, I presented a brief review of incidence, etiology, and classification of CHD, and an overview of the nine most common congenital cardiac anomalies and their management. The exact etiology of CHD is not known and the majority of cardiac defects can be explained by multi-factorial inheritance hypothesis. The CHD may be classified as acyanotic and cyanotic defects and the former is further divided into obstructive and left-to-right shunt lesions. Pathologic, physiologic, clinical and laboratory features of nine most common CHD were described; these are distinctive. Methods of management for each of these defects include transcatheter techniques for most of the acyanotic defects and by and large, surgery for the cyanotic defects. Based on this review, it appears that while the etiology of CHD is not clearly identified, their recognition by clinical evaluation and non-invasive laboratory tests is possible and their treatment with currently available transcatheter and surgical methods is feasible, effective and safe.

In the next section on prevalence and etiology, Sayasathid and associates from Naresuan University, Thailand, discussed epidemiology and etiology of CHD including preventative guidelines for pregnant mothers. They suggested that the number of patients with CHD continues to increase and that epidemiology studies reveal that cases of CHD are underestimated. Huang and Liang of Guangxi Traditional Chinese Medical College, Nanning, China explored molecular mechanisms of CHD. These authors reviewed normal cardiac development and recent discoveries of the genetic causes of CHD. They provided possible strategies for exploring these new developments to improve understanding of the genetic basis of CHD. They support the use of animal biomedical models to understand normal and abnormal function from gene to phenotype and to provide a basis for preventive or therapeutic intervention in human diseases. In the next chapter, Minamisawa and Yokoyama from Waseda University, Japan, presented recent advances in the molecular mechanism of PDA. The authors describe acute and functional closure of the ductus, and discussed complex molecular mechanisms involved in ductal closure. The remodelling that includes the differentiation of vascular smooth muscle cells (SMCs) and endothelial cells, accumulation of extracellular matrix, vascular SMC migration into the sub-endothelial region, impaired elastogenesis, and eventually fibrotic changes due to apoptosis and necrosis were reviewed. The role of PGE_2-EP4-cAMP signal pathway, oxygen, and calcium channels, multiple vasoreactive stimulations in the modulator of vascular remodelling of the ductus arteriosus was also discussed. These authors concluded that this knowledge may help develop novel therapeutic strategies for patients with PDA and ductal dependent cardiac anomalies. Harmelink and Jiao of the University of Alabama at Birmingham, AL, describe bone morphogenetic protein (BMP) signaling pathways in heart development and disease. They review evidence from multiple experimental models that demonstrates the role of BMP signaling pathways in the heart development. Initially, they describe normal heart development in the mice model and then the BMP signaling pathways in general and specific to heart development including that of the mesoderm, myocardial wall formation, valve development, chamber septation, and outflow tract morphogenesis. These authors conclude that BMP signaling pathways are critical regulators of heart development in several species including humans and that mutations in the BMP pathway have been identified in humans with CHD and that this insight may help develop diagnostic tests and therapeutic options for CHD in the future. Vogler et al of Sanford-Burnham Medical Research Institute, La Jolla, CA, described recent advances and findings gained from a Drosophila model for CHD. They begin with comparing Drosophila with vertebrate cardio-genesis and point out their similarities. They then allude to the lessons learned from studying Drosophila heart morphogenesis. This is followed by a discussion of manipulating the heart and genome of a fly. They also suggest that the Drosophila model is useful in elucidating the molecular mechanisms of CHD and cardiomyopathy. They concluded that development of technologies such as time-lapse analysis of heart formation and optical techniques to study function suggest that further studies using this system will provide insights into fundamental cellular mechanisms underlying heart function and disease.

In the next section, three individual cardiac defects were reviewed. Flack and Graham from Vanderbilt University, Nashville, TN, described incidence, natural history, clinical and laboratory features and management of congenitally corrected transposition of the great arteries (CCTGA). These authors allude to the problems associated with dysfunction of left-sided, morphologic right ventricle with or without Ebstein's type of malformation of the morphologic tricuspid valve. Conventional medical management and cardiac resynchronization were discussed. Role of conventional surgical therapy and double-switch operation were also detailed. Follow-up recommendations and pregnancy outcomes were also discussed. They concluded that outcomes, based on long-term follow-up of physiologic vs. anatomic repair for CCTGA, favor anatomic correction. Ríos-Méndez of "El Cruce" Hospital, Buenos Aires, Argentina, presented four cases of double-chambered right ventricle from their institution, discussed significance of these findings and present a literature review. This author concluded that double-chambered right ventricle is a rare cardiac anomaly, VSD is the most commonly-associated defect, echocardiography (trans-thoracic or TEE), performed by a cardiologist familiar with CHDs is the method of choice for diagnosing this condition and that surgical treatment is effective with low morbidity. Pierre et al of Bichat Hospital, Paris, France, reviewed features of anomalous connections of coronary arteries (ANOCOR) and presented a simple classification, point out low prevalence of about 1 percent in the general population, discussed anatomical patterns associated with a risk of sudden death, explored prevention of sport-related fatalities and modalities of cost-effective screening, advocated multi-detector computed tomography (CT) angiography with three-dimensional reconstruction as an accurate diagnostic tool, supported surgery by un-roofing technique in ANOCOR arising from the aorta (and direct aortic implantation for ANOCOR connected with the pulmonary artery), deplored lack of long-term follow-up evaluation after surgery, and supported setting up of registries to determine the outcome of children and young adults (≤ 30-year-old) with high-risk ANOCOR.

Management of CHD was discussed in the next section. Hadzimuratovic discussed evaluation and emergency treatment of critically ill neonates with cyanosis and respiratory distress. This author reviewed some important aspects of normal and abnormal findings in physical examination, ECG, and chest x-ray films of the neonate, and suggested approaches to diagnose and treat neonates with central cyanosis. This author then discussed management of several neonatal issues, namely, heart failure in the newborn infant, HLHS, premature neonates with a large PDA, persistent pulmonary hypertension of the newborn and transient myocardial ischemia. Guzman et al from Cardiovascular Clinic Santa Maria, Medellin, Colombia, present the results of Fontan Surgery performed at their institution. They state that management strategies for functional single ventricle have evolved into staged procedures with a goal to obtain normal ventricular pressures and volumes and normal systemic arterial saturation. They examined the results of total cavo-pulmonary connection (Fontan operation) and concluded that the Fontan operation performed at their institution is safe with a mortality rate (14.3 percent), comparable to previously published large series.

In the next section on international issues, Bode-Thomas of University of Jos, Nigeria, reviewed practical problems encountered in the diagnosis, treatment and prevention of CHDs in the developing countries. This author initially pointed out that there is a paucity of data on the incidence or birth prevalence of CHDs in most developing countries, which in turn under-estimates the burden of CHD, undermining arguments for more resource allocation in the face of the many other competing health care needs. A discussion of peculiarities and challenges of CHD diagnosis and treatment in developing regions followed with a suggestion for establishing treatment centers in developing countries.

The final section includes several miscellaneous issues. Chalajour et al of Stanford University, Stanford, CA, discussed dynamics of myocardial cell populations following birth and the role of cardiac progenitor cells (CPC) in neonatal myocardial tissue expansion and heart growth as well as therapeutic strategies for CHDs. These authors concluded that the presence of resident CPC in myocardium is well supported; however, controversies continue regarding the origin of CPC. Methods for activating resident CPC are still in the early discovery phase and the potential applications of CPC-focused therapies in CHD treatment are likely in the future. Li from University of Alberta, Canada, in a chapter on "Accurate measurement of systemic oxygen consumption in ventilated children with CHD," pointed out inaccuracies of using estimated oxygen consumption values (calculated by predictive equations developed by several workers in the past) in the Fick principle, particularly in children younger than three years of age, whether it be in the Catheterization Laboratory or in the Intensive Care Unit (ICU) postoperatively. This author described the use of respiratory mass spectrometry to accurately measure oxygen consumption and discussed the post-operative physiology following Norwood operation and its management. Itoi from Kyoto Prefectural University of Medicine, Kyoto, Japan, discussed myocardial use of energy substrates in young patients with ASDs, VSDs, and PDAs and presented their data. They concluded that myocardial energy metabolism in acyanotic CHD was sustained by fatty acid oxidation irrespective of workload and there was accelerated glucose use with overload. Lactate seemed to play an important role in maintaining lactate-pyruvate redox potential. When mild myocardial workload (as in ASD), the NADH demand was complemented by lactate oxidation, while with higher workload (as in pulmonary hypertension), lactate production was accelerated to maintain the cellular redox state. Okuneva et al from E.N. Meshalkin Research Institute of Circulation Pathology and A.V. Nikolayev Institute of Inorganic Chemistry, Russia, describe the results of their study to investigate the structure of cardiomyocytes and the content of chemical elements (CE) in infants with TGA. They found that pathologic hypertrophy of myocardium in TGA is reflected by the decreased Zn, Br, Cr, Cl and Se content in myocardium (also Ca) and excess of Copper. They recommend that pregnant women and nursing mothers should get the optimum quantity of micro-elements Cr, Zn, Sr, Ni, Rb, Br and most impotently Se (to protect the myocardium from lipid peroxidation) in order to prevent development of CHDs including TGA, although no data to support this recommendation were presented.

In summary, there are significant advances in the understanding of the molecular mechanisms of cardiac development and of the etiology of CHD. However, these have not evolved to such a degree so as to be clinically useful in preventing CHD at this time. Treatment of the majority of acyanotic and simpler cyanotic heart defects with currently available transcatheter and surgical techniques is feasible, effective and safe. Recent advances in medical and surgical therapy, particularly the application of staged total cavo-pulmonary connection (Fontan), have markedly improved the long-term outlook of children who have one functioning ventricle. There are a number of other developments, some of which were reviewed in this book. These discussions will give a fund of information to the practicing physician caring for infants, children and adults with CHDs, which may help them provide optimal care for their patients.[49]

ATRIAL SEPTAL DEFECT

The author was again requested by InTech to organize and edit a book on ASD; this was accomplished by selecting several investigators from our and other institutions to contribute to this book (Figure 15).[50]

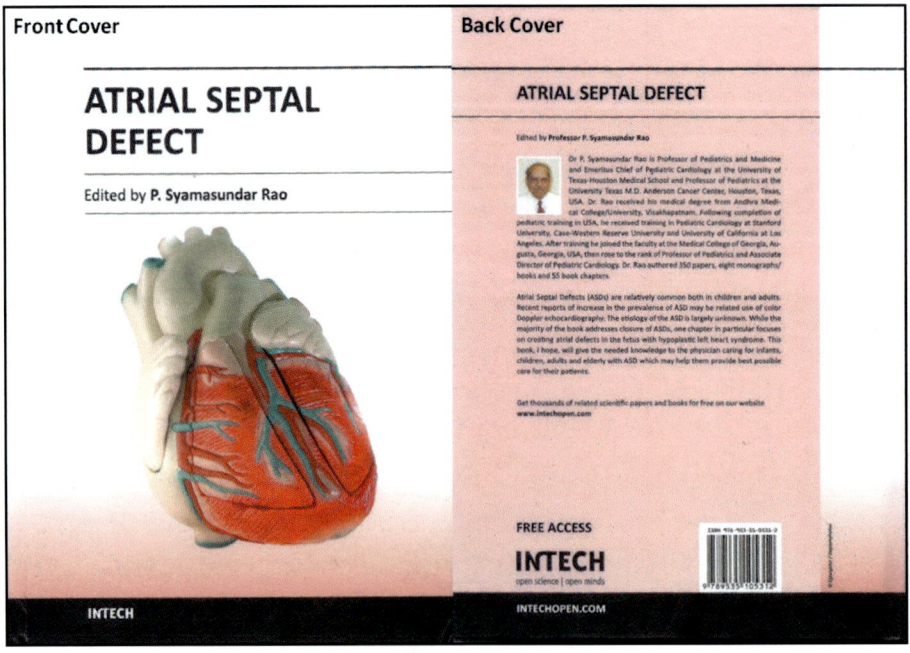

Figure 15. Photograph of book titled "Atrial Septal Defect" published by *InTech* in 2012. Both front and back covers are shown.

Defects in the atrial septum are one of the most common types of CHDs in children and such a defect is the most common CHD in adults. ASDs cause left-to-right shunt because the left atrial pressure is higher than that in the right atrium. This causes volume overloading of the right ventricle. While this is generally well tolerated during infancy and childhood, development of exercise intolerance and arrhythmias in later childhood, adolescence and adulthood, and the risk for development of pulmonary vascular obstructive disease in adulthood make these defects important. The major types of atrial defects are ostium secundum, ostium primum, sinus venosus, and coronary sinus ASDs and PFO.

In the first chapter, I reviewed the clinical features and management of ASDs. Patients with small defects are usually asymptomatic, while moderate to large defects may present with symptoms. Physical findings include hyper-dynamic precordium, widely split and fixed second heart sound, ejection systolic murmur at the left upper sternal border and a mid-diastolic flow rumble at the left lower sternal border. In patients with ostium primum ASDs, an apical holosystolic murmur may also be heard. Clinical diagnosis is not difficult and the diagnosis can be confirmed and quantified by echocardiographic studies. While surgical intervention was used in the past, transcatheter methods are currently used for closure of ostium secundum ASDs. Surgical correction is necessary for the ostium primum, sinus venosus, and coronary sinus defects. PFO is present in nearly one-third of normal population and is likely to be a normal variant and such isolated PFOs do not need intervention. When associated with other CHDs, the PFO facilitates intra-cardiac shunt to allow appropriate egress and/or mixing of blood flow. Hypoxemia in post-surgical residual defects including Fontan fenestrations, right ventricular infarction, and platypnea-orthodexia syndrome may be secondary to right-to-left shunt across PFO and these defects may need closure. PFO, presumed to be the seat of paradoxical embolism resulting in stroke/TIAs is the subject of active investigation. Similarly, the role of PFO in Caisson's disease and migraine is not well-established. There are varying degrees of evidence for benefit of transcatheter occlusion of these PFOs.

In the second chapter, Dr. Balaguru from the University of Texas Medical School, Houston, TX, discussed issues related to ASD in pregnant women. There are remarkable changes in cardiovascular physiology during pregnancy; the cardiac output increases, related to increased stroke volume and heart rate. The systemic vascular resistance decreases; however, concurrent increase in cardiac output keeps blood pressure stable. The blood volume increases (by 1.5 times) by raise in plasma volume; however, this is out of proportion to the increase in red cell mass with consequent relative anemia. These changes are tolerated well because the changes occur gradually. During the third trimester, enlarging uterus compresses the inferior vena cava (IVC) in supine posture leading to decrease in cardiac output and predisposes to deep vein thrombosis. In pregnant women with ASD, there is a greater increase in right atrial and right ventricular size (compared to pregnant women with no heart defect) and a higher incidence of SVT. The probability of paradoxical embolism via the ASD is high, given the predisposition to deep vein thrombosis and hypercoagulable state. If the diagnosis is known prior to pregnancy and the ASD is large and associated with moderate or severe right heart enlargement and is a potential candidate for SVT and thromboembolic events during pregnancy, labor or postpartum, the ASD should be closed prior to planned-pregnancy. Transcatheter or surgical closure can be performed based on the size of the ASD and adequacy of septal rims. When the ASD is diagnosed during pregnancy but the patient is asymptomatic without functional compromise (NYHA Class I and II) and has no heart failure, atrial arrhythmia, pulmonary hypertension or history of stroke, then these women are likely to do well throughout pregnancy and do not require transcatheter or surgical closure. On the contrary, in the presence of any of these issues, transcatheter or surgical closure may be performed. If transcatheter closure is opted, second trimester (between thirteen to twenty-eight weeks) is preferred instead of first trimester to avoid irradiation to the fetus. Local anesthesia with conscious sedation, intra-cardiac echocardiography (ICE) to aid balloon sizing and device deployment and use of long venous sheath; the latter two to avoid or reduces radiation, may be appropriate. If the ASD is unsuitable for transcatheter closure, surgical closure of ASD may be performed in the second trimester with the following precautions: Infusion of high-concentration of glucose (to provide energy for fetus), fetal monitoring, maintenance of high-flow, high mean arterial pressure (60 mmHg) and high hematocrit (> 25 percent) and hyper oxygenation. Dr. Balaguru concludes that the need for closure of ASD during pregnancy is rare and if possible should be avoided. When closure is indicated transcatheter or surgical closure may be performed, taking appropriate precautions.

In the third chapter, Dr. Reller from Oregon Health & Science University, Portland, OR, reviewed the data on the prevalence, associated cardiac and non-cardiac findings and natural history of secundum ASDs, defined as size greater than 4 mm. The prevalence of secundum ASD is estimated to be 10.3 per 10,000 births, prevalence comparable to that of peri-membranous VSDs. The increase in the prevalence of secundum ASD was attributed to evaluation by color flow Doppler echocardiography. The association of secundum ASD with perimembranous VSD and valvar PS is well recognized. The cause(s) of secundum ASD remain largely unknown. Genetic syndromes associated with secundum ASD include Trisomy 21, 13 and 18; Holt-Oram syndrome; chromosome 22q11 deletion in association with DiGeorge syndrome; velo-cardio-facial syndrome; Noonan syndrome; and NKX2-5 gene defect. Patients with secundum ASD are more likely to have a positive family history of CHD. There is higher prevalence of secundum ASD in girls. Secundum ASD is also associated with non-cardiac malformations such as cleft palate and VACTERL association. Fetal alcohol syndrome, cytomegalovirus (CMV) and rubella infections during pregnancy and maternal diabetes are also associated with an increased prevalence of secundum ASD. Lower gestational age (low birth weight), small for gestational age, increased maternal age and multiple gestation pregnancy are also associated with higher prevalence of secundum ASD. With regard to natural history, the ASDs have a tendency to regress in size, including spontaneous closure. Small defects (between 4-5 mm) at the time of initial diagnosis either spontaneously close or regress to a size considered to be insignificant (< 3 mm). Larger defects (> 10 mm) do not close spontaneously and 75 percent of these patients may require surgical or device closure. It may be concluded that secundum ASD is the third most common CHD with incidence similar to peri-membranous VSD, the prevalence of secundum ASD is increasing, the cause of which remain speculative and there is a tendency for spontaneous closure or decreased size, especially in small defects.

Dr. Yamashita and associates from National Centre for Child Health and Development, Japan, in the Chapter 4, described a new approach with an automatic delivery system of high intensity focused ultrasound (HIFU) with real-time two dimensional-ultrasound (2D-US) imaging analysis to establish fetal inter-atrial communications. In the fetus with HLHS and restrictive atrial septum leads to irreversible pulmonary vascular damage. The current approach of ultrasound-guided percutaneous puncture through both the uterine wall and fetal chest wall to create interatrial communications is associated with serious complications such as profound bradycardia, bleeding and hemopericardium and intra-cardiac thrombus formation. In addition, closure of the in utero created ASDs can also occur prior to delivery. They developed a new approach with HIFU to establish fetal inter-atrial communications with potential for minimal adverse effects. HIFU ablation requires highly accurate pinpoint delivery in real-time based on computer-aided auto-tracking of atrial septum. Their system features automatic detection of rate of heart beat, automatic estimation of atrial septal position and automatic generation of HIFU delivery timing. They describe system configuration of computer-aided automatic HIFU delivery, automatic detection of heart beat rates, position of the atrial septum and other procedural details. They performed a feasibility study for creation of an atrial septal defect using the beating heart of four anesthetized adult rabbits, which appear not to be satisfactory. But, these authors interpret that they were able to confirm pinpoint delivery of HIFU to the pulsating atrial septum within beating hearts of anesthetized adult rabbits. The above studies were performed with 2D-US. Three-dimensional-US to track movement of intrauterine fetus may make the procedure more accurate. In conclusion, these workers developed computer-aided automatic delivery system of HIFU for creation of an ASD and further work to improve precision of the focus positioning of HIFU delivery and improvement of HIFU energy efficiency to intra-cardiac tissue is in progress. The concept appears good as is the design of the system. While the current results are far from clinically applicable, the technique has good potential.

In the fifth chapter from our institution, Dr. Alapati and I review the historical aspects of transcatheter closure of ASDs. Since the initial description of ASD occluding devices by King, Rashkind and their associates, a large number of single disc and double disc devices have been designed and tested in animal models followed by clinical trials in human subjects. Feasibility, safety and effectiveness have been demonstrated with most devices. However, design, redesign, testing and re-testing have been the typical path with most devices. Currently, only two devices are approved by the FDA in the US and these are: Amplatzer septal occluder and HELEX septal occluder. Several other devices are in development, some at the stage of animal experimentation and some in clinical trials in Europe or US. We will wait for additional devices to be approved for general clinical use so that the practicing interventional cardiologist will have several devices at his/her disposal so that an appropriate device that suits best for a given patient and his/her defect is available. A brief review of historical aspects of PFO closure was also included. Majority of the ASD devices described in the ASD section, as and when they became available, have also been used to close PFOs; these include King's, clamshell, buttoned, Das-Angel-Wing and CardioSEAL devices. Existing devices were modified to address the anatomic features of the foramen ovale or new devices were designed to specifically address the PFOs and the latter include: Amplatzer PFO occluder, Cardia devices (PFO-Star and several of its subsequent generations), Premere occluder, Coherex Flat stent, PFx Closure System (not a device but employs monopolar radio frequency energy to effect closure of a PFO by welding the tissues of the septum primum with the septum secundum), pfm PFO-R, Solysafe PFO occluder and others. Amplatzer cribriform device was also used on off-label basis to close PFOs.

In the next chapter, Dr. Biliciler-Denktas, also from our institution, describes the role of TEE in percutaneous closure of ASDs. Initially, the embryologic development of the atrial septum was reviewed. Currently used imaging techniques during device implantation, namely, transthoracic echocardiography, TEE, intracardiac echocardiography (ICE) and real time three-dimensional transesophageal echocardiography (3D TEE) were reviewed and relative advantages and disadvantages of each of these techniques were discussed; TEE and ICE are the two most commonly employed techniques. The importance of defined protocols to evaluate the heart, the ASD and the septal rims is stressed. Evaluation prior to device implantation include, examination of the entire atrial septum and its surrounding structures and exclusion of additional defects that may render the defect unsuitable for closure; measurement of the number and size of the defect(s); color Doppler imaging to define the shunt, left to right or right to left; dimensions of the septal rims and measurement of balloon stretched diameter of the defect (when a sizing balloon is used) and identification of other defects while balloon occluding the defect. The echo and the interventional physicians work as a team to decide on the device size to be used for closure of ASD/PFO. Monitoring of the device deployment and verifying for correct position of the device prior to device release are germane. Post-implantation study is performed to detect impingement on valves, obstruction to venous return, and residual shunting. TEE is also useful in the detection of complications of device closure such as device dislodgement and pericardial effusion/tamponade. The author concluded that TEE is of utmost value during percutaneous closure of ASDs and PFOs and is the preferred imaging modality in most catheterization laboratories.

In Chapter 7, Drs. Gonzalez, Cao, and Hijazi of Rush University Medical Center, Chicago, IL, review the role of ICE in transcatheter closure of ASDs. Accurate and precise knowledge of the anatomy of the secundum ASD and the nearby structures is essential for safely performing ASD closure. While the conventional imaging method has been TEE, these authors advocate ICE to guide device closure of ASDs and PFOs because general anesthesia is not needed, risks of anesthesia are avoided and patient discomfort after the procedure is reduced. Ultrasound tipped catheters became available during the 1950s and 1960s and progressed through the current state of the art ICE catheters. Several types of ICE catheters from different manufacturers are currently available and include, Ultra ICE mechanical single-element system (Boston Scientific Corp), AcuNav system (Siemens from Biosense-Webster), Clear ICE system (St Jude Medical), SoundStar Catheter system (Biosense-Webster) and ViewMate Z Intracardiac Ultrasound System and ViewFlex Plus ICE Catheter (St Jude Medical). These authors opine that AcuNav catheter is the most popular ICE catheter currently in use. The AcuNav catheter should be carefully advanced from the groin to the heart under continuous fluoroscopic guidance to prevent inadvertent advancement of the catheter into side branches with potential vessel injury before reaching the right atrium. Their ICE protocol involves obtaining different views (home view, septal view, long axis view and short axis view) along with fluoroscopic images. Then ICE imaging during each step, namely, balloon sizing, deployment of left and then right disks and after releasing the device, is undertaken to ensure appropriate positioning of the device. The authors believe that ICE is more accurate in evaluation ASDs when compared to TEE, apart from avoiding general anesthesia, usually required for TEE. They mention limitations of ICE, which include large shaft size, complications related to ICE catheter placement, cost and non-availability of real time three-dimensional (3D) imaging. They concluded that ICE along with fluoroscopy will improve the safety and outcome of percutaneous closure of ASDs.

In the next chapter, I addressed issues related to why, when and how should ASDs be closed in adults. ASDs in adult subjects should be closed at presentation, electively, irrespective of their age. Evidence was presented to indicate that untreated ASD patients tend to have decreased event-free survival rates when compared to normal population and surgical closure is safe and effective with high event-free survival rates. ASD closure also prevents functional deterioration, improves cardiac function, and increases functional capacity. Consequently, hemodynamically significant (right ventricular volume overload) ASDs in adults should be occluded irrespective of symptomatology. When the effect of age at closure of ASD was examined, the Mayo Clinic data indicated that the actuarial survival rates are lower in patients who had surgery after twenty-four years of age; the earlier the surgery was performed the better were the twenty-seven-year survival rates. Since there is no advantage in waiting beyond twenty-four years of age, the closure should be performed at the time of identification of the case. While surgical closure is safe and effective, device closure has less morbidity, lower number of complications, requires less hospital stay, and is less expensive than surgery. Multiple devices have been investigated over the last few decades, but only Amplatzer and HELEX devices received FDA approval as of this time. The Amplatzer is useful in most ASDs, while the HELEX device is useful in small and medium-sized defects. Surgical repair is largely reserved for ASDs with poor septal rims. ASDs could also be closed surgically when intra-cardiac repair of other defects is contemplated. Some procedural details were mentioned with particular emphasis on the need for test occlusion of ASD in the elderly and testing with vasodilator agents in patients with associated pulmonary hypertension. Approaches taken to occlude ASDs with complex anatomy were also reviewed. Amplatzer device appears to be best available option for closure of ASDs at the present time. Careful attention to the details of the technique is mandatory to achieve successful outcomes.

In the next chapter, Dr. Akagi of Okayama University Hospital, Okayama, Japan, reviews ASD closure in geriatric population. He introduced the subject of ASDs in the elderly ($\geq$ 70 years) by pointing out increasing prevalence of CHD in general and ASDs in particular in this age group. He also states that mortality of CHD in the aged is increasing during past few decades. The clinical features of ASD in the elderly are different from those in children and young adults because they present with hemodynamic abnormalities such as pulmonary hypertension, valvar regurgitation, CHF and LV diastolic dysfunction, atrial arrhythmias and co-morbidities, such as hypertension, chronic obstructive lung disease, coronary artery disease, kidney disease, and others. Dr. Akagi emphasized that there are only a few studies in the aged population regarding the functional results of catheter and surgical closure of ASD and reviewed his experience with catheter closure of ASD in geriatric patients as well as the long-term outcome. Of the 420 patients who had attempted transcatheter closure of ASD at their institution, thirty patients were older than seventy years. Their mean age was 75.8 $\pm$ 3.8 years with a range of seventy and eighty-five years. Mean ASD diameter was 20.3 $\pm$ 6.4 mm and mean pulmonary-systemic flow (Qp/Qs) was 2.4 $\pm$ 0.7. Test balloon occlusion of ASD with measurement of pulmonary arterial wedge pressure was performed in only seven of thirty cases. Device implantation was successful in twenty-eight (93 percent) of the thirty patients. Significant improvement of NYHA functional class in twenty (74 percent) of the twenty-seven patients, significant improvement in plasma Brain natriuretic peptide (BNP) level, decreased resting heart rate, improvement of tricuspid regurgitation in eleven of seventeen patients (65 percent), and cardiac remodeling with improvement in RV end-diastolic dimension/LV end-diastolic dimension (RVEDD/LVEDD) ratio at follow-up were observed. This author concluded that his experience in the elderly patients, while small, indicates that transcatheter closure of ASD can be performed safely and contributes to improvement of NYHA functional class and encourages positive cardiac remodeling.

In the next chapter, Dr. Numan from the University of Texas Medical School, Houston, TX, discussed the role of ASD/PFO in migraine. The incidence of migraine is 13 percent and has adverse effect on social life and potential for development of neurological complications. The age of migraine attacks is said to be twenty to sixty-four years with the majority occurring prior to the age of thirty years. Migraine with aura, also known as "classic migraine" is seen in only 25 percent cases. There is an increased prevalence of PFOs in patients with migraine, but no causal relationship between these two was established. Such association appears to more convincing in patients with migraine with aura. Dr. Numan then described the pathologic anatomy and echocardiographic features of PFO. Trans-cranial Doppler (TCD) has higher sensitivity than Echo (trans-thoracic, TEE or ICE) in detecting the right-to-left shunt across the PFO. This author reviewed several studies examining the effect of occlusion of PFOs with devices; most single institutional, non-randomized studies show improvement in migraine; this improvement is greater in patients with aura. However, Migraine Intervention with STARFlex Technology (MIST), a randomized prospective study with patients blinded for PFO closure did not demonstrate statistical difference between the two groups. Dr. Numan offered several objections to the interpretation of the study, but concluded that the MIST study raises questions to be addressed in future studies. However, it may be concluded that the majority of the studies show benefit to patients suffering from migraine with aura.

In the last chapter, Dr. Daraban and her associates, also from the University of Texas Medical School, Houston, TX, discussed transcatheter occlusion of atrial defects for prevention of recurrence of paradoxical embolism. Stroke is the third most common cause of death in the United States. Cryptogenic stroke, consisting of 40 percent of stroke population may be related paradoxical embolism via PFO or ASD. Therapeutic measures for secondary prevention in this patient population include medical treatment or surgical/percutaneous closure of the PFO/ASD. These authors describe embryology, fetal and postnatal changes of PFO. These authors then described the anatomy and associated anomalies such as atrial septal aneurysms (ASA), Chiari network and fenestrated atrial septum. TEE with or without contrast injection and Valsalva maneuver and TCD are important diagnostic tools in the identification of right-to-left shunt across the PFO. They then go on to describe the rationale for PFO and ASD closure treatment in patients with paradoxical embolism. These authors briefly describe the devices used for occlusion of PFO and describe in detail the procedure of closure using Amplatzer PFO Occluder. A number of randomized clinical studies comparing medical treatment with closure of atrial defect are underway. The authors describe the CLOSURE I, REDUCE and RESPECT trials. CLOSURE I, a randomized trial comparing the safety and efficacy of percutaneous PFO closure with STARFlex device versus best medical therapy. During a two-year follow-up, the rates of stroke or TIA were no different between groups. REDUCE is a FDA approved prospective, randomized, multi-center trial designed to demonstrate the safety and effectiveness of the HELEX Septal Occluder for PFO closure in patients with a history of cryptogenic stroke or TIA. The RESPECT trial is a randomized, multi-center study investigating whether closure of PFOs using the Amplatzer PFO Occluder device is safer and more effective than current standard-of-care treatment in the prevention of a cryptogenic stroke. If the results of these clinical trials, favor device closure, it is likely that percutaneous PFO closure can be used to prevent recurrence of paradoxical embolism and stroke.

In summary, of the major types of atrial defects, namely ostium secundum, ostium primum, sinus venosus, and coronary sinus ASDs and PFO, ostium primum, sinus venosus, and coronary sinus defects usually require surgical closure. Such surgery may be performed at about three to four years of age or if they present later, at the time of presentation. Earlier surgery in infancy is not necessary, unless heart failure is present. Ostium secundum ASDs can be successfully closed with transcatheter methodology and the majority of the book addresses the issues related to such technology. PFOs are ordinarily considered as normal variants, although, sometimes they become the seat of right left shunting, requiring closure. The evidence for closure PFO with potential right-to-left shunt in situations related to paradoxical embolism, migraine and others is equivocal. The studies currently in progress may throw light on this subject. While the majority of the book addresses closure of ASDs, one chapter in particular focused on creating atrial defects in the fetus with HLHS. I envision that the fund of information provided in this book will be useful to the practicing physician caring for infants, children and adults with suspected or known ASDs, which may aid them in providing optimal care for their patients.[50]

A COMPREHENSIVE APPROACH TO MANAGEMENT OF CONGENITAL HEART DISEASES - 2013 AND 2019

Dr. Vijayalaxhmi of Sri Jayadeva Institute of Cardiovascular Sciences and Research in Bangalore, India, requested me to help her in formulating a textbook on the management of congenital heart disease. Following the acceptance of the request, I refined the title of the book, suggested topics for the book, contributed five chapters to the book, and edited a large number of chapters submitted to the book; however, bulk of the work was performed by Dr. Vijayalaxhmi herself. Subsequently, Dr. Reema Chugh of Kaiser Permanente Medical Center Panorama City, CA, joined us to help edit the book. Her valuable expertise in adult congenital heart disease was of immense help in bringing out the book (Figure 16).[51]

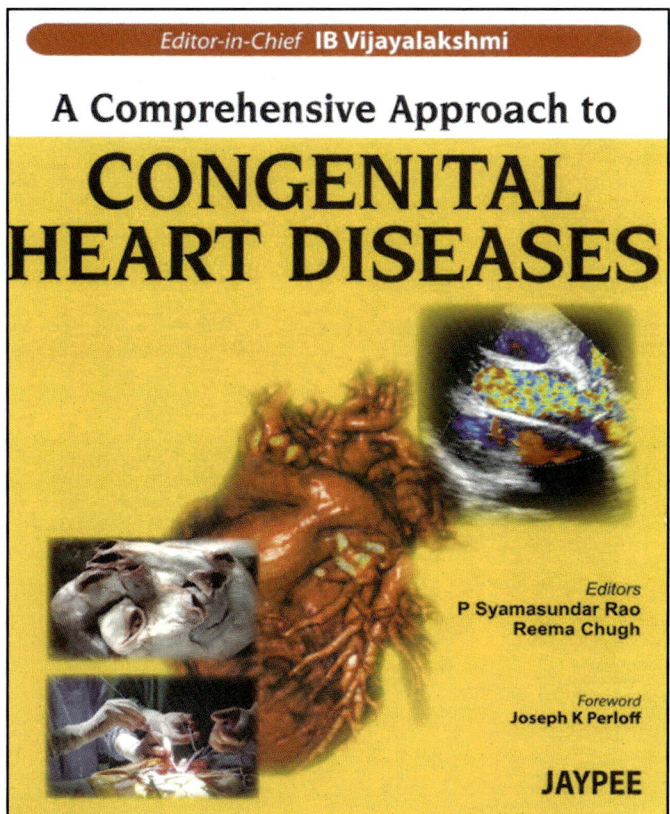

Figure 16. Photograph of book titled "A Comprehensive Approach to Management of Congenital Heart Diseases," published by *Jaypee Publications* in 2013.

Congenital heart disease is the most common birth defect in the neonates worldwide. Advances in pediatrics, congenital heart surgery, anesthesia, internal medicine and obstetrics/gynecology have allowed the majority of these infants to survive into adulthood. Systematic categorization and classifications by embryologists/pathologists had led to a fundamental understanding of these defects and their associated disorders. For a clinician to understand the entire spectrum of CHD from embryology, pathology, clinical manifestations, diagnostics tests, management, and indications for surgical or transcatheter intervention appears to be an insurmountable task. Rapid advances in both catheter-based intervention and surgery for fetus, neonate, children to adults needs a greater understanding of the guidelines and appropriate use of criteria in order to facilitate proper decision-making by combining the best available scientific evidence with the collective judgment of physicians/surgeons. Although there are several textbooks on the various aspects of CHD, there are very few that are focused, yet comprehensive to address all aspects of the care required for this special population. Medical/postgraduate students and practitioners frequently spend a lot of time in referring to various resources in order to gather complete diagnostic and management strategies for one disease. This book titled, "A Comprehensive Approach to Congenital Heart Diseases," is designed to address all the practical aspects that a healthcare provider needs to deliver excellent care to the children and adults with CHD. Multiple distinguished authors from all over the world have made contributions to this book.

In the second edition (Figure 17),[52] the theme and spirit of the initial book[51] was continued, but the advances that occurred in the interim were included.[52]

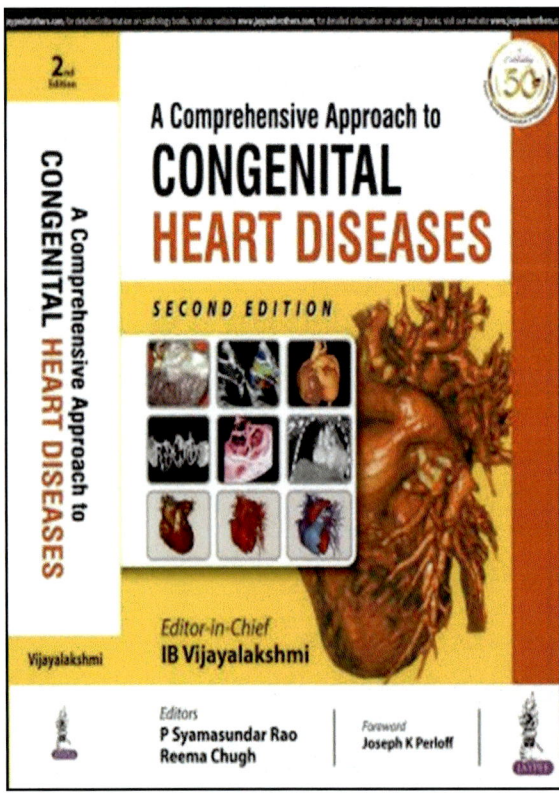

Figure 17. Photograph of book titled "A Comprehensive Approach to Management of Congenital Heart Diseases", 2nd edn., published by *Jaypee Publications* in 2019.

PERINATAL CARDIOLOGY: A MULTIDISCIPLINARY APPROACH

As mentioned above, the monograph "Perinatal Cardiology for The Neonatologist" was intended for local circulation.[47] When Late Dr. Timothy Bricker reviewed the monograph, he strongly felt that this subject material was important and should be available to all physicians caring for the neonates in the USA and abroad and encouraged me to pursue such a goal. Accordingly, I invited Dr. Vidyasagar, an experienced neonatologist from the University of Illinois in Chicago, IL, to collaborate in this effort. Additional neonatology and cardiology topics were added to the existing topics in the monograph on "Perinatal Cardiology for The Neonatologist." Dr. Vidyasagar and I edited the book titled, "Perinatal Cardiology: A Multidisciplinary Approach" (Figure 18).[48]

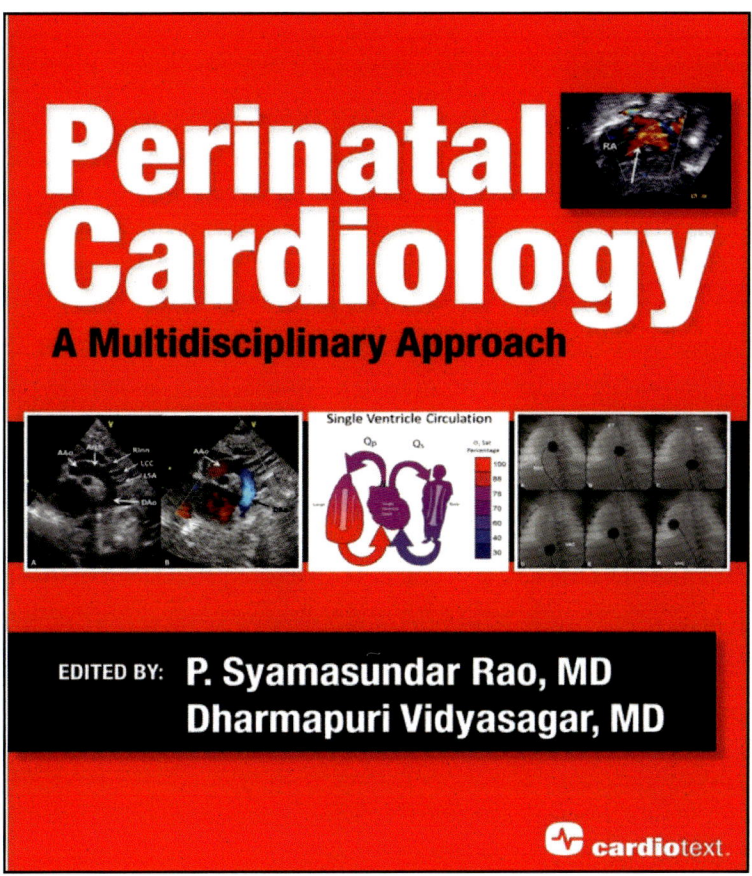

Figure 18. Photograph of book titled, "Perinatal Cardiology: A Multidisciplinary Approach" published by *Cardiotext Publishing* in 2015.

Developments such as early detection of the neonates with serious heart disease and their rapid transport to tertiary care centers, availability of highly sensitive non-invasive diagnostic tools, advances in neonatal care and anesthesia, progress in transcatheter interventional procedures and extension of complicated surgical procedures to the neonate and infant have advanced to such a degree that almost all CHDs can be diagnosed and "corrected." The defects that could not be corrected could be effectively palliated. For achieving excellence in cardiac care, however, close interaction and collaboration of the pediatric cardiologists with neonatologists, pediatricians, general/family practitioners (who care for children), anesthesiologists, and cardiac surgeons is mandatory. Education of physicians caring for the newborn continues to be important in achieving optimal care for the neonate with heart disease. With this in mind, this book was conceived, designed and published.

In the first two chapters, I discussed perinatal circulatory physiology and its role in clinical manifestations and management of neonatal heart disease. Fetal circulation is intended to utilize placenta for gas exchange while postnatal circulation uses lungs for gas exchange. Fetal circulatory pathways, namely, umbilical vessels, ductus venosus, foramen ovale (FO) and ductus arteriosus, high pulmonary vascular resistance and low placental resistance facilitate placental gas exchange and promote distribution of oxygenated blood to the vital organs of the fetus. Mechanical factors, prostaglandins and low PO_2 in the lung maintain the fetal circulatory pathways open. Postnatal circulatory changes are elimination of the placenta, development of pulmonary circulation, and closure of fetal circulatory pathways. Postnatal circulatory changes markedly influence the clinical presentation and clinical course of the neonate with CHDs.

Closure of the ductus arteriosus adversely affects the following: a. The systemic perfusion in HLHS and aortic arch obstructions, b. The pulmonary blood flow in cardiac defects with severe pulmonary stenosis or atresia, and c. Inter-circulatory mixing in TGA. PGE_1 infusion is effective in re-opening the ductus or maintaining its patency. Longer lasting solutions include BT shunts and ductal stents. Spontaneous closure or restriction of PFO adversely affects the following: a. Right-to-left shunting in right heart obstructive lesions and TAPVC, b. Left-to-right shunting in left heart obstructive lesions, and c. Inter-circulatory mixing in TGA. When the FO is restrictive, transcatheter or surgical septostomy is beneficial. Also, pulmonary vascular resistance plays a critical role in patients with large inter-circulatory communications.

In the third chapter, my colleagues at the University of Texas at Houston Medical School, Drs. Biliciler-Denktas and Balaguru and I review embryology of the heart. The fetal heart begins its development in the fourth week of gestation and is fully formed by the tenth week. It is imperative to know the stages in development to understand the normal cardiac structure and the many congenital cardiac malformations. This chapter provides a brief description of cardiovascular development from vasculogenesis to heart tube formation, from looping to septation, to outflow tract and great artery formation, the aortic arch and venous structure formation.

In the next few chapters, my colleagues, Drs. Biliciler-Denktas, Ozcelik and Gupta-Malhotra discuss fetal echocardiography. They state that for the past several decades, fetal echocardiogram became the mainstay in the diagnosis and management of CHDs in-utero. Prenatal diagnosis of CHD is very important for providing optimal care to the mother, fetus and the newborn baby. With advances in ultrasound technology, fetal echocardiogram is proved to be a very important diagnostic imaging test to evaluate the structural and functional abnormalities of the fetal heart. The fetal cardiac evaluation should include the examination of biperital diameter (BPD) for estimation of gestational age, fetal lie and position, fetal visceral situs, cardiac position, four-chamber anatomy, great vessels and their relationships, atrio-ventricular and semilunar valves, aortic and ductal arches, shunting at FO and ductus arteriosus, systemic and pulmonary veins, cardiac chamber dimensions/cardio thoracic index, wall thicknesses, valve/vessel dimensions, fetal heart rate and rhythm, umbilical cord, and pericardial and extra-cardiac spaces for fluid accumulation. The majority of structural abnormalities, particularly the severe cardiac malformations, can be diagnosed with reasonable accuracy and can be used for counseling parents and planning of care of the infant at birth. However, certain lesions are frequently missed by a fetal echocardiogram; the limitations of the scan are its inability to detect small intra-cardiac shunts, minor valve abnormalities (such as a bicuspid aortic valve), systemic or pulmonary venous anomalies (such as partial anomalous venous return) or coronary artery anomalies and these limitations should be clearly explained to the family. Rhythm disturbances are assessed by simultaneous pulse Doppler recordings of ventricular inflow and outflow tract. Since most of these arrhythmias (e.g., premature ventricular contractions [PACs]) are benign and do not cause any hemodynamic compromise, they may be observed throughout the rest of the pregnancy. On the other hand, arrhythmias like SVT and AV block may cause hemodynamic instability and may need medical treatment for control or even may need early delivery of the fetus in some cases. Fetal echocardiography is a very important tool for the diagnosis and follow-up of these arrhythmias. Once a given diagnosis is made, the causes and treatment options should be reviewed and decided upon taking the maternal and fetal factors and side effects into consideration. Pharmacologic management of fetal arrhythmias and hydrops is feasible.

In the next chapter, Dr. Leuthner from the Medical College of Wisconsin reviewed ethical issues in managing fetal and neonatal cardiac lesions. He states that as more "fetal care" or "fetal treatment" centers emerge nationally, and more pediatric sub-specialists participate in the prenatal care of the fetus and woman, understanding the importance of the ethical issues that span from the prenatal to the postnatal period become essential. Differences in obstetrical and pediatric professional cultures both bring important information to the decision-making and are why a multi-disciplinary team approach may best serve prospective parents. When exploring the construct of the "fetus as patient," two surrogate decision-making constructs used in pediatric ethics, "Best Interest" and "Constrained Parental Autonomy," may be useful in eliciting the ethical issues present, as well as aid in decision-making. One conclusion, both these constructs come to is that full support of the pregnant woman's autonomy ultimately must be respected. These theoretic concepts are useful in exploring the ethical issues that exist in frequently encountered perinatal clinical situations, as well as those clinical cases that lead to interventions, innovations and experimentation. Finally, when exploring the decisions around the transition from the fetal to neonatal environment, of utmost importance is consistency in counseling and supporting families in different types of decisions, not only regarding fetal intervention, but as parents of the newborn.

In the chapter to follow, Dr. Bhandankar of the JN Medical College, Belgaum, India, and Dr. Vidyasagar of University of Illinois at Chicago, Chicago, IL, discussed changes in oxygen saturations during first few minutes of life in the delivery room. After birth, the newborn undergoes a series of physiologic changes during the transitional phase in establishing normal extra uterine respiration and simultaneously improving pulmonary circulation, both of which are important in proper oxygenation of blood. Compromised infant unable to establish normal respiration requires resuscitation in the delivery room. Current reliance on clinical assessment of degree of oxygen desaturation (cyanosis) was found to be inadequate. The introduction of non-invasive method of assessment of oxygenation using pulse oximetry has opened the door to accurately assess oxygenation during transition much more. Several studies show that it takes the newborn about four minutes to reach oxygen saturation of 90 percent and six to seven minutes to reach 95 percent. These studies have established the "the reference values" of oxygenation at birth. Infants who do not reach these target levels will require resuscitation. Thus, routine use of pulse oximetry of the newborn in the delivery room will help clinicians to decide the timing of initiation of resuscitation in the delivery room. Hence, routine use of pulse oximetry of the newborn at the time of delivery was strongly recommended. In the succeeding chapter, Dr. Vidyasagar explored pulse oximetry screening for detecting CHDs in the newborn. Major advances in pediatric cardiology and cardiac surgery have occurred during middle and later part of the twentieth century leading to improved survival of infants with CHDs and critical CHD. The main barriers for better outcomes are early diagnosis of critical CHD and timely intervention. Until recently clinical examination complemented with ECG and chest X-ray have been the main tools for the diagnosis of CHD in the newborn. Introduction of echocardiography improved the postnatal diagnosis of CHD and critical CHD. Fetal echocardiography has enabled us to make antenatal diagnosis of CHD. In spite of these advances there are chances of missing critical CHD. A non-invasive, yet simple method of measuring the blood oxygenation, pulse oximetry, had opened the door for a number of things beyond the original goal of measuring oxygen saturation non-invasively. Pulse oximetry detects minimal degrees of desaturation that clinicians cannot detect visually. Early investigators found that pulse oximetry can be used to diagnose CHD, primarily those which are ductus dependent, most of which fall into the category of critical CHD. A study by middle Tennessee investigators found that prior to implementation of pulse oximetry for screening the newborns for CHD, twelve infants with critical CHD were missed. These infants had a negative fetal ultrasound. Investigators concluded that continued postnatal evaluation with pulse oximetry is important to detect all critical CHD. Based on numerous studies, the advantages of pulse oximetry in the neonatal period include: Early diagnosis of critical CHD in otherwise asymptomatic infant, and early medical/transcatheter/surgical intervention and improved survival. Although not mandated since the approval of screening test in the US by the department of Health and Human Services, twenty-six states have adopted pulse oximetry screening in the neonates born in all hospitals. Many more states are considering implementing universal pulse oximetry screening in the newborn. Similarly, use of pulse oximetry screening to detect critical CHD in resource poor countries has a great potential. He summarizes that pulse oximetry is a simple but most valuable non-invasive tool to diagnose critical CHD in the newborn. And, as declared in Lancet: Introduction of pulse oximetry screening for critical CHD is *"A major Mile Stone in the history of cardiology."*

In the next chapter, I presented an approach to the diagnosis of cyanotic neonate for the primary care provider. Cyanosis is a major manifestation of cyanotic CHD in the neonate. A number of cardiac and non-cardiac entities cause cyanosis in the neonate. The majority of patients can be diagnosed based on their well described clinical and laboratory findings. In a few patients in whom a clear-cut diagnosis is not possible, analysis of PO_2 response to 100 percent O_2 and continuous positive airway pressure (CPAP) may help distinguish cardiac from non-cardiac cyanosis. Once diagnosed to be a cardiac baby, careful analysis of pulmonary vascular marking on a chest x-ray may facilitate categorization into subgroups from which additional analysis of ECG and other features may assist in coming up with a reasonably good diagnosis. Echo-Doppler studies can certainly aid in achieving an accurate diagnosis. The exercise presented is an approach that could be taken when echo is not readily available or used prior to the arrival of echocardiographer.

Once a cardiac baby is identified, a detailed Echo-Doppler study should be performed and the diagnosis confirmed. Cardiac catheterization and selective cineangiography are rarely required for diagnostic purposes. In this chapter, a brief review of the principles of Echo-Doppler technique was presented. M-mode and two-dimensional echocardiography, pulsed, continuous wave and color Doppler studies from standard views are recorded; subcostal views are most helpful in making a diagnosis in the neonate. Normalcy of the heart can be confirmed in important non-cardiac causes of cyanosis or respiratory distress such as persistent pulmonary hypertension, neonatal asphyxia, central nervous system disorders, polycythemia, methhemoglobinemia, hypoglycemia, pulmonary hypoplasia, shock and sepsis, maternal drugs, and others. The principles of estimation of pulmonary artery pressure were addressed. Usefulness of echocardiogram in evaluation of infant of a diabetic mother (IDM), PDA in the premature, side of the aortic arch in tracheo-esophageal fistula babies, heart defects in Down syndrome and cardiomegaly was elucidated. Characteristic echocardiographic features of important cardiac defects such as tetralogy of Fallot, TGA, tricuspid atresia, TAPVC, truncus arteriosus, and HLHS were presented. Echocardiographic images of pulmonary atresia with intact ventricular septum, double outlet right ventricle, double inlet left (single) ventricle, Ebstein's anomaly of the tricuspid valve, and interrupted aortic arch were also shown. In a non-distressed infant with simple cardiac murmur, the cause of murmur may easily be detected, whether it is a small VSD, peripheral pulmonary artery stenosis, mild semilunar valve (aortic or pulmonary) stenosis or a functional murmur. Echocardiogram is extremely useful in the evaluation of the neonate with suspected and known heart disease. In the chapter to follow, Drs. Doshi, Jadhav and Gupta explore the role of magnetic resonance imaging (MRI) and computed tomography (CT) in the evaluation of heart disease in the neonates. Cardiac MRI and CT scan technology has evolved significantly over past two decades and their application to image the cardiac defects, particularly in the young infant, has been refined. They are great tools to complement traditional cardiac diagnostic imaging techniques like echocardiography and catheterization with angiography. Appropriate coordination with cardiologist and radiologist is very important to obtain all necessary diagnostic information.

In the Chapter 13, I enumerated principles of management of the neonate with CHD. During the process of identification, transfer to a tertiary care center and work-up, prevention of hypothermia, maintenance of neutral thermal environment, monitoring for and prompt treatment of hypoglycemia, treatment of hypocalcemia, monitoring acid-base status, treatment of metabolic acidosis with sodium bicarbonate ($NaHCO_3$), and management of respiratory acidosis with suction, intubation and assisted ventilation as deemed necessary are important and should be undertaken. In patients with cyanotic CHD, 30-40 percent O_2 is adequate and 100 percent O_2 is not necessary. If ductal dependant CHD is suspected, intravenous infusion of PGE_1 should be started, while waiting for confirmatory diagnosis. After administering the supportive care, the treatment required, by and large, is determined by the specific physiologic and/or anatomic diagnosis. Prostaglandin infusion and modified BT shunt for the neonate with pulmonary oligemia, anticongestive measures with or without banding of the pulmonary artery for babies with pulmonary plethora and transcatheter or surgical relief of inter-atrial obstruction, as needed, should be provided. When feasible, transcatheter and/or surgical correction should be offered. Management of each individual lesion was reviewed briefly.

In the next chapter, I reviewed management strategies to deal with neonatal cardiac emergencies. Emergencies of life-threatening nature involving the cardiovascular system in the neonate are many and complex. Successful management depends upon prompt and accurate diagnosis of the problem in order to institute appropriate therapeutic measures and referral to a specialized treatment center, if necessary. These situations may manifest themselves as severe cyanosis, heart failure, lethargy and lack of spontaneous movement, arrhythmia and special problems seen in post-operative single ventricle physiology babies. Management of these cardiac emergencies was outlined.

In Chapter 15, Drs. Ray and Northrup form our institution reviewed genetics of CHD. The authors state that molecular diagnosis for disease entities improves the understanding of pathology, and opens the door for future therapeutic opportunities to managing or even preventing disease. This chapter provides a systematic approach to categorizing genetic conditions by heart lesion in order to generate a concise differential for accurate diagnosis. Increased suspicion for genetic etiology has become an essential part of standard medical practice. Establishment of an accurate diagnosis provides valuable prognostic and recurrence information for the patient and physician, has the potential to decrease morbidity, and direct further management. It is appropriate for the pediatrician, neonatologist or pediatric cardiologist to begin diagnostic work-up with a chromosome microarray, while referring to a medical geneticist, when a genetic involvement is suspected. Additionally, single gene testing or genetic testing panels for isolated heart lesions such as thoracic aortic aneurysms and arrhythmias as a baseline test for genetic involvement is appropriate.

In the next chapter, Drs. Afolayan and Konduri from Children's Hospital of Wisconsin review pathophysiology and management of persistent pulmonary hypertension (PPHN) of the newborn. PPHN is a complication of neonatal transition in pulmonary circulation. Diagnostic approach for suspected PPHN was discussed and a proposed algorithm for the evaluation and management of a cyanotic neonate is shown. Studies over the last twenty-five years have dramatically improved our understanding of the altered vascular biology in PPHN. This knowledge has led to rapid advances in the application of new pulmonary vasodilators to treat neonates with PPHN. Introduction of inhaled nitric oxide (iNO) has been one of the most important advances in neonatal intensive care over the last fifty years. Inhaled NO has greatly reduced the mortality and morbidity from PPHN, while decreasing the need for invasive rescue therapies like Extracorporeal Membrane Oxygenation (ECMO). Recent evidence also suggests that early use of surfactant for PPHN caused by parenchymall lung disease leads to reduction in the use of ECMO and mortality. Early application of surfactant, iNO and optimal lung recruitment strategies can lead to further reduction in morbidity and mortality from PPHN. Recent development of new signaling targets in PPHN may lead to improved oxygenation in neonates, who are unresponsive to iNO or other currently available vasodilators. These approaches can further decrease lung injury from hyperoxia and barotrauma and improve the long-term outcome for these affected infants.

In the next chapter, Dr. Numan from our institution reviews neonatal rhythms and dysrhythmias. Neonatal rhythm disturbances frequently are benign and self-resolved in few weeks to few months after birth without the necessity of medical intervention. Increased automaticity (Phase 4 of the action potential) is responsible for most of these benign rhythms. Careful evaluation of the ECG and rhythm strips during neonatal tachycardia can reveal the mechanism in most of them. Stabilizing the airways and maintaining adequate tissue oxygenation during the tachycardia are priority in management. This is followed by measures to terminate the arrhythmia. Neonatal bradycardia has higher morbidity than tachyarrhythmia. Assessing the hemodynamics and tissue perfusion is essential to guide the management of these bradycardias.

In Chapter 18, single ventricle physiology was discussed by Dr. Yarrabolu of Texas Tech Health Sciences Center, Amarillo, TX and Dr. Douglas of University of Texas at Houston Medical School. Single ventricle physiology (SVP) encompasses a vast number of diagnoses. However, the strategy of creating a neonatal circulation with unobstructed systemic blood flow and moderately (balanced) pulmonary blood flow results in a relatively small number of procedures most commonly used to palliate neonatal SVP. The majority of patients can be grouped into a few common treatment pathways, all of which are intended to lead towards eventual palliation with a Fontan procedure. Neonatal palliation of SVP still carries a high risk of surgical mortality, especially when compared with surgical correction of many defects with biventricular physiology.

In Chapters 19 through 21, I reviewed various catheter interventional techniques that are currently being used in neonates. There are a number of cardiac defects in which an ASD is beneficial. But, the naturally occurring PFO undergoes spontaneous closure, causing poor mixing and/or obstruction to systemic or pulmonary venous flow. In such situations, the PFO may be enlarged or an ASD created by transcatheter methods (Rashkind balloon atrial septostomy, Park blade atrial septostomy, balloon angioplasty [static balloon dilatation], atrial septal perforation, and stent implantation). The selection of the method used is largely based on the atrial septal anatomy and left atrial size. In the vast majority of the patients, the septostomy procedures are successful in creating an appropriate sized opening. In the rare cases, surgical septostomy may be required. Severe or critical pulmonary and aortic valvar obstruction may occur in the neonatal period and these obstructive lesions can be successfully treated by balloon valvuloplasty techniques. Milder forms of obstruction do not need intervention in the neonate. Aortic coarctation can be successfully relieved with balloon angioplasty in the neonatal period. However, there is a high rate of recurrence. Consequently, surgical repair is the first line therapeutic option in the neonatal period. If recoarctation develops following surgical repair, balloon angioplasty is the method of choice, although the true need for such intervention in the neonatal period is infrequent. Pulmonary valve stenosis associated with complex heart defects, causing hypoxemia can be successfully treated with balloon valvuloplasty and such intervention is used in highly selected cases. In addition to these procedures, perforation of atretic pulmonary valve, occlusion of defects or vessels causing cardiac failure and stents to keep open closing fetal circulatory pathways and vascular stenotic lesions can also be performed. These procedures should complement other medical therapies and surgical interventions. In a given patient, the method selected should be a method that is most likely to provide the best outcome in a given neonate.

In Chapter 22, Dr. Gardiner from the UT Health reviewed in utero intervention for severe CHD. She states that fetal therapy is offered for many disorders diagnosed before birth, but while some are introduced following randomized trials, others enter the clinical arena in a more piecemeal fashion. Cardiac malformations are common with major lesions affecting about 3.5 per thousand pregnancies; however, only a small proportion of affected fetuses are likely to benefit from an intrauterine intervention. Currently, fetal valvuloplasty is offered for severe aortic and pulmonary stenosis, perforation and stenting of the closed or restrictive interatrial septum and pacing for complete heart block, all using a percutaneous approach. Technical success is high for fetal valvuloplasty, but is not matched by biventricular outcomes. This may be attributed in part to the lack of knowledge of the underlying mechanisms and factors affecting disease progression that contributes to the difficulty in patient selection for intrauterine therapy. Published series have proposed retrospective guidelines for selection, but have a level of evidence of three; none compares outcomes in contemporaneous controls with similar pre-procedure anatomy and physiology. Dr. Gardiner goes on to state that the place of fetal cardiac intervention remains uncertain. It is unlikely that a borderline two-ventricle repair is better than a good uni-ventricular repair. It is certain that the problem will be more difficult to resolve than the treatment of twin to twin transfusion syndrome, in part because it is more heterogeneous and rare. There is theoretical potential for important improvement in the rapidly growing heart if fetal therapy is successful and even if antenatal therapy provides only a temporizing measure, some improvement in the fetal circulation and well-being may permit delivery at a more mature gestation and thus improve postnatal management and eventual outcome. This re-emerging field deserves a careful and rigorous investigative approach to provide more information on its likely clinical applications.

In the next chapter, Dr. Ramanathan of Keck School of Medicine of University of Southern California, Los Angeles, California, reviews surfactant therapy and neonatal hemodynamics. He opines that respiratory distress syndrome due to surfactant deficiency is a major cause of morbidity and mortality in preterm neonates worldwide. Surfactant therapy in preterm infants improves lung compliance, decreases pulmonary vascular resistance, and RV afterload. Preterm infants treated with surfactant do not manifest with a higher incidence of hemodynamically significant PDA. Management of PDA remains controversial. Early closure of the ductus arteriosus results in less severe grades of inter-ventricular hemorrhage; however, no long-term neuro-developmental benefits have been demonstrated. In late preterm and term infants, surfactant treatment for hypoxemic respiratory failure secondary to parenchymal lung diseases has been shown to improve survival and decrease the need for ECMO. CHDs that are ductal dependent for pulmonary or systemic blood flows as well as obstructive lesions, such as, obstructed total anomalous venous connections may not benefit from surfactant therapy.

In Chapter 24, Drs. Rafique and Gautam from our institution review anesthesia for the neonate with CHD. They state that considering the complexity of the neonatal clinical condition and the number of interdependent mediating variables, the anesthesiologist plays an extremely important role in achieving a successful cardiac surgical outcome. While there is not a gold standard anesthetic regimen, a balanced common-sense approach to anesthetics, knowledge of underlying pathophysiology, maintenance of high situational awareness, unremitting vigilance and tight coordination with the pediatric cardiac team are absolutely essential for the safe care of the neonate with cardiac disease. In the next chapter, Drs. Yarrabolu, Spicer and Douglas from our institution review issues related to cardiac surgery in the neonate. They state that cardiac surgery is commonly performed in neonates. Some procedures require the use of cardiopulmonary bypass (CPB), while some procedures can be performed without CPB. Many cardiac lesions are ductal dependent and surgeries are typically performed four to fourteen days after birth. Although results are very favorable for certain repairs, many procedures still have extremely high mortality rates. Many lesions can undergo biventricular repairs as a neonate. Many other lesions, including single ventricle and biventricular defects, require palliative procedures. In general, palliative procedures have higher mortality rates, especially those that require CPB. In the succeeding chapter, Dr. Balaguru, again from our institution reviewed perioperative care of newborn with critical heart disease. While there is some overlap between some prior chapters and this chapter, it is believed that this is acceptable to preserve the continuity of discussion. Preoperative management of neonate with critical heart disease entails early recognition and confirmation of diagnosis. Early stabilization includes a combination of fluid resuscitation, prostaglandin infusion, inotropes, respiratory support and treatment of any concomitant pulmonary or other organ dysfunction. After initial stabilization, while on Prostaglandins, changes in hemodynamic state occur as a result of transition from fetal to neonatal circulation. Babies should be closely watched for these changes and appropriate modifications made to the management. Feeding babies while on Prostaglandin infusion, awaiting surgery remains controversial due to increased incidence of necrotizing enterocolitis. However, enteral feeding is generally considered beneficial when optimal conditions exist. Since surgery may be necessary within hours when medical management fails to maintain adequate balance of circulations, it is preferable to manage the baby in a surgical center. Postoperative management also has evolved into a multi-disciplinary approach over the past several decades with good results. Overall mortality from CHD in neonates has decreased significantly from 27 percent in 1987 to 4 percent in 2007. This improvement reflects advances in technology, preoperative management, surgical approach and postoperative management.

In Chapter 27, Dr. Natarajan from the Children's Hospital of Michigan, Detroit, Michigan, discussed feeding strategies in neonates with severe CHD along with comments on necrotizing enterocolitis (NEC). She states that the outcomes of infants with severe CHD may be improved by implementation of a standardized feeding algorithm with the goal of achieving normal growth. Early enteral and oral nutrition should be initiated when the clinical condition allows and should be accompanied by close monitoring for cardiac and gastrointestinal complications. A structured multi-disciplinary approach to evaluation and management of oromotor difficulties in the postoperative period may be beneficial. Continued assessment of growth and nutrition following discharge from hospital is warranted, especially in infants with single ventricle physiology. A higher prevalence of NEC in CHD is well recognized. Standardized feeding algorithms for infants following cardiac surgery indicated reduction in NEC rates in a limited number of studies.

The preceding chapters have mostly addressed the general topics involving entire spectrum of cardiac and pulmonary issues, including CHDs in the fetus and neonate. In the ensuing chapters commonly encountered individual cardiac defects were discussed. TGA is a CHD in which the aorta arises from the RV while the pulmonary artery comes off of the LV. In this condition, the systemic and pulmonary circulations are parallel instead of the normal circulation that is in series. This anomaly is classified into TGA with intact ventricular septum, TGA with VSD, and TGA with VSD and PS. The intact ventricular septum patients present in the very early neonatal period, while the other two may present with symptoms slightly latter. Cyanosis is the major symptom in intact septum patients, while heart failure is the presenting symptom in patients with TGA and VSD. TGA with VSD and PS have a variable presentation. Murmurs are notably absent in intact septum babies, while loud holosystolic or ejection systolic murmurs dominate in the other two groups. While the chest x-ray and ECG are helpful in the diagnosis, echocardiographic studies are confirmatory in the diagnosis and quantification of the associated defects. PGE_1 to open the ductus and/or balloon atrial septostomy to enlarge the PFO may sometimes be required for palliation. Surgical correction by arterial switch (Jatene) procedure for TGA babies with intact ventricular septum and those with VSD and Rastelli procedure for TGA patients with VSD and PS has become standard of care.

In Chapter 29, Dr. Alapati from Texas Tech Health Sciences Center, Amarillo, TX, and I addressed issues related to TOF. TOF is the most common cyanotic CHD beyond one year of age and constitutes 10 percent of all CHDs. In the neonate however, it is less common than TGA. TOF is a constellation of four abnormalities: 1. VSD, 2. PS, 3. Right ventricular hypertrophy, and 4. Dextroposition of the aorta. Because the VSD is large, the systolic pressures in both ventricles are equal and for practical purposes both ventricles act as one functional chamber. The quantity of blood flow into the systemic and pulmonary circuits depends upon their respective resistances. The level of systemic vascular resistance and the resistance offered by the right ventricular outflow tract stenosis determine the flows. The more severe the PS, the less is the pulmonary flow. There are several variants of TOF with differences in presentation in the neonatal period; neonatal TOF may be classified as: Type I, Classic TOF; Type II, TOF with pulmonary atresia; Type III, TOF with multiple aorto-pulmonary collateral arteries (MAPCAs); Type IV, TOF with absent pulmonary valve syndrome. The majority of classic TOF patients are either acyanotic or minimally cyanotic in the neonatal period and do not require surgical intervention as a neonate. The initial management of TOF with pulmonary atresia (ductal dependent) is by prompt infusion of PGE_1 to keep the ductus open. Once the baby is stabilized, a permanent way to provide pulmonary blood flow should be made. In patients whose cardiac defect could not be corrected in the neonatal period, a modified BT shunt using an interposition GoreTex graft between the right or left sub-clavian arteries and the ipsilateral pulmonary artery is the current surgical procedure of choice. The initial management of patients with TOF and MAPCAs depends on the extent of pulmonary blood flow. The majority of patients will maintain acceptable arterial oxygen saturations in the range of 80 percent to 90 percent and may not require intervention in the neonatal period. Patients with decreased pulmonary flow and hypoxemia may need PGE_1 followed by BT shunt. Patients with increased pulmonary flow may need anti-congestive treatment. Some babies may need catheter interventions to improve the baby's clinical status. The definitive management of TOF with MAPCAs includes combined staged approach with surgery and interventional catheterization to establish antegrade pulmonary blood flow from the right ventricle, rehabilitate the pulmonary arteries, and closure of the VSD. Symptomatic neonates with TOF and syndrome of absent pulmonary valve require ventilatory support to stabilize the patient followed by total surgical correction under cardiopulmonary bypass, including closure of the VSD, relief of PS by a trans-annular pericardial patch as necessary, and partial resection and plastic repair of aneurysmally dilated pulmonary arteries.

In Chapter 30, I discuss tricuspid atresia. Tricuspid atresia is the third most common cyanotic CHD. Significant differences in the associated defects and consequent physiology result in varied clinical presentations. The diagnosis is fairly simple and can frequently be made by clinical features and simple studies such as chest X-ray and ECG, which can be confirmed by Echo-Doppler studies. Aggressive treatment to normalize the pulmonary blood flow and to correct associated defects such as coarctation of the aorta should be carried out at the time of initial presentation. Careful follow-up and management in an attempt to preserve (or normalize) cardiac structures and function (for example, pulmonary artery pressure and anatomy, and LV function) should be pursued. Lastly, undertaking staged Fontan (bidirectional Glenn followed by modified Fontan-Kreutzer) operation, before any deterioration of the LV function, should noticeably improve the prognosis for tricuspid atresia patients.

TAPVC was reviewed in Chapter 31. In TAPVC, all pulmonary veins drain into a common pulmonary vein, which is then connected to the left innominate vein, superior vena cava, coronary sinus, portal vein or other unusual sites. TAPVC is the fifth most common cyanotic CHD and the prevalence is 0.6 to 1.2 per 10,000 live births. In all types of TAPVC, the entire pulmonary venous blood is ultimately returned into right atrium, mixes with systemic venous return and is redistributed to the systemic circuit through PFO and to the pulmonary circuit through the tricuspid valve. The TAPVC is classified based on the following: 1. Anatomic site, into which the connecting veins drain, namely, supra-diaphragmatic (supra-cardiac and cardiac) or infra-diaphragmatic, and 2. Physiologic based on obstruction to the pulmonary venous return, namely, obstructive or non-obstructive. The supra-diaphragmatic TAPVC is usually non-obstructive and the infra-diaphragmatic forms are always obstructive. TAPVC to the left innominate vein is the most common type when all TAPVCs at all ages are included, but infra-diaphragmatic type is most common in the neonate. Babies with obstructive TAPVC present within the first few hours to days of life with signs of severe pulmonary venous congestion with evident tachypnea, tachycardia and cyanosis. Examination shows rales in the lung fields and a loud pulmonary component of the second heart sound. Infants with non-obstructive TAPVC, on the other hand, typically present with signs of CHF later in the first month of life. On examination, they are not cyanotic or mildly cyanotic and have clinical signs of heart failure. Other findings are similar to those seen in patients with ASD. Clinical and chest x-ray findings are suggestive of the TAPVC diagnosis and echocardiographic studies are confirmatory. In the obstructive type, initial stabilization by intubation and ventilation with high airway pressure should be undertaken. Then, emergent surgical correction by anastomosis of the common pulmonary vein with the left atrium should follow. In the non-obstructive type, after control of CHF and stabilization of the baby, elective or semi-elective surgery is suggested. Periodic post-surgical follow-up to detect development of pulmonary venous obstruction was recommended.

In Chapter 32, Dr. Balaguru and I reviewed truncus arteriosus, which is one of the conotruncal anomalies with high association with 22q11 microdeletion/DiGeorge syndrome. The diagnosis is relatively simple and can often be suspected on clinical features and confirmed by echocardiography with a rare need for cardiac catheterization and selective cineangiography. Surgical correction by VSD closure and insertion of RV to PA conduit, usually an aortic homograft in early infancy is the current management option. Outcome depends on defect type, pulmonary artery anatomy, aortic arch anomalies and truncal valve function. After surgery, these patients may need multiple re-interventions both for replacement of RV to PA conduit and transcatheter therapy for pulmonary artery rehabilitation and to address conduit dysfunction. Overall, surgical outcome has improved over the past several decades. Risk of recurrence of the genetic and cardiac defect in the offspring depends on genetic testing in the mother. Appropriate counseling should be provided to prospective mothers with repaired truncus arteriosus.

Then, I and Dr. Alapati review HLHS in Chapter 33. HLHS is a constellation of anomalies, which include diminutive left ventricle with poor development of mitral and aortic valves and hypoplastic ascending aorta. A PFO and a PDA are generally present and are essential for survival. Aortic coarctation may be present in some babies. Pulmonary venous blood traverses the atrial septum and mixes with systemic venous blood in the right atrium and from there passed on to the RV and the PA. The systemic and the pulmonary circuits are connected to each other by the ductus arteriosus and the blood exiting the RV is distributed into the lungs through the branch pulmonary arteries and into body across the ductus arteriosus. HLHS encompasses 1.2 percent to 1.5 percent of all CHDs and is uniformly fatal, unless it is promptly recognized, treated with PGE_1 and palliated by surgery. The babies can be identified by prenatal ultrasound and those that are not so detected present shortly after birth with symptoms as the ductus starts to close. The time of presentation is largely dependent on ductal patency, the level of PVR and the degree of atrial level obstruction. The diagnosis can typically be made with Echo-Doppler studies. The initial management of HLHS is by timely infusion of PGE_1 to maintain the ductus open, balancing the pulmonary and systemic circulation to maintain adequate systemic perfusion and ensure adequacy of PFO for easy egress of left atrial blood while waiting for surgery. Ambient O_2 should not be administered. Surgical therapy is either by multistage surgery, comprising of Norwood procedure (Stage I) in the neonatal period, bidirectional Glenn procedure (Stage II) at about six months of age, and Fontan conversion (Stage III) one or two years later or by orthotopic cardiac transplantation. At the present time, the actuarial survival rate of HLHS babies treated with either of these surgical procedures is 70 percent at five years and is comparable to that of infants with other complex types of CHD in whom a two-ventricle repair is not possible.

In the next two chapters, Dr. Balaguru and I discussed pulmonary atresia with intact ventricular septum (PA-IVS) and Ebstein's anomaly of the tricuspid valve. PA-IVS is a complex cyanotic CHD that is characterized by pulmonary valve atresia and varying degrees of RV hypoplasia. Associated lesions include hypoplasia of tricuspid valve, coronary sinusoids and RV-dependent coronary circulation. Neonatal transcatheter intervention has evolved into first line therapy at most institutions. Decision regarding single-ventricle or two-ventricle repair generally needs to be made in the neonatal period. So called, 1.5 ventricle repair option also exists. Outcome for these babies is good except when there is RV-dependent coronary circulation. Ebstein's anomaly is a rare CHD. Clinical manifestations vary depending upon the severity of the lesion. Mild forms may be asymptomatic and may not need any treatment. Moderate forms may be managed with relative ease and improve as the PVR decreases with increasing age. Severe forms of the disease are a challenge to manage and may require surgical intervention. Prognosis depends on severity of the lesion, age at presentation and type of surgical repair. Surgical outcomes have improved over time, but early presentation as fetus and newborn is associated with poor prognosis.

In Chapter 36, I discuss cardiac malpositions including heterotaxy syndromes which have significant association with complex CHD. The prevalence of CHD is significantly higher than normal babies and the incidence varies with the associated viscero-atrial situs. The best approach to diagnosis is segmental analysis. Initially however, dextroposition should be excluded. In segmental analysis, the visceroatrial situs, ventricular location, status of atrioventricular connections, relationship of the great arteries and conotruncal relationship are determined with the use of ECG, chest x-ray and echocardiographic studies and when necessary other imaging studies, including angiography. After the sites of atria, ventricles and great arteries are identified, the associated defects such as ASD, VSD, valvar and vascular stenosis or atresia may be determined by review of the history, physical examination and analysis of chest x-ray, ECG and echocardiographic studies. At presentation, addressing the physiologic abnormality produced by the defect complex, whether it be augmenting pulmonary blood flow or restricting it, is the initial step. Other associated defects should also be addressed accordingly. Biventricular or univentricular repair depending upon the baby's anatomy should be planned.

In the preceding chapters a relatively detailed discussion of a number of cyanotic CHD presenting in the neonatal period was reviewed. In Chapter 37, pathology, pathophysiology, clinical presentation, non-invasive evaluation and management of double outlet right ventricle, univentricular hearts, interrupted aortic arch, l-transposition of great arteries, and mitral atresia with normal aortic root were discussed. By and large the initial management is focused onto normalizing or improving the pathophysiological state produced by the defect complex. The objective is to increase pulmonary blood flow by PGE_1 infusion followed by BT shunt in neonates with pulmonary oligemia, institute anti-congestive measures followed by correcting the defect or banding of the pulmonary artery in babies with pulmonary plethora, transcatheter or surgical relief of interatrial obstruction in infants with obstructed ASD/PFO, resection or bypass inter-ventricular obstruction by Damus-Kaye-Stansel operation in neonates with constriction of inter-ventricular communication (VSD or bulbo-venricular foramen), and relieve of aortic obstruction in babies with aortic coarctation or interruption. When feasible biventricular repair should be attempted; for those who do not have two functioning ventricles, staged Fontan operation should be planned.

In Chapter 38, I reviewed issues related to coarctation of the aorta (COA). COA is a congenital cardiac anomaly consisting of a constricted aortic segment with a prevalence of five to eight percent of all CHD. The classic COA is located in the thoracic aorta distal to the origin of the left sub-clavian artery, at about the level of the ductal structure. Neonates have a higher prevalence of other cardiac defects. Significant hypertension and/or CHF are indications of intervention. Surgical relief of the aortic obstruction and catheter interventional techniques (balloon angioplasty and stents) are available options. Since the introduction of surgical correction by Crafoord and Nylin and Gross and Hufnagal in mid 1940s, surgical therapy has been the treatment of choice for aortic coarctation; multiple surgical techniques including resection and end-to-end anastomosis, subclavian flap angioplasty, prosthetic patch aortoplasty and tubular bypass grafts were used. More recently, balloon angioplasty has been utilized to enlarge coarcted aortic segments. The procedure consists of positioning a balloon angioplasty catheter across the coarctation and inflating the balloon with diluted contrast material. Because of high rate of recurrence following neonatal balloon angioplasty, surgery is the preferred treatment option at most institutions. However, balloon angioplasty is preferred for post-surgical recoarctation, although the need for such intervention in the neonatal period is unusual. Because of problems associated with surgical and balloon therapy, stents have been attempted. But, the stents do not grow as the baby grows and therefore, investigations are needed to test the utility of biodegradable and growth stents.

In Chapter 39, Dr. Bhat from Children's Hospital of Wisconsin, Milwaukee, WI, reviewed issues related to PDA in the premature infant. As stated by the author, the incidence of PDA is inversely related to gestational age. Antenatal steroid use decreases the incidence and respiratory distress increases the incidence. Spontaneous closure rate of PDA is around 34 percent to 40 percent for infants < 1000g and for infants > 30 weeks gestation the spontaneous closure rate is > 98 percent by seven days of age. Size of the ductus as measured by color Doppler echocardiogram along with clinical signs and serum BNP levels can assist in identifying hemodynamically significant PDA (hsPDA) requiring intervention. Prophylactic indomethacin or ibuprofen if administered within 12 hours of birth is effective for preventing PDA, pulmonary hemorrhage and severe intraventricular bleeding, but neither drug alters morbidity (chronic lung disease) and long term outcome, but exposes large number of infants for adverse effects. Thus, prophylactic therapy is not recommended at present. Currently, once the diagnosis is established, patients should be managed with fluid restriction, diuretic therapy and respiratory support as needed before the use of indomethacin or ibuprofen. Indomethacin and ibuprofen given orally or IV are equally effective in closing ductus arteriosus (70 to 80 percent). Oral paracetamol can be an alternate choice, but needs further testing. Ductal closure does not decrease morbidity or neuro-developmental outcome. Surgical closure of PDA should be reserved for infants who have failed conservative medical or pharmacological therapy, and are ventilator dependent, show signs of LV overload or poor organ perfusion or has contraindication for medical therapy. Surgical closure of hsPDA is associated with both short term and long term adverse effects, including neurosensory impairment. Since the publication of the book advances in device closure of PDA in premature infants have occurred and is now one the options to address PDAs in premature babies.

In Chapter 40, Dr. Hines from UT Health in Houston reviewed video-thoracoscopic ductal closure in the premature and newborn. He states that appropriate management of the neonate with a PDA requires a complete understanding of the ongoing physiology of ductal shunting in neonates, and the balance of systemic and pulmonary vascular resistance that determine the shunt, along with the help of echocardiography and pediatric cardiologists to determine the significance of a particular PDA based on size, velocity (gradient) and direction of flow, as well as the presence of absence of signs of left sided volume overload associated with a "significant" left-to-right shunt across a PDA. Similarly, careful analysis of the risks and benefits of attempted pharmacologic closure, open surgical closure and closure with the video assisted thoracoscopic surgical (VATS) technique will help provide each neonate with the best clinical care and long term outcome. While not yet widely applied, the VATS technique for PDA closure has been documented to be safe and to be applicable to the vast majority of patients including extremely low birth weight down to 420 grams. Documented advantages include smaller incisions, less recurrent nerve injury, no chest tube requirement, less pain medication requirement, with equal efficacy (essentially 100 percent closure).

In Chapter 41, I reviewed other acyanotic heart defects, not discussed in the preceding chapters. Severe cyanotic CHDs generally present in the neonatal period, while acyanotic CHD rarely show symptoms in the neonatal period; the latter were reviewed briefly in this chapter. Brief description of the anatomy of the defect, clinical presentation, laboratory findings and management of acyanotic obstructive lesions (valvar PS, critical PS, branch pulmonary artery stenosis, AS, critical AS) and left-to-right shunt lesions (ASDs [ostium secundum, ostium primum, sinus venosus and coronary sinus], PFO, VSD, PDA, and AV septal defect) were presented.

In Chapter 42, Dr. Moulik from UT Houston Medical School reviews neonatal cardiomyopathies. She states that cardiomyopathies are primary disorders of the myocardium resulting in ventricular chamber enlargement and/or hypertrophy in the absence of an identifiable hemodynamic cause and are usually associated with myocardial systolic and/or diastolic dysfunction. Dilated cardiomyopathy and hypertrophic cardiomyopathy are the two most common phenotypes of neonatal cardiomyopathies. The underlying etiologic causes of neonatal cardiomyopathies are varied with a multitude of genetic, metabolic and acquired etiologies. Many neonatal cardiomyopathies have a poor prognosis with cause dependent outcome. A thorough diagnostic evaluation of neonatal cardiomyopathies requires a consistent, multidisciplinary approach and best done at a center with advanced laboratory techniques and sub-specialty support.

In Chapter 43, Eghonghon and Gupta-Malhotra from UT Houston Medical School reviewed systemic hypertension in the premature and the neonate. Neonatal hypertension is commonly diagnosed on routine blood pressure measurements, and majority are due to secondary causes including iatrogenic or perinatal risk factors. Management should be tailored to the specific underlying cause and degree of elevation of the blood pressure. Adequate monitoring and follow-up should be implemented to avoid the risk of end-organ damage.

Management of neonate with critical heart disease entails early recognition and confirmation of diagnosis. Early stabilization, using a combination of fluid infusions, inotropes and/or ino-dilators, ventilation, either spontaneous or artificial and treatment of any concomitant pulmonary disease. After initial stabilization, while on Prostaglandins, changes that are part of transitional circulation in a newborn will require close follow up of hemodynamics. Balancing pulmonary blood flow (PBF) vs. systemic blood flow (SBF) is important. Since the tendency is towards, pulmonary over-circulation with progressive decrease in pulmonary vascular resistance (PVR), controlling PBF and thus, maintaining adequate SBF becomes the main task. Clinical and laboratory parameters are used to follow adequacy of the balance between PBF and SBF. Since surgery may be necessary within hours when such medical management fails with uncontrollable PBF, baby should be transferred to a surgical center, while these management strategies are being addressed. Feeding babies while on Prostaglandin infusion, awaiting surgery, remain controversial due to increased incidence of NEC. However, enteral feeding is generally considered beneficial when optimal conditions exist. Recent advances in medical and surgical therapy, particularly the application of the "Fontan" principle, have markedly improved the long-term outlook of these children. Palliative procedures to normalize the pulmonary blood flow (BT or similar aorta-pulmonary shunt for patients with pulmonary oligemia and pulmonary artery banding for patients with pulmonary plethora) and to relieve interatrial and/or inter-ventricular obstruction should be undertaken promptly. Norwood procedure is required for patients with HLHS. Staged total cavo-pulmonary connection (modified Fontan) to bypass the right atrium and right ventricle by bi-directional Glenn procedure initially followed by extracardiac conduit diversion of inferior vena caval flow into the PAs appears to be the current procedure of choice in the surgical management of single ventricle lesions.

This book, I hope, will give a fund of information to the physicians taking care of babies with suspected or known cardiac disease, which may help them provide better care for their babies.

Book reviews published in *Neonatology Today* and *Congenital Cardiology Today* is shown in figure 19.

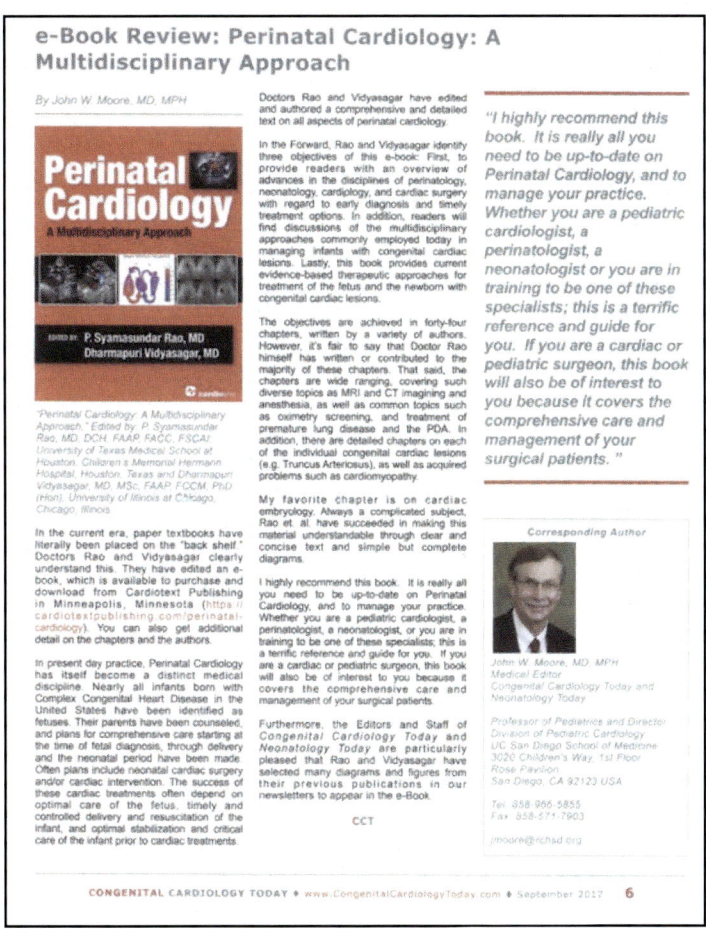

Figure 19. Book review of "Perinatal Cardiology: A Multidisciplinary Approach," published in *Congenital Cardiology Today.*

SEMINARS/SYMPOSIA

I organized and edited several seminars/symposia for a number of journals, which are listed in Table II. Each of these were requested by the Chief Editors of the respective journals; the topics selected largely dependent on the audience of that particular journal. The interested reader may find these papers as listed in Table II.

Table II. Seminars and Symposia That I Edited

1. Rao PS and Linde LM (Guest Editors), "Seminar on Pediatric Cardiology," *Paediatrician*, Vol. 2, No. 5-6, 1973, S. Kargar, Basel, Switzerland.
2. Rao PS (Guest Editor), "Seminar on Pediatric Cardiology," *Paediatrician*, Vol. 4, No. 5-6, 1975, S. Kargar, Basel, Switzerland.
3. Rao PS (Guest Editor), "Seminar on Pediatric Cardiology," *Paediatrician*, Vol. 7, No. 1-3, 1978.
4. Rao PS (Guest Editor), "Pediatric Cardiology Seminar," *Indian Journal of Pediatrics*, Volume 55, No. 1, January-February 1988.
5. Rao PS (Guest Editor), "Pediatric Cardiology Seminar," *Indian Journal of Pediatrics*, Volume 58, No. 485, 1991.
6. Rao PS (Guest Editor), "Cardiac interventions in the pediatric patient," *Journal of Invasive Cardiology*, Vol. 8, No. 7, September 1996.
7. Rao PS, Saxena A (Guest Editors), "Pediatric Cardiology Symposium – Part I," *Indian Journal of Pediatrics*, Vol. 65, No. 1, January-February 1998.
8. Rao PS, Saxena A (Guest Editors), "Pediatric Cardiology Symposium – Part II," *Indian Journal of Pediatrics*, Vol. 65, No. 2, March-April 1998.
9. Saxena A, Rao PS (Guest Editors), "Symposium on Pediatric Cardiology – Part I," *Indian Journal of Pediatrics*, Vol. 69, No. 4, April 2002.
10. Saxena A, Rao PS (Guest Editors), "Symposium on Pediatric Cardiology – Part II," *Indian Journal of Pediatrics*, Vol. 69, No. 5, May 2002.
11. Saxena A, Rao PS (Editors), "Advances in Pediatrics – 1: Cardiology," *Indian Journal of Pediatrics*, New Delhi, India, 2005
12. Balaguru D, Rao PS (Editors), "Special issue: Pediatric Interventional Cardiac Catheterization," *Pediatr Therapeut 2012*, OMICS Publishing Group.
13.13. Rao PS (Guest Editor), "Special issue: Congenital Heart Disease: Recent Advances in the Diagnosis and Management," *Children* 2019 (ISSN 2227-9067), Vol. 6. Available at https://doi.org/10.3390.

BOOK CHAPTERS

I contributed more than 150 chapters to several books over the years; again these chapters were requested by the editors of the respective books The photographs of most of the books in which the chapters appeared are shown in figures 20 and 21.

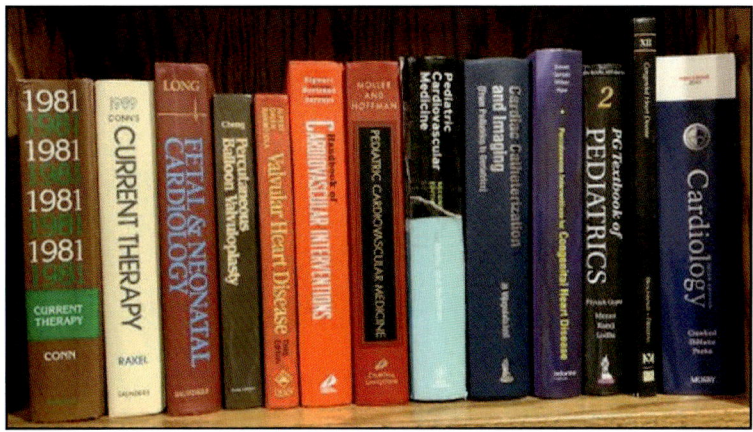

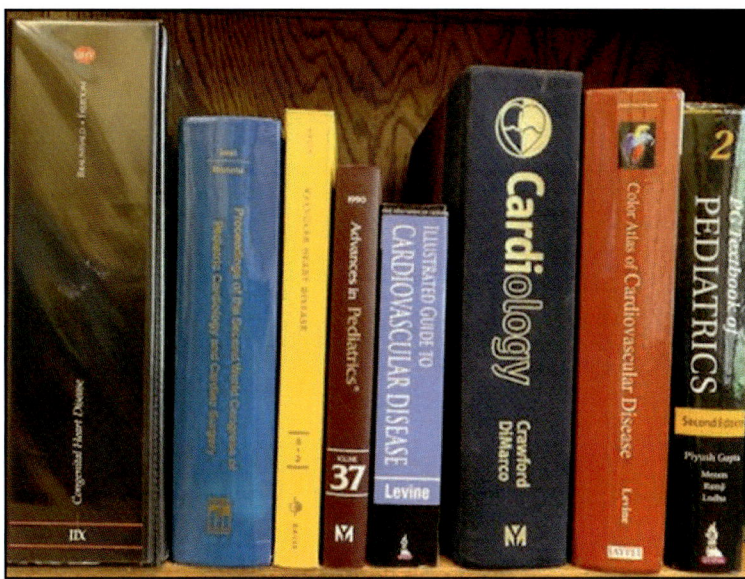

Figures 20 and 21. Photographs of most of the books in which the chapters that I contributed appeared.

The book chapters are listed in Table III for the interested reader.

Table III. Book Chapters I Contributed

1. Rao PS and Strong WB, "Congenital Heart Disease," In: Current Therapy 1981, Conn HF (ed), *W.B. Saunders*, Philadelphia PA, pp. 185-209.

2. Rao PS, "Terminology - Tricuspid Atresia or Univentricular Heart – Chapter 1," In. Rao PS, Tricuspid Atresia, *Futura Publishing Co. 1982,* Mount Kisco, New York.

3. Rao PS, "Demographic Features of Tricuspid Atresia - Chapter 3," In. Rao PS (ed.), Tricuspid Atresia, *Futura Publishing Co. 1982*, Mount Kisco, New York.

4. Rao PS, "Classification of Tricuspid Atresia - Chapter 5," In. Rao PS (ed.), In. Tricuspid Atresia, *Futura Publishing Co. 1982*, Mount Kisco, New York.

5. Kulangara RJ, Boineau JP and Rao PS, "Electrovectorcardiographic Features of Tricuspid Atresia - Chapter 9," In. Rao PS (ed.), Tricuspid Atresia, *Futura Publishing Co. 1982*, Mount Kisco, New York.

6. Covitz W and Rao PS, "Non-invasive Evaluation of Patients with Tricuspid Atresia (Roentgenography, Echocardiography, and Nuclear Angiography) - Chapter 10," In. Rao PS (ed.), Tricuspid Atresia, *Futura Publishing Co. 1982*, Mount Kisco, New York.

7. Alpert BS and Rao PS, "Exercise Electrocardiography in Tricuspid Atresia - Supplement to Chapter 10," In. Rao PS (ed.), Tricuspid Atresia, *Futura Publishing Co. 1982*, Mount Kisco, New York.

8. Rao PS, "Cardiac Catheterization in Tricuspid Atresia - Chapter 11," In. Rao PS (ed.), Tricuspid Atresia, *Futura Publishing Co. 1982*, Mount Kisco, New York.

9. Alpert BS and Rao PS, "Ventricular Function in Tricuspid Atresia - Chapter 13," In. Rao PS (ed.), Tricuspid Atresia, *Futura Publishing Co. 1982*, Mount Kisco, New York.

10. Rao PS, "Natural History of the Ventricular Septal Defect in Tricuspid Atresia - Chapter 14," In. Rao PS (ed.), Tricuspid Atresia, *Futura Publishing Co. 1982*, Mount Kisco, New York.

11. Rao PS, Covitz W, and Moore HV, "Principles of Palliative Management of Patients with Tricuspid Atresia - Chapter 15," In. Rao PS (ed.), Tricuspid Atresia, *Futura Publishing Co. 1982*, Mount Kisco, New York.

12. Rao PS, "Conclusions and Future Directions - Chapter 21," In. Rao PS (ed.), Tricuspid Atresia, *Futura Publishing Co. 1982*, Mount Kisco, New York.

13. Rao PS, "Current Management of Pulmonary Stenosis and Atresia with Intact Ventricular Septum," In: Heart Disease in Neonates and Children, Al Fagih, MR (ed.), *The Medicine Group 1985*, Oxford, England, pp. 109-120.

14. Rao PS, "Doppler Echocardiography in Non-invasive Diagnosis of Congenital Heart disease," In: Current Trends in Pediatrics, Singh M. (ed.), *Vanity Books 1986*; New Delhi, India, pp. 106-144.

15. Rao PS, "Congenital Heart Disease," In: Conn's Current Therapy, 1989 Rakel RE (ed.), *W.B. Saunders 1989*, Philadelphia, PA, pp. 201-213.

16. Rao PS, "Tricuspid Atresia," In: Fetal and Neonatal Cardiology, Long, WA (ed.), *W.B. Saunders 1990*, Philadelphia, PA, pp. 525-540.

17. Rao PS, "Tricuspid Valve Abnormalities Other Than Tricuspid Atresia," In: Fetal and Neonatal Cardiology, Long, WA (ed.), *W.B. Saunders 1990*, Philadelphia, PA, pp. 541-550.

18. Rao PS, "Balloon Valvuloplasty and Angioplasty of Stenotic Lesions of the Heart and Great Vessels in Children," In: Advances in Pediatrics, Barness LA; DeVivo DC, Morrow G, III, Oski F, Rudolph AM (eds.), *Year Book Medical Publishers, Inc., 1990*, Chicago, IL Vol. 37, pp. 33-76.

19. Rao PS, "Percutaneous Balloon Valvuloplasty/Angioplasty in Congenital Heart Disease," In: Percutaneous Valvuloplasty and Related Techniques, Bashore TM and Davidson CT (eds.), *Williams & Wilkins 1990*, Baltimore, MD, pp. 251-277.

20. Rao PS, "Terminology: Is Tricuspid Atresia the Correct Term to Use? Chapter 1," In. Rao PS (ed.), Tricuspid Atresia, 2nd edn., *Futura Publishing Co. 1992,* Mt. Kisco, NY.

21. Rao PS, "Demographic Features of Tricuspid Atresia - Chapter 3," In. Rao PS (ed.), Tricuspid Atresia, 2nd edn., *Futura Publishing Co. 1992*, Mt. Kisco, NY.

22. Rao PS, "Classification of tricuspid Atresia - Chapter 5," In. Rao PS (ed.), Tricuspid Atresia, 2nd edn., *Futura Publishing Co. 1992*, Mt. Kisco, NY.

23. Rao PS, Kulangara RJ, Boineau JP and Moore HV, "Electrovectorcardiographic Features of Tricuspid Atresia - Chapter 9," In. Rao PS (ed.), Tricuspid Atresia, 2nd edn., *Futura Publishing Co. 1992*, Mt. Kisco, NY.

24. Covitz W and Rao PS, "Non-invasive Evaluation of Patients with Tricuspid Atresia (Roentgenography, Echocardiography, and Nuclear Angiography) - Chapter 10," In. Rao PS (ed.), Tricuspid Atresia, 2nd edn., *Futura Publishing Co. 1992*, Mt. Kisco, NY.

25. Rao PS, "Cardiac Catheterization in Tricuspid Atresia - Chapter 12," In. Rao PS (ed.), Tricuspid Atresia, 2nd edn, *Futura Publishing Co. 1992*, Mt. Kisco, NY.

26. Schwartz and Rao PS, "Angiography in Tricuspid Atresia - Chapter 13," In. Rao PS (ed.), Tricuspid Atresia, 2nd edn., *Futura Publishing Co. 1992,* Mt. Kisco, NY.

27. Rao PS, Alpert BS, Covitz W, "Left Ventricular Function in Tricuspid Atresia - Chapter 14," In. Rao PS (ed.), Tricuspid Atresia, 2nd edn., *Futura Publishing Co. 1992*, Mt. Kisco, NY.

28. Rao PS, "Natural History of the Ventricular Septal Defects in Tricuspid Atresia - Chapter 15," In. Rao PS (ed.), Tricuspid Atresia, 2nd edn., *Futura Publishing Co. 1992,* Mt. Kisco, NY.

29. Rao PS, Covitz W, and Chopra PS, "Principles of Palliative Management of Patients with Tricuspid Atresia - Chapter 16," In. Rao PS (ed.), Tricuspid Atresia, 2nd edn., Futura Publishing Co. 1992, Mt. Kisco, NY.

30. Rao PS and Chopra PS, "Modification of Fontan-Kreutzer Procedures for Tricuspid Atresia: Can a Choice be Made? Chapter 19," In. Rao PS (ed.), Tricuspid Atresia, 2nd edn., Futura Publishing Co. 1992, Mt. Kisco, NY.

31. Strong WB, Morera JA and Rao PS, "Sexuality, Contraception, and Pregnancy in Patients with Cyanotic Congenital Heart Disease with Special Reference to Tricuspid Atresia - Chapter 23," In. Rao PS (ed.), Tricuspid Atresia, 2nd edn., Futura Publishing Co. 1992, Mt. Kisco, NY.

32. Rao PS, "Conclusions and Future Directions - Chapter 25," In. Rao PS (ed.), Tricuspid Atresia, 2nd edn., Futura Publishing Co. 1992, Mt. Kisco, NY.

33. Rao PS, "Percutaneous Balloon Pulmonary Valvuloplasty," In: Percutaneous Balloon Valvuloplasty, Cheng T, (ed.) *Igaku-Shion Med Publishers 1992*, New York, pp. 365-420.

34. Rao PS, "Historical Aspects of Therapeutic Catheterization - Chapter 1," In. Rao PS (ed.), Transcatheter Therapy in Pediatric Cardiology, *Wiley-Liss, Inc., 1993*, New York.

35. Rao PS, "Technique of Balloon Valvuloplasty/Angioplasty - Chapter 4," In. Rao PS (ed.), Transcatheter Therapy in Pediatric Cardiology, *Wiley-Liss, Inc., 1993*, New York.

36. Thapar MK, Rao PS, "Mechanism of Balloon Valvuloplasty/Angioplasty - Chapter 5," In. Rao PS (ed.), Transcatheter Therapy in Pediatric Cardiology, *Wiley-Liss, Inc., 1993*, New York.

37. Rao PS, "Balloon Pulmonary Valvuloplasty for Isolated Pulmonic Stenosis - Chapter 6," In. Rao PS (ed.), Transcatheter Therapy in Pediatric Cardiology, *Wiley-Liss, Inc., 1993*, New York.

38. Rao PS, "Balloon Valvuloplasty for Aortic Stenosis - Chapter 7," In. Rao PS (ed.), Transcatheter Therapy in Pediatric Cardiology, *Wiley-Liss, Inc., 1993*, New York.

39. Rao PS, "Balloon Angioplasty of Native Aortic Coarctation - Chapter 10," In. Rao PS (ed.), Transcatheter Therapy in Pediatric Cardiology, *Wiley-Liss, Inc., 1993*, New York.

40. Rao PS, "Balloon Angioplasty of Aortic Recoarctation Following Previous Surgery - Chapter 11," In. Rao PS (ed.), Transcatheter Therapy in Pediatric Cardiology, *Wiley-Liss, Inc., 1993*, New York.

41. Rao PS, "Role of Balloon Dilatation and Other Transcatheter Methods in the Treatment of Cyanotic Congenital Heart Defects - Chapter 13," In. Rao PS (ed.), Transcatheter Therapy in Pediatric Cardiology, *Wiley-Liss, Inc., 1993*, New York.

42. Rao PS, "Balloon Dilatation of Stenotic Bioprosthetic Valves - Chapter 14," In. Rao PS (ed.), Transcatheter Therapy in Pediatric Cardiology, *Wiley-Liss, Inc., 1993*, New York.

43. Rao PS, Thapar MK, "Balloon Dilatation of Other Congenital and Acquired Stenotic Lesions of the Cardiovascular System - Chapter 15," In. Rao PS (ed.), Transcatheter Therapy in Pediatric Cardiology, *Wiley-Liss, Inc., 1993*, New York.

44. Rao PS, Sideris EB, "Transcatheter Closure of Heart Defects: Role of 'Buttoned' Devices. Chapter 18," In. Rao PS (ed.), Transcatheter Therapy in Pediatric Cardiology, *Wiley-Liss, Inc., 1993*, New York.

45. Rao PS, "Transcatheter Retrieval of Intravascular/Intracardiac Foreign Bodies - Chapter 20," In. Rao PS (ed.), Transcatheter Therapy in Pediatric Cardiology, *Wiley-Liss, Inc., 1993*, New York.

46. Rao PS, "Balloon Valvuloplasty/Angioplasty: International Experience - Chapter 22," In. Rao PS (ed.), Transcatheter Therapy in Pediatric Cardiology, *Wiley-Liss, Inc., 1993*, New York.

47. Rao PS, "Conclusions and Future Directions - Chapter 23," In. Rao PS (ed.), Transcatheter Therapy in Pediatric Cardiology, *Wiley-Liss, Inc., 1993*, New York.

48. Wilson AD and Rao PS, "Embryology - Chapter 1," In: Cardiac Anesthesia for Infants and Children, Kambam J (ed.), *Mosby-Year Book 1994*, St. Louis, MO, pp. 1-9.

49. Rao PS, "Fetal and Neonatal Circulation – Chapter 2," In: Cardiac Anesthesia for Infants and Children, Kambam J (ed.), *Mosby-Year Book 1994*, St. Louis, MO, pp. 10-19.

50. Rao PS, Striepe V and Kambam J, "Hypoplastic Left Heart Syndrome – Chapter 27," In: Cardiac Anesthesia for Infants and Children, Kambam J (ed.), *Mosby-Year Book 1994*, St. Louis, MO, pp. 296-309.

51. Buck SH, Rao PS and Kambam J, "Double Outlet Right Ventricle – Chapter 28," In: Cardiac Anesthesia for Infants and Children, Kambam J (ed.), *Mosby-Year Book 1994*, St. Louis, MO, pp. 310-319.

52. Rao PS and Kambam J, "Ebstein's Malformation of the Tricuspid Valve – Chapter 29," In: Cardiac Anesthesia for Infants and Children, Kambam J (ed.), *Mosby-Year Book 1994*, St. Louis, MO, pp. 320-332.

53. Kambam J and Rao PS, "Mitral Valve Prolapse Syndrome (Barlow's Syndrome) – Chapter 31," In: Cardiac Anesthesia for Infants and Children, Kambam J (ed.), *Mosby-Year Book 1994*, St. Louis, MO, pp. 354-360.

54. Kambam J and Rao PS, "Anomalous Origin of the Left Coronary Artery (Bland-White-Garland Syndrome) – Chapter 32," In: Cardiac Anesthesia for Infants and Children, Kambam J (ed.), *Mosby-Year Book 1994*, St. Louis, MO, pp. 361-367.

55. Rao PS. Coarctation of the aorta, In: Secondary Forms of Hypertension, Ram CVS (ed.), Seminars in Nephrology, Kurtzman NA (ed.), *W.B. Saunders 1995*, Philadelphia, PA 15(2):81-105.

56. Rao PS, "Pulmonary Valve in Children," In: Handbook of Cardiovascular Interventions, Bertrand M, Serruys P, Sigwart U (eds.), *Churchill Livingstone 1996*, London, pp. 273-310.

57. Rao PS, "Aortic Coarctation," In: Handbook of Cardiovascular Interventions, Bertrand M, Serreys P, Sigwart U (eds.), *Churchill Livingston 1996*, London, pp. 757-781.

58. Rao PS, "Tricuspid atresia: Anatomy, imaging and Natural history," In: Atlas of Heart Disease: Congenital Heart Disease, Freedom R (ed.), *Current Medicine 1997*, Philadelphia, PA, pp. 14.0-14.4.

59. Rao PS, Sideris EB, Rey C, et al, "Echo-Doppler Follow-up Evaluation after Transcatheter Occlusion of Atrial Septal Defects with the Buttoned Device," In: Proceedings of the Second World Congress of Pediatric Cardiology and Cardiac Surgery, Imai Y, Momma K (eds.), *Futura Publishing Co. 1998*, Armonk, NY, pp. 197-203.

60. Zamora R, Rao PS, Lloyd TR, Beekman RH, III, Sideris EB, "Long-term Results of Phase I FDA Trials of buttoned Device Occlusion of Atrial Septal Defects," In: Proceedings of the Second World Congress of Pediatric Cardiology and Cardiac Surgery, Imai Y, Momma K (eds.), *Futura Publishing Co. 1998*, Armonk, NY, pp. 497-499.

61. Rao PS, "Pulmonary Valve Disease," In: Valvular Heart Disease, 3rd edn., Alpert JS, Dalen JE, Rahimtoola S (eds.), *Lippincott Raven 2000*, Philadelphia, PA, pp. 339-376.

62. Rao PS, "Tricuspid Atresia," In: Pediatric Cardiovascular Medicine, Moller JH, Hoffman JIE (eds.), *Churchill Livingstone 2000*, New York, NY, pp. 421-441.

63. Singh GK, Rao PS, "Left Heart Outflow Obstructions," In: Cardiology, Crawford MH, DiMarco JP (eds.), *Mosby International 2001*, London, pp. 7-11.1 to 7-11.9.

64. Rao PS, "Non-Coronary Uses of Stents in Children and Adults," In: Cardiology Update, 2002, Gambhir DS (ed.), *Cardiological Society of India 2002*, New Delhi, pp. 268-282.

65. Rao PS, "Pediatric Cardiology – a Quarter Century of Progress," In: Hridaya Sangamam – Souvenir – 2002. Manjuran RJ (ed.), *CSI Kerala Chapter 2002*, Kochi, Kerala, pp. 43-48.

66. Rao PS, "History of Atrial Septal Occlusion Devices - Chapter 1," In. Rao PS, Kern MJ. (eds.), Catheter Based Devices for Treatment of Noncoronary Cardiovascular Disease in Adults and Children, Lippincott, *Williams & Wilkins 2003*, Philadelphia, PA.

67. Rao PS, "Buttoned Device - Chapter 3," In. Rao PS, Kern MJ. (eds.), Catheter Based Devices for Treatment of Noncoronary Cardiovascular Disease in Adults and Children. Lippincott, *Williams & Wilkins 2003*, Philadelphia, PA.

68. Rao PS, "Comparative Summary of Atrial Septal Defect Occlusion Devices - Chapter 11," In. Rao PS, Kern MJ (eds.), Catheter Based Devices for Treatment of Noncoronary Cardiovascular Disease in Adults and Children, Lippincott, *Williams & Wilkins 2003*, Philadelphia, PA.

69. Rao PS, "Transcatheter Closure of Atrial Septal Defects with Right-to-left Shunt - Chapter 14," In. Rao PS, Kern MJ (eds.) Catheter Based Devices for Treatment of Noncoronary Cardiovascular Disease in Adults and Children, Lippincott, *Williams & Wilkins 2003*, Philadelphia, PA.

70. Bitar S, Rao PS, "Platypnea-Orthodeoxia Syndrome: Transcatheter Management - Chapter 15," In. Rao PS, Kern MJ. (eds.), Catheter Based Devices for Treatment of Noncoronary Cardiovascular Disease in Adults and Children, Lippincott, *Williams & Wilkins 2003*, Philadelphia, PA.

71. Rao PS, "History of Transcatheter Patent Ductus Arteriosus Closure Devices - Chapter 17," In. Rao PS, Kern MJ (eds.) Catheter Based Devices for Treatment of Noncoronary Cardiovascular Disease in Adults and Children, Lippincott, *Williams & Wilkins 2003*, Philadelphia, PA.

72. Rao PS, "Buttoned Device - Chapter 19," In. Rao PS, Kern MJ. (eds.), Catheter Based Devices for Treatment of Noncoronary Cardiovascular Disease in Adults and Children. Lippincott, *Williams & Wilkins 2003*, Philadelphia, PA.

73. Rao PS, "Summary and Comparison of Patent Ductus Arteriosus Closure Methods - Chapter 25," In. Rao PS, Kern MJ (eds.), Catheter Based Devices for Treatment of Noncoronary Cardiovascular Disease in Adults and Children, Lippincott, *Williams & Wilkins 2003*, Philadelphia, PA.

74. Rao PS, "Newer Stents in the Management of Vascular Stenoses in Children - Chapter 39," In. Rao PS, Kern MJ (eds.), Catheter Based Devices for Treatment of Noncoronary Cardiovascular Disease in Adults and Children, Lippincott, *Williams & Wilkins 2003*, Philadelphia, PA.

75. Rao PS, "Transcatheter Embolization of Unwanted Blood Vessels in Children - Chapter 45," In. Rao PS, Kern MJ (eds.), Catheter Based Devices for Treatment of Noncoronary Cardiovascular Disease in Adults and Children, Lippincott, *Williams & Wilkins 2003*, Philadelphia, PA.

76. Rao PS, "New and Miscellaneous Devices - Chapter 51," In. Rao PS, Kern MJ (eds.), Catheter Based Devices for Treatment of Noncoronary Cardiovascular Disease in Adults and Children, Lippincott, *Williams & Wilkins 2003*, Philadelphia, PA.

77. Kern MJ, Rao PS. Summary and Future Directions, Chapter 53. In. Rao PS, Kern MJ. (editors) Catheter Based Devices for Treatment of Noncoronary Cardiovascular Disease in Adults and Children. Lippincott, Williams & Wilkins, Philadelphia, PA, 2003.

78. Singh GK, Rao PS, "Left Heart Outflow Obstructions," In: Cardiology, 2nd edn., Crawford MH, DiMarco JP, Paulus WJ (eds.), *Mosby International 2004*, Edinburgh, pp. 1317-1326.

79. Gupta ML, Lantin-Hermosa MR, Rao PS, "What is New in Pediatric Cardiology?" In. Saxena A, Rao PS (eds.), Advances in Pediatrics – 1: Cardiology, *Indian Journal of Pediatrics 2005*, New Delhi, India, pp. 10-26.

80. Rao PS, Gupta ML, Balaji S, "Recent Advances in Pediatric Cardiology – Electrophysiology, Transcatheter and Surgical Advances," In. Saxena A, Rao PS (eds.), Advances in Pediatrics – 1: Cardiology, *Indian Journal of Pediatrics 2005*, New Delhi, India, pp. 27-39.

81. Rao PS, "Diagnosis and Management of Acyanotic Heart Disease: Part I - Obstructive Lesions," In. Rao PS, Saxena A (eds.), Recent Advances in Pediatric Cardiology, *Indian Journal of Pediatrics 2005*, New Delhi, India, pp. 1-16.

82. Rao PS, "Diagnosis and Management of Acyanotic Heart Disease: Part II - Left-to-right Shunt Lesions," In. Rao PS, Saxena A (eds.), Recent Advances in Pediatric Cardiology, *Indian Journal of Pediatrics 2005*, New Delhi, India, pp. 17-36.

83. Gupta-Malhotra M, Rao PS, "Current Perspectives on Kawasaki Disease," In. Rao PS, Saxena A (eds.), Recent Advances in Pediatric Cardiology, *Indian Journal of Pediatrics 2005*, New Delhi, India, pp. 99-116

84. Rao PS, Sharma SK, "Management of Patent Ductus Arteriosus with Particular Attention to Transcatheter Therapy," In. Rao PS, Saxena A (eds.), Recent Advances in Pediatric Cardiology, *Indian Journal of Pediatrics 2005*, New Delhi, India, pp. 125-139.

85. Gupta ML, Lantin-Hermoso R, Rao PS, "Recent Advances in Pediatric Cardiology: Part I – Medical Advances," In. Rao PS, Saxena A (eds.), Recent Advances in Pediatric Cardiology, *Indian Journal of Pediatrics 2005,* New Delhi, India, pp. 152-170.

86. Rao PS, Gupta ML, Balaji S, "Recent Advances in Pediatric Cardiology: Part II –Electrophysiology, Transcatheter and Surgical Advances," In. Rao PS, Saxena A (eds.), Recent Advances in Pediatric Cardiology, *Indian Journal of Pediatrics 2005,* New Delhi, India, pp. 171-190.

87. Rao PS, "Pulmonary Valve Stenosis," In: Percutaneous Interventions in Congenital Heart Disease, Sievert H, Qureshi SA, Wilson N, Hijazi Z (eds.), *Informa Health Care 2007*, Oxford, UK, pp. 185-195.

88. Rao PS, "Pulmonary Valve in Cyanotic Heart Defects with Pulmonary Oligemia," In: Percutaneous Interventions in Congenital Heart Disease, Sievert H, Qureshi SA, Wilson N, Hijazi Z (eds.), *Informa Health Care 2007*, Oxford, UK, pp. 197-200.

89. Rao PS, "Coarctation of Aorta," In: Lang F (ed.), Encyclopedia of Molecular Mechanisms of Disease, *Springer-Verlag 2009*, Berlin, Heidelberg, New York, Tokyo. ISBN: 978-3-540-67136-7 (Print), 978-3-540-29676-8 (Online).

90. Sharma SK, Rao PS, "Interrupted Aortic Arch," In: Lang F (ed.), Encyclopedia of Molecular Mechanisms of Disease, *Springer-Verlag 2009*, Berlin, Heidelberg, New York, Tokyo. ISBN: 978-3-540-67136-7 (Print), 978-3-540-29676-8 (Online)

91. Singh GK, Rao PS, "Left heart outflow obstructions," In: Cardiology, 3rd edn., Crawford MH, DiMarco JP, Paulus WJ (eds.), *Mosby Elsevier 2010*, Edinburgh, UK, pp. 1507-1518. ISBN 978-0-7234-3485-6.

92. Rao PS (ed.), Perinatal Cardiology for the Neonatologist, *MHHCS Press*, Houston, TX., April 2011, with the following chapters contributed:

Chapter 1. Rao PS, Perinatal Circulatory Physiology: It's Influence on Clinical Manifestations of Neonatal Heart Disease – Part I.

Chapter 2. Rao PS, Perinatal Circulatory Physiology: It's Influence on Clinical Manifestations of Neonatal Heart Disease – Part II.

Chapter 5. Rao PS, An Approach to the Diagnosis of Cyanotic Neonate for the Primary Care Provider.

Chapter 6. Rao PS, Principles of Management of the Neonate with Congenital Heart Disease.

Chapter 7. Rao PS, Neonatal Cardiac Emergencies: Management Strategies.

Chapter 10. Rao PS, Role of Interventional Cardiology in Neonates: Part I - Non- Surgical Atrial Septostomy.

Chapter 11. Rao PS, Role of Interventional Cardiology in Neonates: Part II – Balloon Angioplasty/ Valvuloplasty

Chapter 12. Rao PS, Role of Interventional Cardiology in the Treatment of Neonates: Part III.

Chapter 14. Rao PS, Transposition of the Great Arteries in the Neonate.

Chapter 15. Alapati S, Rao PS, Tetralogy of Fallot in the Neonate.

Chapter 16. Rao PS, Summary and Conclusions.

93. Preface, In. Rao PS (ed.), Congenital Heart Disease - Selected Aspects, InTech, Rijeka, Croatia, January 2012. ISBN 978-953-307-472-6.

94. "Congenital Heart Defects – A Review, Chapter 1," In. Rao PS (ed.), Congenital Heart Disease - Selected Aspects, InTech, Rijeka, Croatia, January 2012; ISBN 978-953-307-472-6. Available at http:// www.intechopen.com/articles/show/title/congenital-heart-defects-a-review.

95. Preface, In. Rao PS (ed.), Atrial Septal Defect, InTech, Rijeka, Croatia, April 2012; ISBN 978-953-51-0531-2.

96. "Atrial Septal Defect - A Review, Chapter 1," In. Rao PS (ed.), Atrial Septal Defect, InTech, Rijeka, Croatia, April 2012; ISBN 978-953-51-0531-2.

97. "Historical Aspects of Transcatheter Occlusion of Atrial Septal Defects - Chapter 5 In. Rao PS (ed.), Atrial Septal Defect, InTech, Rijeka, Croatia, April 2012; ISBN 978-953-51-0531-2.

98. "Why, When and How Should Atrial Septal Defects Be Closed in Adults - Chapter 8," In. Rao PS (ed.), Atrial Septal Defect, InTech, Rijeka, Croatia, April 2012; ISBN 978-953-51-0531-2. Available at: http:// www.intechopen.com/

99. Rao PS, "Tricuspid Atresia – Chapter 35," In: Pediatric Cardiovascular Medicine, 2nd Edition, Moller JH, Hoffman JIE (eds.), *Wiley-Blackwell/A John Wiley & Sons Ltd. 2012*, Oxford, UK, pp. 487-508.

100. Balaguru D, Rao PS (eds.), "Special issue: Pediatric Interventional Cardiac Catheterization," *Pediatr Therapeut 2012*, OMICS Publishing Group (www.omicsonline.org) with the following papers contributed:

101. Sahu R, Rao PS, "Transcatheter Stent Therapy in Children: An Update," *Pediatr Therapeut 2012*; S5:001. Available at DOI: 10.4172/2161-0665.S5-001.

102. Rao PS, "Historical Aspects of Transcatheter Treatment of Heart Disease in Children," *Pediatr Therapeut 2012*; S5:002. Available at DOI:10.4172/2161-0665.S5-002.

103. Agu NC, Rao PS, "Balloon Aortic Valvuloplasty," *Pediatr Therapeut 2012*; S5:004. Available at DOI: 10.4172/2161-0665.S5-004.

104. Yarrabolu TR, Rao PS, "Transcatheter Closure of Patent Ductus Arteriosus," *Pediatr Therapeut 2012*; S5:005. Available at DOI: 10.4172/2161-0665.S5-005.

105. Doshi AR, Rao PS, "Coarctation of Aorta-Management Options and Decision Making," *Pediatr Therapeut 2012*; S5:006. Available at DOI: 10.4172/2161-0665.S5-006.

106. Rao PS, "Tricuspid Atresia - Chapter 28," In. Vijayalakshmi IB, Rao PS, Chugh R (eds.), A Comprehensive Approach to Management of Congenital Heart Diseases, Jaypee *Publications 2013*, New Delhi, India, pp. 397-413.

107. Balaguru D, Rao PS, "Diseases of the Tricuspid Valve (Ebstein's Anomaly, Tricuspid Stenosis and Regurgitation) - Chapter 29," In. Vijayalakshmi IB, Rao PS, Chugh R (eds.), A Comprehensive Approach to Management of Congenital Heart Diseases, Jaypee *Publications 2013*, New Delhi, India, pp. 414-433.

108. Balaguru D, Rao PS, "Mitral Atresia - Chapter 32," In. Vijayalakshmi IB, Rao PS, Chugh R (eds.), A Comprehensive Approach to Management of Congenital Heart Diseases, Jaypee *Publications 2013*, New Delhi, India, pp. 458-467

109. Balaguru D, Rao PS, "Truncus Arteriosus - Chapter 42," In. Vijayalakshmi IB, Rao PS, Chugh R (eds.), A Comprehensive Approach to Management of Congenital Heart Diseases, Jaypee *Publications 2013*, New Delhi, India, pp. 600-613.

110. Rao PS, Alapati S, "Hypoplastic Left Heart Syndrome - Chapter 47," In. Vijayalakshmi IB, Rao PS, Chugh R (eds.), A Comprehensive Approach to Management of Congenital Heart Diseases, Jaypee *Publications 2013*, New Delhi, India, pp. 662-678.

111. Rao PS, "Pulmonary valve disease: Pulmonary valve stenosis – Chapter 31," In: Sievert H, Qureshi SA, Wilson N, Hijazi Z (eds.), Interventions in Structural, Valvular and Congenital Heart Disease, *CRC Press 2014*, pp. 297-308. Print ISBN: 978-1-4822-1563-2; eBook ISBN: 978-1-4822-1564-9.

112. Rao PS, "Pulmonary valve disease: Pulmonary valve in cyanotic heart defects with pulmonary oligemia – Chapter 33," In: Sievert H, Qureshi SA, Wilson N, Hijazi Z (eds.), Interventions in Structural, Valvular and Congenital Heart Disease, *CRC Press 2014*, pp. 297-308. Print ISBN: 978-1-4822-1563-2; eBook ISBN: 978-1-4822-1564-9.

113. Rao PS, "Non-Surgical Closure of Atrial Septal Defects in Children," In: Atrial and Ventricular Septal Defects: Molecular Determinants, Impact of Environmental Factors and Non-Surgical Interventions, Larkin, SA (ed.), *Nova Science Publishers, Inc.,* ISBN: 978-1-62618-326-1. Available at Softcover: https://www.novapublishers.com/catalog/product_info.php?products_id=37672

Ebook: https://www.novapublishers.com/catalog/product_info.php?products_id=40298
Web: www.novapublishers.com

114. Doshi UH, Rao PS, "Aortic Coarctation – Chapter 46," In: Levine G (ed.), Color Atlas of Cardiovascular Disease, *Jaypee Medical Inc. 2014*, Philadelphia, PA.

115. Rao PS, "What the Adult Cardiologist Should Know About Cyanotic Congenital Heart Disease," In: Chopra HK, et al. (eds.), State of Art CSI Cardiology Update 2014.

116. Rao PS, "Perinatal Circulatory Physiology – Chapter 1," In. Rao PS, Vidyasagar D. (eds.), Perinatal Cardiology: A Multidisciplinary Approach, *Cardiotext Publishing 2015*, Minneapolis, MN.

117. Rao PS, "Role of Perinatal Circulatory Physiology on Clinical Manifestations and Management of Neonatal Heart Disease – Chapter 2," In. Rao PS, Vidyasagar D (eds.), Perinatal Cardiology: A Multidisciplinary Approach, *Cardiotext Publishing 2015*, Minneapolis, MN.

118. Biliciler-Denktas G, Balaguru D, Rao PS, "Embryology of the Heart – Chapter 3," In. Rao PS, Vidyasagar D (eds.), Perinatal Cardiology: A Multidisciplinary Approach, *Cardiotext Publishing 2015*, Minneapolis, MN.

119. Rao PS, "An Approach to the Diagnosis of Cyanotic Neonate for the Primary Care Provider – Chapter 10," In. Rao PS, Vidyasagar D (eds.), Perinatal Cardiology: A Multidisciplinary Approach, *Cardiotext Publishing 2015*, Minneapolis, MN.

120. Rao PS, "Echocardiographic Evaluation of Neonates with Suspected Heart Disease – Chapter 11," In. Rao PS, Vidyasagar D (eds.), Perinatal Cardiology: A Multidisciplinary Approach, *Cardiotext Publishing 2015*, Minneapolis, MN.

121. Rao PS, "Principles of Management of the Neonate with Congenital Heart Disease – Chapter 13," In. Rao PS, Vidyasagar D (eds.), Perinatal Cardiology: A Multidisciplinary Approach, *Cardiotext Publishing 2015*, Minneapolis, MN.

122. Rao PS, "Neonatal Cardiac Emergencies: Management Strategies – Chapter 14 In. Rao PS, Vidyasagar D (eds.), Perinatal Cardiology: A Multidisciplinary Approach, *Cardiotext Publishing 2015*, Minneapolis, MN.

123. Rao PS, "Catheter Interventions in the Neonate: Part I - Non-Surgical Atrial Septostomy – Chapter 19," In. Rao PS, Vidyasagar D (eds.), Perinatal Cardiology: A Multidisciplinary Approach, *Cardiotext Publishing 2015*, Minneapolis, MN.

124. Rao PS, "Catheter Interventions in the Neonate: Part II – Balloon Angioplasty/Valvuloplasty – Chapter 20," In. Rao PS, Vidyasagar D (eds.), Perinatal Cardiology: A Multidisciplinary Approach, *Cardiotext Publishing 2015*, Minneapolis, MN.

125. Rao PS, "Catheter Interventions in the Neonate: Part III – Other Interventions – Chapter 21," In. Rao PS, Vidyasagar D (eds.), Perinatal Cardiology: A Multidisciplinary Approach, *Cardiotext Publishing 2015*, Minneapolis, MN.

126. Rao PS, "Transposition of the Great Arteries – Chapter 28," In. Rao PS, Vidyasagar D (eds.), Perinatal Cardiology: A Multidisciplinary Approach, *Cardiotext Publishing 2015*, Minneapolis, MN.

127. Alapati S, Rao PS, "Tetralogy of Fallot – Chapter 29," In. Rao PS, Vidyasagar D (eds.), Perinatal Cardiology: A Multidisciplinary Approach, *Cardiotext Publishing 2015*, Minneapolis, MN.

128. Rao PS, "Tricuspid Atresia – Chapter 30," In. Rao PS, Vidyasagar D (eds.), Perinatal Cardiology: A Multidisciplinary Approach, *Cardiotext Publishing 2015*, Minneapolis, MN.

129. Rao PS, "Total Anomalous Pulmonary Venous Connection – Chapter 31," In. Rao PS, Vidyasagar D (eds.), Perinatal Cardiology: A Multidisciplinary Approach, *Cardiotext Publishing 2015*, Minneapolis, MN.

130. Balaguru D, Rao PS, "Truncus Arteriosus – Chapter 32," In. Rao PS, Vidyasagar D (eds.), Perinatal Cardiology: A Multidisciplinary Approach, *Cardiotext Publishing 2015*, Minneapolis, MN.

131. Rao PS, Alapati S, "Hypoplastic Left Heart Syndrome – Chapter 33," In. Rao PS, Vidyasagar D (eds.), Perinatal Cardiology: A Multidisciplinary Approach, *Cardiotext Publishing 2015*, Minneapolis, MN.

132. Balaguru D, Rao PS, "Pulmonary Atresia with Intact Ventricular Septum – Chapter 34," In. Rao PS, Vidyasagar D (eds.), Perinatal Cardiology: A Multidisciplinary Approach, *Cardiotext Publishing 2015*, Minneapolis, MN.

133. Balaguru D, Rao PS, "Ebstein's Anomaly of the Tricuspid Valve – Chapter 35," In. Rao PS, Vidyasagar D (eds.), Perinatal Cardiology: A Multidisciplinary Approach, *Cardiotext Publishing 2015*, Minneapolis, MN.

134. Rao PS, "Cardiac Malpositions including Heterotaxy Syndromes – Chapter 36," In. Rao PS, Vidyasagar D (eds.), Perinatal Cardiology: A Multidisciplinary Approach, *Cardiotext Publishing 2015*, Minneapolis, MN.

135. Rao PS, "Other Cyanotic Heart Defects in the Neonate – Chapter 37," In. Rao PS, Vidyasagar D (eds.), Perinatal Cardiology: A Multidisciplinary Approach, *Cardiotext Publishing 2015*, Minneapolis, MN.

136. Rao PS, "Coarctation of the Aorta – Chapter 38," In. Rao PS, Vidyasagar D (eds.), Perinatal Cardiology: A Multidisciplinary Approach, *Cardiotext Publishing 2015*, Minneapolis, MN.

137. Rao PS, "Other Acyanotic Heart Defects – Chapter 41," In. Rao PS, Vidyasagar D (eds.), Perinatal Cardiology: A Multidisciplinary Approach, *Cardiotext Publishing 2015*, Minneapolis, MN.

138. Rao PS, "Summary and Conclusions – Chapter 44," In. Rao PS, Vidyasagar D (eds.), Perinatal Cardiology: A Multidisciplinary Approach, *Cardiotext Publishing 2015*, Minneapolis, MN.

139. Rao PS, "History of Transcatheter Interventions in Pediatric Cardiology," In. Vijayalakshmi IB (ed.), Cardiac Catheterization and Imaging (From Pediatrics to Geriatrics), *Jaypee Publications 2015*, New Delhi, India, pp. 3-20.

140. Rao PS, "Balloon Valvuloplasty for Pulmonary Stenosis," In. Vijayalakshmi IB (ed.), Cardiac Catheterization and Imaging (From Pediatrics to Geriatrics), *Jaypee Publications 2015*, New Delhi, India, pp. 149-174.

141. Rao PS, "Neonatal Catheter Interventions," In. Vijayalakshmi IB (ed.), Cardiac Catheterization and Imaging (From Pediatrics to Geriatrics), *Jaypee Publications 2015*, New Delhi, India, pp. 388-432.

142. Rao PS, "Percutaneous Management of Aortic Coarctation," In. Vijayalakshmi IB (ed.), Cardiac Catheterization and Imaging (From Pediatrics to Geriatrics), *Jaypee Publications 2015*, New Delhi, India, pp. 433-471.

143. Rao PS, "Stents in the Management of Vascular Obstructive Lesions Associated with Congenital Heart Disease," In. Vijayalakshmi IB (ed.), Cardiac Catheterization and Imaging (From Pediatrics to Geriatrics), *Jaypee Publications 2015*, New Delhi, India, pp. 573-598.

144. Rao PS, "Cardiac Malpositions," In: Gupta P, Menon PSN, Ramji S, Lodha R (eds.), PG Textbook of Pediatrics, *Jaypee Brothers Medical Publishers (P) Ltd. 2015*, New Delhi, India, pp.1807-1816.

145. Rao PS, "Tricuspid Atresia," In: Gupta P, Menon PSN, Ramji S, Lodha R (eds.), PG Textbook of Pediatrics, *Jaypee Brothers Medical Publishers (P) Ltd. 2015*, New Delhi, India, pp.1861-1870.

146. Naidu DP, Breinholt JP, III, Rao PS, "Patent ductus arteriosus – Chapter 30B," In. Rajiv PK, Lakshminrusimha S, Vidyasagar D (eds.), Essentials of Neonatal Ventilation, Elsevier 2018, pp. 1-30. ISBN: 978-81-312-4998-7.

147. Beaullieu CC, Lopez SM, Rao PS, "Neonatal limb ischemia due to arterial catheters – Chapter 38B," In. Rajiv PK, Lakshminrusimha S, Vidyasagar D (eds.), Essentials of Neonatal Ventilation, Elsevier 2018, pp. 1-30. ISBN: 978-81-312-4998-7.

148. Rao PS, "Cardiac Malpositions," In: Gupta P, Menon PSN, Ramji S, Lodha R (eds.), PG Textbook of Pediatrics. 2nd edn. *Jaypee Brothers Medical Publishers (P) Ltd. 2018*, New Delhi, India.

149. Rao PS, "Tricuspid Atresia," In: Gupta P, Menon PSN, Ramji S, Lodha R (eds.), PG Textbook of Pediatrics. 2nd edn. *Jaypee Brothers Medical Publishers (P) Ltd. 2018*, New Delhi, India.

150. Rao PS, "Tricuspid Atresia – Chapter 28," In. Vijayalakshmi IB, Rao PS, Chugh R (eds.), A Comprehensive Approach to Management of Congenital Heart Diseases, Jaypee Publications 2019, New Delhi, India.

151. Balaguru D, Rao PS, "Diseases of the Tricuspid Valve (Ebstein's Anomaly, Tricuspid Stenosis and Regurgitation) – Chapter 29," In. Vijayalakshmi IB, Rao PS, Chugh R (eds.), A Comprehensive Approach to Management of Congenital Heart Diseases, Jaypee Publications 2019, New Delhi, India.

152. Balaguru D, Rao PS, "Mitral Atresia – Chapter 32," In. Vijayalakshmi IB, Rao PS, Chugh R (eds.), A Comprehensive Approach to Management of Congenital Heart Diseases, Jaypee Publications 2019, New Delhi, India.

153. Balaguru D, Rao PS, "Truncus Arteriosus - Chapter 42," In. Vijayalakshmi IB, Rao PS, Chugh R (eds.), A Comprehensive Approach to Management of Congenital Heart Diseases, Jaypee Publications 2019, New Delhi, India.

154. Rao PS, Alapati S, "Hypoplastic Left Heart Syndrome – Chapter 47," In. Vijayalakshmi IB, Rao PS, Chugh R (eds.), A Comprehensive Approach to Management of Congenital Heart Diseases, Jaypee Publications 2019, New Delhi, India.

PAPERS IN JOURNALS

As mentioned earlier, my interest in clinical research resulted in publication of more than 390 papers in journals (as first or senior author); photographs of the journals (only the preserved journals) are shown in figures 22 and 23 and collected papers filed in binders are depicted in figure 24.

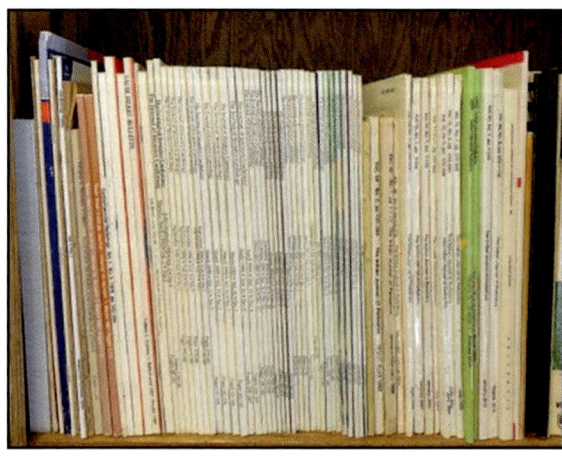

Figures 22 and 23. Photographs of the journals (only the preserved journals) in which my publications appeared.

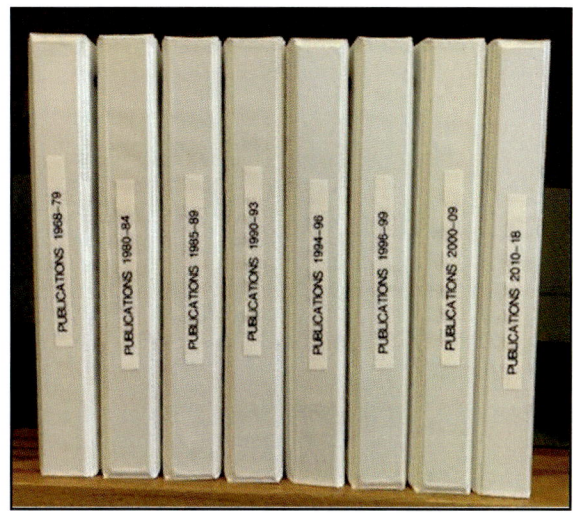

Figures 24. My papers filed in binders.

These papers were referenced in several chapters in this memoir and in the book titled, "Pediatric Cardiology: How It Has Evolved Over the last 50 Years" and will not be reviewed here.

ELECTRONIC PUBLICATIONS

I contributed several electronic publications over the years; again, these were requested by the editors of the respective symposia/publications and are listed in Table IV. The subjects addressed in these electronic publications were reviewed either in the preceding or succeeding chapters in this memoir or in the book titled "Pediatric Cardiology: How It Has Evolved Over the last 50 Years" and will not be reviewed here. The interested reader may however, access them electronically at the indicated website at their discretion.

Table IV. Electronic Publications I Contributed

---

1. Rao PS, "An exchange on septal occlusion devices." http://www.theheart.org/documents/page.cfm?from=590000334&doc_id=204.

2. Rao PS, "Controversy – Aortic Coarctation: Who Should be Dilated? or Operated? First Virtual Congress on Cardiology." http://pcvc.sminter.com.ar/cvirtual

3. Rao PS, "Tricuspid Atresia," In e-medicine – Pediatrics. Available at http://www.emedicine.com

4. Rao PS, "Results of Transvenous Occlusion of Secundum Atrial Septal Defects," Second Virtual Congress on Cardiology. Available at http://www.fac.org.ar/scvc/llave/pediat/rao/raoi.htm

5. Rao PS, "Management of Patent ductus Arteriosus with Emphasis on Transcatheter Therapy." Available at http://www.fac.org.ar/ccvc/llave/c176/rao.php

6. Rao PS, "Faculty of 1000 Medicine: Evaluation of Cowley CG et al. Long-term, randomized comparison of balloon angioplasty and surgery for native coarctation of the aorta in childhood," Circulation 2005; June 28, 111(25):3453-6. Available at http://www.f1000medicine.com/article/id/5019/evaluation

7. Rao PS, "Pulmonary Stenosis," In e-medicine – Pediatrics. Available at http://www.emedicine.com

8. Rao PS, "Hypoplastic left heart Syndrome," In e-medicine – Pediatrics. Available at http://www.emedicine.com

9. Rao PS, "Coarctation of the Aorta," In e-medicine – Pediatrics. Available at http://www.emedicine.com

10. Rao PS, Faculty of 1000 Medicine: Evaluations of Fu YC et al, "Transcatheter closure of perimembranous ventricular septal defects using the new Amplatzer membranous VSD occluder: results of the U.S. Phase I trial," *J Am Coll Cardiol 2006*, January 17, 47(2):319-25. Available at http://www.f1000medicine.com/article/id/13842/evaluation

11. Rao PS, Faculty of 1000 Medicine: Evaluations of Bergersen L et al, "Follow-up results of Cutting Balloon angioplasty used to relieve stenoses in small pulmonary arteries," *Cardiol Young 2005*, December 15, (6):605-10. Available at http://www.f1000medicine.com/article/id/13843/evaluation

12. Rao PS, Faculty of 1000 Medicine: Evaluations of Bartz PJ et al, "Management strategy for very mild aortic valve stenosis," *Pediatr Cardiol 2006*, March-April 27, (2):259-62. Available at http://www.f1000medicine.com/article/id/14150/evaluation

13. Rao PS, "Tricuspid Atresia," eMedicine from WebMD, Updated February 9, 2009. Available at: http://www.emedicine.com/ped/topic2550.htm.

14. Rao PS, Pflieger K. "Pulmonary Stenosis," Valvar, eMedicine from WebMD. Updated July 6, 2009. Available at: http://emedicine.medscape.com/article/891729-overview

15. Rao PS, Seib PM, "Coarctation of the Aorta," eMedicine from WebMD, Updated July 20, 2009. Available at: http://emedicine.medscape.com/article/895502-overview.

16. Rao PS, Turner DR, Forbes TJ, "Hypoplastic Left Heart Syndrome," eMedicine from WebMD, Updated September 22, 2009. Available at: http://emedicine.medscape.com/article/890196-overview

17. Hartas GA, Rao PS, Balaguru D, "Mitral Valve, Double Orifice," eMedicine from WebMD, Updated October 5, 2010. Available at: http://emedicine.medscape.com/article/897322-overview.

18. Rao PS, "Pediatric Tricuspid Atresia," eMedicine from WebMD, Updated October 15, 2011. Available at: http://emedicine.medscape.com/article/900832-overview.

19. Rao PS, Turner DR, Forbes TJ, "Pediatric Hypoplastic Left Heart Syndrome," eMedicine from WebMD, Updated November 10, 2011. Available at: http://emedicine.medscape.com/article/890196-overview.

20. Rao PS, Seib PM, "Coarctation of the Aorta. eMedicine from WebMD," Updated February 1, 2012. Available at: http://emedicine.medscape.com/article/895502-overview.

21. Hartas GA, Rao PS, Balaguru D, "Double Orifice Mitral Valve," eMedicine from WebMD, Updated March 30, 2012. Available at: http://emedicine.medscape.com/article/897322-overview

22. Rao PS, Pflieger K, "Valvar Pulmonary Stenosis," eMedicine from WebMD, Updated June 14, 2012. Available at: http://emedicine.medscape.com/article/891729-overview.

23. Rao PS, Turner DR, Forbes TJ, "Pediatric Hypoplastic Left Heart Syndrome," Medscape Reference, Updated March 22, 2013. Available at: http://emedicine.medscape.com/article/890196-overview.

24. Rao PS, Seib PM, "Coarctation of the Aorta," Medscape Reference, Updated June 10, 2014. Available at: http://emedicine.medscape.com/article/895502-overview.

25. Rao PS, Pflieger K, "Valvar Pulmonary Stenosis," Medscape Reference, Updated June 26, 2014. Available at: http://emedicine.medscape.com/article/891729-overview.

26. Rao PS, "Pediatric Tricuspid Atresia," Medscape Drugs & Diseases, Updated January 5, 2016. Available at: http://emedicine.medscape.com/article/900832-overview.

27. Rao PS, "Pediatric Hypoplastic Left Heart Syndrome," Medscape Drugs & Diseases, Updated January 5, 2016. Available at: http://emedicine.medscape.com/article/890196-overview.

AUDIOVISUAL EDUCATIONAL MATERIAL

I have also participated in preparing audiovisual educational material, which are listed in Table V. The subject material pertaining to "Evaluation of Cyanosis in the Newborn" in the chapter on "Reviews" and will not be repeated. The material related to "Tricuspid Atresia: Anatomy, Imaging and Natural History" may be found in the chapter on "Tricuspid Atresia" in the book titled "Pediatric Cardiology: How It Has Evolved Over the last 50 Years" and will be reviewed here.

Table V. Audiovisual Educational Material that I Participated in Preparing

---

1. Rao PS, Miller MD and Strong WB, "Evaluation of Cyanosis in the Newborn," Distributed by General Services Administration, 1979, Washington, D.C.

2. Rao PS, "Tricuspid Atresia: Anatomy, Imaging and Natural History," In: Slide Atlas of Heart Diseases: Congenital Heart Disease, Volume XII, Freedom RM (ed.), Current Med., Inc., 1997, Philadelphia, PA.

REFERENCES

1. Rao PS, "Preventive aspects of congenital heart disease," *Paediatrician 1973*; 2:224-38.

2. Strong WB, Rao PS, Steinbauch M, "Primary prevention of atherosclerosis: A challenge to the physician caring for children," *Southern Med J 1975*; 68:319-27.

3. Rao PS, "Prevention of pediatric heart disease," *Paediatrician 1975*; 4:320-42.

4. Rao PS, "Preventive aspects of heart disease in infants and children," *South Med J 1977*; 70:728-40.

5. Rao PS, "Prevention of Heart Disease in Infants and Children," Current Problems in Pediatrics, *Yearbook Medical Publisher, Inc.,* May 1977, Chicago, U.S.A., Vol. 7, pp.1-48.

6. Rao PS, Miller EdD, "Medical Examination Review," *Pediatric Cardiology*, Medical Examination Publishing Co. 1980, Inc. New York, U.S.A.

7. Rao PS, "Tricuspid Atresia," Futura Publishing Co. 1982, Kisco, Mount New York.

8. Rao PS, Mardini MK, "Pulmonary valvotomy without thoracotomy: The experience with percutaneous balloon pulmonary valvuloplasty," *Ann Saudi Med 1985*; 5:149-55.

9. Rao PS, "Current management of pulmonary stenosis and atresia with intact ventricular septum," In: Heart Disease in Neonates and Children, Al Fagih, MR (ed.), *The Medicine Group 1985*, Oxford, England, pp. 109-20.

10. Rao PS, Mardini MK and Najjar HN, "Relief of coarctation of the aorta without thoracotomy: The experience with percutaneous balloon angioplasty," *Ann Saudi Med 1986*; 6:193-203.

11. Rao PS, "Transcatheter treatment of pulmonic stenosis and coarctation of the aorta: The experience with percutaneous balloon dilatation," *Brit Heart J 1986*; 56:250-8.

12. Rao PS, "Value of Echo-Doppler studies in the evaluation of the results of balloon pulmonary valvuloplasty," *J Cardiovasc Ultrasonography 1986*; 5:309-14.

13. Rao PS, "Influence of balloon size on short-term and long-term results of balloon pulmonary valvuloplasty," *Texas Heart Institute J 1987*; 14:57-61.

14. Rao PS, "Doppler ultrasound in the prediction of transvalvar pressure gradients in patients with valvar pulmonic stenosis," *International J Cardiol 1987*; 15:195-203.

15. Rao PS, "Balloon angioplasty for coarctation of the aorta in infancy," *J Pediat 1987*; 110:713-8.

16. Rao PS, "How big a balloon and how many balloons for pulmonary valvuloplasty?" (editorial) *Am Heart J 1988*; 116:577-80.

17. Rao PS, Najjar HN, Mardini MK, et al, "Balloon Angioplasty for coarctation of the aorta: Immediate and longterm results," *Am Heart J 1988*; 115:657-65.

18. Rao PS, "Further observations on the effect of balloon size on the short-term and intermediate-term results of balloon dilatation of the pulmonary valve," *Br Heart J 1988*; 60:507–11.

19. Rao PS, Thapar MK and Kutayli F, "Causes of restenosis following balloon valvuloplasty for valvar pulmonic stenosis," *Am J Cardiol 1988*; 62:979-82.

20. Rao PS, Brais M., "Balloon pulmonary valvuloplasty for congenital cyanotic heart defects," *Am Heart J 1988*; 115:1105-10.

21. Rao PS, "Balloon dilatation in infants and children with dysplastic pulmonary valves: Short-term and intermediate-term results," *Am Heart J 1988*; 116:1168-73.

22. Rao PS, Fawzy ME, Solymar L, Mardini MK, "Long-term results of balloon pulmonary valvuloplasty," *Am Heart J 1988*; 115:1291-6.

23. Rao PS, Solymar L, "Transductal balloon angioplasty of coarctation of the aorta in the neonate: Preliminary observations," *Am Heart J 1988*; 116:1558-63.

24. Rao PS and Fawzy ME, "Double balloon technique for percutaneous balloon pulmonary valvuloplasty: Comparison with single balloon technique," *J Interventional Cardiol 1988*; 1:257-62.

25. Rao PS, Solymar L, "Electrocardiographic changes following balloon dilatation of valvar pulmonic stenosis," *J Intervent Cardiol 1988*; 1:189-97.

26. Rao PS, "Value of Echo-Doppler studies in the evaluation of the results of balloon angioplasty of aortic coarctation," *J Cardiovasc Ultrasonography 1988*; 7:215-20.

27. Rao PS, "Balloon angioplasty and valvuloplasty in infants, children and adolescents," *Current Problems in Cardiology*, YearBook Medical Publishers, Inc., 1989, Chicago; 14(8):417-500.

28. Rao PS, "Tricuspid Atresia," 2nd Edition, *Futura Publishing Co. 1992*, Mt. Kisco, NY.

29. Rao PS, "Transcatheter management of heart disease in infants and children," *Pediat Rev Comm 1987*; 1:1-18.

30. Rao PS, "Transcatheter Therapy of Cardiac Defects in Infants and Children," *Indian J Pediatr 1988*; 44:137-140.

31. Rao PS, "Transcatheter treatment of heart disease in infancy and childhood," *Wisconsin Med J 1988*; 87:28-30.

32. Rao PS, "Balloon dilatation in infants and children with cardiac defects," *Cath Cardiovasc Diag 1989*; 18:136-49.

33. Rao PS, "Balloon pulmonary valvuloplasty: A review," *Clin Cardiol 1989*; 12:55-74.

34. Rao PS, "Medical Progress: Balloon valvuloplasty and angioplasty in infants and children," *J Pediat 1989*; 114:907-14.

35. Rao PS, "Balloon angioplasty of aortic coarctation: A review," *Clin Cardiol 1989*; 12:618-28.

36. Rao PS, "Balloon valvuloplasty and angioplasty for congenital and acquired heart defects in children," *Bull Saudi Heart Assoc 1990*; 2:10-22.

37. Rao PS, "Causes of restenosis following balloon angioplasty/valvuloplasty: A review," *Pediatr Rev Comm 1990*; 4:157-72.

38. Rao PS, "Balloon aortic valvuloplasty: A review," *Clinical Cardiol 1990*; 13:458-66.

39. Rao PS, "Balloon valvuloplasty in neonates and children," *Saudi Heart Bulletin 1990*; 1:55-70.

40. Rao PS, "Transcatheter occlusion of cardiac septal defects," *Indian J Pediat 1991*; 58:605-21.

41. Rao PS, "Transcatheter management of cyanotic congenital heart defects: A review," *Clin Cardiol 1992*; 15:483-96.

42. Rao PS, "Transcatheter treatment of pulmonary outflow tract obstruction: A review," *Progress Cardiovasc Dis 1992*; 35:119-158.

43. Rao PS, "Transcatheter Therapy in Pediatric Cardiology," *Wiley-Liss, Inc., 1993*, New York.

44. Rao PS, Kern MJ (eds,), "Catheter Based Devices for Treatment of Noncoronary Cardiovascular Disease in Adults and Children," Lippincott, *Williams & Wilkins 2003*, Philadelphia, PA.

45. Rao PS, "Introduction of Pediatric Cardiology Symposium – I: Pediatric Cardiology," *Indian J Pediatr 2005*, 72:493.

46. Rao PS, Saxena A (eds.), "Recent Advances in Pediatric Cardiology," *Indian Journal of Pediatrics 2005*, New Delhi, India.

47. Rao PS (ed.), "Perinatal Cardiology for The Neonatologist," *MHHCS Press*, April 2011, Houston, TX.

48. Rao PS, Vidyasagar D, (eds.), "Perinatal Cardiology: A Multidisciplinary Approach," *Cardiotext Publishing 2015*, Minneapolis, MN.

49. Rao PS (ed.), "Congenital Heart Disease - Selected Aspects," InTech, Rijeka, Croatia, January 2012; ISBN 978-953-307-472-6.

50. Rao PS (ed.), "Atrial Septal Defect," InTech, Rijeka, Croatia, April 2012; ISBN 978-953-51-0531-2.

51. Vijayalakshmi IB, Rao PS, Chugh R (eds.), "A Comprehensive Approach to Management of Congenital Heart Diseases," *Jaypee Publications 2013*, New Delhi, India.

52. Vijayalakshmi IB, Rao PS, Chugh R (eds.), "A Comprehensive Approach to Management of Congenital Heart Diseases," 2nd edn., *Jaypee Publications 2019*, New Delhi, India.

CHAPTER 11

ADULT CONGENITAL HEART DISEASE

INTRODUCTION

Until recently, the majority of the cardiologists were trained to address coronary artery, myocardial and valvular heart disease without much exposure to congenital heart disease (CHD). Consequently, most cardiologists have developed no interest in addressing CHD; in addition, they are busy in managing coronary artery disease patients. As a result, I was called upon to consult when CHD is suspected in an adult patient beginning my first appointment at the Medical College of Georgia. The same theme continued during my tenure at the University of Wisconsin, St. Louis University, and the University of Texas. In addition, I was involved in performing interventional procedures for non-coronary, congenital heart problems in adults at the last three institutions. In this chapter, I will review my contributions[1-15] to the literature in adult cardiac issues.

INFECTIVE ENDOCARDITIS

A review of fifty consecutive patients with infective endocarditis (IE) seen between 1965 and 1970 at University of California at Los Angeles along with examination of recent developments was presented;[1] this subject was addressed in the section on "Infective Endocarditis" of the chapter on "Reviews" and will not be discussed here.

TRANSCATHETER CLOSURE OF PATENT DUCTUS ARTERIOSUS

I have performed transcatheter closure of patent ductus arteriosus in adults and presented the data in peer-reviewed publications.[2,6] These data were presented in detail in the section on "Buttoned device in Adults" of the chapter on "Patent Ductus Arteriosus" in the book titled, "Pediatric Cardiology: How It Has Evolved Over the last 50 Years" and will not be repeated here.

ECHOCARDIOGRAPHIC EVALUATION OF COARCTATION OF THE AORTA IN ADULTS

In a collaborative review with Dr. Gautam Singh of St. Louis University, echocardiographic evaluation of coarctation of the aorta in adults[5] was discussed. Following a discussion of definition, prevalence, anatomy and associated defects, and pathophysiology of coarctation of the aorta, echocardiographic evaluation was reviewed. Echocardiography is utilized both as a diagnostic and monitoring tool. The morphology of the coarctation segment, severity of obstruction, left ventricular dimensions and function, and associated lesions can be delineated by two-dimensional, pulsed, continuous wave and color Doppler echo studies. Several figures exemplifying the features of coarctation were provided. Advantages of intravascular ultrasound (IVUS) were briefly mentioned. The strengths and pitfalls of the technique were empasized.[5] At the conclusion of the review, ten post-study questions with answer key was also provided.[5]

TRANSCATHETER OCCLUSION OF ATRIAL SEPTAL DEFECT

The results of transcatheter occlusion of atrial septal defects (ASDs) in adults was combined with those of the results in children.[16,23] The results in adult subjects and specific issues related closure of ASDs in adults was reviewed in the section on "ASDs in Adults" of the chapter on "Atrial Septal Defect" in the book titled "Pediatric Cardiology: How It Has Evolved Over the last 50 Years" and will not be repeated here. In addition, issues related to ASD closure in adults was addressed in multiple publications[11-13] for the interested reader.

TRANSCATHETER CLOSURE OF ASD OR PATENT FORAMEN OVALE FOR PREVENTION OF RECURRENCE OF PARADOXIC EMBOLISM

Transcatheter closure of patent foramen ovale (PFO) with the buttoned device for prevention of recurrence of paradoxic embolism was first performed by the author in 1992[24,25] with subsequent reports on larger number of patients.[3,4,16] This subject was reviewed in the sub-section of "PFOs Presumed to be the Seat of Paradoxical Embolism" of the section on "Patent Foramen Ovale" of the chapter on "Atrial Septal Defect" in the book titled "Pediatric Cardiology: How It Has Evolved Over the last 50 Years" and will not be repeated here.

ASDS/PFOS WITH RIGHT-TO-LEFT SHUNT

Adult patients who had prior surgical repair of cyanotic CHDs with residual atrial right-to-left shunts with significant hypoxemia may also be benefited by transcatheter occlusion of their ASDs/PFOs; the results of such studies included both adult and pediatric patients.[26] This issue was reviewed in the subsection of "ASDs/PFOs With Right-To-Left Shunt" of the section on "Patent Foramen Ovale" of the chapter on "Atrial Septal Defect" in the book titled "Pediatric Cardiology: How It Has Evolved Over the last 50 Years" and will not be repeated here.

TRANSCATHETER CLOSURE OF AORTOPULMONARY WINDOW IN AN ADULT

Transcatheter closure with the buttoned device of aortopulmonary window in an adult was reported by me and my associates along with a review of transcatheter occlusion aortopulmonary windows.[7] This was discussed in detail in the section on "Aortopulmonary Window" of the chapter on "Miscellaneous Transcatheter Occlusions" in the book titled "Pediatric Cardiology: How It Has Evolved Over the last 50 Years" and will not be reviewed here.

PLATYPNEA-ORTHODEOXIA SYNDROME: TRANSCATHETER MANAGEMENT

Platypnea-orthodeoxia syndrome (POS) is a rare condition seen in elderly subjects with incapacitating symptoms of dyspnea and arterial desaturation in upright position. Studies on trans-catheter management of POS were published by me and my associates.[8-10] Management of POS was discussed in detail in the section on "Platypnea-Orthodeoxia Syndrome" of the chapter on "Atrial Septal Defects" in the book titled "Pediatric Cardiology: How It Has Evolved Over the last 50 Years" and will not be reviewed here.

WHAT AN ADULT CARDIOLOGIST SHOULD KNOW ABOUT CYANOTIC CHD?

In the past, I have reviewed issues related what an adult cardiologist should know about CHD in adult subjects.[14,15] The prevalence of CHDs in adults has increased during the last two decades such that now there are more adults with CHD than children. On a recent estimate, there were more than one million adults with CHD in the USA alone. Advances in the diagnosis and successful management of CHD appear to be the reason for such a phenomenon. In these review only cyanotic CHD were addressed.[14,15] The majority of these patients are likely to be those that have undergone corrective or palliative surgery, although rarely uncorrected CHD may present for the first time in adulthood. Some patients who had surgical "correction" earlier may have residual abnormalities, which may become significant with time.

Pathophysiologic effects of right-to-left shunt associated with cyanotic CHD were reviewed. Adult patients with uncorrected and palliated cyanotic CHD have intra-cardiac right-to left-shunt with resultant arterial desaturation, cyanosis, clubbing and polycythemia. The latter may in turn cause coagulation abnormalities and symptomatic polycythemia. Other attendant problems are hyperuricemia, gout and uric acid nephropathy. Patients with intra-cardiac right-to-left shunting may also develop brain abscess, cerebrovascular accidents (CVAs) and transient ischemic attacks (TIAs), presumably secondary to paradoxical embolism via the residual atrial or ventricular septal defects.

Brief description of the anatomy of the most common cyanotic CHD, namely, tetralogy of Fallot (TOF), transposition of the great arteries (TGA), truncus arteriosus, total anomalous pulmonary venous connection and tricuspid atresia was presented followed by their management at presentation.

Long-term issues with TOF patient are residual shunts, arrhythmias, residual right ventricular (RV) outflow tract and branch pulmonary artery (PA) obstruction, pulmonary insufficiency, dilated aortic root, and aortic insufficiency. Long-term problems with TGA depend upon the type of surgical correction they had. Patients who had atrial or venous switch (Senning and Mustard) procedures may develop arrhythmias, baffle obstructions, baffle leaks, tricuspid insufficiency and RV dysfunction while those that had arterial switch (Jatene) procedures may have supravalvar aortic stenosis, supravalvar PA and branch PA stenosis, neoaortic dilatation with aortic insufficiency, and coronary artery obstruction. Patients who had Rastelli operation may manifest calcific degeneration of the conduit and valve and develop obstruction of bio-prosthetic RV-to-PA conduits. Left ventricular outflow tract obstruction at the old VSD level may develop in some patients. Patients with truncus arteriosus may in addition develop branch PA stenosis, dilatation of the neo-aorta (old truncus) and neo-aortic valve regurgitation. Patients who had correction of total anomalous pulmonary venous connection may develop obstruction at the site of anastomosis of the common pulmonary vein with the left atrium and pulmonary venous obstruction. Patients who had Fontan correction for tricuspid atresia and other single ventricle defects may develop arrhythmias, obstructed Fontan pathways, cyanosis and CVAs/TIAs, thrombus formation, develop collateral vessels, and protein losing enteropathy. These problems appear to be more frequent with atrio-pulmonary type of Fontan than those who had staged total cavo-pulmonary connection. Diagnosis and management concepts for each of the above were briefly reviewed. Patients who had not previously been corrected may undergo surgical correction, but are likely to have a higher morbidity and mortality than that seen in childhood.[13,14]

REFERENCES

1. Linde LM and Rao PS, "A Modern View of Infective Endocarditis," *Cardiovasc Clinics 1973*, Vol. 5, No. 2:15-34.

2. Lochan R, Rao PS, Samal AK, et al, "Transcatheter closure of patent ductus arteriosus with an adjustable buttoned device in an adult patient," *Am Heart J 1994*; 127:941-3.

3. Rao PS, Ende DJ, Wilson AD, et al, "Follow-up results of transcatheter occlusion of atrial septal defect with buttoned device," *Canad J Cardiol 1995*; 11:695-701.

4. Ende DJ, Chopra PS, Rao PS, "Transcatheter closure of atrial septal defect or patent foramen ovale with the buttoned device for prevention of recurrence of paradoxic embolism," *Am J Cardiol 1996*; 78:233-6.

5. Singh GK, Marino CJ, Rao PS, "Echocardiographic Evaluation of Coarctation of the Aorta in Adults," *Cardiac Ultrasound Today 1977*; 3:111-24.

6. Rao PS, Kim SH, Rey C, et al, "Results of transvenous buttoned device occlusion of patent ductus arteriosus in adults," *Am J Cardiol 1998*; 82:827-9.

7. Jureidini SB, Spadaro JJ, Rao PS, "Successful transcatheter closure with the buttoned device of aortopulmonary window in an adult," *Am J Cardiol 1998*; 81:371-2.

8. Rao PS, Palacios IF, Bach RG, et al, "Platypnea-orthodeoxia syndrome: Management by transcatheter buttoned device implantation," *Cathet Cardiovasc Intervent 2001*; 54:77-82.

9. Bitar S, Rao PS, "Platypnea-orthodeoxia syndrome: Transcatheter management – Chapter 15," In. Rao PS, Kern MJ (eds.), Catheter Based Devices for Treatment of Noncoronary Cardiovascular Disease in Adults and Children, Lippincott, *Williams & Wilkins 2003*, Philadelphia, PA; pp.129-32.

10. Rao PS. Transcatheter management of platypnea-orthodeoxia syndrome (Editorial). J Invasive Cardiol 2004; 16:583-84.

11. Rao PS, "Focus: Atrial septal defects," Structural heart disease in adults (ed.), *J Invasive Cardiol 2009*; 21:A6-A10.

12. Rao PS, "When and how should atrial septal defects be closed in adults?" *J Invasive Cardiol 2009*; 21:76-82.

13. Rao PS, "Why, when and how should atrial septal defects be closed in adults – Chapter 8," In. Rao PS (ed.), Atrial Septal Defect, InTech, Rijeka, Croatia, April 2012, pp. 121-38.; ISBN 978-953-51-0531-2;:121-38.

14. Rao PS, "What an Adult Cardiologist Should Know about Cyanotic Congenital Heart Disease?" J Cardiovasc Dis Diag 2013; 1:104. Available at DOI:10.4172/jcdd.1000104

15. Rao PS, "What the Adult Cardiologist Should Know About Cyanotic Congenital Heart Disease," In: Chopra HK, et al. (eds.), State of Art CSI Cardiology Update 2014.

16. Rao PS, Sideris EB, Hausdorf G, et al, "International experience with secundum atrial septal defect occlusion by the buttoned device," *Am Heart J 1994*; 128:1022-35.

17. Lloyd TR, Rao PS, Beekman RH III, et al, "Atrial septal defect occlusion with the buttoned device: A multi-institutional U.S. trial," *Am J Cardiol 1994*; 73:286-91.

18. Zamora R, Rao PS, Lloyd TR, et al, "Intermediate-term results of Phase I FDA Trials of buttoned device occlusion of secundum atrial septal defect," *J Am Coll Cardiol 1998*; 31:674-6.

19. Sideris EB, Rao PS, "Transcatheter closure of atrial septal defects: Role of buttoned devices," *J Invasive Cardiol 1996*; 8:289-96.

20. Rao PS, Berger F, Rey C, et al, "Results of transvenous occlusion of secundum atrial septal defects with 4th generation buttoned device: Comparison with 1st, 2nd and 3rd generation devices," *J Am Coll Cardiol 2000*; 36:583-92.

21. Rao PS, Sideris EB, "Centering-on-demand buttoned device: Its role in transcatheter occlusion of atrial septal defects," *J Intervent Cardiol 2001*; 14:81-9.

22. Rao PS, Sideris EB, "Buttoned device closure of the atrial septal defect," *J Intervent Cardiol 1998*; 11:467-84.

23. Rao PS, "Buttoned device – Chapter 3," In. Rao PS, Kern MJ (eds.), Catheter Based Devices for Treatment of Noncoronary Cardiovascular Disease in Adults and Children, Lippincott, *Williams & Wilkins 2003*, Philadelphia, PA, pp. 17-34.

24. Rao PS, Wilson AD, Levy JM, Chopra PS, "Role of 'buttoned' double-disk device in the management of atrial septal defects," *Am Heart J 1992*; 123:191-200.

25. Rao PS, Wilson AD, Chopra PS, "Transcatheter closure of atrial septal defect by 'buttoned' devices," *Am J Cardiol 1992*; 69:1056-61.

26. Rao PS, Chandar JS, Sideris EB, "Role of inverted buttoned device in transcatheter occlusion of atrial septal defect or patent foramen ovale with right-to-left shunting associated with previously operated complex congenital cardiac anomalies," *Am J Cardiol 1997*; 80:914-21.

UNPUBLISHED OBSERVATIONS, BOOKS AND BOOK CHAPTERS

INTRODUCTION

Over the years, I have, from time to time, prepared lists of topics worthy of further investigation or review; some of these lists and outlines are shown in figures 1 through 5. Many such other lists existed, but were thrown away during clean up prior to contemplating the publication of this memoir. The data on these topics were collected and preserved, mostly in hand-written or typed format.

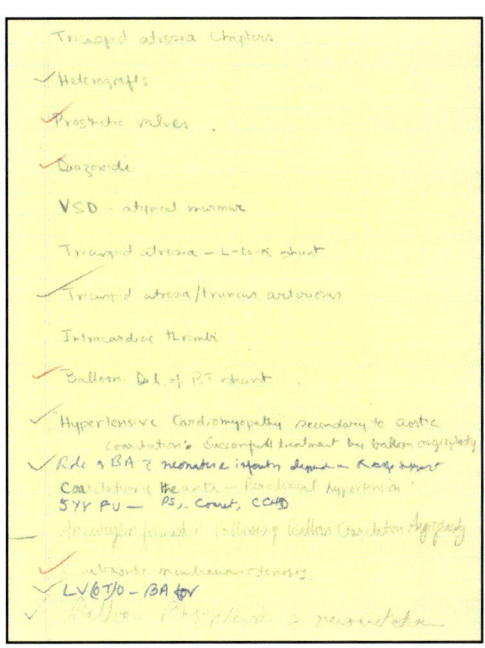

Figure 1. Hand-written notes of topics worthy of further investigation, probably written in late 1980s.

- LVOT obstructive lesions for Seminars in CVD
- Transcath closure for Medical Progress in J Peds — Curr Prob Cardiol
- Reballooning for recurrence of stenosis - AJC
- Balloon dil coarct Umbilical artery approach
- Infant coarctations — comp. c̄ surg
- PDA closure
- Coarct in children
- LT FU of DS & AS
- Trancath closure Clinical Cardiol.
- Subaortic stenosis
- Porcine heterografts - Review Med Progress
- Letter re Ann article - Remodelling
- Umbilical artery Cath - for Coarct dil

Bidirectional Glenn + ASD closure for PA - IVS.
Occlusion LSA, a new complication BA of AC
Stenting RVOT

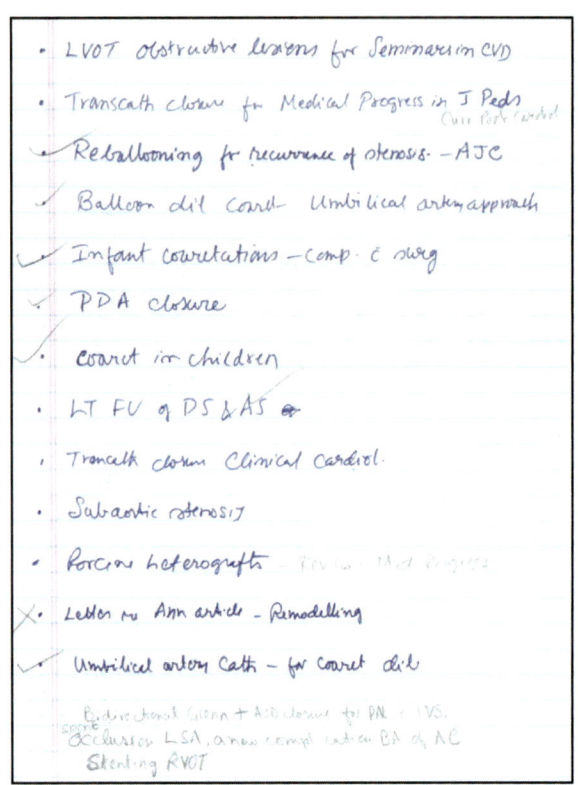

Figure 2. Hand-written notes of topics worthy of further investigation, probably written in early 1990s.

INTRODUCTION

Over the last one and one-half decades, a large variety of interventional pediatric cardiology techniques have been developed[1-3] as alternative methods to surgical therapy. Some of these involve placement of devices either to occlude intra or extra-cardiac defects or to enlarge narrowed blood vessels. Fortunately, either the entire device or major components of the device are radiopaque and can be evaluated by plain chest roentgenogram. The purpose of this review is to familiarize the practicing pediatric radiologists with these new radiographic images to help identify the type of the device and to detect malposition of the device.

For each of major item (as listed below) a brief introductory paragraph should be written. Then, a description of radiologic appearance of the particular device, with examples. Following this, a paragraph or so should be written out to discuss malposition or malfunction of the device.

Outline:

1. Atrial septal defect occluding devices
2. Ventricular septal defect occluding devices
3. Patent ductus arteriosus occluding devices
4. Devices used for occlusion of superfluous vessels
5. Stents
   a) Pulmonary artery stents
   b) Stents in systemic veins
   c) Stents in the aorta
   d) Stents in the ductus

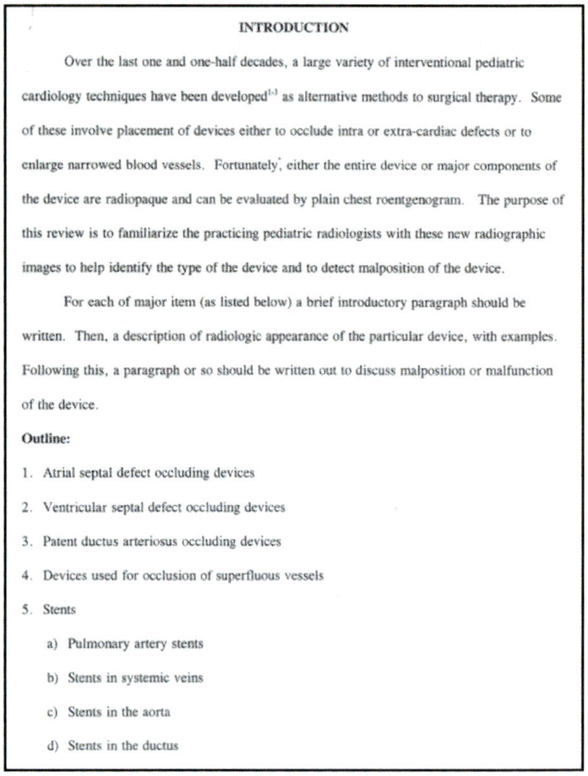

Figure 3. Typed instructions from me to a pediatric radiology fellow regarding a study of radiographic images of transcatheter implanted devices.

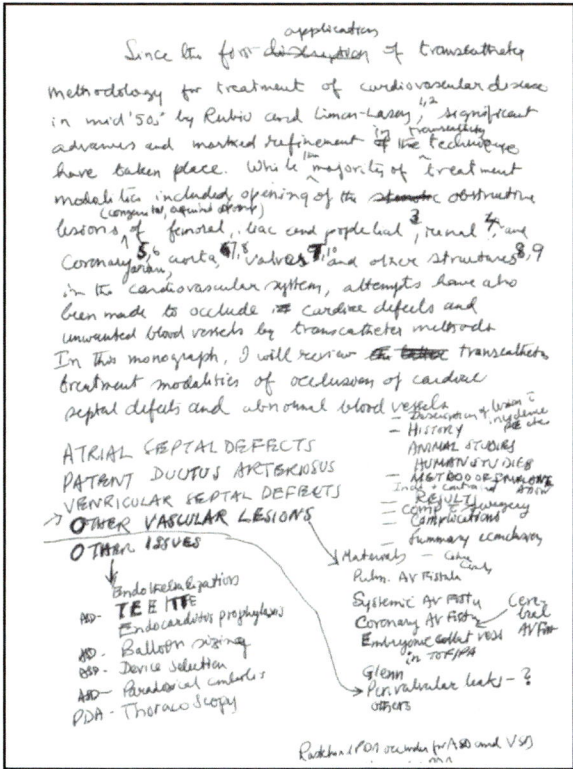

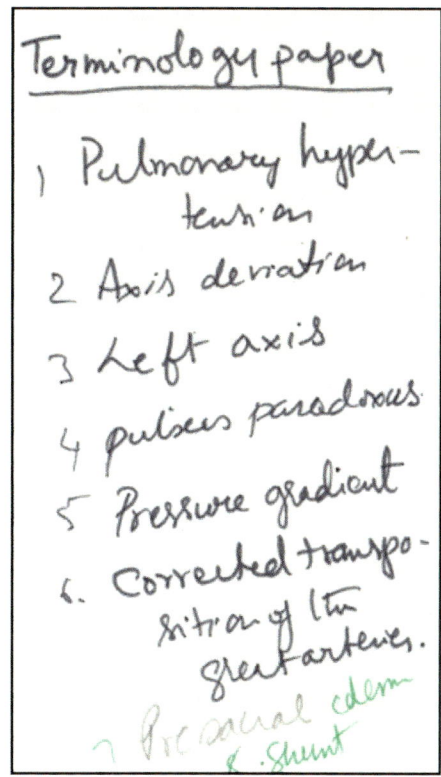

Figure 4. Hand-written notes (probably written in early 1990s) of a review paper/monograph on transcatheter occlusion cardiac defects and unwanted blood vessels in manner similar to that of Rao PS, "Balloon angioplasty and valvuloplasty in infants, children and adolescents," Current Problems in Cardiology, YearBook Medical Publishers, Inc., 1989, Chicago; 14(8):417-500.

Figure 5. Hand-written notes on a review paper on terminology used in pediatric cardiology literature, probably written in late 1980s.

When a given study is completed/published, it is marked off (Figures 1 and 2). Unfortunately, however, not all the selected studies/reviews were completed because of commitments for time for clinical (particularly after advent of interventional pediatric cardiology), administrative (Division Director), teaching, research and other service responsibilities. Some of these topics were presented at local, regional, national or international scientific societies and some were published in abstract form.[1-22] A few of these observations were published recently in *Congenital Cardiology Today*;[23-25] selection of this medium for publication was largely predicated by the prospect of rapid publication and wide distribution to pediatric cardiologists around the world. In this chapter, the unpublished observations will be reviewed; they will be categorized by decades.

1970s

Relationship of Cardiac Arrhythmias with Sudden Infant Death Syndrome

The causes of sudden infant death syndrome (SIDS) are unknown. The major hypotheses include infection, airway obstruction, prolonged apnea, and failure to interrupt apnea. Our recent observations in a three-month old girl suggest cardiac arrhythmia as another possible etiologic factor. This infant had several episodes of paroxysmal supra-ventricular tachycardia (PST) and three episodes of ventricular fibrillation (VF). Features of Wolff-Parkinson-White syndrome (WPW) were also present (predisposing to recurrences of PST) in the electrocardiogram (ECG). On two separate occasions, the infant appeared ill, and was taken to the emergency room where VF was documented. If she had VF at home, it is unlikely that the baby could have survived. We postulated that she had PST at home and developed VF at the time of hospital admission. A third episode of VF occurred while in the hospital. The infant was promptly defibrillated on all three occasions. Recurrence of the arrhythmia was prevented by administration of digitalis and procaineamide. If the episodes of arrhythmia were not initially symptomatic, the infant would have died. Cardiac arrhythmia as one of the mechanisms of SIDS is supported by the following: 1) The findings in this infant, 2) Observations by James of immaturity and electrical instability of the conduction system in early infancy, 3) Increased incidence of cardiac arrhythmias in premature infants, and 4) peak incidence of PST in this age group. The sequence of events appears to be: WPW → PST → VF → Death. Further studies to support this hypothesis is indicated.[1]

Isoproterenol and right ventricular outflow obstruction

We hypothesized that the right ventricular outflow pressure gradients produced by isoproterenol (IP) are due to the differences in the expression of the total fluid energy.[2,3] It should be understood that total fluid energy is equal to the sum of pressure (potential) energy, kinetic energy, and gravitational potential energy. Since the gravitational energy in the pulmonary artery (PA) and the right ventricle (RV) in the supine position is equal, it may be ignored. To provide evidence to support our hypothesis we selected an *in vivo* animal model. The side pressure (with a side hole catheter), the end pressure (end-hole catheter against the direction of the blood stream) and the flow velocity in the PA and the RV pressure were measured in eleven dogs before and after IP. The RV and end PA pressures were equal ($p > 0.05$) and were slightly higher than the side PA pressure in the control state, but increased to markedly higher levels ($p < 0.01$) after IP. IP also increased the velocity of the flow in the PA ($p < 0.01$). The RV and side PA peak systolic pressure difference (mean = 8.82 mm Hg) increased to a mean of 19.09 mm Hg ($p < 0.01$). This change in pulmonary valvar pressure gradient is proportional to the increase in PA flow velocity induced by IP. The side pressure measures only potential energy and the end pressure measures the potential and kinetic energies. In the RV, only potential energy is recorded where kinetic energy is practically non-existent. The gradient between the RV and side PA pressure in this study and the increase in gradient across the RV outflow tract after IP, documented by other workers, is due to partial transformation of the fluid energy into kinetic energy in the PA.[2,3]

Kinetic or flow energy forms a greater proportion of the total energy in the pulmonary circuit than in the systemic circuit and with further increase in flow velocity by IP, the importance of kinetic energy becomes even greater. Thus, the RV outflow tract or pulmonary valvar gradients produced or augmented by IP cannot accurately indicate active obstruction of the RV outflow tract or the severity of pulmonary stenosis. If these gradients exist after accounting for kinetic energy, then and only then, can one draw conclusions that obstruction is produced by IP.[2,3]

Subsequent to this study, I also recorded both end pressure and side pressure in the PA with specially designed catheters in human subjects (during routine cardiac catheterization) and these observations were similar to those stated above. Unfortunately, these studies were not formally reported.

Types of Congenital Heart Disease in Different Genotypes of Down's Syndrome

The association of congenital heart disease (CHD) with Down's syndrome (DS) and the specific types of CHD in DS have been well documented. However, the incidence and type of CHD in different genotypes of DS namely non-disjunction, translocation or mosaic have not been studied, which this study investigates. The records of 420 patients with diagnoses of DS seen at the Medical College of Georgia Institutions were reviewed for the presence and type of CHD and type of chromosomal abnormality. Both clinical and chromosomal data were available in 276 patients of whom eighty (29 percent) had CHD. The genotype distribution was non-disjunction – 90 percent, translocation – 7 percent, and mosaic – 3 percent. The incidence of CHD in these respective genotypes was 23 percent, 29 percent, and 50 percent. The types of CHD in all cases of DS is similar to those reported by others previously: Endocardial cushion defect (ECD) - 35/80, ventricular septal defect (VSD) - 25/80, tetralogy of Fallot - 6/80 and other CHD - 14/80. The type of CHD in non-disjunction and mosaic DS is similar to that described above. But, in translocation DS, three of four patients had ECD and the fourth, patent ductus arteriosus (PDA). Being a persistent fetal structure, PDA may be ignored. The presence of only ECD in translocation DS by contrast to the usual ECD, VSD and other CHD in non-disjunction DS (although could be due to small numbers of translocation DS cases studied) may have some etiologic significance in CHD. These findings may call for chromosomal studies, especially with the newly developed techniques, in ECD patients in order to evaluate minor chromosomal etiology of' CHD.[4]

How to Select Children with Aortic Stenosis for Catheterization by Echocardiographic Criteria

Left ventricular (LV) systolic pressure was predicted from echocardiographic measurements of LV wall thickness and cavity dimension at end systole (S) and end diastole (D) to determine the severity of aortic stenosis in sixteen children aged between two and seventeen years. LV pressure and aortic gradient were obtained by cardiac catheterization on the same day. None of these patients had more than mild aortic insufficiency and none had prior surgery. The correlation with LV pressure using systolic measurements was better than that with two diastolic methods. However, the combination of all three was superior.

A = LVD wall + septal thickness/LVD cavity dimension - $r = 0.64$; $p < 0.01$

B = LVS wal1/LVS cavity dimension - $r = 0.81$; $p < 0.001$

C = LVD mass/LVD volume - $r = 0.62$; $p < 0.01$

Aortic gradient = -327.2A+209.8B+46.96C - 27.92 - $r = 0.86$; $p < 0.001$

When this relationship was applied to separae patients on the basis of a gradient less than or more than 45 mmHg, 94 percent (15/16) correct diagnoses were made. The single error vas a false positive or over-diagnosis. No patient with moderate or severe aortic stenosis was missed. Echocardiography can be utilized to diagnose the severity of aortic stenosis accurately by combining systolic and diastolic wall and mass measurements and is best applied to spare the child with mild stenosis early and repeated catheterizations.[5] At the present time, however, Doppler measurements are considered accurate in estimating severity of aortic valve obstruction.

Natural History of Obstructive Lesions of the Heart

A review paper on natural history of obstructive lesions of the heart was planned and references collected (Figure 6) when I was at the Medical College of Georgia, but this review paper never completed and this is probably related to my move from the Medical College of Georgia to the King Faisal Specialist Hospital.

P. Syamasundar Rao, M.B.
Associate Professor of Pediatrics
Section of Pediatric Cardiology
Medical College of Georgia
Augusta, Georgia
- May 1976 -

Aortic Stenosis

1. Campbell, M.: The natural history of congenital aortic stenosis. Brit. Heart J. 30:514, 1968.
2. Campbell, M.: Calcific aortic stenosis and bicuspid aortic valve. Brit. Heart J. 30:606, 1968.
3. Hoffman, J.I.E.: The natural history of congenital isolated pulmonic and aortic stenosis. Annual Rev. Med. 20:15, 1969.
4. Cohen, L.S., Friedman, W.F. and Braunwald, E.: Natural history of mild congenital aortic stenosis elucidated by serial hemodynamic studies. Amer. J. Cardiol. 30:1, 1972.
5. El-Said, G., Galioto, F.M.Jr., Mullins, C.E. and McNamara, D.G.: Natural hemodynamic history of congenital aortic stenosis in childhood. Amer. J. Cardiol. 30:6, 1972.
6. Mody, M.R. and Mody, G.T.: Serial hemodynamic observations in congenital valvar and subvalvar aortic stenosis. Amer. Heart J. 89:137, 1975.
7. Krovetz, L.J.: Age-related changes in size of the aortic valve annulus in man. Amer. Heart J. 90:569, 1975.

Pulmonic Stenosis

1. Hoffman, J.I.E.: The antural history of congenital isolated pulmonic and aortic stenosis. Annual Rev. Med. 20:15, 1969.
2. Campbell, M: The natural history of congenital pulmonic stenosis. Brit. Heart J. 31:394, 1969.
3. Mustard, W.T., Jain, S.C. and Trusler, G.A.: Pulmonic stenosis in the first year of life. Brit. Heart J. 30:255, 1968.
4. Engle, M.A., Ito, T. and Goldberg, H.P.: The fate of patients with pulmonic stenosis. Circulation 30:554, 1964.
5. Johnson, L.W., Grossman, W., Dalen, J. and Dexter, L: Pulmonic stenosis in the adult-long-term follow-up study. New Engl. J. Med. 23:287, 1159, 1972.
6. Mody, M.R.: The natural history of uncomplicated valvar pulmonic stenosis. Amer. Heart J. 90:317, 1975.

Coarctation of the Aorta

1. Campbell, M.: Natural history of coarctation of the aorta. Brit. Heart J. 32:633, 1970.
2. Maron, B.J. Humphries, J.O., Rowe, R.D. and Mellits, E.D.: Prognosis of surgically corrected coarctation of the aorta: A 20-year post-operative appraisal.
3. Nanton, M.A. and Olley, P.M.: Residual hypertension after coarctectomy in children. Amer. J. Cardiol. 37:769, 1976.

Figure 6. Typed list of references for the planned review paper on natural history of obstructive lesions of the heart.

1980s

Effect of Acute Increase in Stroke Volume on Pulmonary Vascular Impedance

The effect of increased stroke volume (SV) on the pulmonary vascular impedance (PVI) was studied in eleven dogs. After recording control pressure and flow in the main pulmonary artery, an aorta-to-right atrial shunt was created and the data recorded. Fourier analysis was performed and impedance moduli and phase angles as well as other pulmonary vascular parameters were plotted. The control PVI spectrum was comparable that shown in previous reports. The following changes were noted when SV was acutely increased: 1. Impedance moduli at lower frequencies consistently decreased suggesting that the reflection points moved away (toward periphery) from the recording site and 2. The characteristic impedance increased after the shunt even when the SV is only 1.5 to 2 times the control. These results are at variance with our previous studies in the *in vitro* type of pulmonary bed preparation where the characteristic impedance decreased even with SV 2 or 3 times the control SV. In the *in vitro* preparation, the characteristic impedance increased only when the SV was increased four-fold. The difference observed may be related to the type of preparation - *in vivo* vs. *in vitro*. In the *in vitro* preparation, lack of autonomic influence on the pulmonary vasculature may have resulted in the differenced observed in the current studies; 1. The impedance minimum was reached at lower frequencies after the shunt and 2. The terminal impedance also appeared to have decreased. Despite these pronounced changes in impedance patterns, there was an unpredictable change in the pulmonary vascular resistance. These data suggest a marked change in the functional geographic distribution of pulmonary vasculature with increased SV. These may in part be responsible for changes seen pulmonary vascular obstructive disease (PVOD). The PVI studies may be helpful in further understanding the nature and pathogenesis of PVOD and possibly the prediction of impending PVOD.[6]

Syndrome of Absent Pulmonary Valve

This presentation reviews our experience with the syndrome of absent pulmonary valve (SAPV) and suggests that total surgical correction with pulmonary artery (PA) plication, but without pulmonary valve (PV) replacement is the method of choice for correction of this anomaly.[7,8] Ten infants and children with SAPV seen during 1979-84 were analyzed. Their mean age was eleven months with a range of one day to three years. Nine children had associated ventricular septal defect (VSD) and PV ring stenosis, while the remaining infant had an isolated VSD. Five Group I patients (< 6 months) presented with severe tracheobronchial obstruction, cyanosis, and heart failure; five Group II patients (> 6 months) presented with history of recurrent respiratory tract infection and a murmur. Clinical, x-ray, and echo findings were classic for this anomaly. Two-dimensional echocardiographic (ECHO) features included enlarged RV and aorta, aortic override, narrowed PV ring with rudimentary PV leaflets, and markedly dilated main, right and/or left PA.

Nine patients underwent closure of VSD and relief of PV ring stenosis; four of these had additional PA plication and two additional had PV replacement. Two children died after surgery. Plication of PAs was performed as the sole procedure in a five-day-old respirator-dependent infant. Follow-up of the remaining eight patients ranged between 1.5 and 3.5 years and all underwent ECHO and catheterization studies. Symptomatic relief and normalization of cardiac structure and function were greatest in the patients who had plication of PAs as an integral part of total repair as compared with those who had other types of surgical correction. Based on this experience, we recommend total surgical correction along with PA plication, but without PV replacement as the procedure of choice in symptomatic patients with SAPV.[7,8] We did not have the opportunity to prepare a full paper for publication, although one of these cases was reported.[26]

Successful Radical Two-Stage Correction of Pulmonary Atresia with Intact Ventricular Septum, and Right Ventricular and Tricuspid Hypoplasia, using the Fontan-Kreutzer Principle in Childhood

Two patients with pulmonary atresia with intact ventricular septum and tricuspid valvular hypoplasia were presented in whom the initial surgical management was by right ventricular outflow tract enlargement. At subsequent surgery, it was possible in one case to achieve atrial septation with preservation of the tricuspid valve and the re-establishment of normal anatomy.

In the second case, following atrial septation, it was necessary and possible to excise the tricuspid valve and to enlarge the valve annulus allowing forward passive flow; the hypoplastic right ventricle served as a conduit from the right atrium to the pulmonary artery, invoking the Fontan principle. Both cases had a smooth post-operative recovery and were well at four months follow-up. It was concluded that the Fontan concept may be applied if re-establishment of normal anatomy is not feasible.[9]

Immunologic Abnormalities Associated With Asplenia Syndrome.

I had interest in asplenia syndrome[27,28] and collaborated with Dr. Herb Harfi, an immunologist at the King Faisal Specialist Hospital, and developed a project to investigate immunologic abnormalities associated with asplenia syndrome. Our project proposed securing multiple immunological laboratory tests on ten patients with asplenia syndrome, ten children who had splenectomy, and ten patients with cyanotic congenital heart defects (CHDs) and compare and contrast the findings in these three groups of patients. Unfortunately, the project could not be completed since I left the King Faisal Specialist Hospital shortly after the project was initialed.

Doppler Assessment of Function of Blalock-Taussig Shunts.

The aim of the study was to compare and contrast two-dimensional and Doppler (pulsed and continuous wave) echocardiographic findings with those of cardiac catheterization and angiographic data of patient who had Blalock-Taussig (BT) shunts as a palliative procedure for cyanotic CHD in order to assess utility of echocardiographic studies in evaluating BT shunts. However, the project was not completed since I left the King Faisal Specialist Hospital shortly after the project started.

Proposed Book titled "Pediatric Cardiology: Common Problems in Clinical Practice"

I have prepared an outline and proposal for a book titled "Pediatric Cardiology: Common Problems in Clinical Practice" and secured a contract to publish by G. K. Hall Medical Publishers of Boston in 1984. Several chapters were completed including permission to reproduce figures. While I can't truly recall what happened and why the book was not published, becoming busy in the administrative matters and catheter interventional procedures, and move from the King Faisal Specialist Hospital to the University of Wisconsin may have been the reasons for non-completion of the book project.

Randomized Double Blind Study of Hydralazine and Captopril in Refractory Congestive Heart Failure

A randomized double blind study of hydralazine and captopril in refractory congestive heart failure was initiated in collaboration with Dr. Mohinder Thapar. This followed our study demonstrating benefit with use of hydralazine as an afterload reducing agent in infants and children with primary myocardial disease.[29] A summary of the project will be briefed. Efficacy of after load reducing agents in the management of refractory congestive heart failure has been well documented in the adults. However, their efficacy in pediatric patients with refractory congestive heart failure has not been established. Therefore, a double blind randomized study was planned to compare the long-term efficacy of hydralazine and captopril in patients who fail to show adequate response to the conventional decongestive therapy with digoxin and diuretics. Unresponsive patients will receive one of the agent in a randomized double blind fashion. Their response will be monitored by clinical and various non-invasive means, i.e., echocardiogram and Doppler studies and radionuclide techniques. The patients will be evaluated every three months. At that time, their response of these agents will be analyzed and compared. During this period, patients will be monitored for any of the side effects of the drugs administered. The patients who fail to show a satisfactory response to one of the agents, will have a trial of the combined therapy with these two agents. Soon after starting the study, I and subsequently Dr. Thapar left the King Faisal Specialist Hospital.

1990s

Book Chapters in a Book titled "Alternatives in Pediatric Cardiac Surgery"

In April 1991, Dr. Michael Ilbawi, Director of Pediatric Cardiac Surgery at Heart Institute for Children in Oak Lawn, Illinois, invited me to write chapters for his proposed book titled "Alternatives in Pediatric Cardiac Surgery." I have agreed to participate in his project and wrote four chapters:

1. Balloon angioplasty is the best treatment for recoarctation.
2. Balloon pulmonary valvuloplasty as an alternative to shunt procedure.
3. Staged approach with initial balloon angioplasty of native coarctation.
4. Is there a place for transcatheter methods in the management of pulmonary atresia?

Summary and conclusions for these four chapters are as follows:

Balloon Angioplasty Is The Best Treatment for Recoarctation. Since the first human application of balloon angioplasty of the postoperative aortic recoarctation in 1982 by Singer and his associates, this technique has been used extensively by many other workers. Balloon dilatation of aortic recoarctation is next only to valvar pulmonic stenosis with regard to the acceptability by cardiologists. Immediate results seem excellent with an acceptable level of complication rate. The results and risks appear comparable to or better than those seen with repeat surgical intervention. Follow-up results are available in only a limited number of patients, with recurrence and aneurysm formation rates of 25 percent and 9 percent, respectively. These and arterial complication rates are likely to diminish because of progressive improvement of the balloon catheter technology and a greater understanding by cardiologists of the angioplasty technique.

Most cardiologists agree that balloon angioplasty is the treatment of choice for management of aortic recoarctations. A peak-to-peak systolic pressure gradient across the operative site in excess of 20 mmHg with angiographic demonstration of discrete narrowing is an indication for balloon dilatation. Use of heparin, appropriate choice of balloon diameter, and avoidance of manipulation of the tips of the catheters/guide wires in the vicinity of freshly dilated coarctation are important technical features of balloon angioplasty. Periodic evaluation for evidence of renarrowing after angioplasty and for development of aneurysms is necessary; these may be performed by clinical, Echo-Doppler, nuclear magnetic resonance, and angiographic studies.

The mechanism for effectiveness of angioplasty appears to be intimal and medial disruption produced by controlled injury through radial forces of balloon inflation.

Further miniaturization of balloon/catheter systems, a better understanding of the technique of balloon angioplasty, longer duration of follow-up in a larger number of patients than is currently available, and delineation of causes and natural history of aneurysm formation following angioplasty are all important in advancing balloon angioplasty as a successful therapeutic option for the management of postoperative aortic recoarctations.

Balloon Pulmonary Valvuloplasty As An Alternative To Shunt Procedure. Balloon pulmonary valvuloplasty appears to offer excellent relief of pulmonary oligemia and systemic arterial hypoxemia in patients with tetralogy of Fallot type of hemodynamics. Based on the data presented, we recommended balloon pulmonary valvuloplasty to manage patients with cyanotic heart defects and pulmonary oligemia secondary to pulmonary outflow tract obstruction. We recommend this procedure for patients with cardiac defects that are not amenable to total surgical correction at the age and size at the time of their presentation. We believe it is an effective alternative to surgical creation of a systemic-to-pulmonary arterial anastomosis, thus, avoiding potential complications associated with surgical shunts. The procedure is likely to be beneficial if the valvar obstruction is the dominant obstruction. Presence of two or more obstructions in series is desirable to prevent flooding the lungs when the procedure proves successful.

Staged Approach With Initial Balloon Angioplasty of Native Coarctation. The technique of balloon angioplasty of aortic coarctation has been available since 1983 and several workers used this technique in native coarctations. Immediate and intermediate-term follow-up results are generally good with some chance for recoarctation. Complications of the procedure are modest in degree, although arterial complications in the neonate and young infant may be significant.

Although good immediate and intermediate-term follow-up results of balloon angioplasty of aortic coarctation have been reported, recommendations for the use of this technique as a choice of treatment have been clouded by the reports of development of aneurysms at the site of coarctation dilatation. We feel that balloon coarctation angioplasty is the treatment of choice in the neonates and small infants, especially if associated with other significant cardiac defects, including ventricular septal defects. If there is no spontaneous resolution or improvement of the associated defects, further palliation or correction of these defects could be undertaken.

A substantial miniaturization of balloon catheter systems has taken place. Further miniaturization and improving rapidity of inflation/deflation of balloons are necessary for increasing the safety and effectiveness of this technique in infants and children. Meticulous attention to the details of the technique and further refinements of the procedure are likely to further reduce the complication rate.

Is There a Place for Transcatheter Methods in the Management of Pulmonary Atresia? The prognosis for patients who have pulmonary valve atresia with intact ventricular septum is poor with or without conventional surgical intervention. Therefore, we suggested the adoption of a comprehensive medical and surgical treatment program leading to complete surgical correction of the lesion. The objectives of such a program were as follows: 1) To relieve hypoxemia and acidosis by a timely and appropriate procedure to increase pulmonary blood flow at initial presentation (usually in the newborn period); 2) To facilitate adequate egress of blood from the fight atrium; 3) To stimulate the growth of the right ventricle.

The objectives of the program may be achieved by appropriately timed, multiple surgical procedures. Two transcatheter treatment strategies have recently been suggested for the management of these difficult patients: a) primary perforation of the atretic pulmonary valve by transcatheter methods, and b) limited opening of the pulmonary valve at surgery, both followed by balloon valvuloplasty. Both the above approaches are innovative methods and may have clinical utility. Appropriate clinical trials are warranted to assess their effectiveness and safety.

All the four chapters along with illustrations were submitted to Dr. Ilbawi in July 1992. However, proofs of the chapters were never received despite repeated enquiries (May 1993 and December 1996).

Surgical Repair of Common Atrioventricular Septal Defects - Long-term Results Using Single-patch Technique

During a twenty-year period ending 1992, fifty-two children with a mean age of twenty-two months (2 to 180) and an average weight of 9.5 kg (3 to 40) with a diagnosis of complete atrio-ventricular (AV) septal defect, underwent complete surgical correction. Twenty-two babies had Down syndrome. The frequency of the Rastelli types was A-19, B-3, and C-30. Surgical correction was performed under cardiopulmonary bypass and moderate hypothermia down to 28^0C in thirty-seven patients and with deep hypothermia and circulatory arrest in fifteen patients. In all but one instance, a single patch was used to close the atrial and ventricular septal defects with repair and re-suspension of the anterior mitral leaflet, producing excellent relief of mitral insufficiency. Overall hospital mortality was 9.6 percent (five deaths). Three deaths were in patients with major associated cardiac anomalies, and two (4 percent) in children with isolated AV septal defects. The remaining patients were followed from one month to fourteen years. There were five late deaths (9.6 percent). Re-operation was required in three (6 percent) to close residual shunts in two (4 percent) and repair of mitral valve in one (2 percent). Follow-up echocardiograms were available for review in twenty-eight (66 percent) patients, the last study was performed 1 to 156 months after initial surgery. Left ventricular systolic function was normal in all patients. Significant mitral insufficiency was present in only 4 percent of patients. Small atrial (5 percent) and ventricular (2 percent) shunts were detected, but none required surgical intervention. Functional status was evaluated in forty of the surviving patients by clinical examination, and in some by exercise testing. 92 percent remained in NYHA Class I and 8 percent in NYHA Class II. Our data suggested that excellent long-term mitral valve function is possible with total surgical correction using a single patch technique in patients with common AV septal defects.[10]

Aortico-Left Ventricular Tunnel

In early 1990s, when I was still at the University of Wisconsin, we observed two rare cases of aortico-left ventricular tunnel. Dr. Subash Reddy, a clinical fellow with me at that time and I wrote up these cases. The summary of this report is as follows:

Aortico-left ventricular tunnel is a rare type of congenital cardiac malformation with approximately sixty-five cases reported in the English literature as of that date. This malformation is characterized by an abnormal communication between aorta and left ventricular outflow tract. This communication causes paravalvular aortic regurgitation of increasing nature and can lead to left ventricular volume overload and congestive heart failure. Surgery is the treatment of choice. We described these two cases. The first is a three-year-old male, in whom the diagnosis of aortico-left ventricular tunnel was made by transthoracic echocardiography and confirmed by angiocardiography. He underwent successful surgical repair with monitoring by intra-operative transesophageal echocardiography. The second patient is a nine-year-old male, who underwent successful repair at the eight months of age. He has been followed in our clinic over a period of eight-and-a-half years during which he developed increasing aortic regurgitation and left ventricular dilatation. Despite lack of symptoms, his clinical course seems to require either aortic valve repair or replacement in near future. We presented our experience with different imaging modalities that were helpful for the diagnosis in our first case. We also present a collective review on this rare congenital malformation for prevalence of late onset aortic regurgitation following surgical repair, as noted in our second case. Unfortunately, this report was never submitted for publication, presumably related to our busy schedules and my move to the St. Louis University.

Book Chapter titled "Congenital Heart Disease"

In mid-1990s, when I was still at the University of Wisconsin, Dr. Nabil Bittar of the Department of Medicine, Division of Cardiology, requested me to contribute a chapter titled "Congenital Heart Disease" for his book on "Principles of Medical Biology" to be published by Elsevier Science, Amsterdam, Netherlands. The manuscript was submitted, but to the best of my knowledge, the book never got published. However, a large proportion of the material was published later in other forums.[30-34]

Applications of Pediatric Cardiac Interventional Technology to Adults.

A review paper titled "Applications of Pediatric Cardiac Interventional Technology to Adults" was conceived and draft prepared (Figure 7) in late 1990s, while I was at the St. Louis University. The project was never completed.

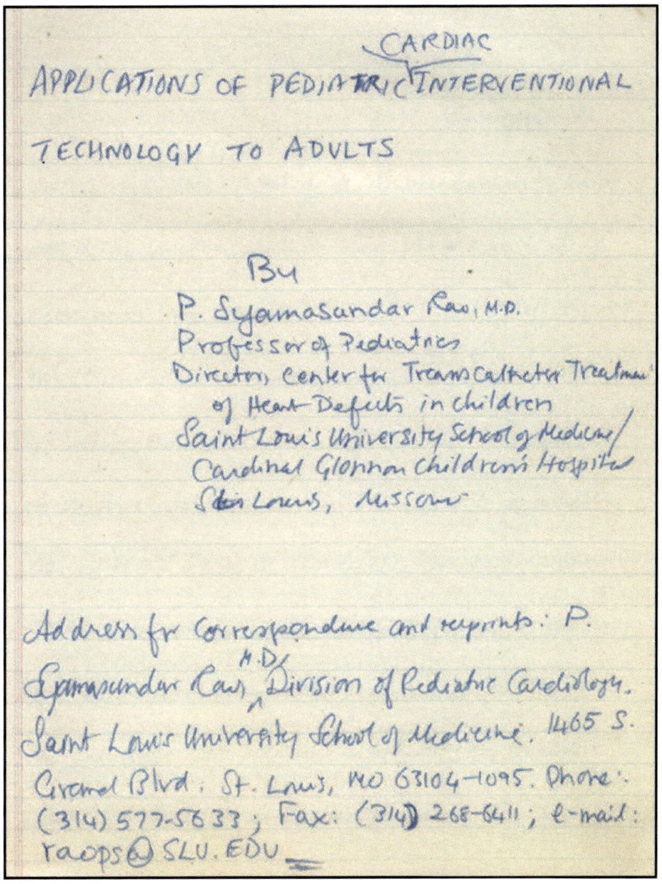
APPLICATIONS OF PEDIATRIC CARDIAC INTERVENTIONAL TECHNOLOGY TO ADULTS

By

P. Syamasundar Rao, M.D.
Professor of Pediatrics
Director, Center for Transcatheter Treatment of Heart Defects in Children
Saint Louis University School of Medicine/
Cardinal Glennon Children's Hospital
Saint Louis, Missouri

Address for Correspondence and reprints: P. Syamasundar Rao, M.D., Division of Pediatric Cardiology, Saint Louis University School of Medicine, 1465 S. Grand Blvd; St. Louis, MO 63104-1095. Phone: (314) 577-5633; Fax: (314) 268-6411; e-mail: raops@SLU.EDU

Figure 7. Hand-written title page (probably written in late 1990s) of a review paper on "Applications of Pediatric Cardiac Interventional Technology to Adults."

2000s

Pressure Recovery and Pressure Gradients in Stenotic Outflow Tract Lesions: A Simultaneous Doppler and Catheter Correlative Study in Pediatric Patients

Despite good correlation between Doppler-derived and catheterization-measured gradients across obstructive lesions of the heart as we observed/reported[35-38] as well as by others, I found significant discrepancies between these values when I was at the University of Wisconsin. To investigate the reasons for such discrepancy, I encouraged my echocardiography colleague, Dr. Allen Wilson to participate in such a study while recording simultaneous catheter and echo measurements in the catheterization laboratory. Shortly after the initiation of the study, I moved to the St. Louis University/Cardinal Glennon Children's Hospital in St. Louis, MO. Here I encouraged another of my echocardiography colleague, Dr. Gautam Singh to participate in such as study. The study was started and data secured and the data were presented to multiple scientific societies,[11,12,16] but neither I nor Dr. Singh completed the study manuscript for publication. The following is a summary of the study and data:

Doppler pressure gradients are routinely used as a surrogate for catheter peak-to-peak gradient (PPG) for referring pediatric patients with aortic stenosis (AS), pulmonary stenosis (PS) and coarctation of aorta (CoA) for intervention, but do not predict the catheter PPG accurately. This results in misclassification of lesion severity and often, inappropriate referral for intervention. Pressure recovery (PR) accounts for much of the discrepancy between Doppler PG and catheter PPG in *in-vitro* experiments and studies in adult subjects. But, the occurrence of clinically significant PR in congenital AS, PS and CoA have not been well studied. Simultaneous Doppler and catheter PPG were prospectively measured in eighty-two consecutive patients (median age: 12.2 months; weight: 7.5 kg), with AS (n=30), PS (n=24), and CoA (n=28) and agreement before and after correcting for PR were analyzed. PR was calculated from the fluid dynamic based equation using echo data. The effect of lesion geometry on the magnitude of PR were also analyzed.

PR-corrected Doppler peak instantaneous gradient (PRcPIG) had significantly better correlation with the catheter PPG (p<0.001) than the uncorrected Doppler peak (PIG) and mean instantaneous gradient (MIG). PRcPIG predicted PPG with high specificity and accuracy in all lesions (95 percent CI: 36-97 percent and 85-100 percent respectively, p <0.05 for both). The PR, which accounted for 4 percent to 42 percent overestimation of catheter PPG by Doppler PIG, was directly related (r = 0.33 to 0.47) to valve area, inversely related (r = -0.22 to -0.34) to downstream vessel area, and was significantly (p < 0.05) more in CoA and PS than in AS. Based on these data it was concluded that significant PR occurs in congenital AS, PS, and CoA accounting for misclassification of lesion severity by Doppler PIG. The PRcPIG reliably predicts the catheter PPG in lesions with area > 0.5cm^2/M^2 and vessel area < 2.75cm^2/M^2. The PR magnitude depends on the geometry of stenotic lesion in pediatric patients.

Recently, a complete manuscript was prepared and submitted for publication and will be referenced should the manuscript get published before this book goes into press.

Buttoned Device Modifications: Influence on Feasibility, Safety and Effectiveness.[13,18]

This issue was reviewed in the chapter on "Atrial Septal Defects" in the book titled "Pediatric Cardiology: How It Has Evolved Over the last 50 Years" and will not be repeated here.

Prenatal Growth of Tricuspid Valve and Right Ventricle Determines the Evolution and Postnatal Outcomes of Tricuspid Atresia (Morphogenetic Insight in Evaluation of Tricuspid Atresia)

Although the prevalent hypothesis is that tricuspid atresia (TA) results from mal-alignment of ventricular loop with atrio-ventricular (AV) canal during embryogenesis, there is paucity of studies on antenatal natural history of TA. We hypothesized that TA may evolve prenatally from tricuspid stenosis (TS) without mal-alignment and sought to identify the prenatal morphological determinants of postnatal outcomes. To elucidate antenatal evolution of TA, ten fetuses diagnosed with "tricuspid stenosis" (TS) [tricuspid valve (TV) z score <-2.0] and normal segmental alignment at 24.5 ± 3.2 weeks gestation were studied by serial echocardiography up to infancy. Cardiac segments were measured and growth curves were developed and compared with those of fifty-one normal fetuses and hundred infants. Serial measurements of ventriculo-atrial septal (VAS) angles in TS fetuses were compared with normal to discern the mal-alignment of ventricular loop with AV canal. Mid-trimester right ventricle (RV) had smaller (p< 0.005) inflow (z-score -3.7 ± 2.0), trabecular (z-score -5.3±2.6) and outflow (z-score -2.3±0.9) segments than normal. Their growth rates were slower (p<0.001) than normal through gestation. VAS angles in TS fetuses were similar to normal initially, but increased with gestation due to increasing left ventricular dimensions. Eight of these ten fetuses were found to have TA, two with severe TS and all with hypoplastic RV at birth. TS fetuses with restrictive ventricular septal defects (VSD) (N=6) became duct-dependent, whereas those with unrestrictive VSD (N=4) had duct-independent postnatal pulmonary circulation. It was concluded that TA evolves from mid-trimester TS without prerequisite mal-alignment of AV canal and ventricular loop. Mid-trimester right heart segment z scores ≤ 2.0 and reduced growth rate predict development of TA and RV hypoplasia. In fetuses with evolving TA, the VSD size may predict ductal dependence of postnatal pulmonary circulation.14,15

Clinical Comparison of Rigid with Flexible Stents in the Management of Vascular Obstructive Lesions in Children.[17]

The study comparing rigid with flexible stents was reviewed in the chapter on "Stents" in the book titled "Pediatric Cardiology: How It Has Evolved Over the last 50 Years" and will not discussed here.

Book Chapters for a Book titled "Congenital Heart Disease in Adults."

The cardiologists and cardiovascular surgeons from the Washington University/St. Louis Children's Hospital, St. Louis, Missouri, planned for the book titled "Congenital Heart Disease in Adults" and requested me to contribute two chapters for their book. The first was the clinical aspects of tricuspid atresia and the second on history of Fontan. Both manuscripts were prepared and sent to them, but the book was never published. The subject material reviewed in these chapters was extensively discussed in the chapter on "Tricuspid Atresia" in the book titled "Pediatric Cardiology: How It Has Evolved Over the last 50 Years" and will not repeated here.

Book Chapters for a Book titled "Fetal and Neonatal Cardiology."

In early 2000s, I was invited by Dr. Charles Klienman of Columbia University in New York, NY, to contribute a chapter titled "Tricuspid Atresia in the Neonate" for a book on "Fetal and Neonatal Cardiology" to be published by W.B. Saunders, Co. This chapter was prepared (Figure 8) and sent to Dr. Kleiman. Unfortunately, however, this book did not seem to get published as planned. This material reviewed in other publications[39,40] and discussed in the chapter on "Tricuspid Atresia" in the book titled "Pediatric Cardiology: How It Has Evolved Over the last 50 Years" and will not repeated here.

TRICUSPID ATRESIA IN THE NEONATE

By

P. Syamasundar Rao, MD
Professor of Pediatrics
Director, Center for Transcatheter Treatment of
Heart Defects in Children
Saint Louis University School of Medicine/
Cardinal Glennon Children's Hospital
Saint Louis, Missouri

For a Book Entitled "FETAL AND NEONATAL CARDIOLOGY"
Editors: Charles S. Kleinman, MD
Joshua Copel, MD
W.B. Saunders, Co.

Address for correspondence: Division of Pediatric Cardiology, Saint Louis University School of Medicine, 1465 South Grand Blvd., St. Louis, MO 63104. Phone: 314-577-5633; Fax: 314-268-6411; e-mail: raops@SLU.EDU

Figure 8. A copy of the title page of chapter titled "Tricuspid Atresia in the Neonate" for a book on "Fetal and Neonatal Cardiology;" the book was not published.

Reliability of Echocardiographic Estimation of Angiographic Minimal Ductal Diameter.[19]

This study was reviewed in the chapter on "Patent Ductus Arteriosus" in the book titled "Pediatric Cardiology: How It Has Evolved Over the last 50 Years" and will not be repeated here. This study was also recently published.[25]

Versatility of Amplatzer Vascular Plug in Occlusion of Different Types of Vascular Channels

Embolization of superfluous vascular channels is a crucial procedure in patients with congenital heart disease. A number of embolic materials have been used to occlude abnormal vascular channels; Gianturco coils were most commonly used in the past. Recently described Amplatzer vascular plug (AVP) has been applied to several cardiac lesions with success. The purpose of this presentation was to describe our experience in a variety of clinical scenarios where the Amplatzer Vascular Plug was successfully used. Between May 2005 and March 2008, seven patients (five male, two female; six months to eighteen years of age) were referred for transcatheter occlusion of a variety of vascular abnormalities. Indications for embolotherapy were similar to those used in the past. Following the definition of the anatomy of the lesion, 6 to 12 mm diameter AVPs were delivered via 5 or 6 F right coronary artery guide catheters. Angiography was performed prior to and ten minutes following implantation of the plug. The technical success rate was 100 percent, with total occlusion of all target vessels or lesions. Examples of AVP occlusion are shown in figures 9 through 15. No complications were encountered. Based on these experiences it was concluded that occlusion of vascular connections in a variety of clinical scenarios is feasible using Amplatzer vascular plug devices. Our experience indicates that the procedure is technically simple with excellent results. It is particularly useful in large vessels and avoids the use of multiple coils. A knowledge of the vascular anatomy, patho-physiologic effects of embolic occlusion of the target lesion and understanding of potential complications is crucial prior to embarking on transcatheter occlusion and these principles are equally applicable to Amplatzer vascular plug occlusion.[20]

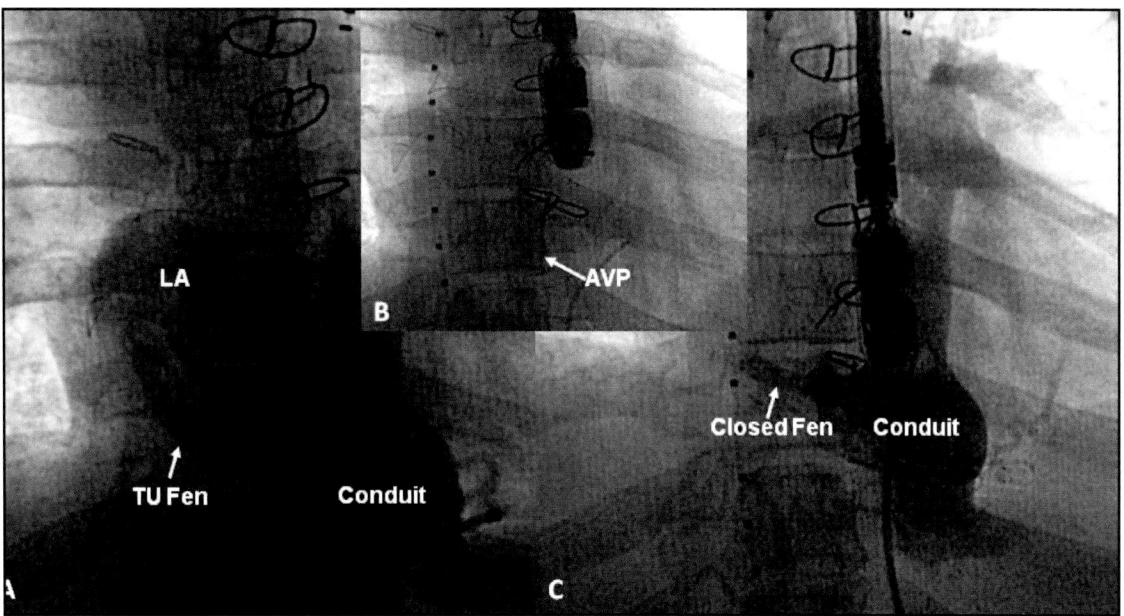

Figure 9. A. Selected cine frame from Fontan conduit cineangiogram in antero-posterior view demonstrating tubular fenestration (TuFen) with opacification of the left atrium (LA). B. The TuFen is closed with Amplatzer Vascular Plug (AVP). C. Follow-up conduit cine angiogram after AVP implantation showing complete occlusion of the TuFen. TEE, trans-esophageal probe. Reproduced from the poster of Reference 20.

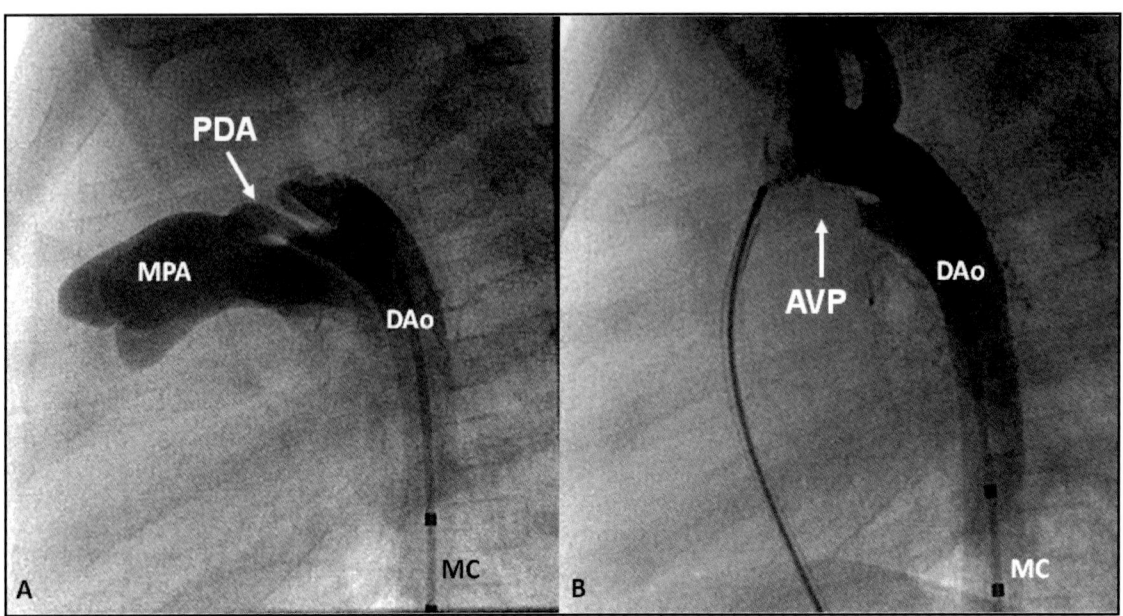

Figure 10. A. Selected cine frame from aortic arch angiogram in lateral view demonstrating a tubular patent ductus arteriosus (PDA). B. An Amplatzer vascular plug (AVP) was positioned across the PDA; note that there is complete occlusion of the PDA with no residual shunt. DAo, descending aorta; MC, marker pigtail catheter; MPA, main pulmonary artery.

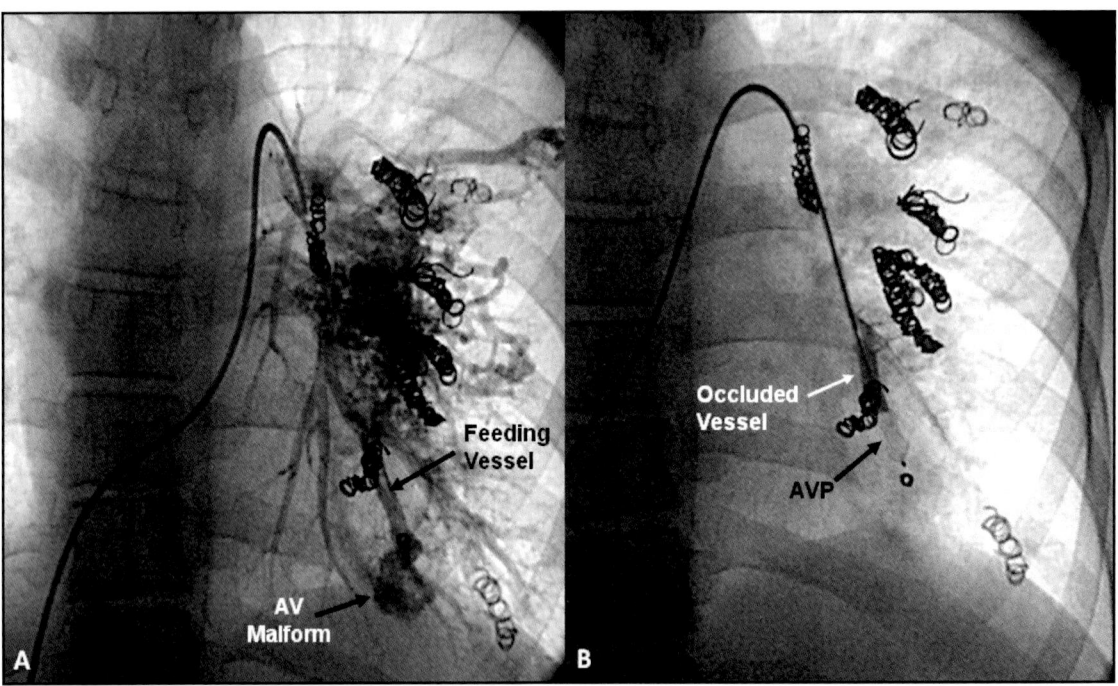

Figure 11. A. Selected pulmonary cinearteriographic frame in posterio-anterior view showing a large pulmonary arteriovenous malformation (AV Malform) in a patient who had multiple coils implanted in prior procedures. B. Implantation of Amplatzer vascular plug (AVP) into the target vessel (TV) resulted in complete occlusion of the pulmonary AV Malform. Reproduced from the poster of Reference 20.

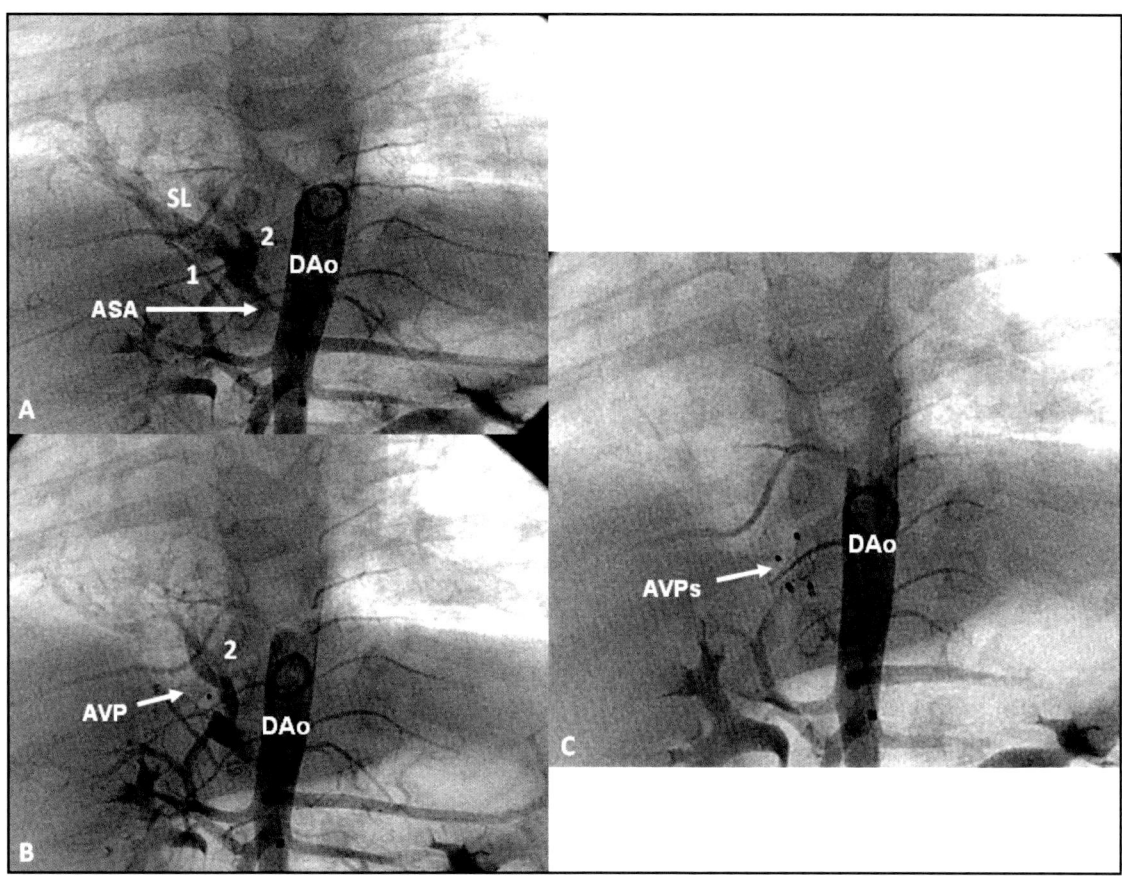

Figure 12. A. Selected cine-angiographic frame from abdominal aortogram (DAo) demonstrating a large anomalous systemic artery (ASA) opacifying a sequestered lung (SL) in an infant with congestive heart failure. The ASA divides into two branches, labeled 1 and 2. B. The ASA was occluded with Amplatzer Vascular Plug (AVP); branch 1 was completely occluded, while branch 2 remained patent. C. A second AVP was implanted in branch 2 resulting in complete occlusion. Following the procedure, the infant improved. Renal collecting systems (not marked) are seen in the lower portions of all three frames. Reproduced from the poster of Reference 20.

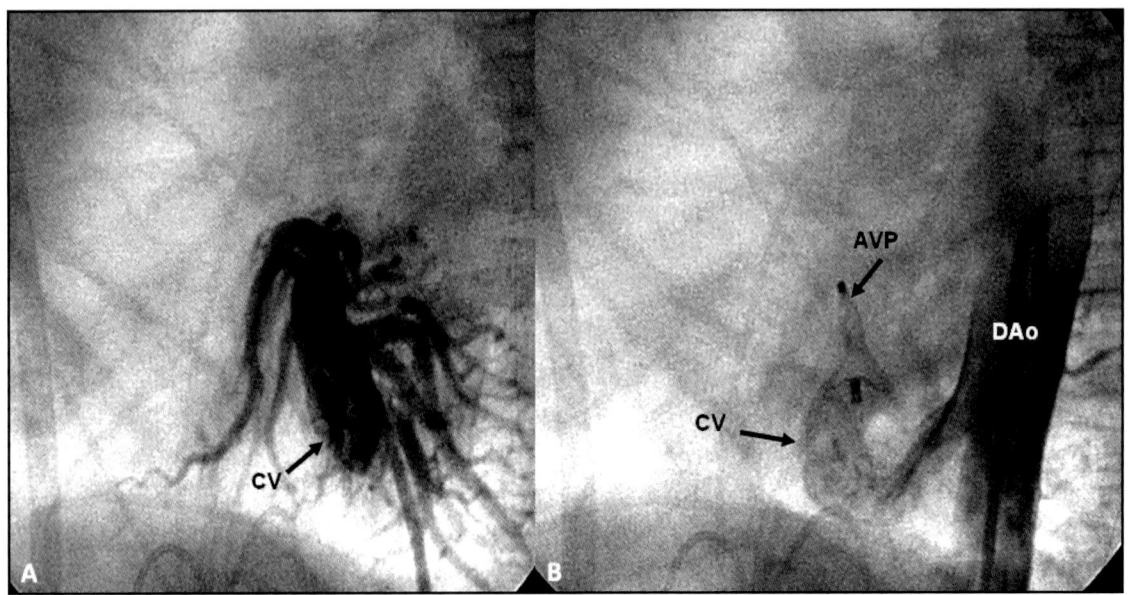

Figure 13. A. Selected cine frame from an angiogram in lateral view from an injection into a persistent embryonic collateral vessel (CV) arising from the descending aorta (DAo) demonstrating opacification of the lung. This infant was in congestive heart failure following a uni-focalization procedure. B. The CV was occluded with an Amplatzer vascular plug (AVP); no residual shunt was seen. The infant improved clinically following the procedure. C, catheter; PC, pigtail catheter. Reproduced from the poster of Reference 20.

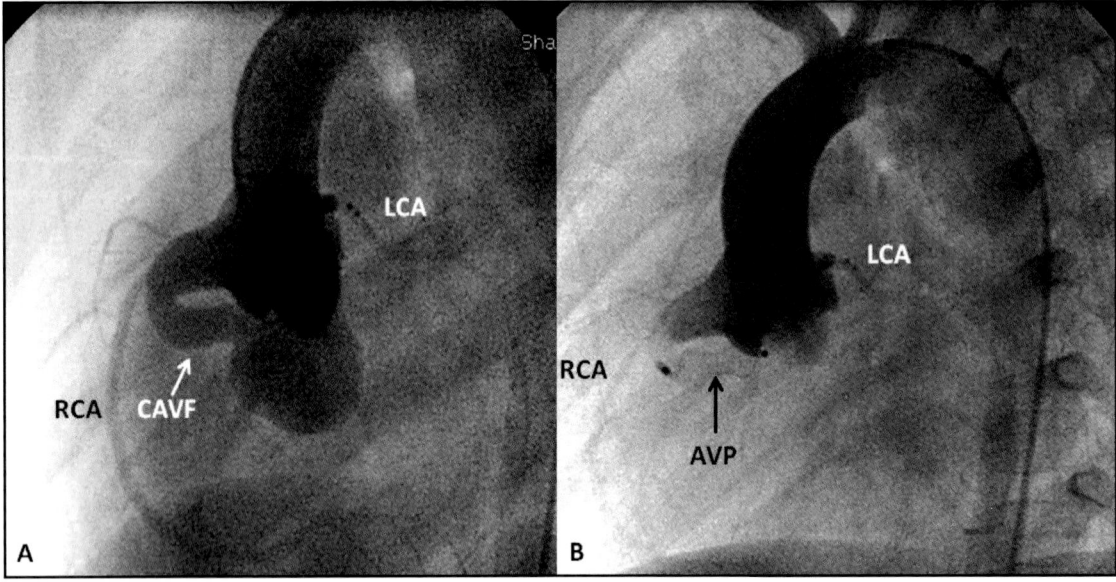

Figure 14. A. Selected cine frame from aortic (Ao) root cine-angiogram in a left anterior oblique projection demonstrating a large coronary arteriovenous fistula (CAVF) in a neonate with heart failure. Both the right (RCA) and left (LCA) coronary arteries were visualized. B. Following occlusion with an Amplatzer Vascular Plug (AVP), no residual CAVF shunt was seen. Both the RCA and LCA were seen as in A. The infant clinically improved following the procedure. Reproduced from the poster of Reference 20.

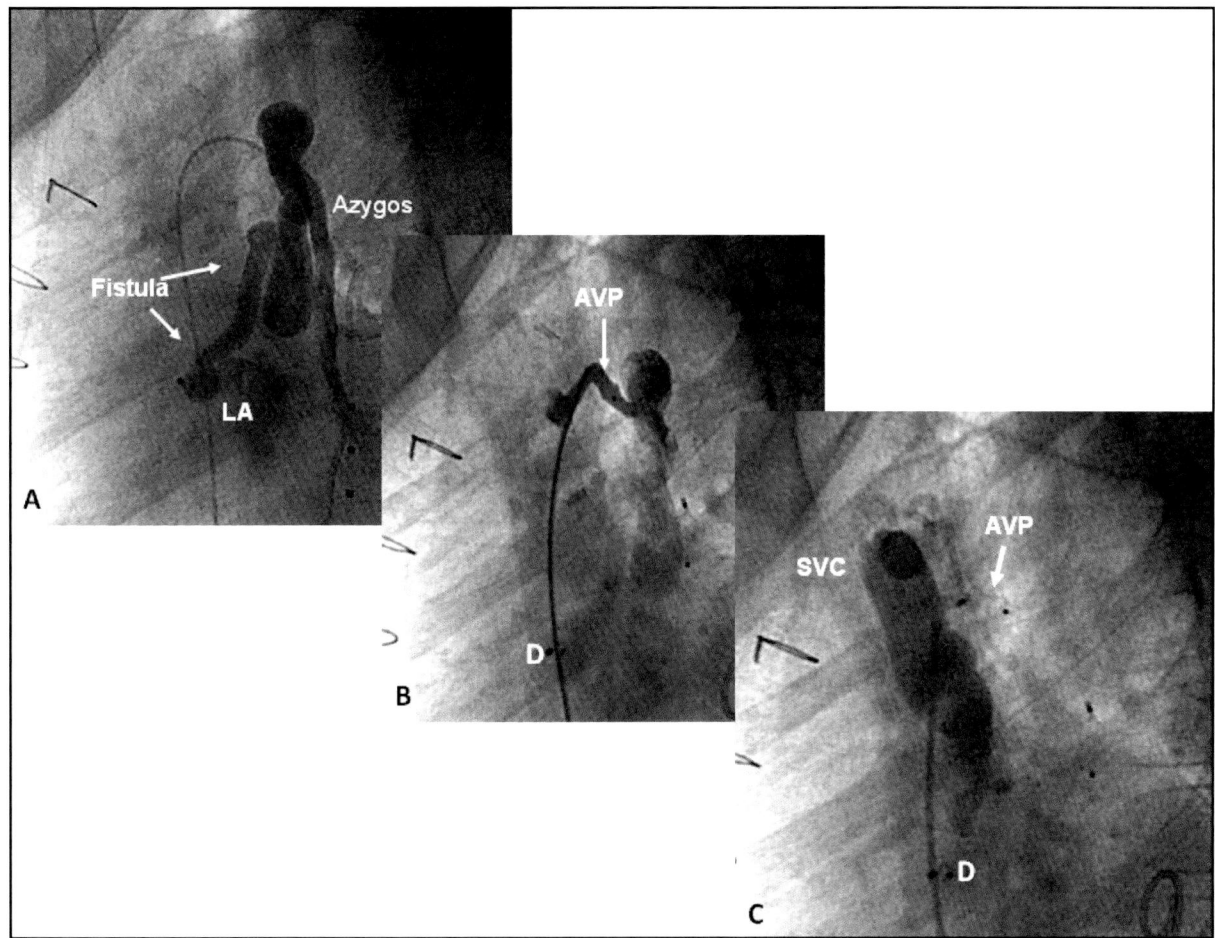

Figure 15. A. Selected cine frame from azygos vein cineangiogram demonstrating fistula in a patient who had Fontan procedure previously. The fistula opens into the left atrium (LA). B. Amplatzer Vascular Plug (AVP) was implanted in the proximal azygos vein. Device (D) across Fontan fenestration closed during a prior procedure is seen. C. Selected cine frame from the superior vena caval (SVC) cineangiogram demonstrating complete occlusion. Reproduced from the poster of Reference 20.

2010s

Intermediate and Long-Term Follow-up after Patent Ductus Arteriosus Closure Using Amplatzer Device.[21]

The results of this study were reviewed in the chapter on "Patent Ductus Arteriosus" in the book titled "Pediatric Cardiology: How It Has Evolved Over the last 50 Years" and will not be reviewed here.

Patent Ductus Arteriosus in Siblings

Sudden death of a twenty-seven-year-old patient prompted referral to us for evaluation of his son, a fourteen-year-old young man. History and physical examination revealed no abnormalities. Echocardiogram revealed a small PDA with left-to-right shunt. It measured 1.4 mm at pulmonary end. While this is unlikely to be related to the issue of sudden death of the father, following detailed discussions with the patient's pediatrician and the mother, it was decided to transcatheter occlude the PDA. Cardiac catheterization and angiography confirmed echocardiographic diagnosis of PDA, which measured 1.5 mm at the pulmonary and 5 mm at the aortic end. Transcatheter closure of PDA was performed using a 0.038 inch Gianturco coil measuring 8 cm x 5 mm. There was no residual shunt at conclusion of the procedure. Ten-year-old brother and eight-year-old sister were also evaluated; the ten-year-old boy had normal findings, while the eight-year-old girl had a grade 2/6 ejection systolic murmur. Echocardiograms of both these children revealed small PDAs without any other abnormalities. Cardiac catheterization and angiography revealed small PDAs (minimal ductal diameters were 1.4 mm and 1.2 mm, respectively). Both the PDAs were occluded with 0.038 inch Gianturco coils. Follow-up echocardiograms revealed no residual shunt and no evidence for symptomatology. Detailed genetic history did not reveal any evidence for PDA in members of the family, but paternal grandfather had myocardial infarction at the age of forty-five years. Usual dietary, yearly BP monitoring and no smoking advice was rendered. Detailed review of the literature revealed prior reports of PDAs in siblings as well as familial occurrence of PDA.[41-43]

Intermediate Follow-up Results of Amplatzer Device Occlusion of Secundum Atrial Septal Defects.[22]

This study was reviewed in the chapter on "Atrial Septal Defects" in the book titled "Pediatric Cardiology: How It Has Evolved Over the last 50 Years" and will not be discussed in this chapter.

Impact of TransCatheter Interventions on Prolonging Life of Right Ventricle to Pulmonary Artery Conduits

One of the graduating fellows, Dr. Durga Naidu and I have examined the role of transcatheter interventions in prolonging the life span of right ventricle to pulmonary artery (RV-PA) valved conduits implanted in infants and young children. A retrospective review of all patients who underwent RV-PA conduit placement from January 2006 to March 2016 was undertaken. RV-PA conduits were implanted on ninety occasions in seventy-six patients. The median age at initial conduit placement was 11.1 months (range 0.1 to 14.8 months). Homografts (aortic or pulmonary) were used in seventy-five patients and xenograft conduits were used in fifteen subjects. Follow-up data was available from 0.1 to 84 months (median of twenty-one months). During this period ninety-two catheter interventions were performed in fifty-four patients (balloon angioplasty [n= 83], stent placement [n= 53]). Catheter interventions prolonged RV-PA conduit life from 0.1 to 193.7 months (median of 25.5 months). Age at initial surgery and diameter of the RV-PA conduits used were not associated with any significant variation in conduit longevity. Longevity of pulmonary homografts (median 24.1 months) was better than aortic homografts (median 10.5 months), but this difference was not statistically significant ($p > 0.05$). On the basis of these data, we conclude that catheter based interventions prolong the longevity of RV-PA conduits by a median of slightly longer than two years. Such prolongation appears to reduce the total number of surgical procedures required over the patient's lifetime. The paper was submitted for publication and will be referenced if published prior to the publication of this book.

REFERENCES

1. Rao PS, Strong WB, Kwon OB, "Sudden infant death syndrome and cardiac arrhythmias," *Pediat Res 1973*; 7:305.

2. Rao PS, Linde LM, Awa S, "Isoproterenol and right ventricular outflow obstruction," *Pediatr Res 1973*; 7:304.

3. Rao PS and Linde LM, "Isoproterenol and right ventricular obstruction," *Proceedings of the XIV International Congress of Pediatrics*, October 1974, Buenos Aires, Argentina, Vol. VIII, Cardiology-Nephrology, pp. 47-49.

4. Rao PS, Salehbhai M, "Congenital heart disease in Down's syndrome - Its genotype distribution," *Pediatr Res 1976*; 10:370.

5. Hayashidera T, Covitz W, Weisman CE, Rao PS, et al, "Echocardiographic selection of children with aortic stenosis for catheterization," *Clin Res*, 26:80A, 1978. Presented at the Southern Society for Pediatric Research Meeting, New Orleans, LA, January 1979.

6. Rao PS, "Effect of acute increase in stroke volume on pulmonary vascular impedance," *Pediatr Res 1980*; 14:449.

7. Rao PS, Mardini MK, Feteih W, et al, "Syndrome of absent pulmonary valve. Abstracts of the International Symposium on Cardiovascular Surgery - 1985," Houston, Texas, September 12-14, 1985, p. 141.

8. Rao PS, Mardini MK, Feteih W, et al, "Syndrome of absent pulmonary valve," *Abstracts of the X World Congress of Cardiology*, September 14-19, 1986, Washington, D.C., p. 475.

9. Reid KG and Rao PS, "Successful radical two-stage correction of pulmonary atresia with intact ventricular septum, right ventricular and tricuspid hypoplasia, using the Fontan-Kreutzer principle in childhood," presented at the Pediatric Cardiology, Symposium: Recent Advances, April 21-22, 1987, Riyadh, Saudi Arabia, *Ann Saudi Med 1987*; 7:258.

10. Chopra PS, Kantamneni V, Wilson AD and Rao PS, "Surgical repair of common atrioventricular septal defects - Long-term results using single-patch technique," presented at the 1st World Congress of Pediatric Cardiology and Cardiac Surgery, Paris, France, June 21-25, 1993, *Cardiol Young 1993*; 3:48.

11. Singh GK, Marino C, Oliver D, Balfour I, Chen S, Jureidini SB, Rao PS, "Pressure gradients in outflow stenotic lesions: A simultaneous Doppler and catheter correlative study in pediatric patients," poster presentation at the 11th Annual Scientific Session of the American Society of Echocardiography, Chicago, IL, June 11-14, 2000, *J Am Soc Echo 2000*; 13:455.

12. Singh GK, Marino C, Oliver D, Balfour I, Chen S, Jureidini SB, Rao PS, "Pressure recovery and pressure gradients in stenotic outflow tract lesions: A simultaneous Doppler and catheter correlative study in pediatric patients," poster presentation at the 3rd World Congress of Pediatric Cardiology & Cardiac Surgery, Toronto, May 27-31, 2001, *Cardiol Young 2001*; 11:184.

13. Rao PS, Sideris EB, "Buttoned device modifications: Influence on feasibility, safety and effectiveness," Poster Presentation at the 3rd World Congress of Pediatric Cardiology & Cardiac Surgery, Toronto, May 27-31, 2001, *Cardiol Young 2001*; 11:279.

14. Singh GK, Marino CJ, Fiore AC, Winn H, Rao PS, "Morphogenetic insight in evaluation of tricuspid atresia," presented at the 13th Annual Scientific Sessions of the American Society of Echocardiography, Orlando, Florida, June 9-12, 2002, *J Am Soc Echo 2002*; 15:547.

15. Singh GK, Balfour IC, Chen S, Ferdman B, Jureidini SB, Fiore AC, Rao PS, "Prenatal growth of tricuspid valve and right ventricle determines the evolution and postnatal outcomes of tricuspid atresia," poster presentation at the 52nd Annual Scientific Session of the American College of Cardiology, Chicago, IL, March 30 – April 2, 2003, *J Am Coll Cardiol 2003*; 41:483A.

16. Singh GK, Balfour IC, Chen S, Ferdman B, Jureidini SB, Fiore AC, Rao PS, "Lesion specific pressure recovery phenomenon in pediatric patients: A simultaneous Doppler and catheter correlative study," poster presentation at the 52nd Annual Scientific Session of the American College of Cardiology, Chicago, IL, March 30 – April 2, 2003, *J Am Coll Cardiol 2003*; 41:493A.

17. Rao PS, Jureidini SB, Singh G.K, et al, "Clinical comparison of rigid with flexible stents in the management of vascular obstructive lesions in children," poster presentation at the 26th Annual Scientific Sessions of the Society of Cardiac Angiography and Interventions, Westin Copley Place, Boston, MA, May 7 – 10, 2003, *Cath Cardiovasc Intervent 2003*; 59:153.

18. Rao PS, Sideris EB, "Buttoned device modifications: Influence on feasibility, safety and effectiveness," poster presentation at the 26th Annual Scientific Sessions of the Society of Cardiac Angiography and Interventions, Westin Copley Place, Boston, MA, May 7 – 10, 2003, *Cath Cardiovasc Intervent 2003*; 59:153.

19. Subramanian U, Hamzeh RK, Sharma SK, Rao PS, "Reliability of echocardiographic estimation of angiographic minimal ductal diameter," poster presentation at the 30th Annual Scientific Session of Society for Cardiac Angiography & Interventions, Orlando, FL, May 9-12, 2007, *Cath Cardiovasc Intervent 2007*; 69:S87.

20. Tsounias E, Rao PS, "Versatility of Amplatzer Vascular Plug in occlusion of different types of vascular channels," poster presentation at the 12th Pediatric Interventional Cardiac Symposium (PICS-X) and Emerging New Technologies in Congenital Heart Surgery (ENTICHS) - 2008, The Bellagio, Las Vegas, NV, July 19-23, 2008, *Catheterization and Cardiovascular interventions, 2008*; Vol. 71, Issue 7, June 2008.

21. Yarrabolu TR, Rao PS, "Intermediate and long term follow-up after patent ductus arteriosus closure using Amplatzer device," poster presentation at the 17th PICS-AICS 2013, Miami, FL, January 2013.

22. Hartas GA, Balaguru D, Brown M, Rao PS, "Intermediate follow-up results of Amplatzer device occlusion of secundum atrial septal defects," poster presentation at the 19th PICS-AICS 2015, Los Vegas, NV, September 2015.

23. Rao PS, "Auscultation is still a valid tool in the evaluation of cardiac defects in children," *Congenital Cardiology Today 2018*; 16(8):1-6.

24. Rao PS, "Transcatheter perforation of atretic pulmonary valve in pulmonary atresia with ventricular septal defect," *Congenital Cardiology Today 2018*; 16(11):1-8.

25. Rao PS, Subramaniam U, "Reliability of echocardiographic estimation of angiographic minimal ductal diameter," *Congenital Cardiology Today 2019*; 17(3):1-7.

26. Rao PS, Lawrie GM, "Syndrome of absent pulmonary valve: Surgical correction with pulmonary arterioplasty," *Brit Heart J 1983*; 50:586-9.

27. Rao PS, Leonard T, "Polysplenia Syndrome," *Cardiology Digest 1976* (March); 11(3):14-22.

28. Rao PS, "Dextrocardia: Systematic Approach to Differential Diagnosis," *Amer Heart J 1981*; 102:389-403.

29. Rao PS, Andaya WG, "Chronic afterload reduction in infants and children with primary myocardial disease," *J Pediat 1986*; 108:530-4.

30. Rao PS, "Diagnosis and management of acyanotic heart disease: Part I - obstructive lesions," *Indian J Pediatr 2005*; 72:496-502.

31. Rao PS, "Diagnosis and management of acyanotic heart disease: Part II - left-to-right shunt lesions," *Indian J Pediatr 2005*; 72:503-12.

32. Rao PS, "Diagnosis and management of cyanotic congenital heart disease: Part I," *Indian J Pediat 2009*; 76:57-70.

33. Rao PS, "Diagnosis and management of cyanotic congenital heart disease: Part II," *Indian J Pediat 2009*; 76:297-308.

34. Rao PS (ed.), "Congenital Heart Disease - Selected Aspects," InTech, Rijeka, Croatia, January 2012; ISBN 978-953-307-472-6.

35. Rao PS, "Value of Echo-Doppler studies in the evaluation of the results of balloon pulmonary valvuloplasty," *J Cardiovasc Ultrasonography 1986*; 5:309-14.

36. Rao PS, "Doppler ultrasound in the prediction of transvalvar pressure gradients in patients with valvar pulmonic stenosis," *International J Cardiol 1987*; 15:195-203.

37. Rao PS, "Value of Echo-Doppler studies in the evaluation of the results of balloon angioplasty of aortic coarctation," *J Cardiovasc Ultrasonography 1988*; 7:215-20.

38. Rao PS, Carey P, "Doppler ultrasound in the prediction of pressure gradients across aortic coarctation," *Am Heart J 1989*; 118:299-301.

39. Rao PS, Alapati S, "Tricuspid Atresia in the Neonate," *Neonatology Today 2012*; 7(5):1-12.

40. "Tricuspid atresia – Chapter 22," In: Rao PS, Vidyasagar D (eds.), Perinatal Cardiology: A Multidisciplinary Approach, *Cardiotext Publishing 2015*, Minneapolis.

41. Martin RP, Banner NR, Radley-Smith R, "Familial persistent ductus arteriosus," *Arch Dis Child 1986*; 61:906-7.

42. Woods CG, Sheffield LJ, "Further family with autosomal dominant patent ductus arteriosus," *J Med Genet 1994*; 31:659.

43. Slavotinek A, Clayton-Smith J, Super M, "Familial patent ductus arteriosus: A further case of CHAR syndrome," *Am J Med Genet 1997*; 71:229-32.

CHAPTER 13

MISCELLANEOUS STUDIES

INTRODUCTION

Although my contributions to the literature were reviewed in multiples chapters in the book titled "Pediatric Cardiology: How It Has Evolved Over the Last 50 Years," which is a companion to this book and in the preceding chapters on case reports, reviews, editorials, monographs and books, adult congenital heart disease, some of my publications were still not included in these deliberations. The purpose of this chapter is to bring together these studies and review them.

USEFULNESS OF CONTINUOUS POSITIVE AIRWAY PRESSURE IN THE DIFFERENTIAL DIAGNOSIS OF CARDIAC FROM PULMONARY CYANOSIS IN THE NEONATE

It is sometimes difficult to differentiate severe pulmonary disease from a cyanotic congenital heart defect (CCHD) in a distressed cyanotic neonate. In mid-1970s, cardiac catheterization and selective cineangiography was required to make this distinction. PaO_2 response to 100 percent oxygen is sometimes helpful, but is not always reliable. A prospective study was undertaken to test the hypothesis that the response of PaO_2 to continuous positive airway pressure (CPAP) with 100 percent oxygen may be useful in making this distinction.[1] Thirty-five neonates admitted to Neonatal Intensive Care Unit (NICU) with a $PaO_2 \leq 50$ tort while in FIO_2 of 0.8 to 1.0 were included in this study. On the basis of clinical, cardiac catheterization and angiography, surgical, and necropsy findings, twenty-one babies were found to have cyanotic CHD, ten infants had pulmonary parenchymal disease (PD) and three cases were categorized as persistent fetal circulation (PFC). The pH, $PaCO_2$ and plasma bicarbonate values were similar (p > 0. 1) in all three groups and did not change following administration of oxygen (FIO_2 of 0.8 to 1.0) and CPAP (See Table 2 of Reference 1). The PaO_2 is similar in FIO_2 of 0.21 to 0.4 in all three groups (Figure 1) and did not increase significantly (p > 0.05) in FIO_2 of 0.8 to 1.0 (Figure 1). Following CPAP, the PaO_2 did not increase in babies with CCHD and PFC. However significant increase in PaO_2 occurred in PD group after CPAP (Figure 1). These data are shown in a slightly different manner in figure 2. The final PaO_2 on 0.8 to 1.0 FIO_2 with CPAP was < 50 torr in the CCHD group and > 50 torr in the PD group. In spite of attaining statistical significance 2 PD infants had no increase in PaO_2 with CPAP. An increase of PaO_2 greater than 10 torr with CPAP suggests PD, and a non-significant increase in PaO_2 does not rule out PD.

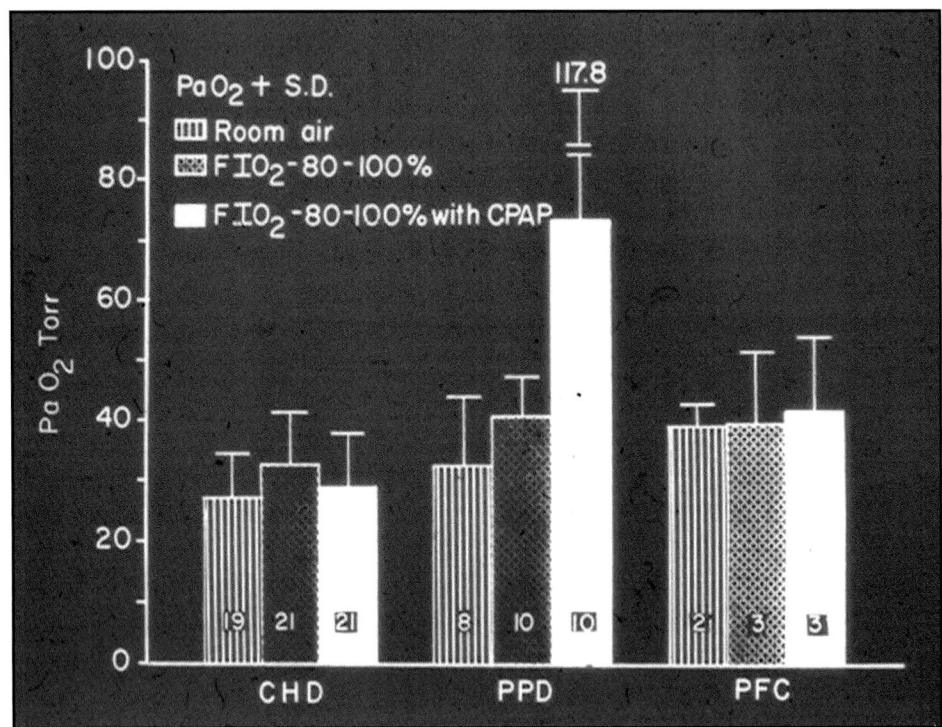

Figure 1. The PaO_2 is expressed as mean + standard deviation. The number of infants in each group is shown in each bar. There was no change in PaO_2 from $F1O_2$ of 0.21- 0.4 to $F1O_2$ of 0.8 -1.0 in all three groups. With additional CPAP, the PaO_2 did not change in babies with congenital heart defect (CHD) and persistent fetal circulation (PFC) groups. However significant increase in PaO_2 occurred in pulmonary parenchymal disease (PD) group after CPAP. Reproduced from Rao PS, et al, *Arch Dis Child 1978*; 53:456-60.

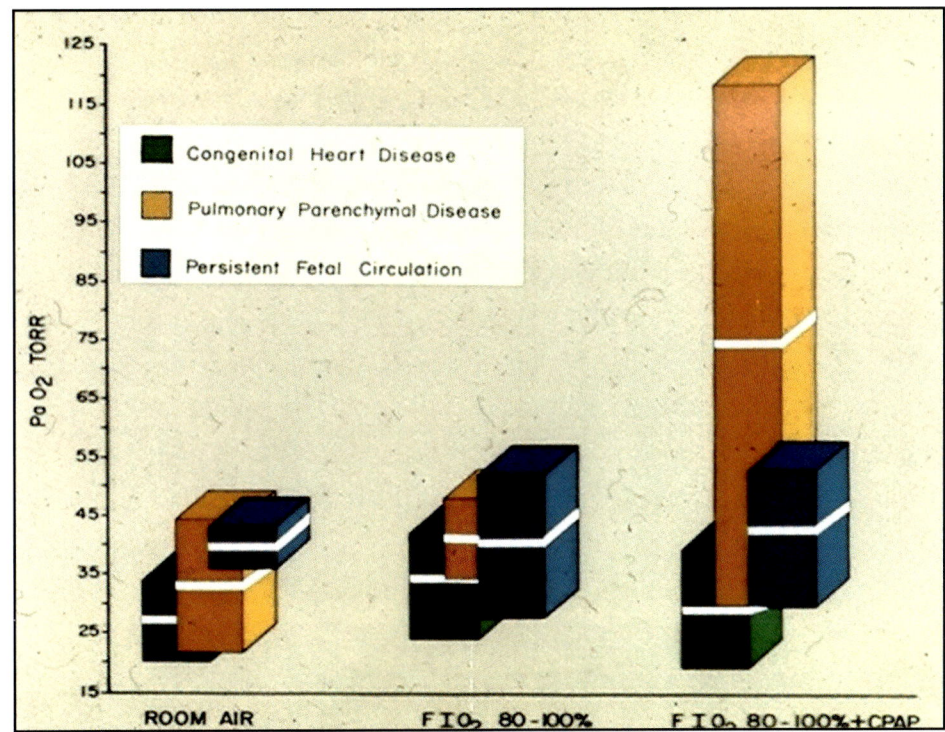

Figure 2. The data are shown slightly differently in this figure and indicate
that PaO$_2$s are similar in room air and in 100 percent O$_2$ in all three groups.
However, the PaO$_2$ is higher in pulmonary parenchymal disease group on CPAP.

It was concluded that: 1. CPAP with 1.0 FIO$_2$ may be used as an adjunct in the differential diagnosis of cyanotic newborn infants, 2. In CHD babies, CPAP does not produce an increase > 10 torr, but such an insignificant change in PaO$_2$ does not rule out PD, 3. In most PD babies PaO$_2$ increases by >10 torr with CPAP and is highly suggestive of PD. A PaO$_2$ response > 10 torr with CPAP practically excludes CHD, 4. Irrespective of the PaO$_2$ in room air and in 1.0 FIO$_2$, the PaO$_2$ with the additional CPAP may be of value in that PaO$_2$ > 50 torr strongly suggests PD and PaO$_2$ <50 torr indicates CHD. However, there are occasional exceptions, and 5. PaO$_2$ response to CPAP in the PFC group mimics the intra-cardiac right-to-left shunting seen in CHD and cannot be distinguished from that observed in CHD.

These results indicate that CPAP may be used as an adjunct in differentiating cardiac from pulmonary disease.[1]

SYSTOLIC TIME INTERVAL CHARACTERISTICS IN CHILDREN WITH DUCHENNE'S PROGRESSIVE MUSCULAR DYSTROPHY

Dr. Sanyal of St. Jude Children's Hospital in Memphis, TN, in collaboration with me analyzed systolic time interval (STI) characteristics of seventeen boys with Duchenne's muscular dystrophy (DMD) and compared them with those of eighty normal boys (control subjects).[2] This study began prior to widespread use of echocardiography. The heart rate decreased linearly with age in normal control subjects (r = - 0.47, p < 0.01). By contrast, heart rate was significantly higher in patients with DMD (p < 0.001) and tended to increase further with age. Each STI variable for normal control subjects increased significantly with age (p ≤ 0.01); QII, left ventricular ejection time (LVET), and pre-ejection period (PEP), in addition, decreased with increasing heart rate (p < 0.05). In DMD patients QII and LVET decreased with increasing heart rate (p < 0.001), but were not influenced by age. None of the other STI values in dystrophic patients was significantly influenced by either age or heart rate. Mean QII, LVET, and QI were shorter and PEP, isometric contraction time (ICT), and PEP/LVET ratio were longer (p < 0.001) for DMD patients than for normal control subjects. In 13/17 patients, QII and LVET were below the 95 percent confidence interval of the normal mean, whereas PEP, ICT, and PEP/LVET exceeded the upper limits of normal in 8, 9 and 11 patients, respectively. For dystrophic patients, the difference (delta) between the observed values and those predicted from regression equations for normal control subjects was lower for QII, LVET, and QI (p < 0.01), but higher for PEP (p < 0.04), ICT, and PEP/LVET ratio (p < 0.001). Delta QII and delta LVET increased with age (p = .001 and .032, respectively). Duchenne's muscular dystrophy is thus documented to be associated with substantial alterations in STI characteristics that suggest a compromised global left ventricular performance. Some of these abnormalities increase with age, probably reflecting the progressive cardiomyopathy characteristics of this disease.[2]

ANTICOAGULANT THERAPY IN CHILDREN WITH PROSTHETIC VALVES

The purpose of this study was to evaluate the effectiveness and complications of several types of anticoagulant therapy in children who had prosthetic valves implanted.[3] During a seven-year period ending April 1985, 130 children aged one to nineteen years underwent left-sided valve replacement. Operative mortality was 3 percent, 5 percent, and 9 percent, respectively, for aortic, mitral, and combined aortic and mitral valve replacement. Among the 123 survivors, thirty-two (26 percent) had aortic, seventy-one (58 percent) had mitral, and twenty (16 percent) had aortic and mitral valve replacement. Follow-up ranged from 2 months to 8.2 years, for a total of 544 patient-years. The survivors were divided into three groups based on anticoagulant treatment: Warfarin sodium, aspirin plus dipyridamole, and no anticoagulants. Among the patients who had aortic valve replacement, thromboembolic complications developed in 2.5 percent (2.5/100 patient-years) of the aspirin plus dipyridamole group and 5 percent of the group given no anticoagulants. Only the warfarin group (4 percent) experienced bleeding complications. Among the patients having mitral valve replacement, thromboembolic complications developed in 4 percent of the warfarin group, 3 percent of the aspirin plus dipyridamole group, and 11 percent of the no anticoagulant group. In addition, 2 percent of patients in the warfarin group experienced severe bleeding (Figure 3).

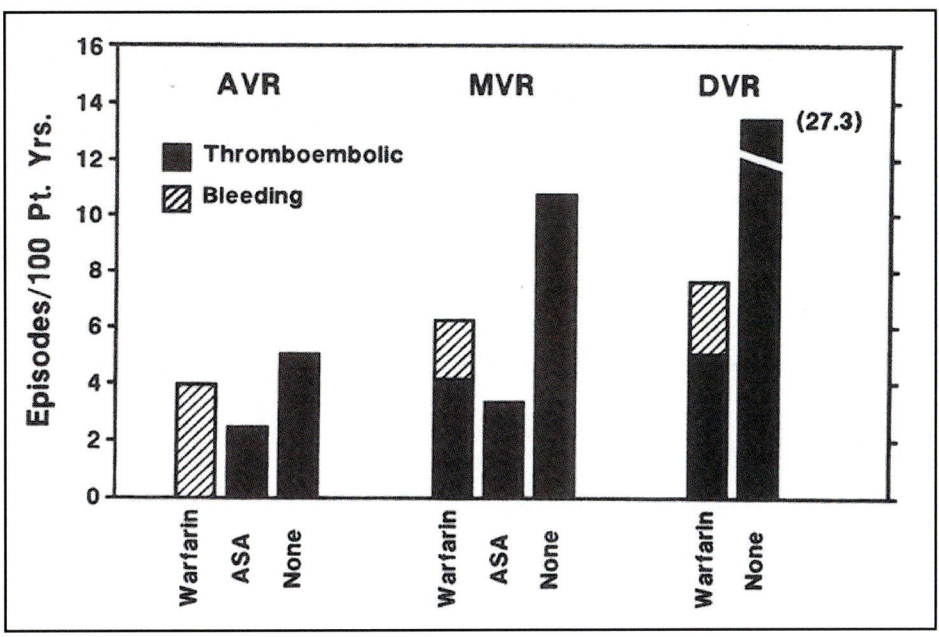

Figure 3. Thromboembolic and bleeding complications, expressed as episodes per 100 patient-years (Pt. Yrs.), based on anticoagulant treatment (warfarin sodium, aspirin plus dipyridamole [ASA], and no anticoagulants) and type of value replacement (aortic valve [AVR], mitral valve [MVR], and double valve replacement [DVR]).

Reproduced from Rao PS, et al, *Ann Thorac Surg 1989*; 47:589-92.

Two fatal cerebrovascular accidents occurred, both in the aspirin plus dipyridamole group. Patients who received a mitral heterograft were not prescribed any anticoagulant medications, and no thromboembolic complications developed. Among patients having double-valve replacement, complications developed in 5 percent of the warfarin group and 27 percent of the group given no anticoagulants. Based on these data, aspirin plus dipyridamole appears adequate for patients having aortic valve replacement, whereas warfarin is required in patients having double-valve replacement. Patients having mitral valve replacement with heterografts require no anticoagulation, but those with mechanical valves may need warfarin anticoagulation. There are not adequate data to evaluate the safety and efficacy of the combined use of warfarin and a platelet-inhibiting drug in children.[3]

LONG-TERM ORAL DIAZOXIDE THERAPY FOR PULMONARY VASCULAR OBSTRUCTIVE DISEASE ASSOCIATED WITH CHDS

This report presents the results of short-term and long-term effects of diazoxide on the pulmonary vascular resistance (PVR) in patients with pulmonary vascular obstructive disease (PVOD) secondary to delayed surgical correction of ventricular septal defect (VSD).[4] Six children, aged four to ten years, who had closure of VSD and who on lung biopsy showed PVOD, received intravenous diazoxide (1, 2, 4, 5, and 6 mg/kg) after measurements of pulmonary artery pressure (PAP), pulmonary flow index (PFI) by a thermo-dilution technique, and PVR were made. The PAP (51 ± 19 mmHg versus 45 ± 16 mmHg) and PVR (11.5 ± 2.7 units versus 8.9 ± 3.8 units) though decreased following administration of intravenous diazoxide, did not attain statistical significance (p > 0.1) (Figure 4). The PFI (3.2 ± 1.1 versus 3.4 ± 0.6 L/min/m²) did not change (p > 0.1).

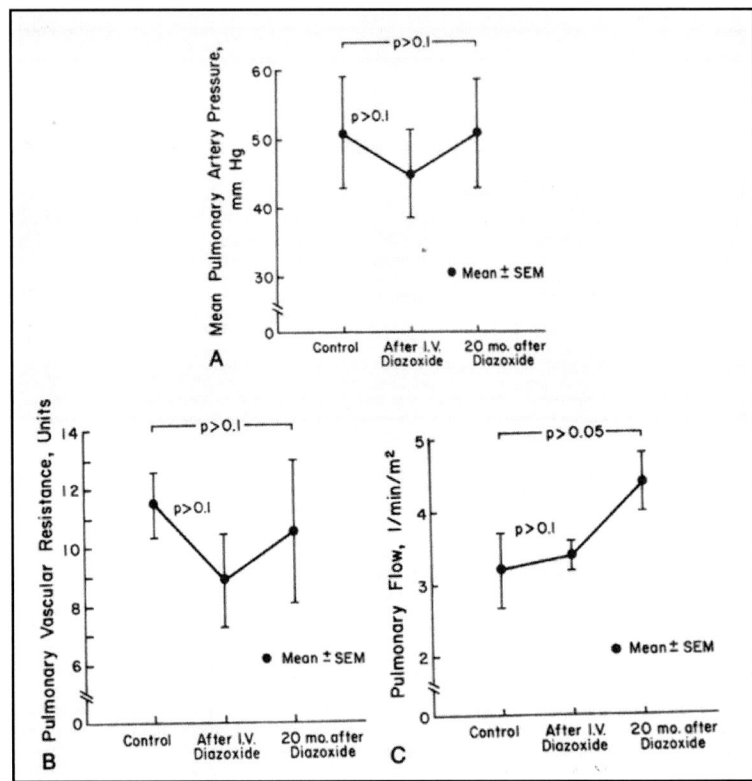

Figure 4. Response of pulmonary artery pressure (PAP), pulmonary vascular resistance (PVR), and pulmonary flow index to intravenous and long-term oral administration of diazoxide. There was a fall in PAP (A) and PVR (B), but this did not attain statistical significance (p > 0.1) following intravenous administration of diazoxide (5 to 6 mg/kg). There was no significant (p > 0.1) change in pulmonary flow index (C). After long-term (mean of twenty months) oral diazoxide, the PAP (A) and PVR {B} remain unchanged (p > 0.1). The pulmonary flow index increased (C), although this increase is not statistically significant (p > 0.05). Reproduced from Rao PS, *Am Heart J 1990*; 119:1317-21.

After oral diazoxide (5 to 10 mg/kg per day) for 20 ± 3.4 months, the PAP (50.8 ± 19 mmHg) and PVR (10.6 ± 5.8 units) did not decrease (p > 0.1), but PFI (4.4 ± 0.9 L/min/m2), though increased, did not attain significance (p > 0.05) (Figure 4 and 5). However, one of these children who had a fall in PVR from 8.5 to 4.5 units following intravenous diazoxide also had a lower resistance (3.9 units) after twenty-months of oral diazoxide therapy (Figure 5) and improved symptomatically. No complications other than hypertrichosis were encountered on long-term therapy. Based on this experience, it is suggested that oral diazoxide therapy may be used to improve PVOD if there is favorable response to intravenous diazoxide.[4] It should be noted that several other, more effective pulmonary vasodilators are currently availble for clinical use.

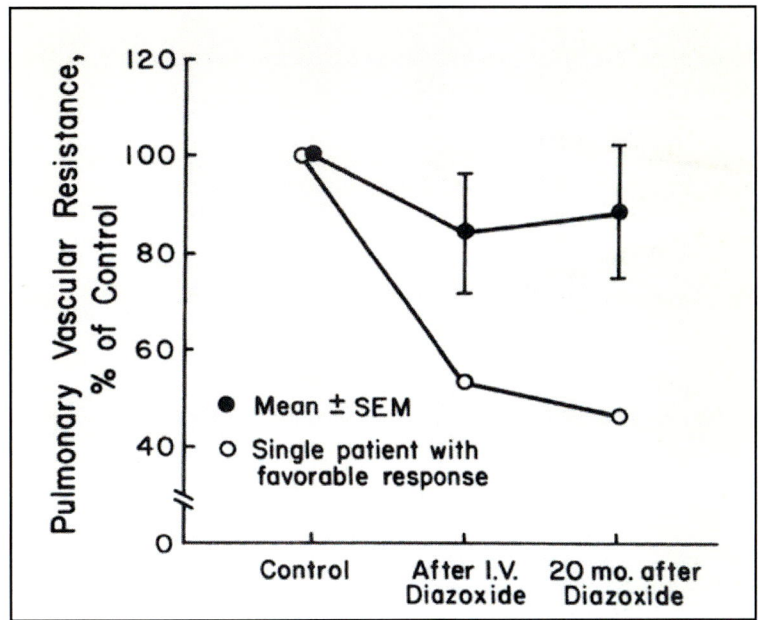

Figure 5. Percent change in pulmonary vascular resistance (PVR) over the short-term following intravenous diazoxide and after long-term oral diazoxide administration are shown. Note that there is no significant change in PVR for the group as a whole (solid circles). In a single patient (open circle), the PVR fell following intravenous diazoxide and remained low after twenty months of oral diazoxide therapy. Reproduced from Rao PS, *Am Heart J 1990*; 119:1317-21.

PROSTHETIC VALVES IN CHILDREN AND ADOLESCENTS

The purpose of this paper was to present short-term and long-term results of prosthetic valve replacement in children.[5] During a seven-year period ending in April 1985, 186 children, ages one to twenty years, underwent valve replacement; there were fifty-five (30 percent) aortic valve replacements, ninety-five (51 percent) mitral valve replacements, and thirty-six (19 percent) multiple valve replacements. 94 percent of the lesions were rheumatic in origin, 4 percent were congenital, and 2 percent were infectious. Of 223 valves replaced, 175 (78 percent) were mechanical valves and 48 (22 percent) were heterografts; the latter were in the mitral position in all but three patients. Surgical mortality rates were 3.6 percent, 4.2 percent, and 19.4 percent respectively for aortic valve, mitral valve, and multiple valve replacements. Five-year and eight-year actuarial survival was 91 percent for aortic valve replacement, 82 percent for mitral valve replacement and 60 percent for multiple valve replacement (Figure 6). Major events included reoperation in thirty-four (with three deaths), progressive myocardial failure that led to death in ten, sudden unexpected death in two, thromboembolic complications in nineteen (death in five), sub-acute bacterial endocarditis in five (two deaths), and bleeding that required transfusion in two patients. Five-year complication-free actuarial survival rates were 83 percent for aortic valve replacement, 63 percent for mitral valve replacement, and 57 percent for multiple valve replacement (Figure 7). The respective eight-year complication-free survival rates were 83 percent, 48 percent, and 43 percent (Figure 7).

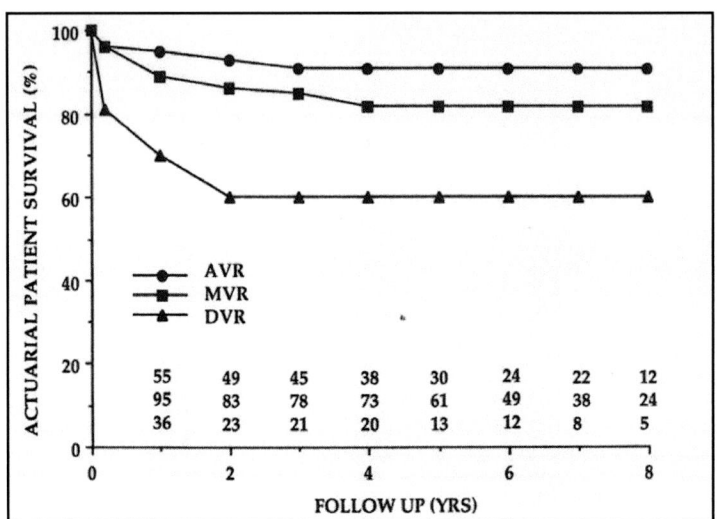

Figure 6. Actuarial patient survival curves following aortic (AVR), mitral (MVR), and multiple (DVR) valve replacement are shown. Note that there is excellent survival in the patients with aortic valve replacement, whereas poor survival is seen in patients with multiple valve replacement. The actuarial survival for MVR is between the AVR and DVR. Reproduced from Solymar L, Rao PS, et al, *Am Heart J 1991*; 121:557-68.

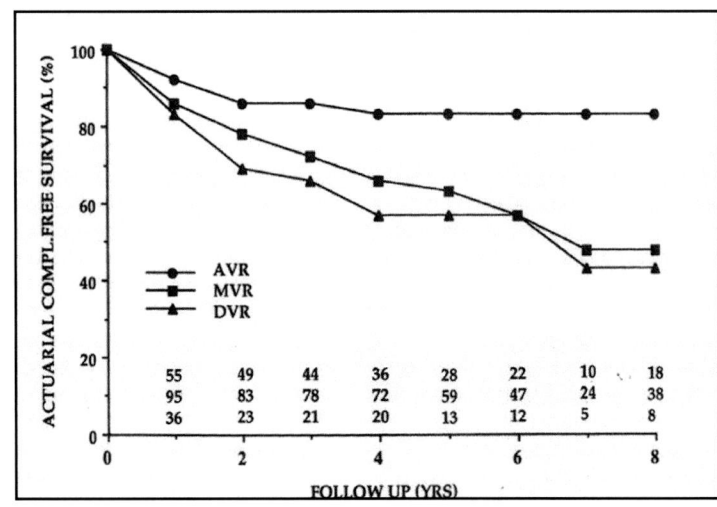

Figure 7. Actuarial major complication-free survival curves for aortic (AVR), mitral (MVR), and multiple (DVR) valve replacement are shown. Complication-free survival rates are better for AVR than for MVR and DVR. Similar complication-free survival rates for MVR and DVR suggest that mitral prostheses are largely responsible for complications. Reproduced from Solymar L, Rao PS, et al, *Am Heart J 1991*; 121:557-68.

Significant morbidity and mortality rates are associated with valve replacement. Therefore, every effort should be made to preserve the native valve by plastic reparative procedures. When prosthetic replacement of mitral valve is contemplated, our data would suggest that heterografts should not be inserted in children fifteen years of age or younger, although heterografts may be used in children over fifteen years of age with the expectation of valve survival comparable to that of mechanical valves.[6] When complications that are associated with anticoagulant therapy were reviewed, platelet inhibiting drugs seem quite satisfactory in patients with aortic valve replacement; patients with mitral valve replacement seem to require warfarin therapy, and warfarin must be used in patients with multiple valve replacement to reduce the risk of thromboembolic complications.[3,5]

REASSESSMENT OF USEFULNESS OF PORCINE HETEROGRAFTS IN MITRAL POSITION IN CHILDREN

The use of porcine heterograft valves in children is restricted because of valve calcification and dysfunction at follow-up. Because of inability to monitor the anticoagulant status or of desire of some teenage girls to get married and get pregnant, several pediatric patients received porcine heterografts. The purpose of this paper is to examine the issue of heterografts in children, based on our experience with children and adolescents, aged one to twenty years, who underwent left heart valve replacement during a seven-year period ending April 1985.[6] Ninety-four percent of the lesions were rheumatic in origin, 4 percent congenital, and 2 percent infectious. Of 168 mitral valves replaced, 54 (32 percent) were porcine heterografts and 114 (68 percent) were mechanical valves. These were divided into four groups, based on type of valve implanted and age at implantation: Mechanical (M), age greater than fifteen years (M > 15), forty-nine cases; heterografts (H) age greater than fifteen years (H > 15), thirty-four cases; mechanical, age less than or equal to fifteen years (M ≤ 15), 65 cases; and heterografts, age less than or equal to fifteen years (H ≤ 15), twenty cases. None of the patients with heterografts received anticoagulation. Five-year actuarial valve survival was 86 percent for M > 15, 96 percent for H > 15, 82 percent for M ≤ 15, and 60 percent for H ≤ 15 (Figures 8 and 9). The respective nine-year valve survival was 86 percent, 72 percent, 75 percent, and 18 percent (Figure 8 and 9). The valve survival data indicate that heterograft valves in patients older than fifteen years are comparable ($p = 0.97$) to mechanical valves (Figures 9), while heterografts in children less than fifteen years do poorly ($p = 0.015$) (Figure 8).

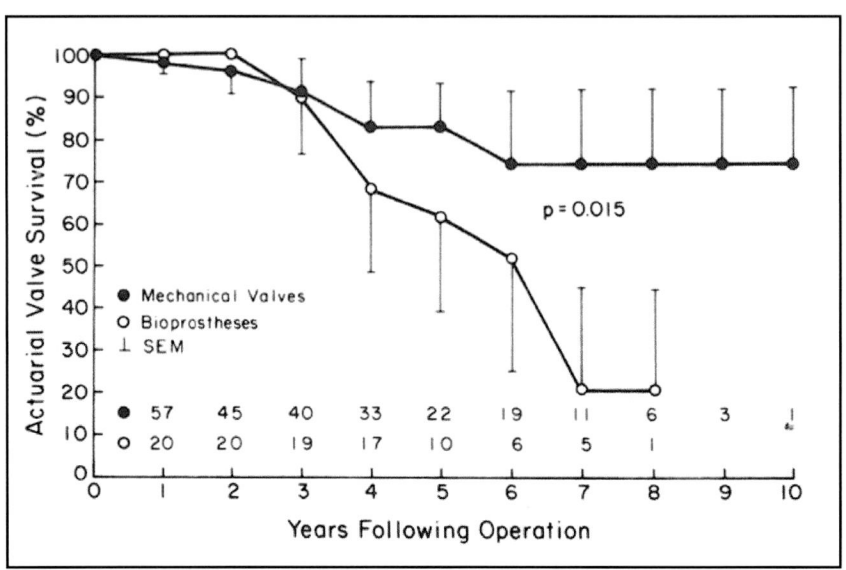

Figure 8. Actuarial valve survival curves for children ≤ 15 years are shown for mechanical and porcine heterografts; note poor survival for heterografts (p = 0.015). The confidence limits are marked on only one side of the curve to clearly discern both the curves. Reproduced from Rao PS, et al, *Pediat Cardiol 1991*; 12:164-69.

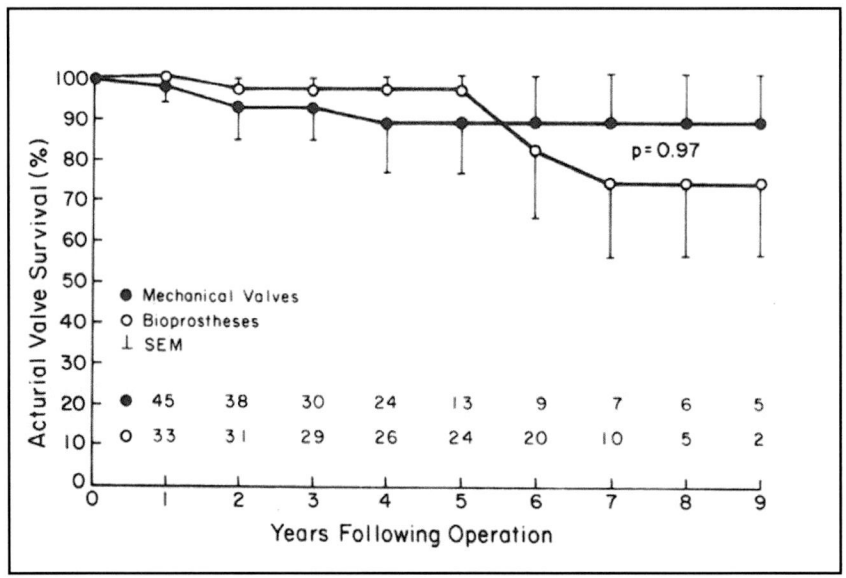

Figure 9. Actuarial valve survival curves for children > 15 years are shown for mechanical and porcine heterografts; the survival curves are similar (p = 0.97). The confidence limits are marked on only one side of the curve to visualize both curves clearly. Reproduced from Rao PS, et al, *Pediat Cardiol 1991*; 12:164-69.

Among the mechanical valves in mitral position, valve survival curves for Beall and Bjork-Shiley valves were similar, while the survival curves for St. Jude Medical valve is slightly better than those in the other mechanical valves (Figure 10).

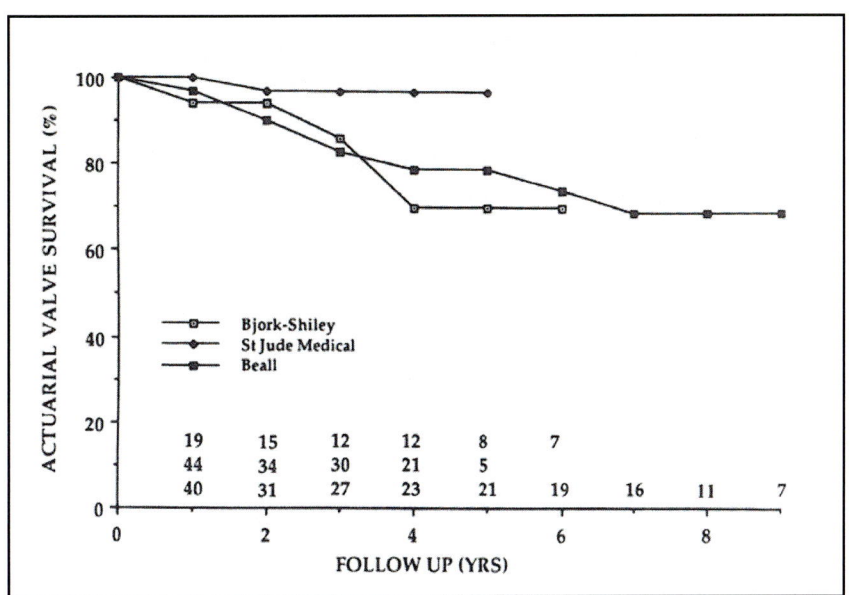

Figure 10. Actuarial valve survival curves for each of the mechanical valves in mitral position. Note similar valve survival curves for Beall and Bjork-Shiley valves. The survival curves for St. Jude Medical valve is slightly better than those in the other mechanical valves. Reproduced from Rao PS, et al, *Pediat Cardiol 1991*; 12:164-69.

On the basis of eight to ten year follow-up data, we recommended that heterografts should not be inserted into children ≤ 15 years of age. Heterografts may be used in children over fifteen years of age with the expectation of valve survival comparable to that of mechanical valves and with little or no threat of thromboembolic complications.[6]

REFERENCES

1. Rao PS, Marino BL, Robertson AF, III, "The usefulness of continuous positive airway pressure in the differential diagnosis of cardiac from pulmonary cyanosis in newborn infants," *Arch Dis Child 1978*; 53:456-60.

2. Sanyal SK, Tierney RC, Rao PS, et al, "Systolic time interval characteristics in children with Duchene's progressive muscular dystrophy," *Pediatrics 1982*; 70:958-64.

3. Rao PS, Solymar L, Mardini MK, et al, "Anticoagulant therapy in children with prosthetic valves," *Ann Thorac Surg 1989*; 47:589-92.

4. Rao PS, "Long-term oral diazoxide therapy for pulmonary vascular obstructive disease associated with congenital heart defects," *Am Heart J 1990*; 119:1317-21.

5.   Solymar L, Rao PS, Mardini MK, et al, "Prosthetic valves in children and adolescents," *Am Heart J 1991*; 121:557-68.

6.   Rao PS, Solymar L, Fawzy ME, Guinn G, "Reassessment of usefulness of porcine heterografts in mitral position in children," *Pediat Cardiol 1991*; 12:164-69.

THE JOURNEY'S FINALE, THE RETIREMENT

INTRODUCTION

In this chapter, the retirement planning and actual retirement, as is occurring while I write this book is reviewed.

RETIREMENT PLANNING

Beginning from training in USA through the rest of the academic career, I have put in sixty to eighty-hours work weeks; however, it has not reached the levels described by the Japanese "Karoshi." The excessive work is largely related to multiple functions that I am called upon to do, which include clinical (outpatient clinics, out-reach clinics, inpatient service, ECG/Echo/other non-invasive study interpretation, cardiac catheterization with selective cineangiography and catheter interventional procedures), administrative (Division Director or Associate Director, Fellowship Director and Committee assignments), teaching (medical students, residents, fellows and continuing medical education), research (resulting in hundreds of publications), and editorial (editorial boards, reviewer for multiple journals, writing editorials and review papers) responsibilities. Largely because of the busy schedule, I have not developed any hobbies other than occasional tennis. Consequently, I planned to slowly reduce work week after I passed the age of seventy-two-years. The plan was go for a four-day work week for the academic year 2014-2015, then go to a three days a week in 2015-2016 and so on. The four-day work week for the academic year 2014-2015 started well in that the Fridays were taken as a vacation day; this was possible because I had a large amount of accumulated vacation time. There was some questioning by the lower level administrators whether such shortened week should be allowed, but higher authorities opined that if there is unused leave, the employees have the right to utilize vacation days as long as it did not unduly disturb the functions of the Division.

The four-day work week for the academic year 2014-2015 began in September 2014 as planned, but in March 2015, I had a severe heart attack requiring placement of six stents in my coronary arteries and balloon pump to support the heart function. On the night of the procedure, I developed paralytic ileus secondary to abdominal and abdominal wall bleeding. These complications snow-balled resulting in acalculous cholecystitis and a total of one-month hospitalization. I then had cardiac rehabilitation, while using sick leave as per FMLA, and subsequently with accumulated sick leave. On days without scheduled cardiac rehab, I came to work reading echocardiograms and ECGs, but stopped seeing patients in the clinic and refrained from performing cardiac catheterizations and catheter interventions. Eventfully, I decided to retire at the end of January 2017. Because of the fact that I have been very busy working for nearly five decades, coming back to work part-time (about two days a week), mostly to interpret echocardiograms and ECGs and teaching of students, resdents and fellows, was thought to be appropriate and was agreed by the respective administrative authorities. Now into mid-2019, this appears to be working well.

Initially, I decided to honor manuscript writing invitations accepted prior to the heart attack, but declined subsequent invitations to write new papers/reviews/editorials. This resulted in publication of several papers.[1-8] But slowly, for one reason or another, I was lulled into accepting invitations to write and edit. These publications[9-20] truly distracted me from timely completion of this book. My initial plan was to complete the book by the end of 2018, but it looks like that it would be completed in late 2019.

RETIREMENT

The retirement began at the end of January 2017, as planned. As mentioned, I formally retired from my professorial position end of January 2017, began working part-time as a Staff Physician in February 2017. However, I retained non-salaried professorial positions in the departments of Pediatrics and Medicine. I started coming to work on Tuesdays and Thursday, mostly to interpret ECGs and echocardiographic studies with fellow-teaching associated with echoes and ECGs as well as infrequent lectures to students, resdents and fellows. I also came to work on couple Mondays a month to attend the Morbidity & Mortality Conference and fellow-teaching. On the remaining days, cardiac rehabilitation type of workout was undertaken either at the local YMCA, treadmill at home or a walk through the streets of Bellaire where we live. In addition, lunch with wife and daughters on most Fridays, playing cards with friends on most Sundays was incorporated into the routine. When there is time, academic work as detailed above, editing chapters for the WebMD (since I serve as the Chief Editor for the Pediatric Cardiology Section of the WebMD) and writing this memoir and a companion book titled "Pediatric Cardiology: How It Has Evolved Over the last 50 Years" were undertaken.

While this appears to work well, some problem surfaced in that I was not able to meet the target dates for completion of the above two books, largely related voluminous amount material to be reviewed and written. Original target date for completion of memoir and the companion book was end of 2108, but it did not happen in that time frame. It is hoped that they will be completed before the end of 2019.

REFERENCES

1. Rao PS, "Is Intracardiac echocardiography essential for monitoring stent deployment across aortic coarctation?" *Echocardiography 2015*; 32:731-3. Available at DOI: 10.1111/echo.12905. Epub 2015 February 13, PMID: 25684662.

2. Yates MC, Gautam NK, Rao PS, "Reactive ductus arteriosus in a nineteen month old patient," *Congenital Cardiology Today 2015*; 13(5): 1-7.

3. Rao PS, "Fontan operation: Indications, short and long term outcomes," *Indian J Pediatr 2015*; 82:1147-56. Available at DOI: 10.1007/s12098-015-1803-6. Epub ahead of print: 2015 June 2, PMID: 26088549.

4. Rao PS, "Editorial: What does the pediatrician needs to know about heart defects in children?" *Indian J Pediatr 2015*; 82:1019-20. Available at DOI: 10.1007/s12098-015-1834-z. Epub ahead of print 2015 September 14, PMID: 26365157.

5. Rao PS, "Prevention of Sudden Death in Athletes," *Pediat Therapeut 2015*, August 20; 5: e129. Available at DOI:10.4172/2161-0665.1000e129.

6. Yarrabolu TR, Thapar MK, Rao PS, "Subpulmonary obstruction from aneurismal ventricular septum in a child with dextrocardia and congenitally corrected transposition of the great arteries," *Tex heart Inst J. 2015*; 42:590-592 eCollection December 2015.

7. Rao PS, "Balloon aortic valvuloplasty (Editorial)," *Indian Heart Journal 2016*; 68: 592-5.

8. Yarrabolu TR, Naidu DP, Pawelek O, Rao PS, "Flash pulmonary edema during pulmonary vasoreactivity testing," *J J Pulmonol 2016*, 2(3):028.

9. Rao PS, "The Journey of an Indian Pediatric Cardiologist," Dr. K. C. Chaudhuri Lifetime Achievement Award/Oration at AIIMS, New Delhi, September 2017, *Indian J Pediat 2017*. Available at DOI 10.1007/s12098-017-2452-8.

10. Rao PS, Harris AD, "Recent advances in managing septal defects: atrial septal defects," *F1000 Faculty Rev:2042, 2017*; 6:2042. Available at DOI: 10.12688/f1000research.11844.1, PMID: 29250321.

11. Rao PS, "Role of echocardiography in the evaluation of preterm infants with patent ductus arteriosus," *Neonatology Today 2018*; 14(1):1-10.

12. Rao PS, Harris AD, "Recent advances in managing septal defects: ventricular septal defects and atrioventricular septal defects," *F1000Res. 2018*, April 26;7. pii: F1000 Faculty Rev-498. Available at DOI: 10.12688/f1000research.14102.1. eCollection 2018, Review, PMID: 29770201.

13. Rao PS, "Role of echocardiography in the evaluation of preterm infants with patent ductus arteriosus," *Congenital Cardiology Today 2018*; 16(4):1-10.

14. Rao PS, "Auscultation is still a valid tool in the evaluation of cardiac defects in children," *Congenital Cardiology Today 2018*; 16(8):1-6.

15. Rao PS, "Transcatheter perforation of atretic pulmonary valve in pulmonary atresia with ventricular septal defect," *Congenital Cardiology Today 2018*; 16(11):1-8.

16. Rao PS, Subramaniam U, "Reliability of echocardiographic estimation of angiographic minimal ductal diameter," *Congenital Cardiology Today 2019*; 17(3):1-7.

17. Rao P.S, "Management of congenital heart disease: State of the art—Part I—Acyanotic heart defects," *Children (Basel) 2019*; 6, 42. Available at DOI:10.3390/children6030042, PMID: 30857252.

18. Rao P.S, "Management of congenital heart disease: State of the art—Part II—Cyanotic heart defects," *Children (Basel). 2019*; 6, 54. Available at DOI:10.3390/children604005, PMID: 30987364.

19. Rao P.S, "Patent ductus arteriosus - A review." *Horizons in World Cardiovascular Research* (In Press)

20. Rao P.S, "Neonatal coarctation of the aorta: management challenges." *Research and Reports in Neonatology* (In Press)